American Red Cross

Foundations for Caregiving

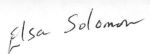 **American Red Cross**

Foundations for Caregiving

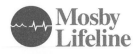 **Mosby Lifeline**

St. Louis Baltimore Boston Chicago London Madrid Philadelphia Sydney Toronto

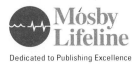

Printed in the United States of America
Composition by The Clarinda Company
Printing/binding by Color Art, Inc.

Mosby–Year Book, Inc.
11830 Westline Industrial Drive
St. Louis, Missouri 63146

Library of Congress Cataloging in Publication Data

Foundations for caregiving / American Red Cross.
    p. cm.
    Includes bibliographical references and index.
    ISBN 0-8016-6515-9
    1. Nurses' aides. 2. Care of the sick. 3. Nurses' Aides— —
education.   I. American Red Cross.
    [DNLM: 1. Caregivers—education—programmed instruction. 2. Home
Nursing—education. 3. Home Care Services—programmed instruction.
WY 18 F7712 1993]
RT84.F68 1993
610.73—dc20
DNLM/DLC
for Library of Congress
                                                            93-3976
                                                              CIP

98 99 00 / 9 8 7 6 5 4

How far you go in life depends on your being tender with the young, compassionate with the aged, sympathetic with the striving, and tolerant of the weak and strong—because someday in life you will have been all of these.

—George Washington Carver

Acknowledgments

The **Foundations for Caregiving** course and materials were developed and produced through a joint effort of the American Red Cross and the Mosby Publishing Company. The effort has been a labor of love by individuals who care deeply about the kind of care they will receive from nurse assistants when they and their loved ones are ill. We hope they will be trained through the American Red Cross Foundations for Caregiving Programs!

Members of the development team at the American Red Cross who designed and wrote these materials included: Cindy Green, M.P.H., and Carolyn Branson, R.N., B.S.N., Project Leaders; Paula Virgin, R.N., B.S.N., Content Specialist/Writer; Linda Wolfe Keister, Managing Editor; Jill Tunick, Assistant Editor; Carol Hunter-Geboy, Ph.D., Instructional Design Consultant; Sharon Dorfman, Education and Evaluation Consultant; Peggy Casey, R.N., Margaret Draganac, R.N., M.P.H., Kathleen Masucci, R.N., Judy Peterson, R.N., B.S.N., Rosemary A. Sullivan, R.N., M.Ed., and Angie S. Turner, R.N., B.S.N., Red Cross Staff Writers; Margaret Callanan, R.N., Deborah Makie Canavan, R.N., B.S.N., Richard S. Ferri, R.N., Ph.D., CRNI, Alexandra Greeley, Pat Hyland, R.N., Rosa Kasper, Jeff Malter, Lisa Malter, Sharon Romm, Joan Timberlake, Barbara E. Tucker, B.S.N., M.P.H., and Ruth G. Wiskind, R.N., M.N., External Writers.

The following individuals provided additional assistance: Esther Silva, R.N., B.S., M.A., Amy Coats, M.Ed., and Meg A. Riley, Artwork Coordinators; Melissa Andrews, Copy Editor; Alison Hilton, Analyst; Venus Ray, Project Assistant/Proofreader; Cynthia Yockey, Desktop Publisher; Lou Ellen Bell, R.N., B.S.N., M.N., Claudette Clunan, R.N., B.S.N., M.A., Fay Flowers, R.N., M.Ed., Genevieve Gipson, R.N., M.Ed., Katherine Graves, R.N., Carole K. Kauffman, R.N., M.P.H., Diane H. Munro, R.N., M.B.A., and Karne J. Peterson, Ph.D., Internal Reviewers; Lynda Ramsey Bradshaw, L.P.N., B.S., and Sandy Johnston, R.N., Technical Reviewers/Assistant Artwork Coordinators; Charles Pierpont, Assistant Source Photographer and Desktop Publisher; and Tara Theodore, Secretary.

The Mosby production team included: David T. Culverwell, Publisher; Richard A. Weimer, Executive Editor; Mary Beth Ryan Warthen and Julie Scardiglia, Developmental Editors; Gayle May Morris, Project Manager; Mary Cusick Drone, Senior Production Editor; Kay Kramer, Director Art and Design; and John Rokusek and Betty Schulz, designers.

Special thanks to Vincent Knaus and Jeanette Ortiz-Osorio, Photographers; and Joe Chovan, Kurt Peterson, Patti Restle, Lisa Petkun, and Michael Cooley, Illustrators.

These materials could not have been completed without the generous assistance in time, materials, and manpower of the Fairfax Nursing Center, Fairfax, Virginia; Grant Park Nursing Center, Washington, D.C.; the National Capital Chapter of the American Red Cross; Peoples Drug, Bailey's Crossroads, Virginia; and Thomas Silva.

The Development Team of Health Care Training extends sincere appreciation to our American National Red Cross paid and volunteer staff for their assistance in completing these materials.

Jan Hodges, M.Ed., M.B.A.
Manager of Paramedical Services
Special Care Home Health, Inc.Monica Lursen,

Sandra Hsieh, R.N., M.S., Ed.
Community Health Nurse/Discharge Planner
San Francisco Veterans Affairs Medical Center
& Consultant, On Lok Senior Health Services

Ann Kobs, R.N., M.S.
Associate Director
Department of Standards
Joint Commission on Accreditation of Healthcare
  Organizations

Renee S. Levesque, Ed.D., P.H.N.
Vice President for Quality and Service
CHAP

Monica Lursen, R.D., L.D.
Registered Dietitian
The American Dietetic Association

Beverly McKeehan, R.N.
Assistant Director of Nursing
Blueridge Haven West

Gail Mott, R.N.-C.
Director of Clinical Services
Hospice Care of DC

Mary Helen Osborn, B.S.
Certified Home Economist
Extension Agent
Virginia Cooperative Extension Service

Bernice Owen, Ph.D., R.N.
Center for Health
University of Wisconsin
School of Nursing

Carole Patterson, R.N., M.N.
Associate Director for Interpretation
Department of Standards
Joint Commission on Accreditation of Healthcare
  Organizations

Cindy Pearson
Program Director
National Women's Health Network

Martha Pelaez, Ph.D.
Associate Director
Southeast Florida Center on Aging
Florida International University

Maryanne Popovich, R.N., M.P.H.
Associate Director
Home Care Accreditation Services
Joint Commission on Accreditation of Healthcare
  Organizations

Joyce Roth, R.N.
Director of Staff Development
Blueridge Haven West

Carlene Russell, R.D., L.D.
Registered Dietitian
The American Dietetic Association

Barbara M. Santamaria, R.N., M.P.H.
Certified Family Nurse Practitioner
Veterans Administration

Denise Shanahan, R.N., M.S.
Quality Assurance Nurse
Chatham Orleans Visiting Nurse Association

Patricia M. Siclari, R.N., B.A.
Program Manager, Professional Development
American Health Care Association

Ellen S. Tishman, R.N., B.S.N.
Director, Professional Development
American Health Care Association

Anna Vicik, R.N., M.S.
Associate Director
Long Term Care Accreditation Services
Joint Commission on Accreditation of Healthcare
  Organizations

Donna L. Yee, Ph.D.
Senior Research Associate
Bigel Health Policy Institute
Heller School, Brandeis University

Contents

Introduction

Welcome to the American Red Cross **Foundations for Caregiving** textbook. Whether you are training to become a certified nurse assistant or a caregiver for a friend or family member at home, this book will be an invaluable resource for you. The authors of this book and accompanying materials believe that caregiving is an art, applied creatively and compassionately, using six principles of care.

The Foundations of Caregiving Program

Foundations for Caregiving continues the focus on providing concerned, individualized care begun in the American Red Cross Nurse Assistant Training Program (NATP) of 1989. The complete **Foundations for Caregiving Program** consists of this textbook and the materials that supplement it: **Skills for Caregiving,** the skills workbook; **Foundations for Caregiving Skills Videos,** volumes 1 to 3; and **The Instructor's Manual for Foundations for Caregiving.** The program meets the federal requirements of the Omnibus Reconciliation Act (OBRA) of 1987 for training nurse assistants. It updates the NATP, endorsed by the National League for Nursing, and adds special information necessary for providing care as a nurse assistant in the hospital setting and in the home.

If you use this book as part of an American Red Cross course preparing you to become a certified nurse assistant, you gain the added benefits of being taught by an American Red Cross–trained instructor; viewing the skills videos, which demonstrate the skills you will learn; using the skills book, which describes step by step how to perform 74 different skills; and being awarded an American Red Cross Nurse Assistant pin and certificate on successful completion of the course.

Six Principles of Care

Focusing on concerned, individualized caregiving, this program continues to adhere to the six principles of care unique to the American Red Cross Nurse Assistant Training Program: safety, privacy, dignity, communication, independence, and infection control.

Patterns of the Book

The textbook is fun and easy to use. Each chapter begins with a list of goals and a scenario and ends with Information Review questions and Questions to Ask Yourself. In between, the chapters include marginal terms, photos, illustrations, boxes, and tables—all of which make learning more interesting.

Goals

The goals provide a road map for the chapter. They tell you which ideas are most important to learn. As you complete each chapter, re-read the goals to see if you grasped the key information.

Scenarios

Each chapter opens with a scenario, depicting an event that has occurred involving a person who is receiving care or a person who is providing care. The characters who appear in the scenarios are purely fictional and represent no persons who are alive or who have lived. They do represent the human aspects of providing and receiving care: health problems, moods, behavior quirks, and opinions. They also demonstrate the need for someone to provide care in a way that makes them feel important, special, and respected. These characters also appear within the chapters and challenge you to be a compassionate caregiver.

Marginal Terms

You will learn many new words as you read this book. To make the words easy to reference and learn, each **bold-faced** term in the text also appears in the margin along with its pronunciation, if necessary, and its meaning.

Look at the way words in the margin are divided into syllables. When saying a word out loud, give the capitalized part of the word the greatest stress. Note how small, familiar words often are used in the pronunciations and how each word is spelled to represent the correct way it should sound. Because every vowel has several sounds, as demonstrated in the chart of vowel sounds, refer to this chart often as you learn to pronounce new words.

For quick reference, all bold-faced, marginal terms also appear in Appendix A, Glossary of Key Words, at the end of this book.

Figures

Figures may be either illustrations, depicting the characters in the scenarios, or photographs. Each figure is positioned on the page near its reference in the text. A description of the figure provides additional information to support the text.

Body Basics

Body Basics boxes provide brief descriptions and illustrations about organs and systems in the human body. They appear in chapters that include information that relates to particular body systems.

Information Review

The Information Review questions, when answered correctly, provide a summary of the chapter. Appendix E, Information Review Answer Key, provides the list of correct answers for each chapter.

Questions to Ask Yourself

The Questions to Ask Yourself boxes pose real-life situations that encourage you to apply your knowledge in decision making. These questions may have several correct answers. They are questions to think about and to talk about with your classmates and your instructor. They are especially useful in classroom discussion.

Appendixes

Appendixes A, B, and C are glossaries that help you develop the special language used by caregivers. Appendix D, Home Safety Checklist, is a tool that you can use to check the safety of your home or the home of the person for whom you are providing care. Appendix E is the Information Review Answer Key.

For the sound of...	As in...	We use...	As in...
short a	apple	ah	**adaptation** (ah-dap-TA-shun)
short a	attend	uh	**assertive** (uh-SER-tiv)
long a	stable	ay	**patient** (PAY-shent)
short e	enter	e	**gender** (JEN-der)
short e	estate	uh	**eliminate** (uh-LIM-uh-nate)
long e	east	ee	**dyspnea** (disp-NEE-uh)
short i	liver	i	**clinic** (KLIN-ik)
short i	chemical	uh	**cuticles** (KYU-tuh-kuhls)
long i	ivy	eye	**IV** (eye-VEE)
long i	ivy	i	**dehydrated** (dee-HI-dray-ted)
long i	ivy	y	**miter** (MY-ter)
short o	obvious	o	**obstetric** (ob-STET-rik)
short o	oven	uh	**suffocate** (SUF-uh-kate)
long o	only	oe	**mobility** (moe-BIL-uh-tee)
long o	only	oh	**obesity** (oh-BEE-suh-tee)
short u	under	u	**custom** (KUS-tum)
long u	dune	ew	**nutrient** (NEW-tre-ent)
long u	human	you	**regulation** (reg-you-LAY-shun)

1

The Art of Caregiving

Goals

After reading this chapter, you will have the information to—

Discuss why caregiving is an art.

Discuss how to put the individual first in caregiving.

Describe the six principles of care and explain why you should practice them.

You walk into Mrs. Agnes Ryan's room to take her for one of her three daily walks. Mrs. Ryan, who is 89 years old, says she isn't ready to go because she is working on her quilt and wants to finish one more section. You remind her that her walk is important to keep her strong, and then you ask her how long it will take to finish the section of quilting. She says it will take about 10 minutes, so you mentally adjust your schedule and decide to change the bed of Mrs. Ryan's room-mate, Mrs. Louise Wang, who is at physical therapy.

As you change the bed, you marvel at how beautifully Mrs. Ryan sews. You ask her how long she has been quilting, and she begins to tell you how her grand-mother made quilts. "When my older sister made our dresses," Mrs. Ryan remem-bers, "she would cut out the pattern and then give the leftover pieces of fabric to my grandmother, who was so happy to receive these scraps of cloth. Bags of gold would not have made her happier. She loved making quilts.

"Grandmother taught me to cut the fabric into different shapes, sort them by color and shape, and stack them neatly on the table. Then we began to sew them together, one stitch at a time. The tiny pieces took on new shapes, sizes, and ar-rangements of color until we had sewn all the little pieces into one piece large enough to cover a bed. Then Grandmother put thick cotton between the pieced top layer and a bottom sheet, and we stitched the layers together to provide soft-ness and warmth for the lucky person who would sleep beneath this masterpiece. It took lots of practice for me to get it just right. The hardest parts were having enough strength to push the needle through the many layers of fabric and the pa-tience to finish all the tasks. My mother always said that Grand-mother sewed the quilts to-gether, not with thread, but with love."

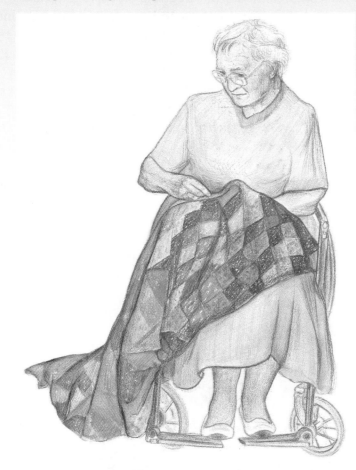

Caregiving Is an Art

Caregiving in a health care setting is like quiltmaking. As a caregiver, you make decisions, fit many pieces of work into a day, pay attention to the details of each person's life, and use personal strength to handle the many complex parts of your job. You work with patience and devotion while helping ill or disabled people feel comfortable, important, and respected.

All of us are caregivers at one time or another when we provide important and necessary care to a friend or family member who needs help because of an illness or disability. Being employed as a trained caregiver, however, requires us to not only provide the best care that we can but also to take on additional kinds of responsibilities.

It takes a special person to provide quality health care in a caring way. As a nurse assistant, you are a valuable and special caregiver who can make a difference in the lives of people receiving care. You blend your knowledge of people and the accurate performance of skills with your caring spirit. Many people learn the skills of caregiving, but not everyone can deliver those skills with kindness and compassion. Skillful care provided in a thoughtful way is an art.

For example, as you made Mrs. Wang's bed, you knew that her delicate skin could be damaged by wrinkled sheets, so you were careful to lay the sheets flat and pull them tight so that there were no wrinkles. You thought about Mrs. Wang as an individual who needed specific care for her skin. You acted as a thoughtful caregiver.

This chapter explores the art of caregiving and also introduces you to the information that you must know to be a skilled caregiver and to make each person feel that he or she has received a gift—the best care possible. As you prepare for your job, whether you are called a nurse assistant, nursing assistant, nurse aide, home health aide, or geriatric aide, you will learn the difference between just getting your job done and providing the quality of care expected from a good nurse assistant. The art of caregiving, the art of treating each person as an individual, makes the difference. Getting to know each person as an individual is the key (Figure 1-1). Each person receiving care is different, as is each situation. This book provides guidelines to help you make the best decisions to provide the best care to each person.

Figure 1-1
The art of caregiving focuses on providing care for each person as an individual. This nurse assistant takes time to listen to a resident's utmost concern—the outcome of last night's televised football game.

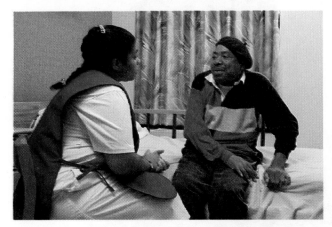

Putting the Person in Your Care First

A generation ago, providing health care was different than it is today. Back then, caregivers believed that the less people in their care had to do for themselves, the better. Caregivers made people stay in bed, fed them, and bathed them. They gave everyone the same care, focusing on treating everyone the same instead of as individuals with special needs and differences.

Over time, health care professionals came to understand that people got better and stronger much more quickly if they were encouraged to do more things for themselves (Figure 1-2). They recovered faster if they were encouraged to do things when and how they liked to do them. People also responded better to treatment if their conditions were explained and if they participated in planning their care.

This discovery has changed the way health care professionals provide care. Although you still **nurture** the people in your care, you no longer do everything for them. You still may have to help them with many things, such as bathing, eating, and using the toilet, but you also encourage them to do as much as possible for themselves.

In caregiving, focusing on the person and her individual needs is important. Daily care must be individualized to meet the needs of each person and should not become routine or automatic. Anything can easily become automatic. For example, have you ever ridden home from your job, walked up to the front door of your home, and suddenly realized that you did not even remember your trip home? What did you miss seeing along the way...the flowers?...budding trees?...a beautiful sunset in the sky? Had your trip home from work become so automatic that you forgot to think about it and to enjoy how special that ride was?

Or have you ever gone to a party where, at first, all the people seemed alike? But, as you met and talked to different people and listened to each one's ideas, they became distinct individuals with various interests. People who receive health care also differ from one another. Each one needs to receive individualized care.

As a nurse assistant, you must see each person as an individual with special needs. That person is more than a body or a disease that you fit into your schedule. Your schedule may make you feel comfortable, but that isn't as important as what makes the person feel comfortable. You need to remember that each person, like Mrs. Ryan, is a human being who has routines of her own. She needs to bathe when she wants to bathe, not when you have written her into your schedule. She needs to use the toilet when she needs to, not when you have time to help her. You must readjust your schedule and put your own needs aside to take care of her needs, because, in good caregiving, the person always comes first.

For example, let's say you have been providing care for Mrs. Ryan. You thought you finally had figured out what Mrs. Ryan's bathing schedule was, and you had worked it very nicely into your daily

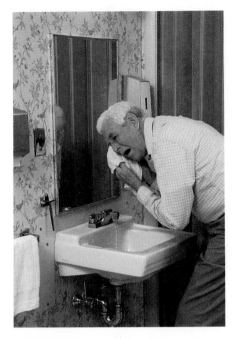

Figure 1-2
Completing even the smallest task gives a person a sense of accomplishment.

nurture
(NUR-tyur)   To promote and encourage good care.

schedule. Then, last week, when you went into Mrs. Ryan's room, prepared to help her with her bath, you discovered that she had changed her mind about what she wanted. Your schedule got all turned around. You felt upset about this change, but, instead of saying some angry words to Mrs. Ryan, you put your anger aside and juggled your schedule. If a person's needs change from day to day, then so must your schedule, because the individual needs of the person receiving care come first.

You must always put your personal thoughts, feelings, and troubles second to those of the person in your care, even though it may upset you. You can *have* your own feelings, but you cannot *act on* them or let your mind rest on your own concerns while you provide care for someone. When you are distracted by your personal thoughts, you can't give good care to an individual. If your thoughts and feelings get in the way of your work, talk to a co-worker, your supervising nurse, or someone else who may be able to help. You may need to continue to work for a while before you get a chance to talk, but, often, making the decision to talk with someone helps you clear your mind so that you can focus on the person in your care.

For example, if you are focusing on something else, you may not hear Mrs. Ryan say that her birthday is tomorrow. Thinking about something else gets in the way of thinking about what this special day means to her.

Practicing the Six Principles of Care

Because you focused on Mrs. Ryan and her needs yesterday, you know that today is her 90th birthday. She asked you to help her with an early morning bath, so you adjusted your schedule for today so that Mrs. Ryan could be dressed and ready for her birthday as early as possible. By 10:00 A.M. you had helped her use the portable commode, served her breakfast, wheeled her to the tub room, assisted her with her bath, helped her button her dress, smoothed out her newly styled hair, and helped her apply her makeup.

principles of care
(PRIN-suh-puls)   Basic rules of caregiving that guide caregivers in making decisions about providing individualized care for each person.

You worked hard to help Mrs. Ryan get ready for an important day, and you let the six **principles of care**—safety, privacy, dignity, communication, independence, and infection control—guide every decision that you made and every action that you took. Look at Box 1-1 to find out how you practice each principle.

The principles of care help you remember to put the person first when you provide care. When making decisions about the person in your care, always ask yourself the following: Is the person safe? Am I protecting her privacy? Am I promoting her dignity? Does she want to talk? Do I need to say something to her? How can I encourage her to be as independent as possible? Would a particular action prevent the spread of germs? These principles also help you by providing guidelines to perform caregiving skills with consideration for the whole person.

Although the care you provided for Mrs. Ryan may seem ordinary,

Box 1-1   **Practicing the Six Principles of Care**

To learn more about these principles, read the chapters indicated in parentheses.

Safety: Keep a person free from harm by preventing injuries (Chapter 6, Keeping People Safe).

Privacy: Keep a person's private business private, and do not allow private things to be seen or overheard by other people (Chapter 3, Protecting People's Rights).

Dignity: Treat each person with respect at all times (Chapter 3, Protecting People's Rights). Report information about the person to your supervising nurse.

Communication: Be available to talk, listen, and respond to a person's thoughts and feelings. Tell the person about the care you plan to provide. Report information about the person to your supervising nurse (Chapter 5, Communicating with People).

Independence: Encourage each person to do as much as possible (Chapter 3, Protecting People's Rights; Chapter 5, Communicating with People).

Infection Control: Help control the spread of germs (Chapter 7, Controlling the Spread of Germs).

you had many opportunities to practice the principles of care. Let's revisit Mrs. Ryan's birthday and look more closely at how you applied these principles.

Today is Mrs. Ryan's 90th birthday. Yesterday, she asked you to help her with an early morning bath, so you adjusted your schedule for today so that she could be dressed and ready for her birthday as early as possible. This morning, at 8:00 A.M., you knocked on Mrs. Ryan's door. When you didn't hear a response, you knocked again. Then you heard her say, "Come in." Closing the door behind you, you gently grasped Mrs. Ryan's hand, looked at her identification bracelet, identified yourself, and said, "Happy Birthday, Mrs. Ryan. I've come early to help you get ready for your birthday." She wanted to use the toilet first, so you washed your hands before helping her onto the portable commode. You made sure the curtain was closed and stood outside the curtain in case she needed your help. Afterward, you helped Mrs. Ryan wash her hands and then washed your own hands again before helping Mrs. Ryan put on her bathrobe and slippers. You helped her move into the wheelchair, locked the brake, and put the call signal nearby while you left the room to get her breakfast tray.

Before serving Mrs. Ryan breakfast, you washed your hands again. After she ate her breakfast, you wheeled her to the tub room, where you closed the door as you helped her with her bath. She needed you to wash her back. After the bath, you put the dirty bath linens in the dirty laundry bag, washed your hands, and then wheeled Mrs. Ryan to her room. She said she wanted to wear the new pink dress that her daughter sent. You suggested that it might be too cold to wear that dress, but Mrs. Ryan insisted. So, you encouraged her to wear a warm slip underneath her dress. After asking Mrs. Ryan how she would like to style her hair, you combed out her hair according

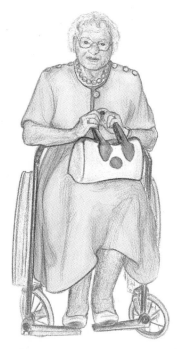

Figure 1-3
Mrs. Ryan feels proud as a she waits for the arrival of her birthday visitors.

to her directions. While you combed Mrs. Ryan's hair, you listened with interest as she talked about her past birthdays.

As you were getting ready to leave Mrs. Ryan's room, you asked if there was anything else you could do to help. Mrs. Ryan said she wanted to wear makeup for her birthday, so you helped her. While putting powder on her face, you noticed a small red patch on her cheek. (You would report that to your supervising nurse as soon as you finished with Mrs. Ryan's personal care.) As you prepared to leave the room, you checked to make sure the wheelchair brakes were locked, made sure the call signal was within her reach, picked up the comb and hair pins that Mrs. Ryan had dropped on the floor, and asked her if she wanted her door opened or closed. As you walked out into the hallway, you looked back through the open door and saw Mrs. Ryan sitting in her wheelchair, proud as a peacock, waiting for the arrival of her birthday visitors (Figure 1-3).

Let's look at how you practiced the principles of care.

Safety:	Looked at her identification bracelet
	Waited outside the curtain while Mrs. Ryan used the portable commode
	Locked her wheelchair brakes
	Put the call signal within her reach
	Picked up things on the floor that people could trip on
Privacy:	Closed the door when you entered Mrs. Ryan's room
	Closed the curtain while she used the commode
	Closed the door while she bathed
	Left the door open at Mrs. Ryan's request
Dignity:	Knocked on the door
	Waited for Mrs. Ryan's response before entering her room
	Called Mrs. Ryan by her title instead of calling her Agnes
	Identified yourself
	Asked her permission to provide personal care
	Asked her what she wanted to wear
	Respected her wishes about what she wanted to wear
	Combed her hair the way she wanted to wear it
	Asked her if she wanted the door opened or closed
Communication:	Greeted Mrs. Ryan warmly
	Introduced yourself
	Asked her permission to provide personal care
	Talked with her about past birthdays
	Observed a new condition on Mrs. Ryan's face and planned to report it

Independence: Asked permission to help with Mrs. Ryan's personal care

Stood outside the curtain so that she could use the toilet by herself

Asked her what she wanted to wear

Infection Control: Washed your hands before and after helping Mrs. Ryan

Helped Mrs. Ryan wash her hands after she used the portable commode

Washed your hands after helping her use the portable commode

Washed your hands before serving her breakfast

Put dirty linens in the dirty laundry bag

Washed your hands after handling dirty linens

The principles of care were the guiding force as you helped Mrs. Ryan. When you applied the principles of care to caregiving, it was like Mrs. Ryan's grandmother sewing cotton into her quilt to provide substance and warmth. By applying the principles of care, you provided substance and warmth to the everyday skills of caregiving.

Questions to Ask Yourself

1. What are your reasons for wanting to become a nurse assistant or a home health aide?

2. What do you think your duties will be in this job?

3. What do you think will be the rewards of this work?

4. What do you think will be the challenges of this work?

5. How would you feel if your friend or family member received thoughtful care from a nurse assistant who practiced the principles of care?

2

Working in Health Care

Goals

After reading this chapter, you will have the information to—

Explain three health care settings where you may work.

List five members of the health care team and explain their roles.

Describe the people who receive care in one health care setting.

Describe what it is like to work as a nurse assistant in one health care setting.

Describe your role and responsibilities as a nurse assistant.

It was raining when 72-year-old Alma Garcia went outside to get her morning newspaper. As she walked back toward the front door, she slipped and fell. She lay unnoticed until a neighbor walked by and saw her lying on the porch. The neighbor phoned for an ambulance, which took her to the hospital. There, a doctor examined her and gave her the bad news: she had broken her hip.

After she began to recover from surgery, Mrs. Garcia worked with a physical therapist, who helped exercise her hip so that she could later learn to use a walker. Nurse assistants helped her bathe and get out of bed and worked with the supervising nurse to provide the best possible care. Over time, she got stronger and no longer needed hospital care, but she wasn't well enough to go home. A hospital staff member referred her to a nursing home.

At Morningside Nursing Home, Mrs. Garcia received nursing care and physical therapy to help strengthen her hip and help her learn to walk with a walker. Nurse assistants helped with bathing, dressing, and walking and also assisted her with special exercises that she learned from the physical therapist. As time passed, she became stronger and more independent and walked longer distances with her walker.

After several weeks, Mrs. Garcia was walking well enough to go home, but she needed assistance at home until she regained total independence. Her doctor referred her to a home health care agency. A registered nurse from the agency visited Mrs. Garcia at her home, evaluated her condition, and continued to check her health regularly. Under the nurse's supervision, home health aides helped Mrs.

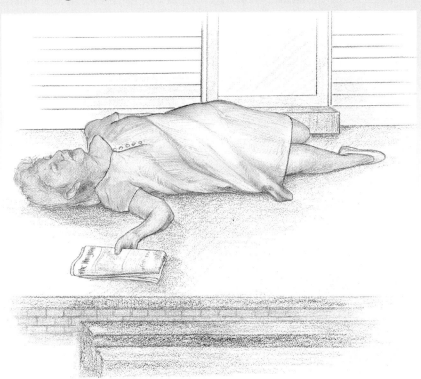

Garcia bathe, dress, and prepare meals. A physical therapist continued Mrs. Garcia's exercises until she could walk without help. After several months, Mrs. Garcia was able to live in her house by herself just as she did before the fall, and she no longer needed the services of the home health care agency.

❖   **Working in the Health Care System**   ❖

Nurse assistants work with a variety of health professionals, such as nurses, physical therapists, and dietitians. These health care workers provide many kinds of health care, depending on the needs of the person receiving care. For example, health care workers in a hospital clinic provide regular medical checkups to help healthy people stay well and avoid health problems.

Health care workers in a hospital find and treat problems, such as high blood pressure, before they become serious. They also help injured people, like Mrs. Garcia, to get better. Health care professionals cannot cure some health problems, such as diabetes, but they can help people learn to live with them and keep them under control. When people have health problems from which they cannot recover, health care workers strive to make them as comfortable as possible.

People choose health care services depending on where they live, the kind of care they need, and how they will pay for their care. In the United States, people pay for health care in a variety of ways. Some people receive health insurance through government programs like Medicare and Medicaid. Others have insurance through their employment or organizations. Some people do not have any health insurance because they cannot afford to pay for it.

The health care system has many parts, each with a special function. Mrs. Garcia used three parts of the system—the hospital, a nursing home, and home health care—to meet her health care needs. Nurse assistants usually work in one of these health care settings.

The Health Care Team

No matter where people go, they want to receive skilled, compassionate, and individualized care. In every place where care is provided, many staff members work together to meet people's needs. Each staff member has special training and skills that contribute to the kind of health care being provided. Along with the person receiving care, these staff members form a **health care team** that plans and provides the necessary services (Figure 2-1). People often think

health care team
A group headed by the person receiving care. Includes doctors, nurses, nurse assistants, therapists, secretaries, and other people involved in the caregiving process.

Figure 2-1
Often health care team members discuss a person's care during a special meeting called a team conference.

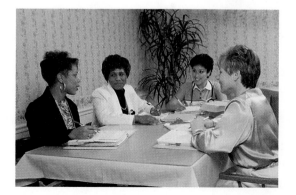

The Health Care Team

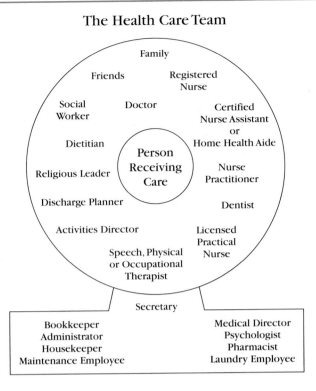

Figure 2-2

that the team includes only a doctor and nurses. Although doctors and nurses have important positions on the team, other people work with them to help meet the needs of the person receiving care. This person is the "captain" of the team. Whenever Mrs. Garcia received care, she was in charge of the team and the care she received, even though she was disabled. The other people on the team worked for Mrs. Garcia. If she had not been able to make decisions or be in charge, the team would have worked for her family.

Wherever you work, you will be part of a health care team. The specific members of your team will vary, depending on where you work. In Figure 2-2, the person receiving care is surrounded by members of the health care team who have the most direct contact with her. Team members in the base of the figure may not have much contact with the person, but they support the health care team, and the work they do is important to the caregiving process.

Next, look at Table 2-1 to learn about the part or role each team member plays in different health care settings.

Your Role as a Team Member

Regardless of where you work, you are part of a team providing health care for ill, hurt, or disabled people. Your role of caregiving is the same in all parts of the system, but the people you help may be more or less ill, more or less independent, and more or less able to recover fully. Your tasks vary, depending on the needs of the people in your care and the requirements of your employer. Your role as a nurse assistant includes four important parts: providing direct care, promoting the six principles of care, providing emotional support, and participating as a team member.

Table 2-1   What Health Care Team Members Do

Team Member*	Role	Setting
Person receiving care (patient, resident, client)	Is the "captain" of the health care team; is in charge of the care she receives; works with the team, which helps her make decisions about needed care	Hospital Nursing home Home health care
Family members and friends	Should be encouraged to help with care if the captain wants them to help; often are important sources of emotional support; may decide about the kinds of care the person receives, if the person turns this responsibility over to them	Hospital Nursing home Home health care
Registered nurse (RN)	Supervises the nursing care team members as they plan and provide care	Hospital Nursing home Home health care
Licensed practical nurse (LPN) or licensed vocational nurse (LVN)	Helps plan and supervise some types of care under the direction of a registered nurse	Hospital Nursing home Home health care
Certified nurse assistant (NA) or home health aide (HHA)	Helps plan care and assists with care under the supervision of a registered or licensed nurse	Hospital Nursing home Home health care
Doctor	Determines the person's illness or condition and supervises medical care; writes medical orders and prescribes medication when needed	Hospital Nursing home Home health care
Discharge planner (or continuing care nurse)	Meets with members of the health care team to develop a plan that will meet the patient's medical needs after she is discharged; often works with the social services department to make appropriate referrals	Hospital
Nurse practitioner	Is a registered nurse with advanced evaluation skills who gives people physical exams; monitors their health and care plans; and helps teach them about their illnesses or conditions	Hospital Nursing home Home health care
Activities director (or recreational therapist)	Plans and coordinates activities that provide opportunities for socializing, spiritual support, creativity, entertainment, exercise, and citizen activities, such as voting	Hospital Nursing home
Dentist	Provides dental care	Nursing home
Housekeeper	Makes sure rooms and other parts of the facility are cleaned each day	Hospital Nursing home
Laundry employee	Washes and mends linens, bedding, and clothing	Hospital Nursing home
Maintenance employee	Makes repairs in the facility and takes care of the grounds around the facility	Hospital Nursing home
Dietitian	Talks with the person/family about food and nutrition; serves as a resource for staff members	Hospital Nursing home Home health care

Providing Direct Care

activities of daily living
Daily self-care activities that help keep a person independent and healthy.

As a nurse assistant, you help people with **activities of daily living**, such as walking, eating, bathing, and dressing, when they cannot complete these activities by themselves (Figure 2-3). You also provide a safe, comfortable environment for the person in your care. You will learn the skills to help with these activities later in this book.

Table 2-1   **What Health Care Team Members Do—cont'd**

Team Member*	Role	Setting
Social worker	Helps admit people to and discharge them from a hospital, a nursing home, or home health care; works with people and their families to make sure their needs are met	Hospital Nursing home Home health care
Medical director (physician)	Serves as the head of the medical staff	Hospital Nursing home Home health care
Psychologist	Provides mental health assessment services	Hospital Home health care Nursing home
Pharmacist	Provides medications ordered by the doctor and keeps a record of all medications	Hospital Nursing home
Religious leader (priest, minister, rabbi)	Provides spiritual support, as needed and requested, for the person receiving care, her family, and staff members	Hospital Nursing home Home health care
Administrator	Directs the overall operation of the facility or agency	Hospital Nursing home Home health care
Bookkeeper	Takes care of paperwork for paying all bills and salaries	Hospital Nursing home Home health care
Secretary	Helps staff members in different departments to communicate with one another; often interacts with the public and family members over the phone; often keeps people's charts in order	Hospital Nursing home Home health care
Speech therapist	Helps people improve their speech and language; helps people who have trouble swallowing	Hospital Nursing home Home health care
Physical therapist	Helps people improve their ability to move their bodies	Hospital Nursing home Home health care
Occupational therapist	Helps people regain their independence in daily living tasks	Hospital Nursing home Home health care

*This list of team members represents only some of the many people on the health care team. The team varies from one facility to another and from one setting to another and includes many different specialists and assistants.

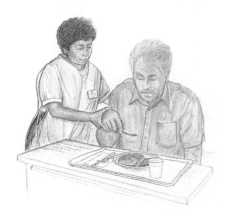

Figure 2-3
Sometimes all you have to do is steady a person's hand so that he can feed himself.

compassion
(kum-PASH-un)   A feeling of sorrow for another person's hardship that leads to help.

Promoting the Six Principles of Care

The ill, injured, or disabled people in your care need more than your assistance. They need your assistance delivered with **compassion** and thoughtfulness, according to the six principles of care. When you keep people's safety in mind, treat them with respect, provide them with privacy, communicate with them, encourage them to do things for themselves, and practice infection control, you are providing more than assistance. You are providing the best care possible.

Providing Emotional Support

You can show thoughtfulness and compassion for people by listening and paying attention to them. The people in your care have health problems, but they also have all the other day-to-day worries and concerns we all have. Often they just need to talk to someone who listens to them. Listening may seem like a simple thing, but it is one of the most important parts of good caregiving (Figure 2-4).

Figure 2-4

By giving Mr. Rivera her full attention, the nurse assistant lets him know that she is interested in what he is saying.

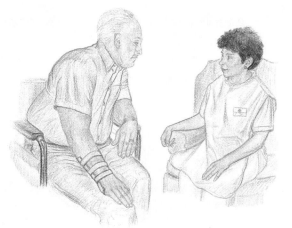

Participating as a Team Member

The nurse assistant is often the eyes and ears for the rest of the health care team. Because of the amount of time you spend with a person, you may see and hear things the rest of the team does not. For example, if someone is afraid of having a test or procedure done, you can relay her fear to your supervising nurse, and together you can help comfort the person. You may also notice that someone doesn't eat. Your supervising nurse may not be aware of this situation. It is your responsibility to tell your supervising nurse your concerns.

When you help the person in your care, you also are assisting your supervising nurse, who helps and supports you by giving you your assignments, receiving your reports, and answering your questions. Your supervising nurse may be called the charge nurse, head nurse, primary nurse, supervisor, or team leader.

Regardless of where you work, your employer provides you with a list of basic tasks and procedures, called a job description. Job descriptions vary from employer to employer, so you must always read

Box 2-1   **Sample Job Description**

As a nurse assistant, you—

1. Assist with the activities of daily living for the person in your care. This includes providing assistance with complete and partial baths, mouth care, skin and nail care, dressing, using the toilet, and exercise.

2. Use safe and correct techniques to assist the person with moving, walking, and positioning.

3. Provide nutritional care, which includes delivering food trays and other nourishment, helping people eat, observing and recording a person's ability to take nourishment, and reporting anything unusual to your supervising nurse.

4. Practice universal precautions and isolation techniques.

5. Take and write down the person's blood pressure, temperature, pulse rate, and respirations. Measure intake, output, height, and weight.

6. Assist with the collection of urine, stool, and sputum specimens for lab tests.

7. Help a person with admitting, transferring, and discharging.

8. Observe the person's general physical and emotional condition and report significant observations, reactions, or changes in the person to your supervising nurse.

9. Respond to call signals to determine the person's needs. Communicate these needs to appropriate health care team members.

10. Provide your supervising nurse with written and/or oral reports of the person's status, nursing care, and services provided. Record information on appropriate nursing forms, bedside charts, flow sheets, and progress/nursing notes.

11. Cooperate with all members of the health care team to provide quality care.

12. Participate in staff and care conferences.

13. Participate in nursing education programs designed for nurse assistants.

14. Respect the person's rights, provide privacy, and maintain confidentiality.

15. Respond properly to emergencies and know how to perform all safety procedures.

16. Follow your employer's policies when using and caring for equipment.

17. Follow all of your employer's policies.

each new job description carefully to make sure you know your responsibilities. Perform only the tasks listed in your job description. Look at the sample job description for nurse assistants in Box 2-1.

Who Can Be a Good Nurse Assistant?

It takes a special person to be a good nurse assistant. Box 2-2 lists these basic qualities.

No matter where you work, your primary role is to assist the people in your care to do the things they cannot do for themselves. Your special qualities of caring, compassion, respect, and kindness are the greatest strengths for this job.

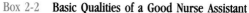

Box 2-2   Basic Qualities of a Good Nurse Assistant

Health/Hygiene

A good nurse assistant—

Eats a well-balanced diet.

Gets plenty of rest.

Has good posture.

Never takes alcoholic beverages
or illegal drugs
before or during work.

Cares about his or her appearance.

Bathes frequently enough so that
he or she has no body odors.

Shampoos often, uses deodorant,
and wears clean clothing.

Exercises.

Wears comfortable shoes
that provide support.

Social

A good nurse assistant—

Is able to get along
with other people.

Is a good listener.

Is able to talk
with families and
other staff members.

Is able to tell someone
when he or she
has a problem
or needs something.

Character

A good nurse assistant—

Keeps private information to himself or herself; does not gossip about a person
with staff or other people.

Is truthful.

Is polite to everyone.

Treats others with respect.

Respects and protects people's personal belongings.

Is dependable; does what he or she is supposed to do.

Is reliable; reports to work as scheduled and on time.

Behaves in a professional manner; uses good judgment when asked to give advice
to the person receiving care.

Never accepts money or a gift as a bribe for special treatment.

Is energetic—has lots of energy to put into his or her job and to give to the
people with whom he or she works.

Information about working in a hospital appears in the next section, which is followed by sections about working in a nursing home and home health care. Each section describes the health care setting, the people who receive care in the particular setting, and what it is like to be a nurse assistant in that setting.

❖   Working in a Hospital   ❖

When Mrs. Garcia woke up in her hospital room after surgery, she looked up and saw some strange-looking equipment beside her bed. She felt afraid. She was in pain and wondered how long it would take to get better. She did not like being in this unfamiliar place. What were those sounds she heard? She just wanted to be back home. Then, someone gently took her hand and said, "Hello, Mrs. Garcia. I'm your nurse assistant. How can I help you feel more comfortable?" (Figure 2-5)

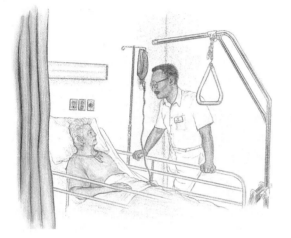

Figure 2-5
You will have many opportunities to comfort and reassure the people in your care.

What Is Hospital Care?

When Mrs. Garcia needed surgery to repair her broken hip, her doctor admitted her to a hospital. A hospital provides care for people who require surgery, have major illnesses, need tests to find out if they have an illness or disease, or get sick suddenly. To keep serious illnesses from occurring, hospital clinics promote wellness through health maintenance and health education. When Mrs. Garcia receives care in the hospital, she is called a **patient**. Part of your job as a nurse assistant is to help patients feel comfortable, as well as to assist nurses and other members of the health care team in providing care for patients.

People who stay overnight in a hospital receive **inpatient** care. Not all hospital patients stay overnight, however. Some people have regular doctor appointments at a hospital **clinic**. They may also go to a clinic to see another health professional, such as a physical therapist, speech therapist, or dietitian. A hospital may also have a surgery clinic, where people go for same-day surgical procedures that do not require them to stay overnight. At a **walk-in clinic**, people can come in without an appointment. Individuals visiting hospital clinics receive **outpatient** care.

Two major types of hospitals are specialized hospitals and general hospitals. A **specialized hospital** provides services for only one type of health care need. Look at Table 2-2, which lists several types of specialized hospitals and the care each provides.

patient
(PAY-shent)   A person who receives health care in a hospital.

inpatient
A patient who must stay overnight in a hospital.

clinic
(KLIN-ik)   A hospital department that provides care to patients who do not need to stay overnight.

walk-in clinic
A hospital department that provides care for patients who do not need appointments.

outpatient
A patient who receives care in a hospital but does not need to stay overnight.

specialized hospital
A facility that provides care for people with certain types of diseases or illnesses.

Table 2-2   Examples of Specialized Hospitals

Type of Hospital	Service and Care Provided for
Obstetric	Pregnant women and those with newborn babies; women with diseases of the reproductive system
Orthopedic	People with broken bones; people with diseases of bones or joints
Pediatric	Children with illnesses or injuries
Psychiatric	People with emotional problems

general hospital
A facility that provides care for people of all ages and with almost any type of illness or injury.

admit
To sign someone into a health care facility.

A **general hospital** usually provides care for patients of all ages and with almost any type of illness or injury. It also provides outpatient care, surgical services, emergency care services, health education classes and testing procedures to identify illnesses. Mrs. Garcia woke up in the orthopedic department of her local general hospital. She had been **admitted** when she arrived at the emergency room. The staff then moved her to the operating room, where the surgeon fixed her hip.

Most general hospitals provide this wide variety of care through individual departments, which help their staffs to focus primarily on one type of patient or illness. This focus allows staff members to become experts in providing specialized care. Look at Table 2-3 to see examples of departments that are common in general hospitals.

Table 2-3   Examples of Departments in a General Hospital

Department	Service and Care Provided for
Medical	Patients who do not need surgery
Surgical	Patients who need surgery
Cardiology	Patients with heart diseases
Clinic	Patients who need medical care but who do not need to stay overnight at the hospital
Emergency	People with emergency medical needs
Intensive care unit	Patients with life-threatening illnesses or conditions
Nursery	Newborn babies
Obstetric	Pregnant women and newborn babies
Oncology	Patients with cancer
Operating room	Patients who undergo surgery
Orthopedic	Patients with bone and joint problems
Pediatric	Children up to 18 years of age
Psychiatric/mental health	Patients with mental or emotional problems

Who Are the People in Hospitals?

Hospital patients vary in age from infants to very old people. The biggest group of people admitted to hospitals are those from ages 15 to 44. Children under 15 years of age make up the smallest group admitted to hospitals.

People in different age groups have different problems that require them to be admitted to the hospital. Children may have respiratory infections and injuries, such as broken bones and burns. Young adults admitted to the hospital may deliver babies, heal from injuries, or get treatment for mental problems, including drug and alcohol abuse. For middle-aged adults, heart disease and cancer are the most common causes of hospital admission.

As a nurse assistant working in a hospital, you provide care for a variety of people. The type of patient in your care depends on the department in which you work. Your patient may be—

❖ An 18-year-old Spanish-speaking woman who has a kidney infection.

❖ A 65-year-old retired lawyer who was recently diagnosed as having diabetes.

❖ A 38-year-old businesswoman who has just delivered her first baby.

❖ A 4-year-old boy who caught his finger in a bicycle chain and requires surgery (Figure 2-6).

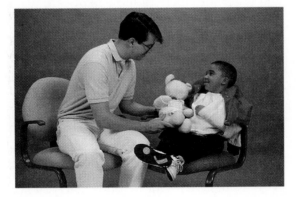

Figure 2-6
Because of the variety of patients in a hospital, you must get to know the people in your care. The hospital can be a scary place for a young child. This nurse assistant knows that using a familiar toy will help the little boy understand what is happening.

The patient in your care may live with a loving and supportive family or may be homeless. This admission to the hospital may be your patient's first, or it may be her fifth admission in 1 year. No matter why she is in the hospital, she needs your compassion and care to feel better while beginning the healing process.

What Is It Like to Work in a Hospital?

Working in a hospital can be exciting, since it is an intense place, full of vigorous activity. Because most patients do not stay a long time, the people in your care may change fairly often. Patients may have

Not Covered

fairly serious illnesses or injuries. The staff, equipment, and facilities of a hospital are expensive, so patients usually are discharged to their own homes or to nursing homes as soon as they no longer require the kind of care a hospital provides.

A hospital can be a difficult place in which to create comfortable, familiar surroundings. Often there is not much space for personal items, and patients are encouraged to leave anything of value at home. Sometimes, for safety reasons, even flowers are not permitted.

Most hospitals have some single rooms, but patients usually share a room with one or more people. Team members can pull curtains around a space so that others cannot see the patient, but it is hard to keep conversations private. Hospitals permit all but the most seriously ill people to have visitors. The visitor's age, the number of visitors, and visiting hours may be limited so that patients can receive the care and rest they need.

For all these reasons, a nurse assistant working in a hospital must have a special ability to form good relationships quickly with people who are under stress. You become an important person for patients who may be afraid of having surgery or tests or who may be in pain. Family or friends may not be around when the patient needs comfort and support. Things happen quickly in a hospital, and patients ask many questions that they may not have had a chance to ask other members of the health care team. Perhaps something was explained to them, but they do not remember what they heard or do not understand. Family members and friends may have similar concerns, and other members of the health care team may not be available to talk with them during visiting hours. It is important for you to tell your supervising nurse about any questions and concerns the patient or the patient's family may raise with you.

Part of the nurse assistant's job in a hospital is practicing the six principles of care: safety, privacy, dignity, communication, independence, and infection control. Remember that each patient is unique and should be treated as a person, not as an illness. The compassionate care you provide can make a difference in how a patient feels about her time in the hospital.

As a nurse assistant in a hospital, you are a vital member of the health care team. You may provide basic patient care under the supervision of a licensed nurse, or you may assist the nursing staff in a certain department by transporting patients to and from the department or helping with examinations. Your duties vary, depending on the department in which you work. Some of these departments are: obstetric, pediatric, orthopedic, and surgical.

While working in the **obstetric** department, you provide care to two patients: the mother and her newborn baby. Your patient may be having her first child, or she may already be a mother. She may be a teenager or a woman in her 30s or 40s. Whatever her situation, she needs encouragement and support. She may be excited, happy, or worried. She may be nervous about the great responsibility of

obstetric
(ob-STET-rik) A type of medicine or care provided for pregnant women, women who have just delivered babies, and their newborn children. The obstetric department includes the maternity ward.

parenting. You help the nurse to teach the mother techniques to provide care for her newborn, including bathing, **umbilical cord** care, diaper changing, and bottle or breast feeding. (You will read about these techniques in Chapter 21, Providing Care for Mothers and Newborns). You also encourage the mother to talk about her concerns and to ask questions so that you can communicate her needs to your supervising nurse.

When you work in the **pediatric** department, you provide care for patients under 18 years of age. Knowledge of the normal stages of growth and development helps you provide better care for these patients and recognize any delays or abnormalities in growth and development. (You will read about growth and development in Chapter 4, Understanding People.) In the pediatric department, the staff encourages parents to participate in providing care for their children. Most hospitals make sleeping arrangements so that at least one parent can be with a child as much as he or she wants. A parent may sleep in the same room as the child or come early in the morning and stay until late at night. With a parent nearby, the child may be less frightened.

In the **orthopedic** department, you provide care for patients who are having difficulty with bones or joints or who are wearing casts. You work with many kinds of specialized orthopedic equipment that aids in the healing process and helps patients move around more easily and independently.

Before and after surgery, patients need special care. In the surgical department, you provide care for patients who may have specific devices or equipment. You will read about working in the surgical department in Chapter 20, Providing Care for People Having Surgery.

What Is It Like to Work in a Hospital Clinic?

In the hospital clinic, you assist the doctors and nurses as they provide patient care. While on duty you—

❖ Follow your supervising nurse's directions.
❖ Tell patients about the clinic, show them around, and help them feel comfortable while they wait to see another health professional.
❖ Help patients prepare for their physical examinations or medical procedures and assist them with dressing.
❖ Assist the doctor or nurse with physical examinations and procedures.
❖ Check and maintain the inventory of instruments and other supplies and restock them.
❖ Take and write down patients' blood pressure, temperature, pulse rate (Figure 2-7), and respirations. Measure intake, output, weight, and height.
❖ Assist with the collection of urine, stool, and sputum specimens for lab tests.

umbilical cord
(um-BIL-uh-kuhl)   A tubelike structure arising from an unborn baby's navel that connects it to the placenta inside the mother. It carries nourishment to the baby and waste out of the baby.

pediatric
(pee-de-AT-rik)   A type of medicine or care provided for children under 18 years of age.

orthopedic
(or-tho-PEE-dik)   A type of medicine or care provided for people who have problems with their bones or joints.

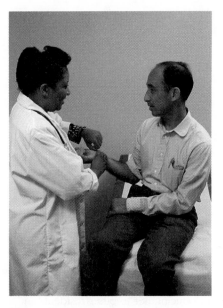

Figure 2-7
Measuring vital signs is an important part of most clinic procedures. Because vital signs are usually taken in the first part of the visit, health care workers can set the tone of the visit by being friendly and efficient.

❖ Provide comfort and safety measures for patients.

❖ Communicate patients' needs and concerns to the appropriate caregivers.

❖ Provide preoperative care for surgical patients. (See the section in Chapter 20 on surgical skills.)

Nurse assistants work in all areas of the hospital. Different departments of the hospital require specific knowledge and skills in addition to the basic skills for providing patient care. Some of this information appears later in this book and in the skills book. You will continue to learn additional information and skills after you begin working in a hospital.

To learn about working in a nursing home, please read the next section of this chapter. To learn about working in home health care, please read the section following the nursing home section. If you choose not to read either of the next two sections, turn to the end of the chapter to read "Information Review" and "Questions to Ask Yourself."

❖   Working in a Nursing Home   ❖

On a sunny day in March, you helped Mrs. Garcia pack the small suitcase her children brought to the hospital. She was feeling much better, and her hip was getting stronger since she started the exercises recommended by the physical therapist. Still, she needed more care before she could return home, so she was going to continue her recovery at a nursing home. As she prepared to go to Morningside Nursing Home, Mrs. Garcia had many questions: "Who else lives in the home? Will I make friends? (Figure 2-8) What will I do with my time? Will the nurses be nice to me? Will I get the kind of treatment I need? Will they treat me with respect?" Her children also had questions: "Will we be able to visit? Will they take good care of Mother?"

Figure 2-8
Showing a new resident around and introducing her to other residents and staff help her to feel at home.

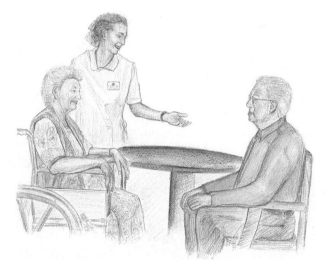

What Is Nursing Home Care?

A **nursing home** provides care for people who do not need to stay in a hospital but require medical care and assistance they cannot get at home (Box 2-3). Some people may stay in a nursing home for a few days or for a few weeks to regain their physical and emotional health through **rehabilitation**. Others may stay there for the rest of their lives if they need care that cannot be provided by their relatives or other caregivers. In the nursing home, Mrs. Garcia is called a **resident**. As a nurse assistant, you work with the health care team to provide daily care and help residents live as fully and independently as possible.

The people who need nursing home care want to know that they will receive good care. To guarantee that people receive a certain level of care, federal and state governments established standards for staffing and operation that all nursing homes must meet. In 1990, new federal nursing home requirements became effective. When working in a nursing home, you hear people talking about these "OBRA" requirements.

nursing home
A facility that provides care for people who do not need to stay in a hospital, but who need medical care and assistance they cannot get at home.

rehabilitation
(re-huh-bil-e-TAY-shun)   The process of regaining physical health.

resident
(REZ-e-dent)   A person who receives health care in a nursing home.

Box 2-3   **Other Terms for Nursing Home**

Assisted-living community	Nursing center
Care center	Nursing facility
Convalescent center	Nursing and rehabilitative treatment center
Geriatric center	Rehabilitation center
Health center	Residential care facility
Health care center	Skilled care center
Long-term care center	

What Is OBRA '87?

In 1987, the United States Congress passed a law to improve the quality of health care in this country. This law is known as **OBRA '87** because it was part of the 1987 **O**mnibus **B**udget **R**econciliation **A**ct.

OBRA **regulations** emphasize respect for a person's independence and rights. Examples of these rights are the right of people in nursing homes and home health care to be treated with dignity and the right to make choices. (You will read about these rights in Chapter 3, Protecting People's Rights.) OBRA regulations led to the requirement that you must be **certified** as a nurse assistant to work in a nursing home or as a home health aide to work in home health care. This certification means that you take a test to demonstrate your

OBRA '87
(OH-brah)   An abbreviation for the 1987 **O**mnibus **B**udget **R**econciliation **A**ct, which provides certain standards for nursing homes and home health care.

regulation
(reg-you-LAY-shun)   A rule that must be followed.

certified
(SER-te-fide)   Having skills that have been tested and approved.

knowledge and skills. OBRA also emphasizes the responsibility of nursing homes and home health agencies to provide residents with the most comfortable and fulfilling lifestyle and to promote their physical, mental, emotional, and spiritual well-being to the highest possible degree.

In addition, OBRA has very important requirements for nurse assistant training. The training ensures that a nurse assistant or home health aide—

❖ Promotes peoples' independence and respects their rights.
❖ Knows about peoples' mental health and social service needs.
❖ Has good communication and interpersonal skills.
❖ Knows safety procedures and can properly respond to emergencies.
❖ Practices infection control.
❖ Knows basic nursing skills, including how to provide personal care.
❖ Knows about basic **restorative services**.
❖ Knows how to provide care for people with **cognitive impairment**.

restorative services
(re-STOR-uh-tiv) Activities or devices that help a person improve, maintain, or regain physical functions.

cognitive impairment
(KOG-nuh-tiv/im-PARE-ment) A condition that decreases a person's ability to think clearly.

Who Are the People in Nursing Homes?

The average age of nursing home residents is 85 years. Of these residents, more than twice as many are women as are men (Figure 2-9). How would you feel about living in a place with twice as many women as men?

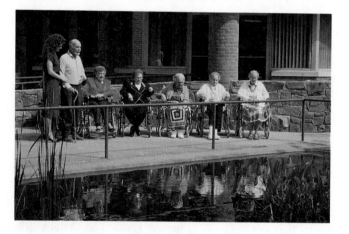

Figure 2-9
Residents in a nursing home may be similar in age and medical condition but have a wide variety of experiences and accomplishments.

Why do you think these very old people, mostly women, live in nursing homes? Almost all people in nursing homes go there because of one of the following conditions: cognitive or emotional disorder (including Alzheimer's disease), circulatory disease (including heart disease and stroke), diabetes, cancer, hip or other fracture, or musculoskeletal system disorder (including arthritis). More residents go to nursing homes to receive care because they are mentally unable to take care of themselves than for any other reason. These residents have some type of cognitive impairment. The most common cause of cognitive impairment is Alzheimer's disease. (You will read about this disorder in Chapter 18, Providing Care for People who have Alzheimer's Disease.) Many people also go to nursing homes because they cannot function alone as a result of circulatory disease.

Most residents have more than one medical condition. For example, a resident may have heart disease and a cognitive or emotional disorder. The heart disease may be the reason for admission, but the resident also needs care because of the cognitive impairment.

The effects of these medical conditions on some people, rather than the conditions themselves, often lead to the need for nursing home care. For example, someone who has arthritis may no longer be able to get in and out of bed, to the toilet, or dressed without help. Or, someone with Alzheimer's disease may be physically able to function but may need constant reminders to eat, get dressed, and stay out of danger because she cannot remember to do these things. Most people in nursing homes require help with activities of daily living (Box 2-4).

Box 2-4   **Activities of Daily Living**

Eating	Using the toilet
Bathing	Walking/moving
Dressing	Communicating
Grooming	

You may be surprised to learn that some children and younger people live in nursing homes. A child or a younger person may live there because of an injury to the head, neck, or back (called a spinal cord injury); a mental disability; or a serious, disabling handicap. No matter how old or young they are, all residents in nursing homes have one thing in common: They cannot take care of themselves completely and have special health care needs that cannot be met at home.

Think for a moment about residents in nursing homes: Most are very old, sick, and disabled people who need help in taking care of themselves. It may be hard to think of these people as "captains" of a health care team. What can you do in your role as a nurse assistant to help a resident be as involved as possible?

What Is It Like to Work in a Nursing Home?

In a nursing home, you have the same responsibility that all nurse assistants have: to provide basic nursing care. In addition, you do certain things that are specific to working in a nursing home. For example, one of the residents' most important needs is having people to talk with. You have time to talk with them as you provide care. Most people like to be asked about their lives, accomplishments, and families. Often nursing home residents do not have family members nearby who can come to visit regularly. You can fill some of their needs by talking with them and encouraging them to talk with each other and to get involved in activities.

You also are a key person to help a resident achieve or maintain her highest level of independence. Sometimes it may be easier and faster for you to do things for the resident, such as with Mrs. Garcia, who moves slowly because of her healing hip. But it means much more to her if you encourage her to do things alone, give her the time to do the tasks, and provide help when she needs it.

To learn about working in home health care, please read the next section of this chapter. If you choose not to read the next section, turn to the end of the chapter to read "Information Review" and "Questions to Ask Yourself."

❖ Working in Home Health Care ❖

Mrs. Garcia is happy to be back at home. She likes sleeping in her own bed and enjoys being alone. She gets in and out of bed by herself, fixes her own simple meals, and even manages to get dressed by herself.

But Mrs. Garcia needs help with bathing, changing the bed linens, and shopping for groceries. She also needs help with doing the exercises recommended by the physical therapist (Figure 2-10). The **home health aide** visits with Mrs. Garcia twice each week to help her with these tasks.

home health aide
A nurse assistant who works in home health care.

Figure 2-10
By helping Mrs. Garcia with her hip exercises, the home health aide is helping her reach her goal of living independently.

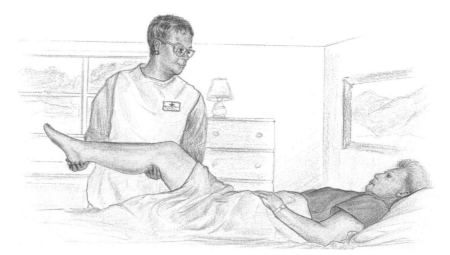

What Is Home Health Care?

After Mrs. Garcia's walking improved, she was discharged from the nursing home and sent home to receive assistance through a home health care agency. A **home health care agency** provides health care services to people in their homes so that they safely get the care they need, while feeling secure within their own homes and with their families. When Mrs. Garcia receives home health care, she is called a **client**. Typically, clients receive home health care from a registered nurse, who **monitors** their health and plans their care, and from a home health aide, who helps them with their daily care.

For many years people were afraid to go to the hospital. They thought that they would get better care at home. As time went on, it became more common for people who were very sick to get health care in a hospital. Today, **home health care** is again popular because it doesn't cost as much as hospital care, and it encourages people to receive individualized care in their own homes. Two purposes of home health care are to help people get better and to promote independence while in the comfort of their homes. Home health aides, who work in this part of the health care system, have training similar to that of nurse assistants and provide the same basic nursing care.

When people are ill or injured or have medical conditions that require them to have professional health care for only part of the day, they may choose to receive that care at home. The rest of the day, they can be alone or have family or friends provide care for them. A client with a **chronic illness** may choose to be cared for at home. A client with a **terminal illness** is not expected to recover and may also use home health care. Many elderly people require some assistance because they are frail and not able to do certain things for themselves. Sometimes home health care workers teach family members or friends to provide care for their loved ones at home.

The people who require home health care want to know that they will receive good care. To guarantee that people receive a certain level of care, federal and state governments established standards for staffing and operation that all home health agencies must meet. In 1987, new home health requirements, which state that home health agencies are responsible for providing good care to their clients, became effective. When working in home health care, you hear people talking about these "OBRA" requirements. (To read about OBRA, turn to "What Is OBRA '87?" in the nursing home section of this chapter.)

Who Are the People Receiving Home Health Care?

Clients receiving home health care can be young or old, male or female, and of any race, religion, or ethnic background. They all have special medical problems that require different kinds of care in their homes to maintain or recover their health.

Examples of clients who may receive home health care include—

home health care agency
A health organization that employs home health aides and others who provide health care and other services to people in their homes.

client
(KLY-ent)   A person who receives health care at home.

monitor
(MON-e-ter)   To check regularly for the quality of a person's physical or emotional condition.

home health care
Health care provided in private homes to people who do not need to stay in hospitals or nursing homes.

chronic illness
(KRAHN-ik)   A long-lasting condition or illness that may occur again.

terminal illness
(TER-muh-nul)   A serious illness or condition from which a person is not expected to recover.

❖ A 5-year-old boy with cerebral palsy who needs help with feeding himself and personal hygiene.

❖ A 39-year-old client with **AIDS** who needs emotional support and help with the basic activities of daily living (Figure 2-11).

❖ A 72-year-old woman who fell and broke her hip and needs personal care and physical therapy.

AIDS

An abbreviation for **a**cquired **i**mmune **d**eficiency **s**yndrome. AIDS is caused by the **h**uman **i**mmunodeficiency **v**irus (HIV), which results in a breakdown of the body's defense systems.

Figure 2-11

A person with AIDS may feel isolated and may depend on the home health aide for comfort and support.

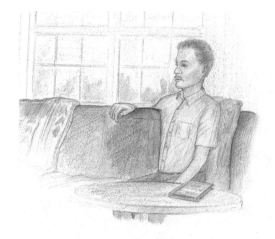

How to Get Home Health Care

After Mrs. Garcia received physical therapy and other rehabilitative care at the nursing home, her doctor decided that her walking had improved and that she could go home. But he also decided that she would still need some assistance, so he referred her to a home health care agency. This **referral process** allows one member of the health care system to let other members know that a person requires their kind of specialized care.

referral process

(re-FER-uhl)   A set of procedures that allows one member of the health care system to inform other members that a person needs their kind of specialized care.

Although the doctor or nurse typically makes a home health care referral, anyone in the community can call a home health care agency and ask for services. The home health care agency evaluates each case to see if they can provide services.

Clients pay for home health care in a number of different ways: through Medicare, Medicaid, private insurance, and private pay. Rules and regulations govern how each of these methods of payment covers the cost. Because these rules differ from agency to agency, a client should check with a local home health care agency for the rules that apply in her state.

What Is It Like to Work as a Home Health Aide?

Because home health aides fill a very important need, the law states that they must take a test to be certified to work in people's homes. To be a good home health aide, you also must be professional and mature. This requirement includes not discussing the client's condition with others either during or after work hours. While you work, no one stands over your shoulder and tells you what to do, but duties and responsibilities are clearly outlined in your job description and the client's care plan.

Depending on your client's needs, your responsibilities will include providing personal care, such as bathing and grooming, and making sure your client is safe. Some clients may need help cooking a meal, or they may need you to prepare the entire meal. Other clients may have to be reminded to take their medications. Still others may need you to do light housekeeping to help them maintain a clean and safe environment.

As a home health aide, you may also need to reinforce the teachings of other health care team members. For example, you might remind a new mother how to change a diaper. It may be better to talk her through the procedure while she demonstrates, rather than tell her how to do it. Or if the physical therapist teaches a client in the morning to use a walker, when you help that client in the afternoon, you can ask her to show you what she learned. You then have the opportunity to encourage her if she learned correctly or to suggest any changes.

Many home health aides typically provide care for only one client at a time. For example, you know that you have 2 hours to be at Mrs. Garcia's home. In those 2 hours, you focus your attention on Mrs. Garcia and not on your other clients.

All nurse assistants deal with families, but in the home health care setting you talk with household members in their own environments. Sometimes you may find working in their homes to be a warm and rewarding experience. At other times you may not like how some people behave. You may be exposed to values that are different from your own.

If your client's home is a caring and safe place, it will probably be a pleasant setting for caregiving. However, some people may not keep their homes as clean as you keep your own. You may also observe or suspect alcohol abuse, drug abuse, physical abuse, or illegal activity while you are providing care in the home. You should report any concerns you have about your client's well-being to your supervising nurse, who will help you decide what to do.

Many families have pets. Pets often are very important to clients (Figure 2-12). If you are afraid of animals or are allergic to them, you may have to ask the family to put the animal in another room during your visit.

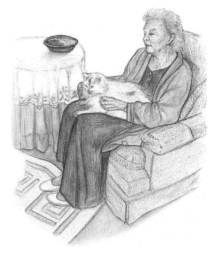

Figure 2-12
Mrs. Garcia missed her cat's companionship while she was away. Pets can help people from becoming lonely.

The Role of a Homemaker

A **homemaker** works through the home health agency to help clients perform basic housekeeping tasks and provide companion services to people in the community. A trained homemaker does not provide personal care. Only a certified nurse assistant, home health aide, or nurse may provide personal care; but often when a home health aide provides care for a client in her home, he or she provides both personal care as a home health aide and household main-

homemaker
A home health agency employee who helps clients perform household tasks.

tenance as a homemaker. Both jobs are important in promoting independence and in helping someone stay at home safely rather than go to a nursing home.

Responsibilities of a homemaker include—

❖ Doing light housekeeping (vacuuming, dusting, mopping floors, cleaning the kitchen and bathroom, changing beds, washing dishes) and other activities, as they are assigned, that keep the client's home clean and orderly.

❖ Performing household duties such as laundry, shopping, and running personal errands.

❖ Preparing and serving nutritious meals, following diet plans.

❖ Observing the client's general physical, emotional, and mental condition and reporting any changes to your supervising nurse.

❖ Noting the care provided on the assignment sheet (Figure 2-13).

❖ Reminding the client to take medication, as assigned.

❖ Being kind and patient in meeting the social needs of the client.

❖ Keeping equipment and supplies clean, safe, secure, and in good working order.

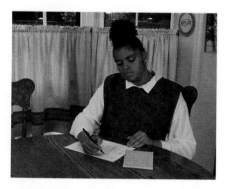

Figure 2-13

Because a homemaker or home health aide often works alone providing care to the client, she must carefully document her activities and observations.

It is important to remember rules about what a homemaker *cannot* do for a client. A homemaker cannot provide personal care. Neither a homemaker nor a home health aide may *give* medications. Only a licensed nurse may give medication. A homemaker or home health aide may remind or "cue" a client to take medication, but he or she cannot give medication. This requirement means that you can open the bottle and bring it to the client with a glass of water. You *cannot* remove the medication from the bottle or touch the medication in any other way.

Your Home Health Care Supervisor

As a home health aide, you work under the direction of the supervising nurse, or supervisor, in charge of your client's care. While you work in a client's home, your supervisor may be miles away in an office or seeing another client, although you can always call the agency to talk with someone who can help you or give you advice. The supervisor in charge of your client's care regularly evaluates the care you provide by coming to see you at your client's home. This visit may be a good time to ask any questions you may have.

One of the hardest facts about not having your supervising nurse with you at the home is that nobody is "down the hall" to help you if something happens or if you have questions. For example, you may arrive for work and find your client sweating and complaining of sharp chest pain. Because this situation could be a life-threatening emergency, you immediately call emergency medical service (EMS), stay with the person until help arrives, and then call your agency to let them know what has happened and to get further instructions.

Using Community Resources

Many services in the community help people get well, help them learn to adapt to their illnesses, or offer emotional support. Some organizations provide information about particular illnesses or conditions, such as cancer, diabetes, or cystic fibrosis, to people in the community. Others also offer community lectures and support groups for people with specific needs. Some community services offer rides to and from doctors' appointments, deliver meals to people's homes, and provide child care. Check with your supervising nurse or the social worker if you think someone in your care would benefit from one of these community services. In addition, AIDS service organizations and **hospices** offer special care and sometimes offer special training programs for nurse assistants and home health aides.

hospice
(HOS-pis)   A program of good medical and emotional care and support for people who are dying, as well as for their families.

Information Review

Circle the correct answers and fill in the blanks.

1. Three parts of the health care system in which nurse assistants may work are ___hospital___, ___Nursing home___, and ___Home health care___.

2. The "captain" of the health care team is the—
    a. Doctor.
    b. Registered nurse.
    c. Administrator.
    d. Person receiving care.

3. A health care worker who helps people learn about what they eat is a—
    a. Nurse practitioner
    b. Dietitian.
    c. Pharmacist.
    d. Physical therapist.

4. In addition to helping the person in your care, you assist your ___Nurse___ ___supervisor___, who gives you your assignments, receives your reports, and answers your questions.

Hospitals

1. A person receiving care in a hospital is called a ___patient___.

2. A person goes to a hospital ___clinic___ when she requires care but does not need to stay overnight.

3. Signing a person into a health care facility is called—
    a. Certifying.
    b. Referring.
    c. Admitting.
    d. Discharging.

4. The department in which you provide care for people with broken bones or diseases of the bones and joints is the—
   a. Orthopedic department.
   b. Pediatric department.
   c. Surgical department.
   d. Obstetric department.

Nursing Homes

1. Some people stay in nursing homes for a short period of time to regain their physical and emotional health. We call this situation—
   a. Activity of daily living.
   b. Cognitive impairment.
   c. Rehabilitation.
   d. Chronic illness.
2. A person receiving care in a nursing home is called a
   _____resident_____.
3. The law passed by Congress that ensures that residents receive the best care possible is known as _____OBRA_____.
4. The condition that affects most residents living in nursing homes is _____Cognitive_____ _____impairment_____.

Home Health Care

1. A nurse assistant who provides care in people's homes is called a—
   a. Maintenance employee.
   b. Home health aide.
   c. Nurse practitioner.
   d. Social worker.
2. A person receiving health care at home is called a
   _____Client_____.
3. The law passed by Congress that ensures that clients receive the best care possible is known as _____OBRA_____.
4. One thing a nurse assistant working in home health care is *not* permitted to do is—
   a. Give medication.
   b. Prepare medication.
   c. Provide personal care.
   d. Remind the person to take medication.

Questions to Ask Yourself

1. What are some of the most important qualities a nurse assistant should have?

2. What special qualities would you bring to your work as a nurse assistant?

3. Think of someone you know who received care in one of the three major parts of the health care system. What did the person think of the care he or she received?

Hospitals

1. You are the first person Mrs. Garcia sees when she wakes up after surgery. She is afraid of the equipment attached to her arm and wants you to remove it. What would you say to her?

2. Mrs. Roberts has just been admitted to your floor in the hospital. She insists that she cannot possibly share a room with Mrs. Garcia. How would you handle this situation?

3. In the cardiology clinic, Mr. Smith will not undress for his examination unless you leave the room. Yet he is very weak and requires constant support while standing or sitting. How would you respect his privacy and make sure he is safe?

Nursing Homes

1. At Morningside Nursing Home, Mr. Flanagan spends a lot of time holding a picture of his wife. Sometimes he talks to the picture. Every day he tells you that he wants to go home. How would you respond?

2. Mrs. Landers dearly loves the fresh flowers her daughter brought her and wants to keep them on her bedside table. But her roommate is allergic to flowers. What would you do?

3. In the activities lounge, two residents are arguing over which television show to watch. What would you say when they ask you, "Who is right?"

Home Health Care

1. Whenever it rains, Mrs. Garcia will not go out to the front porch to get her newspaper. She says she will fall and break her hip again. How would you help Mrs. Garcia regain her independence?

2. When you arrive each Thursday to help Mrs. Rose, she is always glad to see you and says, "You are my only friend." She always wants you to stay all day, but several other clients need your attention on Thursday. How would you make sure Mrs. Rose's needs are met and still provide care for your other clients?

3. Mrs. Gilbert, the wife of one of your clients, has asked you to help her wash and wax the kitchen floor. This task is not on Mr. Gilbert's care plan, but Mrs. Gilbert is old and cannot get around very well. What would you do?

3

Protecting People's Rights

Goals

After reading this chapter, you will have the information to—

Explain what legal rights are and how they came into being.

Give five examples of the rights of people receiving health care.

Explain the difference between legal and ethical responsibilities.

Discuss your role as a caregiver in protecting rights and behaving in an ethical manner.

Describe what you should do if you suspect that a person in your care is being neglected or abused.

At 11:00 A.M., you knock on Mr. Rivera's door. You listen carefully for his response, because he has difficulty speaking as a result of right-sided paralysis from a stroke. "Come in," says Mr. Rivera. When you walk in, you are surprised to see Mrs. Rivera sitting on the edge of the bed. Mrs. Rivera normally visits her husband every day around 2:00 P.M.

Not only is Mrs. Rivera there, dressed up in a pretty purple suit, but she has already served up two plates of homemade food on the overbed table. A red balloon that says, "I love you," floats above the nightstand. This is not what you were expecting. You had already scheduled Mr. Rivera's bath for 11:15, just as you do every day.

"It's the 60th anniversary of the day we met," explains Mrs. Rivera. "Victor and I met at my cousin's 15th birthday party. When I saw him, I knew he was the right man for me." Mrs. Rivera smiles at her husband, who is sitting up in bed against some pillows. She touches his face gently and then starts to cut his food.

You ask Mr. Rivera if he would still like to take his bath at 11:15. Mr. Rivera nods his head from side to side as he chews his food. "Not today," he finally replies, after swallowing. Then he pats Mrs. Rivera on the hand.

Mr. O'Reilly, Mr. Rivera's roommate, has physical therapy from 11:00 to 12:00, so you usually make his bed before assisting Mr. Rivera with his bath at 11:15. As you start to make Mr. O'Reilly's bed, however, Mr. Rivera clears his throat a couple of times. "Mrs. Rivera and I would like some time alone to celebrate our special day," he says with difficulty.

At first you feel a little annoyed. "Why didn't Mr. Rivera tell me about this change so that I could schedule my day differently?" you wonder. Your routine normally works so well.

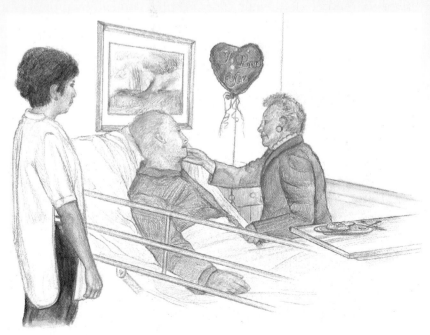

Then you try to put yourself in Mr. Rivera's place. This room is his home, after all, and today is a very important day. You also know that Mr. Rivera has a right to his privacy.

"Congratulations," you say as you close the door on your way out. "I'll be down the hall if you need me."

Do you know what the word "right" means? You probably have heard people using the word all your life. If you look in a dictionary, you will find many different meanings for the word "right." In your work as a nurse assistant, three meanings will be important to you:

❖ "Right" means correct and true, based on some standard of quality or correctness. For example, if you have to take Mr. Rivera's temperature, you want to be sure you take it the right way. Only then will you get a correct reading.

❖ "Right" also means a privilege that belongs to a person and is protected by law. For example, does Mr. Rivera have the right not to take his bath? Or to refuse the medication ordered by his doctor? He has the legal right to refuse his bath and the medication, even though he needs the bath to stay clean and the medication to stay healthy. Legal rights vary from state to state, and you must check with your supervising nurse to make sure you understand how **legal rights** are defined in the state where you work.

❖ "Right" also means good and virtuous, based on the concepts of justice and morality. For example, what if another nurse assistant tells you that she is wearing one of Mrs. Wang's necklaces today? The nurse assistant tells you that Mrs. Wang has so many necklaces that she won't miss this one for just 1 day. The right thing for you to do is to take steps to make sure the necklace is returned to its rightful owner as soon as possible.

Throughout this book you will read about the right way to do different nursing procedures so that you can provide care that meets the standard for quality. In this chapter, you will read about the legal rights of the people in your care and how you can help protect those rights. You also will read about your **ethical** responsibility to do what is morally right when providing care for people.

legal right
(LEE-gul)   A privilege that is protected by law.

ethical
(ETH-e-kuhl)   That which is morally and professionally correct.

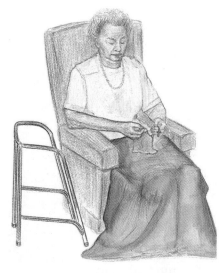

Figure 3-1
The Bill of Rights guarantees a person's right to practice her own religion. As a nurse assistant, you are responsible for helping to protect this right for the people in your care.

abuse
(ah-BYOOS)   Harm that occurs when a person is purposely hurt or mistreated.

The Rights of People Receiving Health Care

Citizens in the United States have certain individual rights. These rights are guaranteed by law, and no one can take them away. The Constitution and the Bill of Rights guarantee U.S. citizens the right to speak their thoughts freely, worship in any way they want (Figure 3-1), gather together in groups, and decide freely what to print.

During our nation's history, many people have fought for legal rights by writing letters, carrying signs and shouting in front of government buildings, and marching down city streets. Because people are free to demonstrate for something they believe in, situations change. Some changes brought about by demonstration are: Today's women have the right to vote; African-Americans have rights to equal education, jobs, and housing; children have the right to be protected from **abuse**; and minorities and the elderly have the right to be protected against discrimination.

A person's rights are protected by law because rights are crucial to a person's freedom. People who receive health care have the same rights and privileges that you have. And, because they are dependent on others for care, they have additional rights that are protected by special laws. These laws guarantee that people in health care have the right to competent, considerate care that is delivered with respect. They have the right to know the kind of care they will receive and the cost of that care, as well as to help decide about the care and who will provide it. In addition, people receiving health care now have the right to confidentiality and privacy and the right to be free from restraints and abuse. These rights about health care exist as law because many people, including families, friends, and health care professionals, fought for and won them.

Today, each hospital, nursing home, and home health care agency has a list of rights, called a **bill of rights**, which it offers to its patients, residents, or clients. The lists differ slightly from one setting to another and from state to state.

In 1975, the American Hospital Association developed the "Patient Bill of Rights" in response to consumers' wishes to know more about what they could expect while they were in the hospital. Today many hospitals voluntarily use this document or develop a similar one.

As more people in our society grew older, the need increased for places to provide care for older people who could not take care of themselves due to mental and physical disabilities. Nursing homes evolved to fill this need. Initially, these facilities were not regulated, and families began to report that their loved ones were being tied in chairs, developing bedsores, and experiencing other difficulties. Many of these problems occurred either because there were not enough caregivers or because the caregivers were not trained properly to provide the care needed by people in the facilities.

Because of consumer concern, in 1987 the federal government passed a law that protects the rights of residents in nursing homes and clients in home health care. In 1990, the federal government issued a mandate requiring nursing homes and home health agencies to provide lists of rights to people receiving care. In 1991 the federal government legislated the Patient Self-Determination Act, which requires all provider organizations that receive Medicare and Medicaid funds to make patients, residents, and clients aware of their rights to make decisions concerning medical care. These rights include the right to accept or refuse care and to develop advanced directives.

Protecting the rights of people receiving health care is one of your most important responsibilities as a nurse assistant, and you can help ensure that the person in your care does not give up any of his rights. The person receiving care, his family, and all members of the health care team need to know what these rights are, how to protect them, how to promote them, and how to report situations in which they have been violated. For example, Mr. Rivera knew he had the right to spend time alone with his wife. And you, as the nurse assistant, knew the importance of protecting that right. So you changed

bill of rights
A list of rights and expectations of health care provided to a patient, resident, or client. A bill of rights may include the person's right to receive information about his care in a language he can understand, the right to refuse treatment, and the right to privacy, confidentiality, and continuing care.

your plans to help Mr. Rivera with his bath, and you decided to make Mr. O'Reilly's bed later in the day.

If someone is unclear about his rights, you can remind him, as well as his family members, to meet with the social worker or supervising nurse, who will give the person a copy of his rights and explain them. Examples of a person's legal rights, along with specific things you can do to protect them, are listed in Table 3-1.

People who receive health care also have the right to name someone to make health care decisions for them if they become **incapacitated**. You and other members of the health care team are responsible for telling each patient, resident, or client about this right. Anyone can use a legal document called a **health care proxy** to name a

incapacitated
(in-kuh-PAH-se-tay-ted)   Being unable to act for oneself.

health care proxy
(PROKS-ee)   A legal document that names a person to make health care decisions if the person receiving care is unable to.

Table 3-1   Respecting and Protecting Rights

A Person Has the Right to. . .	You Can. . .
Know his rights.	Remind the person to meet with your supervising nurse or the social worker to get a copy of the rights and discuss them.
Receive considerate care. Be treated with dignity and respect without discrimination because of race, color, sex, culture, sexual orientation, disability, or diagnosis.	Call the person by name. Explain the care that you are going to provide. Get permission to provide care. Involve the person in his own care.
Have his needs met.	Do everything possible to take care of the person's needs. Communicate the person's needs to the other team members.
Be told about his condition and what the doctor recommends for treatment. (This is called informed consent and involves the right to know the choices in medical or surgical care.)	Encourage the person to ask questions of the appropriate person.
Know the cost of care.	Refer the person to the social worker or the accounting department of a hospital. Encourage the person and family members to ask the doctor about fees. Provide any literature about cost.
Refuse care or treatment and be given information about what may happen because he has refused treatment. Refuse to be part of experimental treatments.	Encourage the person to ask questions. Suggest getting a second opinion, if the person has the resources to pay for one. Offer to come back at a better time. Talk to your supervising nurse about changing the care plan. Work with her to rearrange scheduling to meet needs. Ask her to meet with the person to talk about what may happen if he does not receive his treatment.
Keep records private and confidential and be able to see his own clinical record.	Keep information about the person to yourself when talking with people in or out of the hospital who are not involved in the person's care. Show the clinical record only to those who are involved with the person's care.
Know, and have in writing, the services and items that are covered or not covered by Medicaid or Medicare.	Encourage the person to talk with the social worker and ask questions.
Be treated by the doctor and caregivers of his choice.	Make sure your supervising nurse knows which caregivers the person prefers.
Know about his medical condition and be given current and complete information about the diagnosis, treatment, alternatives, risks, and prognosis.	Encourage the person to talk with your supervising nurse or the doctor and ask specific questions.

friend or family member to make health care decisions for him if he is too ill to decide about his own care.

Josie Miller decided to have a **living will**. A person can use this legal document to state how she would like her health care to be managed if she is too ill to choose for herself. She may state in the living will that she does not want any life support systems, such as a breathing machine, if she becomes too ill to breathe on her own. In some states, a person may need to have both a health care proxy and a living will (Figure 3-2).

Another right of the person receiving health care is the right to voice concerns and complaints. For example, Mrs. Wang's granddaughter and her three children visit every Wednesday afternoon.

living will
A legal document, prepared by a person receiving care, that states how he would like his care to continue if he becomes unable to make health care decisions.

Table 3-1   **Respecting and Protecting Rights—cont'd**

A Person Has the Right to. . .	You Can. . .
Know about all services and the frequency of visits, as well as help plan his care and treatment.	Involve the person and family members in writing the care plan. (Remember, the person is the head of the team.)
Make a complaint or suggest changes in health care services or staff without being threatened or discriminated against.	Communicate a complaint to your supervising nurse and modify care to meet the person's needs.
Be free from abuse.	Treat everyone with dignity and respect. Report incidents of abuse.
Be free from restraints.	Never use restraints without a doctor's order.
Be told in writing if care is going to be denied, changed, or ended. An appeal when this situation occurs (in a nursing home or home health care setting).	Remind the person that he has the right to appeal and that someone who is not involved with the original decision will be reviewing the case.
Privacy.	Get permission to provide care. Keep the person covered and pull the curtain when providing care. Ask permission to open bedside drawers and closets. Talk about the person's medical condition or personal affairs only with others who are involved with the person's care.
Manage his own money matters.	Never take money or gifts from the person in your care. Never discuss the person's finances. Refer the person to the social worker if he has concerns about finances.
Send and receive mail that has not been opened.	Deliver unopened mail to the person. Offer to help open or read mail.
Practice his religion.	Help the person get to religious services. Call the clergy of his choice, if requested.
Use his own clothing or possessions.	Make sure the person gets clean clothes every day. In a nursing home, make sure the person's possessions are marked with his name.
Be alone with his partner or spouse.	Provide privacy. Help the person plan visiting time.

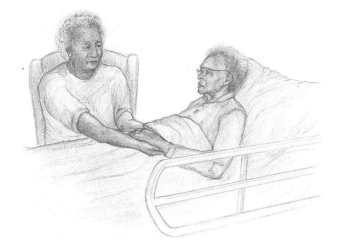

Figure 3-2
Josie Miller tells her sister Arlene about her living will, which states her decision not to be put on life support systems. Josie made this difficult decision so that Arlene wouldn't have to decide for her.

ombudsman
(OM-buds-man)   A person who acts as a mediator between a resident and the nursing home. The ombudsman listens to the resident's concerns and complaints and resolves conflicts with the health care provider.

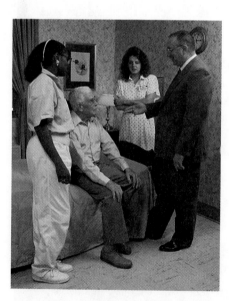

Figure 3-3
This ombudsman is helping to resolve a conflict about a room change.

The lively chatter annoys Mrs. Wang's roommate, Mrs. Ryan, who likes to nap after lunch. Mrs. Ryan complained to you about the noise. As a nurse assistant, you can help resolve this problem by negotiating with the two roommates. (Read about negotiating skills in Chapter 5, Communicating with People.)

If a resident in a nursing home thinks that his rights are being violated, he can talk with his resident representative. The resident representative acts as an **ombudsman**, a person who listens to people's concerns and complaints, investigates their problems, and then tries to correct them. An ombudsman takes care of all types of problems, including legal and ethical ones. The federal government requires each state to have an ombudsman program that serves nursing homes. After an investigation of a problem, the ombudsman informs the right person or agency so that the problem can be resolved. People receiving health care, their families, and caregivers like yourself can take their problem or concern to an ombudsman. The people or their families must give the ombudsman permission to investigate any concerns or complaints, regardless of who reported the complaint (Figure 3-3). After receiving permission, the ombudsman talks with those involved to find out what happened and asks questions to find out what action the nursing home has taken to ensure that the incident doesn't happen again. The ombudsman has the same goal that you have: to make sure the needs and rights of the people in your care are met.

Some hospitals have people on staff, called patient representatives or patient advocates, who are available to talk with patients and their families about their concerns or complaints. If a hospital doesn't employ a person in this capacity, a patient can talk with the nurse or hospital administrator. In the home health care setting, no ombudsman is available to mediate problems. You, as a health care professional and clients or people representing clients must take on the role of advocate and report problems to the agency director.

When Your Responsibility Goes Beyond Protecting Rights

As a nurse assistant, you have a legal responsibility to protect a person's rights, which are guaranteed by law. If you do not protect these rights, you are breaking the law and may be sued or have other actions taken against you.

When providing care for someone, you have another responsibility: to do what is right, meaning what is good or moral. As a caregiver, you must uphold the standards of health care workers, which are to help those in their care and to do no harm. Nurse assistants follow these standards when they practice the six principles of care. When you do what is right (that is, when you act in an ethical manner), and practice the six principles, you go beyond what is legally required.

Any behavior that could cause harm to a person, either physically or emotionally, is unethical. You may have to decide the right thing to do in situations involving people in your care. For example, one day Mr. Rivera is slightly injured when another nurse assistant gets Mr. Rivera's finger caught in the brake on his wheelchair. The nurse assistant does not report the incident, so you have to decide whether to report it. If you do not report it, you may not be committing a crime. However, you will be acting in an unethical manner. Because you have witnessed Mr. Rivera's injury and the nurse assistant's failure to report it, you find yourself in an **ethical dilemma**.

Have you ever heard or read about an ethical dilemma in health care? Ethical dilemmas are problem situations in which health care workers must decide what solution is best for a person in their care (Figure 3-4). Some ethical dilemmas may have more than one good or moral solution. For example, ask yourself what you would do if Mr. Rivera's call signal came on 5 minutes before you had to leave for an inservice training. You know that he wants to use the toilet and that it will take at least 10 minutes. One option is to ignore the light, but that would violate Mr. Rivera's safety, dignity, and independence. Another option is to have him use the urinal. This would be a safe solution that also would allow you to get to the inservice training on time. The option Mr. Rivera prefers is using the bathroom toilet. This would provide for his safety, as well as his dignity and independence, but you would be late for the training. Another option is to ask a co-worker to take him to the bathroom. This option would provide Mr. Rivera with safety, dignity, and independence and would also allow you to get to the inservice training on time. In each option, you follow the six principles of care to help solve this ethical dilemma.

In your role as a protector of people's rights, you have both a legal and an ethical responsibility. Health care workers who do not act in legal and ethical ways may be held responsible for their actions in a court of law. Not only can they be prosecuted for illegal acts, they can be sued for **neglect** or incompetence. To fulfill your legal re-

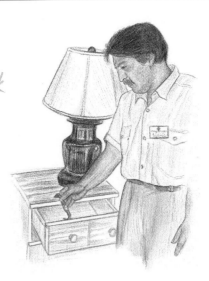

Figure 3-4
There are many possible reasons why this nurse assistant is taking Mr. Lightfoot's watch from his drawer. For example, he may be taking it to the lock box for safekeeping, or Mr. Lightfoot may have asked him to bring it to him in the dayroom. Or he may be stealing it. If you saw this nurse assistant taking someone's watch, what would you say to him?

ethical dilemma
(ETH-uh-kuhl/de-LEM-uh)   A problem or situation in which a nurse assistant must decide what is the correct, moral, and professional thing to do.

neglect
(nuh-GLEKT)   Failure to provide proper care for someone.

sponsibilities as a nurse assistant, you should know the legal rights of those in your care, and to help make decisions about your ethical responsibilities, you should use your knowledge of the principles of care. In Table 3-2 you can see examples of ethical situations that might arise. In each case, you can decide the right thing to do based on the principles of care.

Sometimes a situation will occur that is both illegal and ethically wrong. For example, you may see another nurse assistant pinch someone because he does not do what the nurse assistant wants. Not only is it ethically wrong to do anything to hurt a person intentionally, but this action denies the person's right to be free from abuse and is illegal.

It also is both illegal and ethically wrong to take anything that belongs to the person in your care, his family, or your employer. In your job, you must protect the person in your care, as well as his belongings. What if you see someone else take something? If you do not report the incident to your supervising nurse, you may not be doing anything illegal, but you are doing something unethical, since your job also includes protecting the person in your care from other people's actions.

When you see a person's rights being violated, you should report the incident to your supervising nurse right away. If you work in a

Table 3-2   **Ethical Decisions**

Situation	What You Should Do	Principle
You are in a rush. Your hands are chapped and you decide not to wash them just this once.	Always wash your hands. If your hands are chapped, use hand lotion and wear disposable gloves.	Infection control
Your friend Sue unintentionally drops Mrs. Compton's dentures. Only a small piece chips off one tooth.	Remind Sue to report every incident.	Safety, dignity
You decide to ask a person to use a bedpan instead of the bathroom, because it is convenient for you.	Plan your care around the best interests of the person, not around your schedule or the amount of work involved.	Independence, dignity
A person tells you he hides his pills and does not take them. He shows you his stash because he trusts you.	Tell the person that you must report that he is not taking his pills. Tell him to discuss his medication with his doctor so that they can agree on what he needs and what he will take.	Safety, communication
Your day was busy, and several emergencies happened. You ran out of time to finish one person's exercise. You are new, and you do not want to admit that you did not finish that one task.	Report that you did not finish the person's exercise so that the nurse assistant on the next shift can finish it.	Communication
You are visiting a neighbor, who is also friends with your patient in the hospital where you work. The neighbor asks you what is wrong with her friend.	Tell your neighbor that you cannot give her this information.	Privacy

nursing home and the problem continues, you should call your state
ombudsman and report it. You may take this action without giving
your name. Although the ombudsman usually investigates when he is
contacted by a person or his family who believes the person's rights
are being violated, you also can call the ombudsman to protect a person in your care. As a nurse assistant, you can do many other things
to see that the rights of the person in your care are always respected
and protected.

Your Role in Reporting Abuse

One of a person's rights is freedom from abuse. For many people it
may be difficult to imagine that caregivers or family members would
abuse someone who is dependent on them for care. When someone
is hurt physically or emotionally by being treated unkindly, this action is called abuse. If someone is hurt because his caregiver fails to
provide needed care, this lack of action is called neglect.

You probably have heard or read about child abuse and know that
it is a terrible thing. Sometimes it is hard to believe that people
would abuse children. Children are **physically abused** by people
who hit, bite, push, or kick them. They are **physically neglected** by
parents or caregivers who deny them food, water, clothing, shelter,
or human contact. Children are **emotionally abused** by people
who repeatedly yell at them, call them names, put them down, or
threaten to hurt them. And they are **sexually abused** by others who
fondle their breasts, buttocks, or genitals or force them to have sexual activity of any kind.

Children are not the only people who are abused. Adults also are
abused. Anyone who depends on someone else for physical or emotional care is especially vulnerable, or open to being hurt. When you
provide care for someone, you share the responsibility for keeping
that person safe from abuse. It is your responsibility to report abuse
or neglect if you observe or suspect it (Figure 3-5).

Abuse happens in all parts of society. Abusers and victims of abuse
can be male or female. They can be any age, be members of any
race, or practice any religion. Their families can have any cultural
background, educational level, or income. If you are working in a
hospital or nursing home, be alert for signs of abuse in patients or
residents. They may have been abused by employees or by other patients or residents. If you are working in someone's home, be alert
for signs of abuse to any member of the household, including your
client. The abuser could be someone living in the home or a friend
or relative living outside the home.

As a nurse assistant, you have a legal responsibility to report abuse
if you observe it or suspect that it is happening. Most states have laws
that require you to report abuse that you witness or suspect. To be
able to report it, you must know how to recognize signs of abuse.
Table 3-3 lists types of abuse, as well as signs that might tell you that
someone is being abused.

physical abuse
(ah-BYOOS)   Harm that occurs when a
person's body is purposely hurt.

physical neglect
(ne-GLEKT)   Failure to provide proper
physical care for someone.

emotional abuse
(e-MO-shun-uhl/ah-BYOOS)   Harm that
occurs when one person's words or
actions make another person feel bad
about himself.

sexual abuse
(SEK-shue-al/ah-BYOOS)   Harm that
occurs when a person's body is mistreated for sexual reasons.

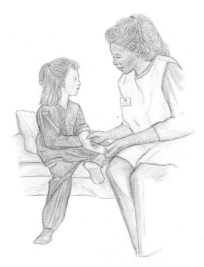

Figure 3-5
If you suspect that someone is being
abused, carefully observe the patient's
injuries and behavior so that you can
give your supervising nurse accurate
information.

Table 3-3   Recognizing Abuse

Types of Abuse	Signs of Abuse
Physical Abuse	
Actions that include pushing, shoving, hair pulling, biting, kicking, choking, and hitting.	A person who is physically abused may have burns, bruises, reddened areas that do not go away, scratches, cuts, or bite marks. A person can be physically abused and not have any of these signs.
Emotional Abuse	
Words and actions that produce mental and emotional stress. These include verbal threats to harm or kill a person.	A person who is emotionally abused may not make eye contact; may be withdrawn, sad, or fearful; or may shield himself.
Sexual Abuse	
Actions that include rape; physical handling of the victim's breasts, buttocks, or genitals; or forced sexual activity of any kind.	A person who is sexually abused may have bruises, scratches, and cuts around the breasts, buttocks, or genitals; may have vaginal or rectal bleeding; or may refuse personal care.

Neglect

Neglect is a specific form of abuse. Neglect is not something someone does to a person. Instead, it is something someone fails to do to or for a person. Neglect occurs when a person does not receive proper food, clothing, shelter, health care, supervision, or human contact. Certain forms of neglect, such as ignoring someone or denying him adequate food, can cause just as much physical and emotional pain as other forms of abuse.

You also must know how to recognize neglect. A person who is neglected may have poor personal care: dirty hair, body odor, dirty fingernails, crusty eyes, bleeding gums or lips, or food in his teeth. His clothing or bedding may be dirty, he may be depressed and withdrawn, and he may refuse food or personal care.

Exploitation

exploit
(eks-PLOYT) To take advantage of someone.

Someone in your care may be **exploited**. For example, you are in the lunch room listening to music on a radio. You ask another nurse assistant in the room about the radio. She says she borrowed it from Mr. Rivera's room while he was sleeping and intends to take it back. She is exploiting Mr. Rivera because she is using his property, not for his advantage but for her own. Using another person's money is another form of exploitation. You might see or hear something that makes you suspect that a person in your care is being exploited. If you do, you should report your suspicions to your supervising nurse.

Whenever you see or hear something that makes you suspect possible abuse, neglect, or exploitation, you must report it immediately to your supervising nurse. She will keep your report confidential and will make sure the information gets to the right people. Because abuse and neglect are both illegal and unethical behaviors, it is your legal and professional responsibility to report suspected abuse or neglect.

Abuse and neglect are very disturbing situations. You may be afraid to report your suspicions about them, but it is important that you do. You may be helping the person in your care out of a dangerous situation. The abuser also needs help to learn not to try to control others by harming them. By reporting the abuser, you may be preventing future abuse of others. If you discover a situation like any of the ones described here, you might want to spend some time talking about your feelings with your supervising nurse or staff social worker.

You always want to do what is best for the person in your care. Sometimes doing your best may mean waiting patiently while the situation is being investigated, and that may take a long time. Try not to be too frustrated by the amount of time it takes to find out what is really going on. Abuse and neglect are serious charges and must be investigated carefully.

Restraints

Another specific form of abuse may be the use of physical and chemical restraints. A person has the right to be free from any form of restraint.

A **physical restraint** is anything that restricts a person's movement and does not allow normal movement. Health care providers once believed that using physical restraints was a good way to protect people from harming themselves or others. People were tied to their beds or chairs so that they would not fall or wander around and injure themselves. Medical researchers have studied the use of restraints and have found that being restrained can injure people emotionally, as well as physically.

Physically restraining a person can cause harm to his body. People who are restrained can injure themselves by struggling to get free. For example, a person may tip his chair over, causing injuries to his arms and head as he struggles to get out of a restraint around his chest. Restraints also rob a person of his dignity and independence. People who have been restrained have said things like, "Being tied was the worst thing they could have done to me. They tie mad dogs, you know."* Think about being tied to your chair or bed. How would you feel? What would you do?

Today, the use of physical restraints is considered a form of abuse, unless it is ordered by a doctor. Physical restraints may be appropriate to stop a disoriented patient in a hospital from removing lifesaving tubes or a person with multiple sclerosis from falling out of his wheelchair. Restraints are never appropriate if they are used to make caregiving more convenient for the health care professional. They must never be used to discipline any person in health care. A doctor

physical restraint
(re-STRAYNT)   A device that prevents a person from moving freely.

---

*From Downs M: Free-to-be in Vermont. In *Untie the elderly,* Kennett Square, Pa, 1990, The Kendall Corporation, p 1.

chemical restraint
(KEM-e-kuhl/re-STRAYNT)　A drug or medication that calms a person and changes his behavior.

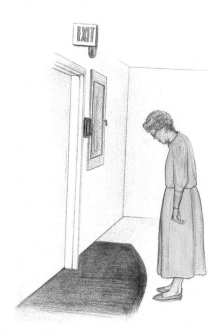

Figure 3-6
Instead of using restraints, the staff in this nursing home painted a black band in front of each exit door to prevent a confused person like Shirley McDay from wandering outside.

will order restraints only as a last resort, after other measures have failed to protect someone from harming himself or others.

Chemical restraints are medications that change a person's behavior, usually by calming him and decreasing his ability to move or respond normally. Just as with physical restraints, chemical restraints should never be ordered for the convenience of the staff or to discipline those receiving care. The doctor will order medication that has a calming effect only if the person has a medical condition that requires such medication.

It is important for you to find out and understand your employer's policy on the use of restraints. If a person in your care is being restrained, talk with your supervising nurse about the situation. You can keep a person safe without using restraints (Figure 3-6). Read Chapter 19, Finding Alternatives to Restraints.

Information Review

Circle the correct answers and fill in the blanks.

1.　A privilege that belongs to a person and is protected by law is called a _____rights_____ .

2.　A person in your care says he doesn't understand the medical procedure he is supposed to have tomorrow. You should—
　　a.　Tell him not to worry about it.
　　b.　Tell him it will be painless.
　　c.　Tell your supervising nurse about his concerns.
　　d.　Tell your supervising nurse that he is afraid of the procedure.

3.　When you bring mail to the person in your care, it should be—
　　a.　Unopened.
　　b.　Opened.
　　c.　Read to him.
　　d.　Tossed on the pile with other mail.

4.　A _____Health Care proxy_____ is a legal document in which a person names a friend or family member to make health care decisions for him if he becomes too ill to decide for himself.

5.　The person who is charged with the responsibility to listen to, investigate, and correct problems at a nursing home is an _____Ombudsman_____ .

6.　If you do what is right based on the six principles of care, you are acting in an _____Ethical_____ manner.

7.　Threatening to hurt a child is a form of _____emotional_____ _____abuse_____ .

8. You arrive on your first visit to provide care for a young woman who is recovering from broken bones she suffered in a fall. While helping her bathe, you notice that her breasts and genitals are scratched and bruised. She closes her eyes and turns her head away when you ask about these injuries. You suspect that she has been—
   a. Physically abused.
   b. Physically neglected.
   c. Emotionally abused.
   d. Sexually abused.

9. A person who is deprived of food, clothing, shelter, or human contact suffers from _Neglect_.

10. Only a doctor can order _physical_ or _Chemical_ restraints.

Questions to Ask Yourself

1. What would you do if you overheard another nurse assistant telling her friend about Mrs. Davis, for whom she is providing care?

2. You are providing care for Miss Eller in her own home. She is dying. She says she would like for you to have the expensive ring that is lying on her dresser. What would you say?

3. You see a co-worker slapping a person in her care. What would you do?

4. You meet some people in the grocery store who recognize you as the nurse assistant who is providing care for their cousin, May. They ask you specific questions about her medical condition. How do you reply?

5. A woman receiving care in the nursing home has been wandering into other residents' rooms. Your supervising nurse tells you to strap her into a wheelchair so that she can't wander. What would you do?

6. Today, when you provide care for Mrs. Morelli, a patient who has multiple sclerosis, you notice that she is covered with bruises. When you ask her how she got the bruises, she begins to cry and begs you to promise not to tell anyone. What would you do?

7. Jimmy London, a 7-year-old boy who has a serious breathing problem, has no toys, books, or pictures in his bedroom. Today you bring him a new teddy bear. His mother grabs it from you and says she will report you for interfering with her son's life. What would you do?

8. Mr. Rivera says that his stroke was God's way of punishing him. You don't agree with his idea. What would you say to him?

4

Understanding People

Goals

After reading this chapter, you will have the information to—

Recognize factors that can influence the way human beings behave.

Describe characteristics and behaviors that occur during stages in the life cycle.

Identify five basic human needs and give examples of each.

Provide caregiving that meets the basic needs of people in your care.

Discuss the factors that make up human sexuality.

Describe sexual feelings and behaviors that characterize stages in the life cycle.

Handle situations in which sex is an issue.

Describe cultural diversity and how culture may influence behavior.

Recognize and respect differences among people in your care.

Today you are on a crowded bus, riding home after a long workday at Morningside Nursing Home. You are surrounded by people you have never met, and you wonder what they're like. You watch what they're doing: Some are reading, some are dozing off to sleep, one woman is knitting, and two young people are kissing. You think: Why do people do what they do? You often ask this question about the people in your care: Why does Mrs. Wang look down when you enter the room? Why does Josie Miller insist that everyone call her by her first name? Why do Mr. Lightfoot and Mr. Wilson argue about when each will have time alone in their shared room? It seems you have to deal with someone's behavior every day.

You overhear two people arguing loudly about money. This situation reminds you of two residents arguing today about whose turn it was to buy the newspaper. They were arguing in the dayroom where everyone could hear them. You noticed that some people in the dayroom continued what they were doing as if nothing was happening, while others seemed to be embarrassed as they shifted uneasily in their chairs.

As you look around, you see many people who appear to have different ethnic backgrounds. You also see people wearing business suits, uniforms, and jeans. Some people carry briefcases, tote bags, and lunch boxes. Some wear wedding rings and some don't. Some look relaxed, while others look upset. You wonder what has happened in their lives that makes them who they are today. The people in your care also have different ethnic backgrounds and behave differently from one another. One woman likes to dress every day in her finest clothes and jewelry, while another woman refuses to wear anything but her nightgown and robe. One man has visitors several times each week, but his roommate has never had a visitor. Some people smile and talk pleasantly, others grumble or lie in bed and moan. You wish you knew more about why people do what they do.

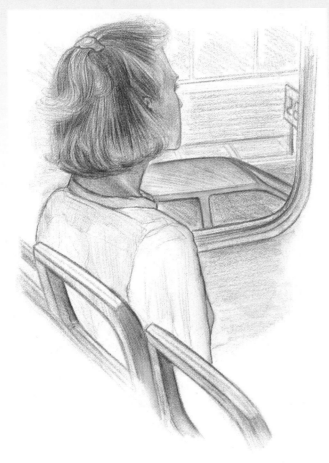

Human Behavior

Have you ever asked yourself, "Now, why did I do that?" Or have you wondered why someone else did something? Behind every **behavior** is a reason. You may never know the exact reason why someone does something, but when you understand some general factors that can influence behavior, you will know how to respond appropriately and how to provide better care.

What is behavior? Behavior is what people do. As a nurse assistant, you see different kinds of people who behave in many different ways. An example of simple behavior is a newborn baby sucking on a nipple or finger. A child who cries and asks for a peanut butter sandwich is behaving in a more complicated way. And a nursing home resident who steals money from his roommate's nightstand or wanders into another resident's room in the middle of the night is behaving in an even more complicated manner. What in a person's life might influence him to behave in these ways?

Some of the factors that influence the way people behave are: physical, social, emotional, and cognitive.

The way a person behaves may be influenced by **physical** factors. Each person's body affects his behavior, and his behavior affects his body. (See Body Basics, Our Bodies and Behavior.) Some behaviors are automatic, such as coughing, yawning, and blinking. Others are responses to physical needs. For example, when the child cried and asked for the peanut butter sandwich, he was responding to a physical need for food (Figure 4-1). Other physical needs include sleep, air, water, and exercise. A later section of this chapter describes these physical needs in greater detail. Biological factors such as heredity, **handedness**, and **gender** are also physical reasons for behavior, as are certain illnesses, which you will read about in Chapter 16, Providing Care for People with Specific Illnesses.

Social factors also influence a person's behavior. A child who is a patient in a hospital may cry when his parents leave his bedside. Or a teenager may be hospitalized for an overdose of alcohol because his friends dared him to drink an entire bottle of vodka in a short period of time. Other people may behave in certain ways because they want approval from their parents, teachers, or co-workers, or because they want to impress a spouse or life partner.

A strong social factor that influences a person's behavior is family. When Mr. Rivera lived at home, his family ate large amounts of fried foods, which was not good for their health. But, even after the doctor told Mr. Rivera to change his diet, he continued to eat the same things because that's what his family had always eaten.

A person's behavior also may be influenced by **emotional** factors, by the way he feels. The resident who stole money from his roommate may have felt upset because the next day was his grandson's birthday, and he didn't have money or a gift to give him. Another person may feel angry and throw a plate of food on the floor, and still another may feel sad and curl up in his bed.

When the resident stole the money, his behavior was also influ-

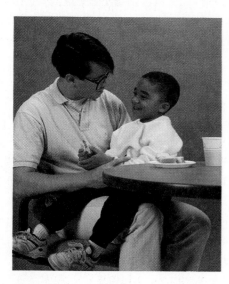

Figure 4-1

By offering a familiar food, this nurse assistant is comforting the child, as well as meeting his physical need for food.

behavior
(be-HAYV-yur)   The way a person acts or conducts himself.

physical
(FIZ-uh-kul)   Relating to the body.

handedness
The tendency to use one hand more frequently than the other.

gender
(JEN-der)   A person's sex.

social
(SO-shul)   Relating to the way people interact with each other.

emotional
(ee-MO-shun-uhl)   Relating to how a person feels and how he expresses himself.

BodyBasics

❖   Our Bodies and Behavior   ❖

Our bodies and how they function impact our behavior. If our bodies are strong, we can work and exercise. If they look good, friends and strangers notice and admire us. When our bodies are in proper working order, we can take walks, enjoy meals, watch movies, and do hundreds of other activities. But, when we are ill or our bodies are injured, our behaviors change.

Ten systems of organs work together to make the body function. Each system plays an important part in daily activities. The bones of the *skeletal system* give structure to the body. The *muscular system* moves the body in many different directions. The skin or *integumentary system* protects the body from cold and germs in the outside world. Food moves through the *digestive system* to nourish the body and to rid it of indigestible material. The *urinary system* rids the body of harmful wastes. The lungs work in the *pulmonary system* to bring oxygen into the body. The heart and blood work together in the *cardiovascular system* to distribute oxygen from the lungs, as well as nutrients from food, to every cell in the body. The *reproductive system* gives the body the ability to produce children. The *nervous system* and *endocrine system* coordinate the other systems. For example, hormones from the endocrine system act on organs in the reproductive system as part of the process of menstruation.

Our bodies change as we age. Aging is an ongoing, natural, and expected process. Throughout life, our bodies replace old cells with new ones. As we age, this process of cell replacement slows down, resulting in body systems that don't work as they used to. Our body systems grow and change until they reach their peak, and then they start to decline. Each system reaches its maximum ability at different times during life. For example, the muscular system reaches its peak of ability when we are in our 20s.

Aging is a normal part of life, not a disease. Some people appear to grow older more rapidly than others because of heredity, and others age faster because they live in an unhealthy environment or ignore their health. Positive behaviors like exercise and nutritious eating can slow down the aging process, but nothing can make it stop. You can keep your body healthy by adopting positive behaviors. And, by encouraging positive behaviors among the people in your care, you can help keep them as healthy as possible.

Throughout this book, the Body Basics boxes present information about each system. The information appears in the chapter that closely relates to that system. For example, the cardiovascular and pulmonary systems are described in Chapter 8, Measuring Life Signs, which explains measuring heart and breathing rates.

---

enced by **cognitive** factors. He *remembered* that his grandson was coming to visit him. He may have *known* the roommate kept cash in the nightstand drawer. He may have *thought* no one was watching him. And he may have *believed* it was okay to take some of his roommate's money without asking.

Four other factors influence behavior: growth and development, needs, sexuality, and culture. Each of these factors is discussed in greater detail in the following paragraphs.

cognitive
(KOG-nuh-tiv)   Relating to thinking, understanding, remembering, believing, learning, and creating.

How Human Growth and Development Influence Behavior

All people move on the same basic track through life. They begin as infants, then grow into children, develop into teens, mature into

BodyBasics

❖ The Nervous System ❖

The nervous system coordinates our responses to what goes on in the world around us, as well as what is happening inside of us. No other animal can think, speak, or act like a human because the human nervous system is more complicated than that of any other creature.

Our window to the outside world is our senses. We see with our eyes, hear with our ears, smell with our noses, and taste with our tongues because these organs have nerves that carry sensations to our brains. Nerves located in our skin give us a sense of touch and balance.

An adult's brain weighs about 3 pounds. It is made up of several types of cells, including neurons, which look like flowers on a stem. Resembling a large, gray acorn squash divided by many hills and valleys, the brain processes all information from the outside world, as well as sensations from inside the body, such as pain and hunger.

The brain sends information about how the body should respond. Messages travel through nerves that go to the spinal cord, a bundle of nerves protected by bones called vertebrae, or the backbone. More nerves run from the spinal cord to the arms, legs, chest, and abdomen. We get messages from the brain that tell us to run, kick up our heels, eat a hamburger, or respond in any of a million other ways that make us human.

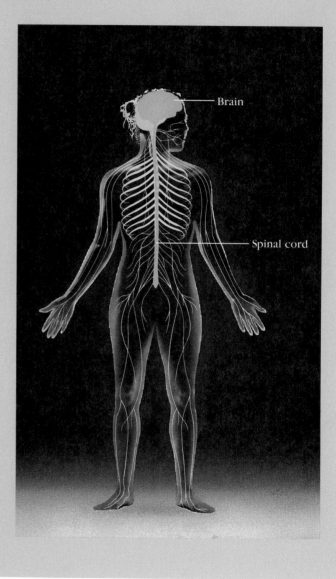

Brain

Spinal cord

stage
(STAYJ)   A defined and predictable period.

life cycle
(SI-kuhl)   The stages of aging and development experienced as a person grows older.

adulthood, and become old. The movement people make from one **stage** to the next is called the **life cycle**, and the changes they go through are called human growth and development (Figure 4-2).

BodyBasics

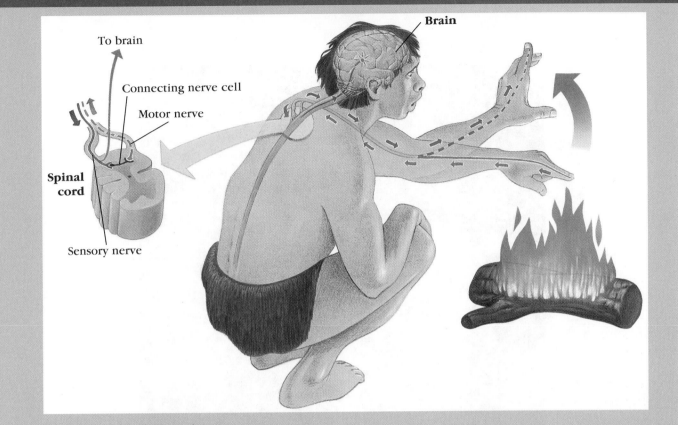

Labels: To brain · Connecting nerve cell · Motor nerve · Spinal cord · Sensory nerve · Brain

How the Nervous System Ages

A person is born with as many neurons as he will ever have. After age 25, the body experiences a slow, but steady, loss of nerve cells. That loss causes no changes in behavior or function unless a person has an injury, disease, or poor nutrition. The rate at which messages are sent from the body to the brain also slows down, causing the body to react more slowly. For example, it may take longer for the hand to receive the message that it is on something hot. The rate of learning may also slow down.

Fascinating Fact

Nerve cells coming together at junctions called synapses do not actually touch. The transmission from one cell to another is carried out by chemicals that "ferry" the impulse across the synapse.

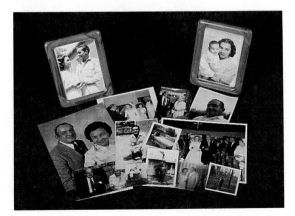

Figure 4-2
When you provide care for older people, remember that they have experienced all the previous life stages.

BodyBasics

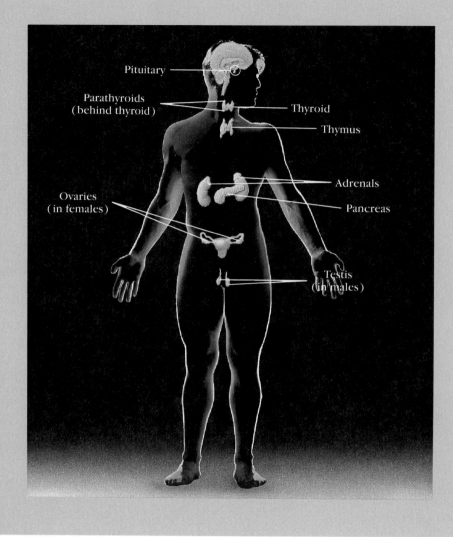

Pituitary

Parathyroids
(behind thyroid)

Thyroid

Thymus

Adrenals

Ovaries
(in females)

Pancreas

Testis
(in males)

adolescence
(add-uh-LES-ense)   The period between the ages of 12 and 20 when a
person becomes more interested in sex
and begins to have relationships with
other people.

human development
(HUE-men/de-VEL-up-ment)   The physical, social, emotional, and cognitive
changes a person experiences as he
grows older.

infancy
(IN-fan-see)   The first stage of life. The
word "infant" means "unable to speak."

Human growth refers to physical changes, such as growing bigger
and cutting teeth in infancy or growing taller and developing breasts
or a beard in **adolescence**. These physical changes occur in the size
and structure of the human body as it ages. The endocrine and nervous systems regulate the body's growth. (See Body Basics, The Nervous System and The Endocrine System.)

   Human development refers to all the changes that occur in the
way a person looks, relates to others, feels, and thinks as he grows
from **infancy** to old age. These changes are called social, emotional,
and cognitive. Social changes occur in the way a person relates to
other people. Emotional changes occur in the way a person feels and

BodyBasics

❖ The Endocrine System ❖

Many glands, located throughout the body, make up the endocrine system. Each gland secretes one or more substances called hormones. Hormones travel through the blood or through specific tubes called ducts to an organ called the "target." Hormones tell their targets just what to do, when to do it, and how much they should do.

The endocrine system cannot work alone, however. It works closely with several other body systems. The nervous system, for example, regulates glands by letting them know how much hormone to secrete, and the cardiovascular system helps carry the hormones to their targets.

The largest gland is the pancreas, located in the abdomen near the stomach. Scattered throughout the pancreas are cells called islets of Langerhans, which secrete insulin, the hormone that regulates the amount of sugar in the bloodstream. If the pancreas doesn't secrete enough insulin, the body develops diabetes.

A group of glands—the four small parathyroid glands and the larger thyroid gland—is located in the neck in front of the windpipe. Parathyroid hormone controls the level of calcium in the blood and bones. Thyroid hormone is the key in regulating metabolism, which is the rate at which the body turns food into energy.

Two other glands that influence metabolism are the adrenal glands, situated on the top of each kidney. Adrenal hormones control the amount of salt, potassium, and water in the body and constrict blood vessels and make the heart pump faster.

Men's testes secrete androgens, the hormones responsible for male sex characteristics. Women's ovaries secrete estrogen and progesterone, the hormones that influence menstruation and pregnancy. Testes and ovaries are part of the reproductive system, but the hormones they secrete are part of the endocrine system.

The pituitary, the master gland situated deep in the brain, controls all other glands in the body.

How the Endocrine System Ages

In the endocrine system, the most striking effects of aging are seen in women. The ovaries stop producing the hormones estrogen and progesterone, and women have their "change of life," or menopause. They no longer menstruate, and their ability to have children ends. Androgen production in men slows with aging but doesn't stop. Most other hormones are not affected by aging.

Fascinating Fact

Growth hormone is one of the hormones secreted by the pituitary gland. General Tom Thumb, the midget attraction in P.T. Barnum's circus, was a dwarf who did not have enough growth hormone. As an adult he reached only 40 inches in height.

how he expresses his feelings. Social and emotional changes are closely linked and often are considered together. Cognitive changes occur in the way a person understands the world: the way he thinks, remembers, believes, solves problems, learns, and creates.

We can predict differences in behavior that occur at certain stages in a person's life and recognize the differences in the things he does. For example, adult women ages 50 to 60 differ from teen and young adult women in many ways. The most notable difference is that they generally do not have babies. Physically most women are not capable of becoming pregnant after about age 55 because they no longer menstruate. Emotionally, socially, and cognitively they focus on other things, such as careers, volunteer interests, friends, older children and grandchildren, and leisure activities.

How Do Growth and Development Occur?

Certain things about human growth and development apply at every stage in the life cycle. Human growth and development are continuous processes that occur in the same order and follow the same pattern for all human beings. All people must go through each stage in the same order because each stage includes progress that is needed for the next stage. However, people may go through stages at different ages because people grow and develop at different rates.

Human growth and development move from head to foot. Newborn babies' heads, for example, are much larger than any other part of their bodies. Later, their bodies begin to grow faster than their heads. Growth and development also move from the simple to the complex. Preschoolers learn to jump with both feet before they can hop on one foot alone. When developing language, they use one word by itself at first, then put two words together, and then speak in whole sentences.

Each stage of human development emphasizes a particular type of behavior. For example, school-age children seem to spend most of their time and energy practicing physical skills, such as building, playing sports, and making crafts. Young **adolescents**, on the other hand, are much more focused on practicing social skills, such as dancing, talking with their friends, and getting into, or out of, relationships (Figure 4-3).

Human growth is influenced by physical changes inside the body. For example, growing taller and walking are influenced mostly by physical changes. Human development is influenced by conditions in which people live. For example, social skills and problem solving are influenced mostly by a person's learning experience and other factors in his environment.

The process of learning to walk is influenced by both growth and development. Physical factors and external factors must work together. Some of the major physical factors that must be present before a person can walk are a functioning nervous system, adequate muscle strength in the lower body, and well-formed spine, legs, and feet. The growing need to be independent, the encouragement of caregivers, and other external factors contribute to a person's developmental readiness to walk.

Scientists who study human growth and development divide the process into eight separate stages: infancy, toddlerhood, preschool age, school age, adolescence, young adult years, middle adult years, and older adult years. They define each stage of growth and development by certain distinctive characteristics. These characteristics are guidelines to help you understand a little about each stage in the life cycle. Depending on where you work in the health care system, you may provide care for people of all ages, for adults only, or mostly for

adolescent
(add-uh-LES-ent)   A person between the ages of 12 and 20.

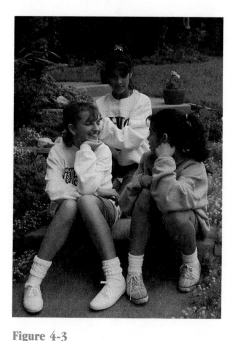

Figure 4-3
To a young adolescent, acceptance by her friends is so important that she may go to great lengths to look, act, and talk the same way they do.

Box 4-1   Characteristics of the Eight Stages of Human Growth and Development

Infancy (birth to 1 year). When babies are born, they have been growing and developing since conception, about 9 months. At birth babies are called neonates, and by the time they are 1 month old, they are called infants, which describes this first official stage of growth and development—infancy.

Areas of Change	During Infancy a Person. . .
Physical	Triples weight and increases length by 10 inches at 1 year. Begins to control body movement: Lifts head at 1 month; holds and throws objects and puts them in mouth; rolls over, sits up, crawls, climbs, takes first steps with assistance; and stands at 1 year. Begins cutting teeth and taking solid food at 6 months.
Social/Emotional	Cries to communicate. Begins to smile between 1 and 3 months. Recognizes caregivers and trusts them at 6 months. Cries at the sight of strangers at 7 months.
Cognitive	Uses sight, touch, hearing, smell, and taste to explore the world. Prefers to look at bright colors, sharp lines. Sees well at 2 months. Uses eyes to follow moving objects at 3 months. Explores with fingers and mouth at 5 months. Can say a few short words at 1 year.

Toddlerhood (1 to 3 years). Toddlers are children who, at the beginning of this stage, are not very steady on their feet. By their first birthday many young children are not yet able to stand alone. However, by age 3, these same children are climbing, running and jumping, feeding and dressing themselves, and talking in sentences.

Areas of Change	During Toddlerhood a Person. . .
Physical	Usually walks alone by 15 months. Does many things that require coordination of large muscles in arms and legs: runs, jumps, and climbs. Plays with toys. Has 6 to 12 baby teeth and eats regular table food. Learns to use the toilet and eats, drinks, and dresses with little or no help. Needs to rest frequently during the day.
Social/Emotional	Does not share toys. Likes to play alone or side by side with another child. Doesn't like to take orders. Learns to be independent. Throws temper tantrums when desires are not met. May be afraid when left alone.
Cognitive	Responds fairly well to adult language. Points to objects named by adults. Follows simple instructions when given slowly and clearly. Begins to put words together to make short sentences. Understands that objects taken out of sight still exist. Likes to choose own activities and toys.

Continued.

very old people. But, because most people have friends and family that may be in any stage of the life cycle, it is helpful to understand something about the characteristics of each stage. At the same time, it is important not to confuse "ages" with "stages," because there is no definite time when someone can or should be able to do something. Box 4-1 provides a description and the basic characteristics of each stage according to the kinds of changes that occur—physical, social/emotional, and cognitive. It is important to remember that these characteristics are general guidelines, not rules.

Although the "older adult years" is a normal stage in the life cycle, it is the last stage. As people move through their older adult years, they typically wrestle with certain necessities as the end of life approaches. If you work with this age group, it is important for you to know that older adults struggle with accepting the reality of being old, fulfilling their responsibility to themselves and others as they

Box 4-1   Characteristics of the Eight Stages of Human Growth and Development—cont'd

Preschool Age (3 to 5 years). Preschool children seem like miniature adults at times. They can do most things for themselves, have friends, may go to nursery school or kindergarten, can hold very interesting conversations, and spend a great deal of time "pretending" to be grown-ups. However, they still see the world through young children's eyes and imagine and fear things adults know cannot be possible.

Areas of Change	During Preschool Age a Person. . .
Physical	Has improved large-motor skills. Has more control over small-motor skills like drawing and writing. Combines several motor skills into one project or activity. Does many things to take care of himself like dressing, eating, and using the toilet.
Social/Emotional	Has a strong sense of who he is. Responds to messages about himself received from parents and other adults. Is more independent than a toddler. Makes his own choices. Plays easily with other children and enjoys games involving sharing and taking turns. Looks up to and imitates adults. Likes routine and may feel insecure if schedule is changed too often.
Cognitive	Knows many words and names of people, places, and things. Learns new words quickly. Begins to read some words before age 5. Counts and enjoys learning things with numbers. Groups objects that are alike. Picks out objects that do not fit with others. Follows directions. Has strong curiosity and imagination. Asks many questions. Has a strong, self-oriented point of view and sometimes is unable to understand others' points of view.

School Age (5 to 12 years). School-age children come in all sizes and shapes and behave in many different ways. During school years children develop skills and grow at different rates. Because no two children have the same experiences, they behave differently.

Areas of Change	During School Age a Person. . .
Physical	Grows steadily. (Females usually reach adult height by age 12.) Is physically well coordinated. Uses large muscles for games and sports, cycling, and dance. Develops muscle tone, balance, strength, and endurance. Uses small muscles to write, draw, and do crafts. Enters puberty at about age 10 to 12 for girls and age 12 for boys.
Social/Emotional	Begins to form lasting relationships with friends. Spends more time away from parents. Forms small, close-knit groups that exclude other children, especially those of the opposite sex. Begins to understand that other people also have feelings. Has many emotions and sometimes has difficulty expressing them. May have dramatic mood swings that accompany hormonal changes when going through puberty.
Cognitive	Pays attention longer, remembers longer, and follows more complex directions. Thinks logically and makes decisions about the "real" world. Starts to organize new information in meaningful ways. Behaves more responsibly. May question and resist adult decisions.

approach the end of life, and exercising their rights in spite of their age.*

In accepting reality, an older adult such as Mr. Rivera struggles as he gets used to his physical limitations, develops new relationships when his loved ones die, asks for and accepts help, and prepares for death. He fulfills responsibilities by planning for his survivors, bud-

*From Ebersole E, Hess P: *Toward healthy aging: human needs and nursing response,* St. Louis, 1985, Mosby, p 573.

Box 4-1   **Characteristics of the Eight Stages of Human Growth and Development—cont'd**

Adolescence (12 to 20 years). During adolescence, children leave their childhood ways behind and gradually move into adulthood. Their bodies reach full size during these years, and their minds begin to work like those of adults. Social and emotional experiences are intense because this is a time to deal with strong friendships and early love relationships. Some adolescents begin parenting children of their own.

Areas of Change	During Adolescence a Person. . .
Physical	Reaches reproductive maturity and is capable of having children. (Breasts grow to adult size, hips widen, pubic and underarm hair appears, and menstruation begins about age 12, if the person is female. Penis and testes grow to adult size, ejaculations begin, pubic and facial hair develops, voice deepens, and neck and shoulders grow, if the person is male.) If a girl, tends to be taller than boys of the same age at the beginning of the age range and tends to be shorter at the end.
Social/Emotional	Feels awkward around adults and strangers because of recent changes in his or her body. Gets embarrassed easily if he or she has to undress in front of an adult or talk about body, growth, or sexual development. Assumes more responsibility for own behavior. Often rebels against adult authority.
Cognitive	Thinks logically. Learns about and deals with the abstract or possible. Thinks about himself or herself privately. Plans for the future. Imagines alternatives when making a decision, which makes decision making more difficult. Becomes more self-conscious. Tries to change physical image. Imagines an ideal world and ideal self. Is easily disappointed and discouraged. May set unreasonable goals.

Young Adult Years (20 to 45 years). For most people, the young adult years are years filled with beginnings: living on one's own away from parents, starting a career, beginning a sexual relationship with someone who may be a life partner, and marrying or living with one person. Many couples and some single adults begin a family by having or adopting children.

Areas of Change	During the Young Adult Years a Person. . .
Physical	Has all body functions fully developed by age 23. (Most women are fully grown by age 17; about 10 percent continue to grow until age 21. Most men are fully grown by age 21; about 10 percent continue to grow until age 23.) Reaches peak of muscular strength between ages 25 and 30 and then strength begins to decrease. Has best small-motor skills until about age 35, then these skills decrease. Has sharpest senses at about age 20, then senses gradually decrease. Is healthiest of population. Gets sick infrequently. Recovers more quickly. Continues to menstruate and may bear children, if female.
Social/Emotional	Establishes lasting and intimate relationships with friends and partners. Makes commitments. (Most men and women marry by age 30. Many adults become parents. Some struggle with infertility. Some voluntarily choose not to become parents.)
Cognitive	Functions at higher level than children and adolescents, although some young adults continue to think and reason much like adolescents and children. Is able to put himself in another's place and imagine how the other feels. Has better-developed moral reasoning.

Continued.

geting his income and energy to meet everyday needs, choosing how to spend the rest of his life, and assuming as much responsibility for his own care as possible. At the same time, Mr. Rivera must exercise his right to move at his own pace, have privacy (even when he is being cared for by another person), be treated with respect and dignity, refuse certain kinds of care or treatment, and participate in plans and decisions about his life.

Box 4-1 Characteristics of the Eight Stages of Human Growth and Development—cont'd

Middle Adult Years (45 to 65 years). Middle-aged adults experience the satisfaction of enjoying what they began in their 20s and 30s. Their careers are often at their peak, children are growing or grown, finances may be secure enough to allow for more leisure time, and health and vitality have not yet begun to fade. For many people, the middle adult years are the "prime" years of their lives.

Areas of Change	During the Middle Adult Years a Person. . .
Physical	May develop chronic illnesses. (Some find that existing health conditions disappear or become less problematic.) Has slight sensory ability loss. Has slight loss in physical strength and coordination. Has occasional difficulty sleeping and eating certain foods. Goes through menopause between the ages of 45 and 55, if the person is female.
Social/Emotional	Begins to feel anxious about aging. Begins to become aware of mortality and death. Feels more satisfied by work. If female, may become depressed as children grow up and leave or may delight in the new freedom.
Cognitive	Increases in mental growth and has high levels of intellectual performance. Can learn new skills. Finds this is often the most creative time of life and may pursue adult education.

Older Adult Years (65 years and older). In our society, older adults often are called "senior citizens," "golden agers," or the "elderly" in an attempt to avoid calling them "old." Even though most older adults still lead healthy, productive lives, being old often is seen as a negative experience, and few people want to admit to being old.

Areas of Change	During the Older Adult Years a Person. . .
Physical	Is likely to experience more chronic illnesses, such as high blood pressure. Is generally healthy enough to continue normal physical activities. Has decrease in vision, with loss of night vision and less depth and color perception. Experiences some hearing loss and a decreased sense of smell and taste. Has less strength and balance and is prone to accidents and falling. Is noticeably shorter because of spinal column shrinkage. Adjusts less quickly to cold.
Social/Emotional	May experience old age as positive and feel increased energy, productivity, and creativity, although the negative attitudes of younger generations can make this stage less than pleasant. May have strong desire to make a will and have strong attachment to familiar objects. May have increased awareness of time and life cycle. May be less confident and have lower self-esteem due to loss of loved ones, work roles, and physical and sensory capabilities. May have more clearly defined personality and values and has continued need for friendships and other relationships. May have a need for the companionship of a pet. Continues sex life if he or she was sexually active earlier.
Cognitive	Generally maintains intellectual abilities, although may not process information as quickly. Makes decisions with less speed. Is able to learn new information and skills but needs more time to learn. May experience some memory loss due to external conditions, such as medication or the need to move to a new residence, or because of physical or emotional reasons, such as poor nutrition, depression, or illness.

Why Nurse Assistants Must Understand Human Growth and Development

As a nurse assistant, you come into contact with people at all ages of life and all stages of growth and development. You may respond differently to someone's behavior when you understand what stage of development may be influencing that behavior. For example, you are not surprised when a 2-year-old child occasionally throws temper tantrums and shouts "No" when you try to do something for him. You also expect an adolescent to be very concerned about what his friends will think and you will take these feelings into consideration when providing care. Because a 30-year-old husband and father has different responsibilities than an 85-year-old man, you might anticipate the younger man to react differently to a diagnosis of chronic arthritis and foresee a need for special services and counseling for him.

How Basic Human Needs Influence Behavior

Mrs. Ryan is one of the easiest residents to provide care for, even though she is one of the oldest. Her health is good and she eats well, drinks a lot of water, uses the bathroom regularly, exercises, gets lots of fresh air, and rests and sleeps well. She enjoys living at the nursing home, dresses and grooms herself every day, socializes with the other residents, and enjoys talking with several friends and relatives who visit her each week. She also prides herself on her quiltmaking, as well as on the number of books she reads each month. She may be 90 years old, but she still enjoys life.

On the other hand, Josie Miller, who is 9 years younger than Mrs. Ryan, is very **frail**. Some days she refuses to eat because she says she is too tired. Yet, at night, she doesn't sleep well. Because she is frail and often tired, she doesn't exercise much and seldom goes outside for fresh air. She spends much of her time in her room or dozing off in the dayroom. She doesn't socialize as much with the other residents as she once did, except for Jake Wilson, who has become her special friend. When Josie's friends and relatives visit, she often dozes off, so now they don't come as often as they once did (Figure 4-4).

To live and to be healthy and happy, people need certain things, such as food, sleep, and air. These things are called **human needs.** How these needs are met varies from person to person. For example, both Mrs. Ryan and Josie need food, but each responds differently when you bring her food tray. Mrs. Ryan smiles, says, "Thank you," and begins to eat with enthusiasm. Josie turns her head away and says, "I just want to sleep." Mrs. Ryan eats her full meal, and Josie usually picks at her food. Both are responding to their need for food, but in different ways.

Many years ago, Abraham Maslow, a famous psychologist, studied how people feel and behave. He spent many years trying to find out what people need to live and be happy and to grow in a healthy way. He developed a **theory** about people and their needs. Maslow's theory is only one theory on human needs, and it focuses on what motivates people. Some of what he learned appears in Figure 4-5.

Maslow learned that people have needs on different levels, beginning with physical needs and moving to self-fulfillment needs. People need to have the lower-level needs met before they can think about higher-level needs. When people struggle to have their physical needs met, they put their higher-level needs in the back of their minds. For example, you may come to class one day feeling very tired. If the need is great enough, you might fall asleep. You may be somewhat concerned about whether your action upsets your instruc-

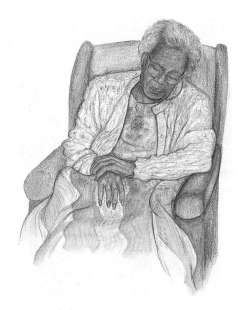

Figure 4-4
Josie uses all her energy just to try to manage her activities of daily living—eating, bathing, dressing, moving, and using the bathroom—so she has little energy left for socializing or pursuing other interests.

frail
Very slender and fragile.

human need
A basic requirement that enables a person to live healthily and happily.

theory
(THEE-o-ree)   An explanation based on observation and reasoning.

Maslow's Hierarchy of Needs: Basic Needs of All People

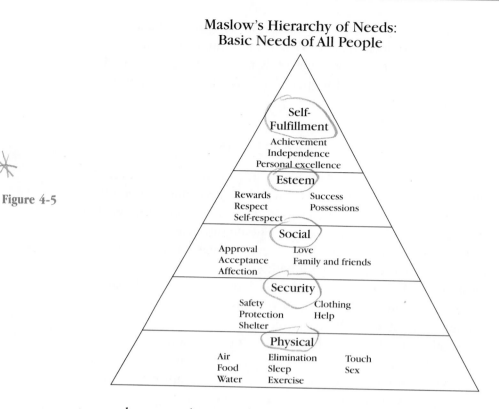

Figure 4-5

tor or classmates, but your basic physical need is more important at that time than your social need.

The people in your care have physical needs. They, too, do not concern themselves with higher-level needs until their physical needs are met. For example, a person who needs to use the toilet immediately may not worry about being polite to others. A person who feels nauseated probably does not care about going to physical therapy.

As a nurse assistant, you play a large role in helping people meet their physical, security, social, and esteem needs. As these needs are met, the person turns inward to meet the self-fulfillment need on his own.

Physical Needs

Physical needs are a person's most basic bodily needs and are what he needs to be able to live. The most important physical needs are air to breathe, food to eat, and water to drink. Everyone also needs to sleep, exercise, eliminate body waste, and experience human touch.

If you stay up late several days in a row, you know how much you need sleep and rest. And if you've ever been sick in bed for a week or more, you know how hard it is to begin to move around and exercise when you get better. The people in your care also need exercise, rest, and sleep. As a health care worker, you can help those in your care meet these needs by making sure that they exercise and participate in activities during the day and by providing them with quiet time in the evening. You can provide a person with a comforting item, such as an afghan or pillow, or a favorite teddy bear for a child. You can further enhance a person's sleep time by giving a back massage, turning lights down or off, and creating a quiet environment with closed doors and limited noise and discussion at the nurse's station.

Another basic human need is going to the bathroom or eliminating wastes from the body. Satisfying other basic needs may be put off for a day or longer, but eliminating body wastes cannot be put off for a long time.

Being touched by another person is also a physical need. Think of a time when you had a bad day. Nothing went right. You were feeling really bad. Then a friend came along and gave you a big hug. How did you feel then? The people in your care also need to receive a hug, a pat on the arm, or a squeeze of the hand. This physical need for touch is one that people often forget about. To live and to be well, people need the touch of others.

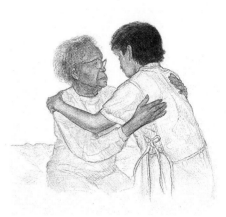

Figure 4-6
This nurse assistant knows how important touch and affection are to Josie and gives her a hug.

Health care workers know that, even if healthy babies get enough food, water, rest, and exercise, they get sick and eventually die if they are left alone and not held. Babies need to be held and touched. Sick people in hospitals and older people in nursing homes also get well sooner and stay healthier when they are touched by other people. They have a need to be touched by health care workers, family members, and friends (Figure 4-6).

Touch is important, but it is also very personal. Some people do not like to be touched by anyone outside their families or circles of close friends. People from certain cultures may have strong feelings about being touched. For example, in Southeast Asia, touching a child on the head is a **demeaning** act, while in the United States such an act can be a sign of affection or approval. When you provide care to people, ask them how they feel about being touched, and then ask what kind of touch is acceptable.

demeaning
(duh-MEEN-ing)   Something that lowers someone's dignity.

Human beings also have another physical need—a sexual need. Even sick, disabled, old, and dying people have sexual needs. Sexual needs do not end when people reach a certain age. They do not end when people lose the use of their legs or develop illnesses. People don't need to express their sexual feelings daily, but, like the need for food and water, sexual needs are always there. The best way you can help people in your care meet their sexual needs is to provide privacy and have an accepting attitude.

Table 4-1 contains examples of ways you can help people in your care meet their physical needs.

Even though all people have the same physical needs, they don't have them at the same times. One person may be hungry and need to eat, while someone who feels nauseated needs to eat but doesn't want to. One person may need to go for a walk, while someone else may need to sleep. It is part of your job to find out the physical needs of each person in your care.

Security Needs

People whose basic physical needs are reasonably well met begin to want their needs for security met. For most people, security means

Table 4-1 Meeting Physical Needs

To Help Meet the Need for. . .	You Can. . .
Air	Tell your supervising nurse if a person is having trouble breathing.
Food	Serve a person's meals. Check the temperature of the food.
Water	Refill a water glass.
Elimination	Answer a person's call signal immediately.
Sleep	Tell your supervising nurse if someone is having trouble sleeping.
Exercise	Help a person with prescribed exercises. Help someone walk.
Touch	Touch a person on his arm and make eye contact as you pass by. Encourage family members to touch the person and hug him.
Sex	Provide the person with privacy.

feeling safe and comfortable. We all need shelter, clothing, safety, and someone who can help when we need assistance. What would make you feel more secure in your own life? Table 4-2 contains some examples of ways you can help people in your care meet their needs for security.

You must find out what makes each person in your care feel secure. For example, Mrs. Garcia may want to keep her door closed so that strangers do not look in. Mr. Rivera may want his door open so that people can hear him if he calls. Each person feels more secure when you provide what that person needs. When you help a person meet his individual security needs, that person begins to trust you.

Table 4-2 Meeting Needs for Security

To Help Meet the Need for. . .	You Can. . .
Safety	Lock a person's wheelchair brakes when the chair is not moving. Answer a person's call signal as quickly as possible. Make sure a person wears his eyeglasses if he needs them.
Protection	Check often on a person who cannot get around by himself to see if he needs anything.
Shelter	Close a person's door if he wants privacy. If a person's home has no heat, report this situation to your supervising nurse.
Clothing	Make sure a person wears the right clothes for the weather.
Help	Keep a person's door open if he thinks he needs to be able to call for you.

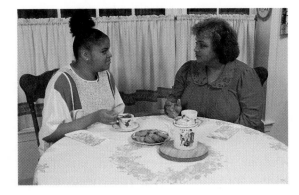

Figure 4-7
Sometimes when a person is receiving health care at home, few friends and visitors may call. The home health aide often plays an important role in meeting a client's social and physical needs.

To find out what makes a person feel secure, ask the person, his family, or your supervising nurse.

Social Needs

When their needs for security are fairly well met, people become interested in meeting their social needs. Even as people are seeking to have their social needs met, however, they still need to have their physical and security needs met.

What are social needs? Think for a moment about the people in your life. Think about family members, friends, a special person you love, and people you work with. What things do you need from them to feel good? Most people need to be liked, loved, and accepted by individuals and groups. These are social needs. No one wants to be ignored, to feel left out, or to feel unloved or lonely. As a nurse assistant, you can help meet the social needs of people in your care many times each day. You can be especially helpful when a person's family and friends cannot be with her (Figure 4-7). Table 4-3 contains examples of small but important things you can do to help people meet their social needs.

Table 4-3   **Meeting Social Needs**

To Help Meet the Need for. . .	You Can. . .
Approval	Show a sincere interest when a person talks about his past accomplishments.
Acceptance	Introduce people to one another. Talk to people in a friendly way. Listen to people in a way that shows you really care.
Affection	Give people smiles and hugs.
Love	Tell a person that you care about him.
Family and friends	Encourage a person's family and friends to visit as often as they can. Help a person dial a phone number to talk with a friend. Help a person spend time with other people he likes.

Being sick, disabled, or elderly can be lonely. To people who are old or ill, it often seems like everyone else is healthy, able-bodied, and young, which may make it difficult for them to seek out new friendships and social opportunities. Your role in meeting the social needs of the people in your care is very important. What other things can you do to help meet someone's social needs?

Esteem Needs

esteem
(es-TEEM) A high regard for someone.

People whose social needs are met may be interested in having their needs for **esteem** met. They need to feel good about themselves and also to feel that others respect them. At the same time, they still need to have their physical, security, and social needs met.

What do you do that makes you feel good about yourself? What do you do so that others respect you? Your answers to these questions show how you meet your needs for esteem. What do your family and friends do to help meet your needs for esteem? Do they compliment you, encourage you, and say you are important to them?

Some people who are sick, old, or disabled feel that they are no longer important. They don't feel good about themselves because they can't do what they once were able to do. Table 4-4 contains examples of ways you can help people meet their needs for esteem and let them know that you think they are important.

People who are ill, disabled, or old often don't have the opportunity to reap the pleasures of success. As a nurse assistant, you can increase their opportunities by noticing small accomplishments and

Table 4-4   **Meeting Needs for Esteem**

To Help Meet the Need for. . .	You Can. . .
Rewards	Give a person recognition in the form of hugs, handshakes, and other physical signs, if touching is acceptable to him. Congratulate a person when he accomplishes something he has been trying to do.
Respect	Use a person's correct name and title when speaking to him. Listen to what a person has to say so that he knows it matters to you.
Self-respect	Help a person do whatever he can for himself so that he can become more independent. Encourage a person to remember and talk about times in his life when he was held in great esteem.
Success	Help a person share his successes with others. Praise a person if you notice improvement in what he is trying to do.
Possessions	Compliment a person when he is wearing clothing that you know he is proud of.

talking about them. Your role in meeting the needs for esteem of the people in your care is very important. What other things can you do to help meet these needs?

Self-Fulfillment Needs

People whose basic four needs are met satisfactorily can seek self-fulfillment. Self-fulfillment means that a person feels satisfied with himself. Each person needs to strive to satisfy his own self-fulfillment needs. The only way you can help is by helping to meet the other four needs. Maslow, who talked about the levels of needs, explained self-fulfillment as the highest level of human need. He said that when people satisfy their self-fulfillment needs, they believe that they are doing what they are best suited to do (Figure 4-8). For example, a person may experience self-fulfillment by writing a great book, working toward finding a cure for a disease, becoming a terrific parent, or working to provide good care for the elderly. Because each person excels in one area of his life, each person's self-fulfilling experience will be different. When you talk with the people in your care, you can help by encouraging them to talk about their needs for self-fulfillment.

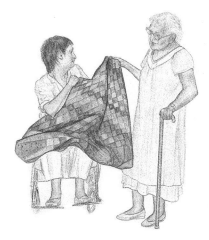

Figure 4-8
Mrs. Ryan has been quilting for many years and is proud of her accomplishments.

Why Nurse Assistants Must Understand Human Needs

When you work as a nurse assistant, you provide care for many people with many different needs. When you understand the levels of needs, you can provide better care. For example, Mrs. Ryan looks forward to dressing every day. If she says she doesn't want to get dressed today, this statement is a clue for you that something may be wrong. A change in a person's usual pattern of behavior may mean that one or more of her needs have not been met.

The Needs of a Nurse Assistant

Did you spend some time thinking about your own needs as you read about other people's needs? Just like them, you also have human needs. For example, one of the reasons you work is to help meet your own physical survival needs. The air is free, but just about everything else you need to live and be happy costs money. You also may work because being in the workplace meets a social need for you.

Many people choose to be nurse assistants because they need to help others and provide care for them. Think about your needs for social belonging, esteem, and self-fulfillment. You may feel like you are part of something important as you learn to become a nurse assistant. How do you feel about becoming part of the health care system that is responsible for the lives and well-being of so many people in hospitals, nursing homes, and their own homes? Do you feel like what you do is important? Are you doing the best you can do? Are you learning to be the best you can be? (Figure 4-9)

When you work hard, it may be difficult to have your own needs met, especially if you also are trying to help meet the needs of others in your life. It may be difficult some days to find time to eat breakfast

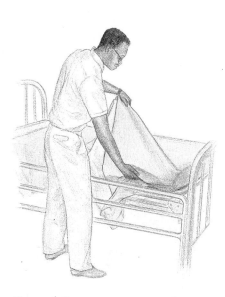

Figure 4-9
Learning new skills can make you feel good about yourself and help you as you help meet the needs of others.

before coming to work. Then you have a need for food. It may be difficult to buy a comfortable pair of shoes. Then you have a need for physical comfort. You may forget to lock your door at home one day. Then you worry about your security. If your needs are not met, you may have a hard time doing your job well.

How Human Sexuality Influences Behavior

One day when you go to Stephen Lightfoot's room to help the 83-year-old man get dressed, you overhear his conversation with his roommate, 79-year-old Jake Wilson.

"What do you mean when you say you like Josie Miller?" Mr. Lightfoot asks Mr. Wilson. "I like her, too. Everyone likes her."

"I mean I like her, well, special," says Mr. Wilson, peering through his thick glasses. "If we weren't living here, I'd ask her to go out dancing with me."

"Maybe she don't dance," Mr. Lightfoot says, adjusting the tube that feeds oxygen into his nose.

"She does too," says Mr. Wilson. "She told me about some beau years ago who gave her a gold necklace and who could dance better than anyone."

"Did she marry him?" Mr. Lightfoot asks.

"No, she said he married her best friend and that they were married for 49 years until he died. She seemed kinda sad. I was wishing I had a beautiful necklace to give to her."

"Well, you can give her something else," says Mr. Lightfoot. Mr. Wilson grasps his cane and slowly hobbles over to Mr. Lightfoot, leans over, and speaks directly into his face.

"I did. I gave her my package of wheat crackers. And I squeezed her hand."

"This sounds serious," says Mr. Lightfoot.

"Could be," says Mr. Wilson, rubbing his chin. "Could be."

What do you think of when you hear the word "**sexuality**"? As with most people, you may be more familiar with the word "sex." To many people, sex means having sex, or sexual intercourse. But sex is only part of the word "sexuality," only the first three letters of a bigger and more complicated term. Sexuality includes sensuality, intimacy, sexual identity, reproduction, and sexualization.

Sensuality

The part of people that lets them feel pleasure from the way their bodies look, feel, and behave is called their sensuality. Sensuality enables people to feel attractive when they look at their bodies in the mirror (Figure 4-10). It allows them to experience pleasure when they touch or rub certain parts of their bodies. It also makes it possible for them to enjoy the release of sexual tension known as sexual climax, or orgasm.

Sensuality lets people feel good about other people's bodies, too. It is what makes one person feel attracted to another person. Sensu-

sexuality
(sek-shue-AL-uh-tee)   A basic human need for sexual pleasure and sexual expression.

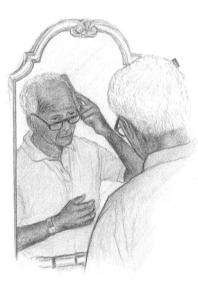

Figure 4-10
Mr. Wilson feels more confident when he is pleased with his appearance.

ality lets each person feel pleasure when he or she is touched by a special person. It also makes people want to be touched and held by other people they know, not just in a sexual way but in loving, caring ways.

Knowledge of sensuality is important in your work. As a nurse assistant, you help people with their personal care. You help them bathe, dress, and comb their hair. They may behave differently, depending on how they feel about themselves. Part of a person's healthy sexuality is having a good **body image**. When you provide care for a person, it is important when you—

body image
(IM-ij)   A person's attitude toward his body.

❖   Notice some small difference—a new shirt or hair cut—and comment on it, complimenting the person on his appearance.
❖   Ask the person what he wants to wear, encouraging him to make choices.
❖   Focus on the positive things about a person's appearance—his smile or sparkling eyes—things that do not degenerate with disease or age.

You must be sensitive to someone who does not feel comfortable with his body image because of a disease, disability, or disfigurement or because he is very old. You help this person by looking beyond the physical features and seeing the person inside.

You also have to be aware that any person you provide care for may get pleasure by touching and rubbing his or her **genitals**. This person may be a baby, teenager, adult, or older person. Many people touch themselves to achieve an orgasm and release sexual tension. This touching is called masturbation.

genitals
(JEN-uh-tuhls)   The external sex organs between the legs.

Some people have been taught by parents or their religion that masturbation is a wrong way to behave. If that belief is what you were taught, it's okay for you to believe that idea. However, you must remember that some people in your care may believe that masturbation is an acceptable action. They may want privacy to engage in masturbation. No matter how you personally feel about masturbation, providing privacy for the person is one way of showing respect and promoting dignity.

There may be times when a person who is in your care may be physically, or sexually, attracted to you. You may even be attracted to someone in your care. Feelings of sexual attraction for someone, even for the person in your care, can happen anytime. It is okay for you to acknowledge these feelings to yourself, but you should not act or comment on these feelings when you are with the person.

Likewise, if a person in your care is attracted to you, he or she should not act on these feelings. If a person in your care makes sexual advances toward you, you should refuse them firmly but gently. You can say something like—

"I really like you as a person, but I don't like it when you touch me that way."

"I really enjoy providing care for you, but I feel uncomfortable when you talk to me that way."

"I want you to stop touching me like that. Please do not do that again."

Let the person know that you do not want the sexual behavior but that you still like him or her.

You must be careful not to misread something that may look like sexual attraction. For example, when you are bathing or washing a male, he may have an **erection**. When a male has an erection, this physical change does not necessarily mean that he is attracted to you or that he is thinking about you sexually. Erections are normal and happen to teenage boys and men for many different reasons. An erection may mean the person has a full bladder, is thinking about something that is sexually exciting, is feeling afraid, or is feeling pleasure. You may feel embarrassed if someone in your care has an erection, but he also may feel embarrassed. To make the situation more comfortable, you may want to talk about something unrelated or simply continue the task without talking.

erection
(uh-REK-shun)   A stiffening of the penis.

Intimacy

The need and ability of a person to feel close to another human being and to have that closeness returned is called intimacy. Intimacy is all those good feelings that people have for one another, such as liking, loving, sharing, and caring (Figure 4-11). To express their feelings of intimacy, people may kiss, hug, touch, or hold hands. Intimacy may include a sexual relationship, or it may not.

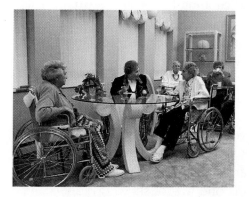

Figure 4-11
To help nursing home residents become intimate with one another, you can encourage them to sit together at a meal or special activity.

Intimacy can affect your job as a nurse assistant. For example, in your relationship with someone in your care, you can be emotionally close even if the person does not respond to you at first. You can decide to make an emotional investment in that person and to show how much you care for him. You can let a person know that you like him. Your emotional investment may or may not lead to an intimate relationship in which the person also makes an emotional investment.

In addition, you can respect the person's intimacy with a partner or spouse, family members, and friends. Be accepting of behaviors such as holding hands, touching, kissing, and hugging. Romance or sex may or may not be part of this intimate relationship. Since many people might be embarrassed to ask the nurse assistant to provide privacy for themselves and their partner, you must look for cues that a couple may want to be alone. When a couple is together, you should excuse yourself and say what time you will be back. As always, you should knock on the person's door and wait for a reply before entering.

Sexual Identity

The way a person feels about who he or she is sexually, including his or her maleness or femaleness, is called sexual identity. Sexual identity may seem complicated. But, if you think of it as three pieces of a puzzle that fit together, it makes more sense. The three pieces of sexual identity are (1) recognizing that we are male or female; (2) learning how males and females are expected to behave; and (3) knowing whether we are attracted to the other sex, the same sex, or both.

Most children recognize whether they are male or female by the age of 2. They know by looking at their bodies whether they are girls or boys.

People learn how men or women should behave by watching the groups in which they grow up. Families and cultures have strong opinions and have made "rules" about what men and women can and cannot do. For example, some people have rules about whether women with children should work, whether men should cry, whether women should play certain sports, and whether men or women should hold certain jobs. Some people learned the "rule" that only women, and not men, should have jobs as nurse assistants (Figure 4-12). How do you feel about this idea? What rules about being men and women did you hear when you were growing up?

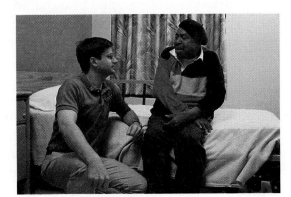

Figure 4-12
In the past, few men worked as nurses and nurse assistants. Today that has changed.

A person can be attracted to someone of the opposite sex, the same sex, or both. A person who is mostly attracted to a person of the opposite sex is called heterosexual (some people say "straight"), and a person who is attracted to someone of the same sex is called homosexual (some people say "gay" or "lesbian"). A person who is attracted to people of both sexes is called bisexual.

About 10 percent of all people are attracted only to someone of the same sex, which means that homosexuals are in a minority. Some people may not understand homosexual people, just as they may not understand other minority groups. They may be afraid of them, may not want to associate with them, and may even want to harm them. This kind of fear and harm is called discrimination. Have you ever been discriminated against or mistreated because of something special or different about yourself? How did you feel?

As a nurse assistant, you provide care for all people, including homosexuals. It is important to think about what you have been taught about homosexuality and how you feel about gay and lesbian people. Regardless of what you feel, you must treat all people with the same respect and consideration when you provide care.

The person in your care may have a partner of the same sex. Whether you believe that homosexual relationships are right or wrong, you may feel uncomfortable observing intimate behavior, such as hugging and kissing, between people of the same sex. And, because a person's attraction to other people of the same or opposite sex often lasts a lifetime, you may be providing care to an older homosexual couple. Sometimes it is difficult to think about older people being sexually active. It may be even more difficult to think about the sexually active couple being homosexual. No matter what you feel about the couple's relationship, you must respect the right of the partners to be together, provide them with the privacy they may want, and provide them with the best possible care.

Some situations in your job as a nurse assistant also may be affected by sexual identity. For example, you may provide care for people who have very different ideas about the roles that men and women should play. A man in your care may believe that only a male nurse assistant should give him a bath. A person in your care may believe that only males should take charge in an emergency. You, too, may have your own ideas about male and female roles, but you must put these ideas aside so that you can fulfill the responsibilities of your job as a nurse assistant.

Reproduction

The physical and emotional aspects of getting pregnant, having babies, and avoiding pregnancy are part of reproduction. Having sex is a part of reproduction, as are the growth and development of the reproductive organs during puberty. (See Body Basics, The Reproductive System, on pages 74 and 75.)

The way people feel about sexual intercourse is related to how they feel about sex and sexuality. People usually have strong attitudes about sex and sexuality, including their attitudes toward their genitals, how private they feel about their bodies, and whether they think marriage is necessary before sexual intercourse. People's feelings and attitudes about sex and sexuality develop from the messages they receive from family, friends, religion, school, and the media.

As a nurse assistant, you might have to deal with some things related to reproduction. For example, you may provide care for a woman who is menstruating and acts embarrassed about it. When you provide care for her, you also may feel embarrassed about changing her sanitary napkins or washing her genital area, but it is part of your job to make the woman feel comfortable. You must be sensitive to how she may feel. You must reassure her that her menstrual needs are natural and that helping her is part of your job.

You also may provide care to a woman just before or after she has given birth to a child. As a result of her delivery, you may need to give special attention to the area where the baby was delivered— either the genitals or the abdomen, in the case of a cesarean section. You also may need to provide special care for her breasts, especially if she is going to nurse her baby.

You may feel uncomfortable when you see a woman's genitals or breasts. Those feelings are okay, but you still must do your job. Part of your job is to help the woman feel more comfortable. It also is part of your job to help a new mother relax so that she can nurse and provide care for her baby.

Sexualization

Using sex or sexuality to control other people is called sexualization. Some people use sexuality to get other people to do what they want. For example, a teenager may say to a date, "If you really loved me, you'd have sex with me." Or an adult who is upset with a spouse or sexual partner may respond to sexual advancements by saying, "Not tonight. I have a headache." Sexual abuses, such as rape and incest, are extreme forms of sexualization.

One form of sexualization that happens on the job is called **sexual harassment** (Figure 4-13). Sexual harassment often happens to women and sometimes to men. For example, a boss or supervisor may demand that a person have sex with him or her in order for that person to get a raise or promotion. This demand is illegal. If this situation ever happens to you, you should report it immediately to your supervising nurse or personnel office or to a civil rights organization.

Another form of sexual harassment happens on the job when someone creates a sexually **hostile** or threatening workplace. Telling "dirty" jokes, showing pornographic material, touching, or giving unwelcome attention not only makes the workplace uncomfortable but also can be illegal.

Sexualization also affects the elderly and disabled when others deny them their right to sexual expression. This denial is called sexual oppression. For example, someone may refuse to close the door to provide privacy for a person's sexual activities.

Situations in your job as a nurse assistant might involve sexualization. For example, you may provide care to a person who has been sexually abused, such as an adult or a child who has been raped. Although you may feel angry about the abuse, you must provide care for this person in the same way that you provide care for anyone, with kindness and gentleness. Often a social worker is assigned to

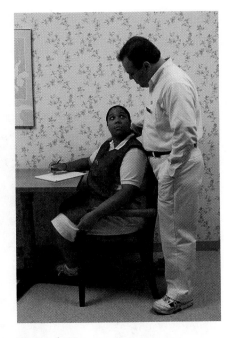

Figure 4-13
If a co-worker does something that makes you feel uncomfortable, let him or her know how you feel. If you need to, speak with your supervising nurse or personnel office.

sexual harassment
(SEK-shew-uhl/HAIR-as-ment) Purposely annoying or threatening someone by not respecting his sex or sexuality.

hostile
(HOS-tuhl)   Unfriendly.

BodyBasics

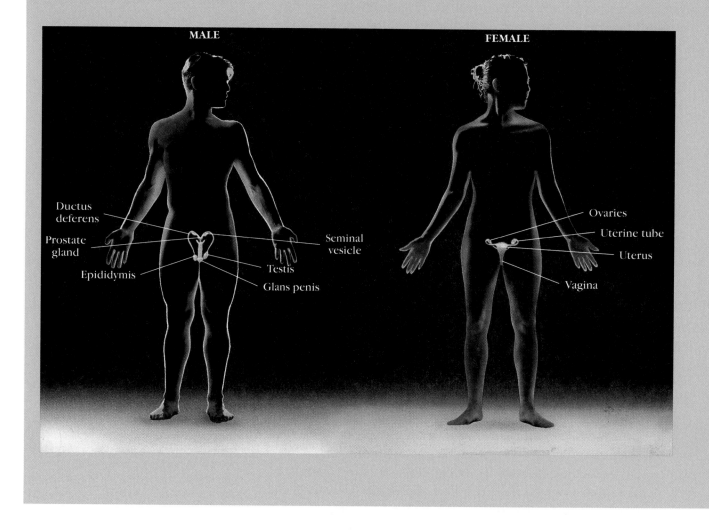

talk with someone who has been abused. You can talk with the social worker about your own feelings about the person's abuse. There may be a time when you suspect that someone has been sexually abused. You must report your suspicions to your supervising nurse. (Refer to Chapter 3, Protecting People's Rights.)

You may be approached on the job by a person who wants you to have sex with him or her. Or you may be bothered by a person who may want to touch, hold, or fondle you in a certain way. If the person is putting pressure on you, you must report such actions immediately to your supervising nurse or to your personnel office.

BodyBasics

❖ The Reproductive System ❖

Humans reproduce when the man's sperm joins with the woman's egg. The resulting embryo grows for 9 months in the woman's uterus before it makes its appearance in the world. The process may sound simple, but the human reproductive system is a complex set of organs inside and outside of the male and female bodies.

The male reproductive organs are situated mostly outside the body. The penis is a finger-shaped organ between a male's legs. Behind the penis hangs the scrotum, a pouch of loose skin that holds the testes, the inch-and-a-half long, bean-shaped organs that produce sperm and hormones. Loose channels inside the penis fill with blood when it is erect. Urine is carried from the body through a tube in the penis, the urethra. When a man ejaculates, semen, the fluid that carries sperm, also flows through the urethra. Urine and semen do not flow through the urethra at the same time.

Inside a woman's abdomen, separate from her digestive tract, is the uterus, the growing baby's home for 9 months. Nearby are two ovaries that produce eggs and hormones. The cervix, a narrow, thick-walled structure, separates the vagina from the uterus. Outside, near the opening of the vagina, the woman has a clitoris, a small organ that gives sexual pleasure.

How the Reproductive System Ages

As the body ages, the most important change that may occur in the male reproductive system is the enlargement of the prostate gland, which squeezes the urethra and interferes with the passage of urine. A man also may have increasing difficulty maintaining an erection and produce fewer sperm and less seminal fluid, but he can still father a child in later years. A woman, on the other hand, stops producing eggs and hormones when menstruation ceases in menopause. This change occurs naturally from the mid-to-late 40s to the early 50s, or earlier if the woman has had her ovaries and uterus surgically removed. Both men and women can enjoy sexual activity well into old age.

Fascinating Fact

The total amount of blood in a pregnant woman's body increases by 25 percent by the time her baby is born. The total amount of water carried in her body increases by about 3½ quarts.

Why Nurse Assistants Must Understand Human Sexuality

Learning about and understanding human sexuality are important to you as a nurse assistant, because you have to deal with sexual behaviors and feelings in your work. For example, when someone in your care make hints about wanting to be alone in his or her room, because you know about and understand human sexuality, you will respect that need. Or, when someone in your care is sexually attracted to you, you will know how to respond to his or her behavior in a professional way.

You may want to spend some time thinking about what you have just read about human sexuality. Talk about these ideas with friends and family members. Much of this information may be new to you. Since we all learn many myths about sex and sexuality when we are growing up, it is sometimes hard to sort the facts from the fiction. But what you have learned can be useful in your everyday life. If you have children, you can help them learn about their sexuality in a positive way. And, if you have a sexual partner, you may discover a new understanding of him or her.

How Culture Influences Behavior

You are concerned about Louise Wang, an 83-year-old woman in your care. On today's report, you read that she is refusing her medicine. And this morning, when you deliver her breakfast tray, she refuses to eat. She says she wants only a cup of hot water for her tea—a special herbal tea that her sister brought yesterday. Mrs. Wang tells you that the tea has great healing powers and that it comes from the country where she grew up. When you try to encourage her to eat so that she can keep up her strength, she says that she cannot eat food while she is taking the special tea. Because she is such a small woman, you try again to convince her to eat, and she simply removes her hearing aid so that she can't hear what you are saying.

Unless you are a Native American, you or your family or one of your **ancestors** came to America from another part of the world. Possessions, ideas, and beliefs that you and your family hold explain who you are and define your **culture**.

What Is Culture?

Culture is a combination of what you believe (religion), what you consider to be acceptable social forms (behavior and values), and how you express yourself through material things (food, clothing, art, and music). As a family or group repeats these cultural expressions, they become **customs**. As families pass these customs from one generation to another, they become **traditions** (Figure 4-14). People whose parents, grandparents, or great-grandparents were born in another country may try to keep all or some of the traditions and values of their homeland. Being "American" means being a mixture of the old and the new. The culture that people are "born into" is their **heritage**, or inherited culture. All people have a national, racial, or tribal heritage that connects them by a shared language, **ancestry**, and religion, and often by physical characteristics, to other people with the same heritage.

Our inherited culture helps us understand who we are and how we fit into our society. Together with our environment, it tells us how to think about being male or female, being young, growing up, marrying, aging, becoming ill, and dying. These ways of thinking feel natural, comfortable, and "right" to us. Problems may arise when we experience the differences of other people's inherited culture. We sometimes fear these differences and decide that our way is right and their way is wrong.

ancestor
(AN-ses-ter)   A distant relative from whom a particular family descended.

culture
(KUL-tyur)   The racial, ethnic, social, and religious principles that shape a person's thoughts and beliefs.

customs
(KUS-tums)   Actions or practices that are done regularly by a group or family.

tradition
(tra-DISH-uhn)   An inherited ritual or pattern of doing things.

heritage
(HAIR-uh-tij)   The culture passed on to a person through birth.

ancestry
(AN-ses-tree)   A family's history.

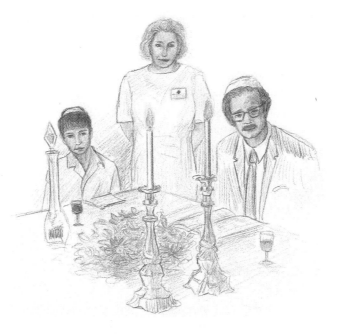

Figure 4-14
Working with people of different cultures gives you an opportunity to learn about their customs and traditions.

Imagine that you are in a foreign country where people dress differently and eat strange-looking and odd-smelling food. You do not understand what people are saying to you, and they do not understand you. If you get sick and need medical attention, how might you feel?

Some people in hospitals and nursing homes feel as if they are in a foreign country. They do not understand the language. They are served food that they do not like or cannot eat because of social or religious customs. They are required to wear gowns that reveal more of their bodies than their customs permit.

You provide nursing care for people who may have inherited a culture that is different from yours. You must accept and respect their cultural differences and not pass judgment on them. Their inherited culture and yours may be different, but that difference does not make one right and the other wrong. Your culture is right for you, and the other person's culture is right for him. Picture each culture as a different color of thread that is woven into a beautiful piece of cloth that becomes the fabric of our society. Everyone is different, and even people from the same culture can have different beliefs.

If you provide care to someone in his home, and that person is from a different culture, you may feel strange and perhaps a little uncomfortable when you first go into the home. You may see personal belongings that look different. The person's family might speak a language that is different from yours, and they might have different personal and dietary habits. Once you are accustomed to being in the home, you can use this opportunity to learn about your client's culture, since you must include your client's cultural practices, as well as his personal needs, wants, and desires, in his care.

Two important things to remember are that our world is a diverse place made up of many people and many cultures and that each person's culture is important to him.

Why Nurse Assistants Must Understand Cultural Differences

When you work as a nurse assistant, it is important to understand how culture influences behavior and to respect each person's culture and individuality.

You have your own cultural background that influences your actions on the job. You need to be aware of your feelings and how they may affect the person in your care. Ask yourself the following questions, answer them, and then think about how someone else might answer them differently:

❖   What do you believe about being healthy? Do Mrs. Wang's beliefs about being healthy differ from yours?

❖   Why do people get sick? How would someone you know answer this question in a different way?

❖   How do people in your family respond to pain? How do your friends respond in a different way?

❖   What are your personal health practices? Think of someone who has different personal health practices.

❖   What are your beliefs about food and health? Do Mrs. Wang's beliefs differ from yours?

❖   What are your beliefs about medical care? Think of someone you know who has different ideas about medical care.

❖   What do you believe about family? What is your family culture like? What cultural differences do you notice when you think about someone else's family?

❖   What are your beliefs about birth and death? Think of someone whose beliefs about birth and death are different from yours.

It is not always easy to accept what other people believe. In fact, you do not have to. What you must do, however, is respect people's beliefs while helping them learn what they need to learn to get better or adapt their lives to a lifelong illness.

Table 4-5 lists some areas in which you may see cultural differences among the people in your care. Next to the differences is a list of suggested actions you can take when you help plan the care for these people.

To provide the best care possible for people, you must learn to see the beauty of each person, each family, and each culture. By appreciating each person within his or her family and culture, you understand the person's needs better. And, in understanding the needs of the people in your care, you may assist in reducing the amount of stress people and their families may be feeling about illness, disability, or old age.

Table 4-5   **Handling Cultural Differences**

To Help Bridge the Cultural Difference Gap. . .	You Can. . .
Language	Ask clear, short questions. Point to pictures or use flash cards. Watch facial expressions and nonverbal language to understand what the person may be feeling, understanding, or trying to communicate.
Diet	Gather information about the person's likes and dislikes. (Some cultures or religions have rules about food. This information needs to be part of the person's care plan. See Chapter 12, Healthful Eating.) Ask if the person has a special diet.
Religion	Ask if the person would like to see clergy. Report a request to see clergy to your supervising nurse. Provide privacy for visiting clergy, as well as for religious practice, such as prayer.
Illness	Respect rituals as long as they do not interfere with the care plan or anyone else's well-being.
Death	Ask the family if they want a special ritual before death or immediately after. Ask them if special treatment of the body is required.

Information Review

Circle the correct answers and fill in the blanks.

1. Four factors that influence how a person behaves are
   ___physical___, ___social___,
   ___emotional___, and ___cognitive___.

2. Human development occurs in the same
   ___order___ and follows the same
   ___pattern___ for all human beings.

3. You are providing care for 13-year-old Kathy Harrison at her home while she is recovering from injuries caused by a car crash. She has stitches along her forehead and across one cheek and sits in a wheelchair for much of the day. Her friends call, but she doesn't want to see them. She may be worrying that—
   a. Her friends want her to go to the mall.
   b. Her friends will think she is ugly.
   c. Her mother won't let them come over.
   d. Her friends will bring her schoolwork.

4. Mrs. Wang's niece is discouraging her aunt from learning how to knit. She tells you that her aunt is too old to learn anything new. You could tell the niece that—

   a. Older people can still learn things, but it may take a little longer than it once did.

   b. She is right, and you will take the knitting needle from her aunt so that she won't frustrate herself.

   c. She is right. Knitting is too complicated for an older person to learn.

   d. She should not be concerned about what her aunt wants to learn.

5. Mr. Jameson always talks about his days as a leader in his union, but he hardly ever talks about the present. When he starts to talk about the past, you could—

   a. Tell him not to dwell on the past.

   b. Tell him how interesting it must have been in those days and ask him some questions about it.

   c. Change the subject by asking him what he would like to do today.

   d. Ignore him.

6. According to Abraham Maslow, the five basic needs are

   ___physical___ , ___security___ ,
   ___social___ , ___esteem___ , and
   ___self fulfillment___ .

7. If your ___needs___ are not met, you may have a hard time doing your job as a nurse assistant.

8. Having a good body image is part of a healthy person's ___sexuality___ .

9. One of the people you provide care for starts to speak to you in a whisper. As you bend over to listen closely, the person tries to grab your bottom and kiss you. You should—

   a. Pull back and slap the person's hand.

   b. Tell the person firmly, but gently, that you do not like to be touched like that.

   c. Use the call signal to get help.

   d. Shout at the person to stop.

10. Mrs. Goldstein has recently been diagnosed with diabetes and must eat meals at regular intervals. Today is a fasting day in her religion. She knows that she needs to eat because of her disease, and she knows that her religion says that sick people don't have to fast. Yet, when you serve her food, she tells you that she feels funny about eating. You could—

    a. Tell her that she shouldn't feel bad.

    b. Avoid talking about religion and serve her food without saying anything.

    c. Tell her that she doesn't really have to eat if she doesn't want to.

    d. Tell her that you can understand that it must feel strange to eat on a fasting day and encourage her to talk about it.

Questions to Ask Yourself

1. Mr. Smith enters the hospital where you are working. His family says he is usually cheerful and talkative, but he has hardly said a word since his admission. Why do you think he is not talking?

2. What are the care needs of an 80-year-old woman? Of a 30-year-old woman? Which needs are the same? Which are different?

3. How is providing care for a 1-year-old child different from providing care for a child of 4? Which child do you think is easier to provide care for? Which do you prefer to provide care for?

4. How can you find out exactly what a person needs? What can you look for? What can you do?

5. Think of a time when you had a special need that was met. How did you feel when that need was met?

6. How can you help a very shy woman become less embarrassed about having her genitals washed?

7. If you found a nursing home resident masturbating in the dayroom, how would you feel? What would you do?

8. How would you feel about providing care for a homosexual man in the home where he and his partner live? How do you think you would act?

9. You are providing care for a woman who believes it is wrong for anyone to view her unclothed body. She has the right to refuse a bath, but she needs one, and it is part of your job requirement. What would you do?

10. The person in your care is a vegetarian. A dish of beef stew is on his supper tray. What would you do?

5

Communicating with People

Goals

After reading this chapter, you will have the information to—

Understand communication and how it works.

Use communication skills to interact with all people in your care, influence a person's behavior, interact with families, and teach.

Use medical terminology, including abbreviations.

Use your senses to make observations.

Communicate accurate observations about people to other health care workers.

When you knock on Rachel Morgan's door, you brace yourself to deal with this new resident, who has not spoken to you since she was admitted yesterday to Morningside Nursing Home. Mrs. Morgan is just 45 years old, but as you read on her chart, she often has double vision, weakness, and loss of balance caused by multiple sclerosis. Sometimes her hands shake and often she has sudden, uncontrollable outbursts of anger or crying. She can no longer live alone safely.

You are surprised when Mrs. Morgan says, "Come in," and are even more surprised when she looks up at you and smiles.

You say, "Hello, Mrs. Morgan," introduce yourself, and check her name band as you give her a firm, but gentle, handshake. "I've come to help you get ready for bed."

"Thank you," she says, "for introducing me to Agnes Ryan. She is such a dear woman. I was sitting in this chair, thinking how I don't belong in a nursing home with a bunch of old people—I'm too young and I should be in my own home, with my own friends, surrounded by my own things.

"At that point, I had never felt so alone. I was crying, when I felt a gentle touch on my shoulder. I looked up and saw Agnes. She kept patting my shoulder and saying, 'There, there.'

"Then she explained that you had introduced us yesterday when I was coming in. She said she'd stopped by to see how I was doing and to let me know that everyone missed seeing me at dinner.

"I was amazed. I wasn't seeing too well when I came in yesterday. And I didn't

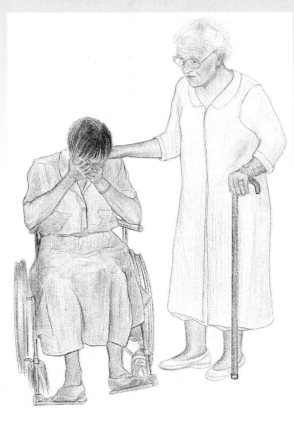

go to any meals today because I'm embarrassed about my weak, shaky arms. But I just couldn't believe what I was hearing: They missed seeing me at dinner!"

You tell Mrs. Morgan you're glad to hear that Mrs. Ryan stopped in to see her. You mention that 90-year-old Mrs. Ryan makes beautiful quilts.

"Do you think she would show me one?" Rachel asks.

You tell her "yes" and suggest that Mrs. Morgan ask her during lunch tomorrow in the dining room. "I think I *will* talk with her tomorrow at lunch," Mrs. Morgan says, and smiles.

Using Communication to Interact with Others

As you read in the previous chapter, people can be hard to understand. But they do not have to be a mystery if you talk with them and listen to their stories. When you interact with the people in your care, you learn many things about them that help you understand them better. To do this well, you must understand **communication**, how it works, and how you can use it effectively in your work.

Communication is the principle of care that you use when you follow all the other principles. You communicate to help keep people safe, to respect their privacy, to give them dignity, to promote their independence, and to help maintain infection control.

Your ability to send and receive messages helps other people understand you and makes it possible for you to understand others. You may think that communication takes place only when you talk or write, but much communication takes place in the expressions on your face, the grip of your handshake, or the tilt of your head.

How Communication Works

You probably know from personal experience how common it is for people to misunderstand one another. When you talk and someone misunderstands you, you may react by thinking, "What's wrong with her? Why didn't she understand me? What I said was so clear!"

Effective communication requires more than just one person talking or providing information. Table 5-1 shows how five important parts or elements of communication work together to get a message across.

Look at how these five elements worked together when Mrs. Morgan talked with you about Mrs. Ryan.

You tell Mrs. Morgan that she could ask Mrs. Ryan about her quilt-making tomorrow during lunch. Mrs. Morgan says she thinks she will do that. You are the *sender*. The suggestion to talk with Mrs. Ryan at lunch is the *message*. You use verbal communication as the *channel*. Mrs. Morgan is the *receiver*. *Confirmation* occurs when Mrs. Morgan says that she thinks she will talk with Mrs. Ryan tomorrow.

communication
(kuh-myou-nuh-KAY-shun)   The process of giving and receiving information.

Table 5-1   **Five Elements of Effective Communication**

Communication Element	Description of the Element
Sender	The person who wants to communicate information
Message	The information the person sends
Channel	The way the message is sent—verbally (talking), nonverbally (facial expressions, body movements), or in writing
Receiver	The person to whom the message is sent
Confirmation	The way the receiver lets the sender know that he has received the message

If these five elements work together for clear communication, why do people misunderstand one another? Sometimes the message itself may not be clear. Other times the sender may be using the wrong channel. For example, a man who talked to a nurse about the care his mother received became so upset that he didn't make sense when he spoke. His message might have been understood better if he had calmed down before he spoke or if he had communicated through a different channel, such as a letter.

Other times, misunderstanding occurs when the receiver does not confirm the message to the sender by telling the sender what she thinks the message means. If you are the receiver, confirm the message by repeating, in your own words, what the sender said. If you are the sender and you have to ask the receiver for confirmation, ask an **open-ended question**, not a **close-ended question**. For example, the man who was talking to the nurse about his mother could have said, "Do you understand?" (a close-ended question) and the nurse could have said, "Yes," even if she didn't understand. However, if the man had said, "What do you understand about the situation that I just explained?" (an open-ended question) the nurse would have answered by repeating the man's message in her own words if she understood him.

Good communication requires much thought, careful attention, skill, and cooperation. It also has many benefits, including increased understanding among people.

Choosing Communication Channels

As a nurse assistant, you use three channels of communication: Verbal communication is words spoken for the receiver to hear, nonverbal communication is actions and expressions for the receiver to observe, and written communication is words or symbols written on paper or some other medium for the receiver to read. The channel that you choose to send your message depends on the message and the receiver. For example, you would choose verbal communication to send a message to someone who cannot read or who is blind. In certain situations, you might use more than one channel to send your message. For example, you could explain something (verbal communication) and then write it down (written communication) as a reminder (Figure 5-1). Or you could demonstrate a skill (nonverbal

open-ended question
A question that requires more than a simple "yes" or "no" answer. An open-ended question encourages a person to talk.

close-ended question
A question that requires a simple "yes" or "no" answer.

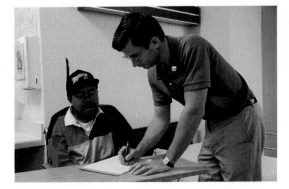

Figure 5-1
A written reminder can be especially helpful if your message is complicated or if the person in your care has trouble remembering things.

communication) and describe what you are doing (verbal communication) at the same time.

Verbal communication.   Verbal communication has two important parts: (1) what you say and (2) how you say it. Effective verbal communication requires that you have useful information to share, speak clearly, and express your thoughts well.

When you talk with a person in your care or with your co-workers, use the following verbal communication skills:

❖ **Get the receiver's attention before you start talking.** If the person is doing something, and your message is not urgent, it may be better to talk with her later.

❖ **Use words that the receiver understands.** When communicating with people in your care, be careful about using medical terms that may not be familiar to them. Because some people may feel shy about asking what you mean, they may not get the message.

❖ **Choose the right volume.** Speak loudly enough to be heard but not too loudly. How loudly you speak depends on how well the receiver can hear, how much noise is around you, and whether you are discussing personal information. If a person is having trouble hearing you, move closer to her.

❖ **Speak slowly and clearly.** Talk slowly enough to express your thoughts clearly and to give the receiver time to hear and think about what you are saying, as well as the opportunity to respond or ask questions.

❖ **Be aware of your tone of voice.** Listen to how you sound to be sure that your tone of voice matches what you are trying to say. Sometimes, when you are in a hurry or have something else on your mind, you say things in a tone of voice that is not **appropriate** for the situation. For example, if you are thinking about an unpleasant conversation you experienced with the bus driver today, you may reflect your anger at the bus driver when you speak to the person in your care.

❖ **Listen to the receiver.** By asking receivers to respond and by listening to what they say, you receive confirmation that they understand your message. If they don't understand, you may have to send the message again in a different way.

appropriate
(ah-PRO-pree-it)   Right or correct for a given situation.

Nonverbal communication.   A performing mime never speaks. He uses only actions—nonverbal communication—to send a message. Information and feelings often are shared through body movements and facial expressions. Sometimes these actions are called body language.

To communicate effectively, you need to understand two different elements of nonverbal communication: receiving information and sending information. When you look at people, you notice their facial expressions and how they hold their bodies. The information you receive from their faces and bodies affects how you interpret their messages. If you talk to a woman whose arms are folded tightly across her chest, you may think she is angry or upset. You interpret this message not by what she says, but by how she holds her body. However, her arms may be folded because she is cold. A person's background and culture also can affect nonverbal expression. For example, looking a person in the eye is a form of respect in some cultures, but it is offensive in others. When you receive information through nonverbal communication, ask the sender if you are interpreting it correctly (Figure 5-2).

On the other hand, you must be careful about the information you send. Sometimes you have to keep your feelings inside so that they don't show on your face. For example, when you provide care to someone who has an infection that neither looks nor smells nice, you must keep a calm look on your face so that the person does not feel afraid or rejected. If a situation really bothers you, you may need to excuse yourself, get a breath of fresh air, and return. Be aware of how you hold your body and what you are doing so that you communicate the right message. For example, if you are pleased about something, make sure your facial expression (perhaps a smile) and body (standing erect), as well as your words, communicate your pleasure.

The same nonverbal clue can signal many possible messages, which the receiver needs to check out. Consider the following aspects of nonverbal communication:

- ❖ **Personal appearance.** When you look professional—by wearing clothing without stains, wrinkles, or holes and by polishing your shoes, keeping your hair clean and neat, and trimming your nails—you send the message that you care about yourself and the people that you are with (Figure 5-3).
- ❖ **Facial expressions.** The meaning of facial expressions can vary. For example, a smile can be a sign of welcome or a sign of approval. A frown can suggest unhappiness or annoyance. The look in a person's eyes can show understanding or confusion.
- ❖ **Touch.** A caring touch, such as a hand on a shoulder, a pat on the back, or a hug, is often a good way to make someone feel

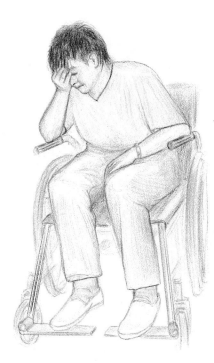

Figure 5-2
You have already read some things about nonverbal communication. If you saw this woman sitting alone and crying, you might conclude that she is sad and wonder what you could do to make her feel better. In response to what you see, you can approach her and offer help.

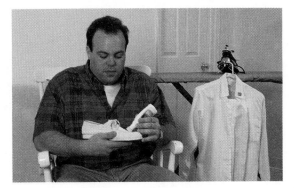

Figure 5-3
It takes effort to present a neat, professional appearance on the job. Having a good personal appearance is important to your own self-esteem and also sends a positive message to others.

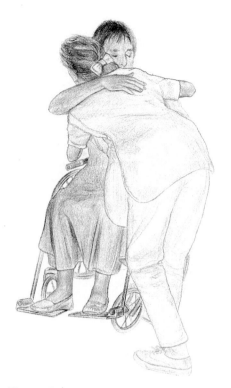

Figure 5-4
Mrs. Morgan recently arrived at the nursing home. The nurse assistant doesn't know her very well, so, before touching Mrs. Morgan, she asks, "Can I give you a hug?"

comfort zone
(KUM-fert) The distance between one person and another that feels comfortable when communicating.

special or emphasize what you are saying (Figure 5-4). As you know, touching is not appropriate in all cultures, and some people simply don't like to be touched.

Sometimes, because of how you feel, it is not appropriate to send a message by touch. If you feel angry, tense, or impatient, you may want to grab, slap, or shake a person, but you must never touch a person in this way. If something is bothering you, talk about it right away with your supervising nurse or with someone else you trust.

❖ **Body position and movement.** People in your care communicate how they feel physically and emotionally by the way they move, stand, and sit. For example, a person who usually sits up straight may be slouching in his chair today. His slouched position may indicate that he is in pain, tired, or feeling depressed.

You also send messages when you move, stand, and sit. Move toward people slowly so that you don't startle them and so that they don't think that you are in a hurry or that you don't want to be bothered with them. *Where* you stand or sit in relation to another person also is important. Every person has a **comfort zone**. Your own comfort zone may allow you to stand very close to others, but some people in your care may find your closeness uncomfortable and back away. Or you may need a lot of personal space, but someone in your care may think that the distance means you do not like her. Be aware of each person's comfort zone, and find a distance that feels right to you and the other person.

Written communication.   In your work, you often communicate by writing telephone messages for co-workers, reminders for people in your care, and information for your co-workers about the people in your care. (See Learning the Language of Caregiving and Communicating About the People in Your Care later in this chapter.)

Before you write a message for someone in your care, find out if she will be able to read it. Her ability to read may be a source of pride or embarrassment. Although she communicates well verbally, she may not be able to read because she never learned, she doesn't read English, or she has problems with her eyesight. To find out about her reading ability and protect her dignity, talk to her or her family members.

When you communicate in writing, use the following written communication skills:

❖ **Write neatly.** If your handwriting is hard to read, print instead.
❖ **Choose the best size and colors for your letters.** If you write something for a person with limited eyesight, use large letters and a black or dark blue pen or crayon on white paper.
❖ **Draw pictures.** Sometimes a picture says more than words, and it communicates well to a person who can't read.
❖ **Choose simple words.** Use the simplest words you can to get the message across.

❖ **Be specific.** For example, if you are noting the time, be sure to write "A.M." or "P.M." If two people with the same last name are in your care, write additional information with their last names, such as their first names or their room numbers.

❖ **Be thorough.** Make sure that your message is complete.

❖ **Spell correctly.** If you are not sure of the spelling, look it up or ask.

❖ **Include your signature.** Always sign your note so that people know who wrote it.

❖ **Double-check your message.** To make sure that you have not made any mistakes, check over what you have written before you deliver the message.

Whether you use verbal, nonverbal, or written communication as the channel for sending a message, you want to do your best to make sure the message that you intend is the message that you send.

Using Clear Communication When Providing Care

In your work as a nurse assistant, your ability to communicate can have a positive impact on the health and well-being of the people in your care. At the beginning of the chapter, when you went to Mrs. Morgan's room to help her get ready for bed, you used verbal and nonverbal communication as you interacted with her. Look at Table 5-2 to see the positive meaning that your messages carried.

Table 5-2   **Clear Communication in Caregiving**

Your Message	Channel	Positive Meaning
Knock on the door.	Nonverbal	You show respect for Mrs. Morgan and her privacy.
Greet her and call her by her title (Mrs.) and last name.	Verbal	Your greeting is friendly, and you show respect for her dignity.
Introduce yourself.	Verbal	You help Mrs. Morgan to remember your name by introducing yourself each time you see her.
Check her name band.	Nonverbal	You care about her safety.
Shake her hand firmly yet gently.	Nonverbal	You care about her and are sensitive to her needs; you also are confident about yourself and your work.
Ask permission to help her get ready for bed.	Verbal	Mrs. Morgan still has control over her life.
You tell Mrs. Morgan that Mrs. Ryan makes quilts.	Verbal	You confirm that you listened to Mrs. Morgan's story.
You suggest that Mrs. Morgan talk with Mrs. Ryan at lunch.	Verbal	You want to help Mrs. Morgan make friends and be happy at the nursing home.

Using Assertiveness When Communicating

If you deliver your message firmly and with confidence, it sounds strong, and the receiver is more likely to agree with you. If you deliver your message weakly and in a way that sounds as if it's not important to you, the receiver may not respect what you have to say (Figures 5-5 and 5-6). The difference between the examples in the figures is that, in the first example, you are using **assertiveness** to communicate.

assertiveness
(uh-SER-tiv-nes)   Communication that firmly expresses what the communicator wants.

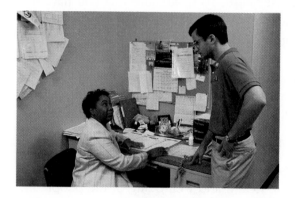

Figure 5-5
If you stand tall, speak in a firm voice, and look into your supervising nurse's eyes when you say, "I need to take off one day next week to take care of some important personal business," she probably will try to rearrange your schedule so that you can take care of your needs.

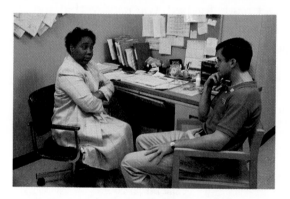

Figure 5-6
If you hunch over, shuffle your feet, mumble, and look at the floor when you say, "I don't suppose I could take off some time one day next week," your supervising nurse will probably say "no."

Being assertive can be an effective way to let people know what you want. Of course, you may not always get what you want because other people may say "no." For example, no matter what you say, a person in your care might refuse your assistance. Or, no matter how you ask, your supervising nurse may not approve your request for time off. Sometimes, however, being assertive can change someone else's mind.

At times people do not want to be assertive because they think other people may not receive it well. It may make other people angry. Also, some people may confuse being assertive with being pushy or aggressive. In some cultures, people learn not to be assertive, and in other cultures, assertive behavior is considered to be rude, manipulative, and too direct. So, use assertive communication selectively, always considering how the receiver might feel about how you send your message. Table 5-3 gives examples of how to take assertive action to send a strong message.

Table 5-3   **Using Assertiveness Effectively**

Situation	Assertive Action	Ineffective Action
A person says "no" to your request.	Decide whether it is important to keep trying to get what you want and, if so, keep trying.	Give in right away.
You decide a denied request is worth pursuing.	Tell the person you understand her position (if you do).	Tell the person her idea is wrong or silly.
	Repeat what you want and explain why it is important.	Repeat what you said and demand to know why your request was denied. If that doesn't work, whine.
	Speak in a firm voice, look into the person's eyes, and stand tall.	Glare at the person and shout.
	Keep your hands by your side or hold them in your lap.	Make angry gestures and pound on the table.
You must refuse someone's request.	Say "no" firmly and explain why.	Say "No. That's that. The case is closed."
The person asks again.	Listen carefully to what the person says, then say "no" politely.	Yell, "Didn't you hear me? I said 'no'!"
The person asks again.	Ask the person to stop pressuring you.	Ask, "Are you deaf?"
The person asks again.	Excuse yourself and walk away from the situation.	Tell the person to leave you alone.
The person asks why you don't like her.	You say you are rejecting her request, not her.	You say it's because she annoys you.

Using Communication in Special Situations

As a nurse assistant, you provide care to people who are different from you, and you may not feel comfortable talking with them about some things. You also communicate with people who cannot see or hear well, with people who speak different languages, and with children. In addition, you use the telephone, which requires you to use your best verbal skills.

Communicating About Difficult Subjects

The people in your care and their families look to you for answers to their questions and talk to you about difficult situations. Most of the time you probably can provide answers. Sometimes, however, you may not know how to respond. These situations happen to everyone.

When you have a good relationship with the person in your care, as you hope to have with Mrs. Morgan, she trusts you enough to express private and personal thoughts. For example, a person might say, "My family doesn't care about me anymore." A family member might say, "I wish she would just die." These messages may make you feel uncomfortable.

When a person says such things, you may feel afraid, nervous, or unsure about how to respond. You may have the same uncomfortable feelings about messages that a co-worker might send when he or she confides in you about problems at work or at home.

Sometimes you may feel so uncomfortable with such messages that you may want to do things to get out of the conversation, such as leave the room quickly, change the subject, tell a "little white lie" that might help the person feel better, or make a comment like, "You don't really mean that," or "Don't be silly."

While these responses may get you off the hook, they cut off communication with the person who is sending the message. Because part of your job is to listen and talk with the person in your care, it is important to keep lines of communication open (Figure 5-7), even when you feel uncomfortable with the message.

The suggestions explained below may help you handle difficult messages better.

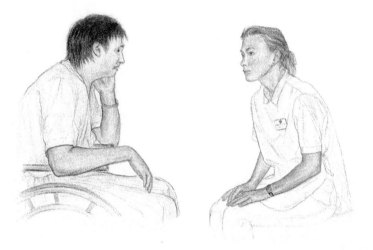

Figure 5-7

Often an upset person doesn't want to be cheered up or offered advice or solutions. She may just want you to listen to her.

Pause for a few moments. To calm yourself, stop to figure out how you feel and why you feel that way. Then, instead of focusing on your uncomfortable feelings, think about the feelings of the sender and how she is trying to communicate with you.

Nonverbally show your interest. Show the person that you care about her feelings by stopping what you are doing, paying full attention, and making eye contact. If it is appropriate, hold or gently squeeze her hand or touch her on the shoulder. If she feels your interest and concern, your silent support can sometimes help more than words.

Verbally encourage the person to talk. Ask a question such as, "How do you feel?" Or ask a question to confirm the person's message:

"Are you saying that you miss being close to another person?" Or, confirm the message by repeating it in your own words: "It sounds like you miss seeing and hearing from your family."

Listen.   Sometimes all a person needs is someone who listens. If she needs answers that you are unable to provide, rather than a listening ear, let another member of the health care team handle the situation or concern. Tell the person that you will talk with someone who can help. Then be sure to follow through.

Talk about your feelings.   To help you understand your feelings, clear your mind, and gain confidence in handling a similar situation, talk with your supervising nurse or someone else you trust.

Communicating with People Who Are Visually Impaired

You may provide care for people who have impaired sight. Some people may only need reading glasses, while others may be blind. Visual impairment may be caused by many factors. For example, Mrs. Andrews has cataracts, a clouding of the lens of the eye that causes a gradual decline of sight. Cataracts may be caused by aging, injury, or other diseases and may develop in one eye or in both eyes. Mrs. Andrews, whose vision is blurred, says she feels as if she has a film over her eyes. Mr. Wilson has diabetes, which caused changes in his eyes, resulting in blurred vision.

Imagine what it must be like for Mrs. Andrews and Mr. Wilson. They cannot move around at will because they can't see clearly what is in front of them. They are unable to read a newspaper or watch television comfortably. When planning care for a person with vision problems, the important points to consider are safety and communication. You can improve safety and communication by remembering that he may not see you, by being sensitive to his surroundings, and by using your voice, words, and touch to help him see.

Remember that a visually impaired person may not see you.   Knock on the person's door or tell him right away that you are there so that you don't startle him. Stand where he can see you, and call him by name: "Good morning, Mr. Wilson." Then tell him who you are.

Be sensitive to a visually impaired person's surroundings.   If a visually impaired person wears eyeglasses, keep them clean and within his reach. Keep the room well-lighted by opening the curtains to let in daylight and turning on the lamps in early evening. Describe his surroundings and tell him what is going on. Describe the people or events in a way that helps him create a picture: "Mr. Wilson, your daughter Susan is here, and she's wearing a beautiful red dress." Or, "It's sunny today, and the patio door is open if you would like to go outside." Keep furniture and belongings in the same place all the time to help him keep a mental picture of where things are and to avoid mishaps (Figure 5-8). If he is in a hospital or nursing home

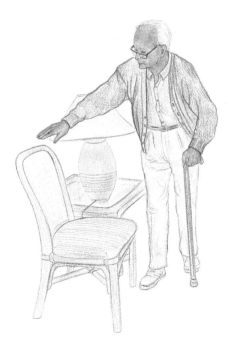

Figure 5-8
Mr. Wilson has impaired vision. He knows that this chair is always in the same place and has no trouble finding his way around it.

and if the facility has raised numbers or symbols on the doors, help him find them.

Use your voice, words, and touch to help a visually impaired person see.   Describe what you are going to do: "It's time for dinner, and I'm going to help you get to the dining room." When serving food, describe the items on the table or tray by location, using a clock as a reference point: "Your meal is chicken, green beans, and potatoes. The chicken is at 12 o'clock on your plate, the potatoes are at 4 o'clock, and the beans are at 8 o'clock." Identify the placement of food or drinks that are not on the plate: "Here is your hot tea. I'm putting it at the top of your plate at 1 o'clock."

When helping a person move around, encourage him to hold your arm just above your elbow for support, describe where you are going, and mention things that are in your path: "We're going up three steps now." When using a piece of equipment, describe it to the person. If it doesn't cause an infection control risk and if he is interested, let him touch what you are holding. Check with your supervising nurse about available aids for people who are visually impaired.

A vision problem is often a chronic condition that doesn't go away. So, keep your focus on safety and on how well you communicate so that the person's life is as pleasant and safe as you can help to make it.

Communicating with People Who Are Hearing Impaired

You provide care for Mrs. Wang, who is hearing impaired and wears a hearing aid. Sometimes she becomes depressed about losing her hearing. Her speech has changed because she cannot hear herself talking. She often appears self-conscious or embarrassed and doesn't want to be around other people. Sometimes she tries to dominate the conversation to avoid the embarrassment of giving the wrong answer to a question. As you help plan Mrs. Wang's care, you emphasize how to communicate effectively with her.

Some people who are hearing impaired may be deaf, while others may have problems hearing certain sounds. Hearing aids improve some hearing problems, as with Mrs. Wang, but just because someone has a hearing aid does not mean she can hear well. Because hearing-impaired people still need to communicate, learn what the people in your care can and cannot hear. You can improve communication with a hearing-impaired person by remembering that she may not hear you, by being sensitive to her surroundings, and by using your face, hands, body, and words to help her hear.

Remember that a hearing-impaired person may not hear you.   Gently touch her on the hand or arm to gain her attention before speaking. Always approach her from the front, and face her so that she can see your moving mouth and facial expressions (Figure 5-9). If she has a hearing aid, encourage her to wear it whenever she is awake, and ask her from time to time if it is working well. Help her use the

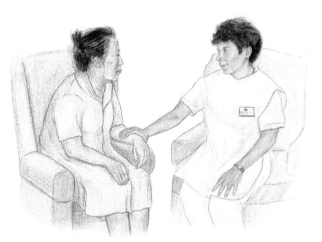

Figure 5-9
If a person in your care is hearing-impaired, adjust your position so that you are face to face with her, not standing over her.

hearing aid properly, care for it according to the manufacturer's directions, and store it in the same place when she is not using it.

Be sensitive to a hearing-impaired person's surroundings. Reduce background noise as much as possible, because television or radio sounds can be very distracting to the hearing-impaired person during conversation. Avoid talking and laughing in front of her unless you include her in the conversation, because she may think that you are talking about her or laughing at her.

Use your face, hands, body, and words to help a hearing-impaired person hear. If the person doesn't seem to understand what you say, change your words, not the volume of your voice, unless you may have spoken too softly. Shouting sometimes creates more distress for the person, and she still may not understand what you are saying. Don't cover your mouth while speaking, because hearing-impaired people often learn to read lips and rely on watching your mouth move. Pronounce your words slowly and clearly, without saying words unnaturally, exaggerating syllables, or shouting. Speak in short sentences.

If a hearing-impaired person hears more clearly in one ear than the other, find out which ear is better and position yourself near that ear when you talk. Use gestures and body movements to help explain what you are saying. Or, if she can read, write messages on paper. When you have important information to get across, make sure that she understands you by asking for confirmation. Ask your supervising nurse about available special devices that can help some hearing-impaired people.

When you make the effort to communicate with a person who has a hearing loss, she may feel more comfortable about communicating her needs and feelings to you.

Communicating with Children

Children communicate in a variety of ways, depending on many factors, such as their ages and their physical conditions. Sometimes it can be easier to communicate with children than with adults, because children tell you exactly how they are feeling and what they want. On the other hand, a child who is sick or hurt may be even more afraid and confused about his situation than an adult and may not trust you. You can improve communication with children if you gain their trust and send them clear nonverbal and verbal messages.

Learn about the child.   To make it easier for you to communicate with children who are shy or unhappy, learn what they like to talk about. Also, ask parents to tell you about their children. Parents appreciate your interest in their children and may tell you how their children communicate in everyday situations.

Send nonverbal messages.   Smile in a friendly way or sit beside a child to gain his trust. When you speak to him, think about your nonverbal message. Stoop or sit so that you are on his level (Figure 5-10).

Figure 5-10
This nurse assistant's body language lets the child know that he is friendly and trustworthy. The nurse assistant's nonverbal message influences the child to respond in a cooperative way.

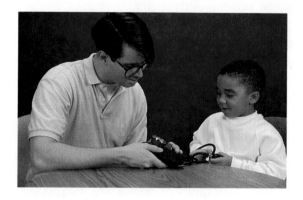

Provide short, simple explanations.   To explain what is happening to a child, use simple explanations and few details. If the child asks questions, he is probably curious and wants to know more. Give him a little information at a time, then pause and ask for confirmation. If the child seems confused about what you said, say it again in another way.

Even though talking to a child can be quite different from talking to an older person, the child wants and deserves the same attention, respect, and caring as an adult.

Communicating with People Who Speak a Different Language

People who speak a language other than English have the same needs and desires for communication as anyone else. In fact, in a nursing home or hospital, their needs may be greater because they have few people to talk with. In addition, they may not have materials written in a foreign language that they can read. You can improve communication with a person who speaks another language by building trust and sending nonverbal messages.

Build the trust of a person who speaks a different language.   Try to find out how much English the person speaks. Be sensitive to her possible embarrassment about making mistakes, as she may not want to try speaking. When she does speak English, praise her efforts.

Send nonverbal messages.   Draw pictures, point, and use facial expressions. Encourage her also to use nonverbal communication so that she can point to what she wants or show you the location of her pain.

If a language barrier makes it seem impossible to get important information across, try to find someone who speaks and understands both English and the language of the person in your care. Ask this person to serve as a translator. This person may be a family member, a friend, or someone who works for your employer. When you communicate through a translator, make sure that both the translator and the person in your care understand your message.

Communicating by Telephone

In your work, you may talk on the telephone with many different people, such as the family and friends of people in your care, doctors, and other health care professionals. Because the person on the other end of the telephone cannot see you, you must speak clearly and choose your words carefully. Most employers have strict rules about what you can and cannot tell various people. If you are unsure about what to do in a specific situation, ask your supervising nurse. In all situations, use a professional manner, common sense, and the following suggestions when talking on the telephone.

Be professional.   Know how to use the telephone system to make outgoing calls, answer incoming calls, put someone on hold, transfer a call, and use any other features. If you make a professional call, identify yourself as soon as someone answers the telephone. For example: "This is nurse assistant Anna Li calling from Metropolitan Hospital Center. May I speak with Mrs. Jones?"

Be courteous.   Answer the telephone as soon as you hear it ring. Speak slowly and clearly. In a hospital or nursing home, tell the caller your location, your name, and your position. For example: "Metropolitan Hospital Center, B wing. This is nurse assistant George Casey speaking. How may I help you?" (Figure 5-11) In someone's home, you might say, "This is the Garcia residence." Check with your supervising nurse to find out how you should answer the telephone.

If you have to put a call on hold, do it for only a short time. If the wait is going to be longer than a minute, get back on the line to let the caller know. Offer to take a message.

Take accurate messages.   If you are asked to take a message, write it down carefully and repeat it to the caller to make sure the informa-

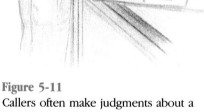

Figure 5-11
Callers often make judgments about a health care facility based on the way staff members answer the phone.

tion is correct. Include the date and time of the call on the message, and sign your name. Put the message where the receiver is most likely to find it.

Respect privacy.   Callers may ask questions about someone's health or may request other personal information. Do not provide any information unless you are sure that your employer permits it, and be sure that any information you provide is correct.

Using Effective Communication to Influence Behavior

As you read earlier, many factors influence behavior. What you say and do can influence other people's behavior in either a positive or negative way. At times, you may influence the people in your care to increase appropriate behaviors that improve their health and well-being. At other times, you may influence them to stop or reduce **inappropriate** behaviors that may be harmful.

Communication sends messages to let people know if their behaviors are liked or disliked. Sometimes, people respond to these messages by continuing behavior that is liked and stopping behavior that is not liked. Your messages may help influence the behaviors of the people in your care.

Increasing Appropriate Behaviors

The people in your care need to do what is in their **care plans**. Part of your job involves helping them do these things correctly and regularly. One of the items in the care plan may be the encouragement of certain appropriate behaviors, such as eating without assistance and taking walks. A special kind of communication called **social reinforcement** helps increase the likelihood that people repeat these appropriate behaviors. Look at Table 5-4.

Each type of verbal social reinforcement helps people increase their appropriate behaviors, especially if you combine the reinforcement with a physical expression of approval, such as a hug, handshake, or touch on the shoulder. Look at the following formula for increasing appropriate behavior to see how verbal and nonverbal reinforcement work together to influence behavior:

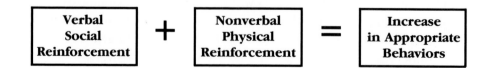

No single type of reinforcement is always successful with the same person or in the same situation because people behave in certain ways for many reasons. For example, a person may not try to walk with a walker because she doesn't understand or is afraid. If what you are doing to reinforce a positive behavior is not working, try to

---

inappropriate
(in-uh-PRO-pree-it)   Not right or correct for a given situation.

care plan
A form used to record overall health care information.

social reinforcement
Encouragement that emphasizes appropriate attitude and behavior.

Table 5-4   **Verbal Social Reinforcement**

Type of Verbal Social Reinforcement	Example
Praise	"Mrs. McDay, I really like the way you styled your hair."
	"Congratulations, Mrs. Garcia. The physical therapist said you walked 10 feet farther than you did last week."
Appreciation	"Thank you, Mr. Lightfoot, for helping me."
	"Mrs. Ryan, thank you for helping Mrs. Morgan feel more at home here."
Encouragement	"Keep trying to touch your shoulder, Mr. Rivera. You're doing a little better every day!"
	"You're doing a great job walking today, Mrs. Wang. I know you can make it another 2 feet to the dayroom."
Approval	"That's right, Josie. You're doing it exactly right."
	"I think that was a good choice, Mr. Rivera."
Recognition	"Everyone, Mrs. Morgan has joined our group today. Let's welcome her."
	"Let's all thank Mrs. Ryan for the beautiful wall hanging she quilted for our dayroom."

figure out why the person is not responding and, with the rest of the health care team, try a different approach.

Reducing Inappropriate Behaviors

Most of the people in your care appreciate what you do for them and try to cooperate. At times, however, a person may yell, spit, or curse at you, or someone may make a racist or sexist remark.

These inappropriate behaviors could be harmful to the person or someone else, and they are difficult to handle. Some people think that those who behave in such inappropriate ways should be punished. But it is never acceptable for you, as a nurse assistant, to punish people in your care. Your response, even to inappropriate behaviors, must uphold the six principles of care. An appropriate response to an inappropriate behavior always allows for safety, privacy, dignity, communication, independence, and infection control. An appropriate response also never violates a person's rights. When a person in your care behaves in an inappropriate way, it is natural for you to feel upset, angry, embarrassed, or frustrated. It is understandable that you feel this way, but it is never all right to act the way you feel if that action is not an appropriate response.

If it seems appropriate, you may leave a negative situation and come back when you and the person feel calmer. When you return, tell the person that you noticed that she seemed upset about something. By communicating in this way, you make it possible for her to talk about what is troubling her, which may stop or reduce negative or harmful actions.

When a person in your care behaves in an inappropriate way, try to ignore the behavior. Sometimes a person uses inappropriate behavior to attract attention. If you pay much attention to these behaviors, she may repeat them. If you think someone in your care is trying to attract attention through inappropriate behavior, pay more attention to her when her behaviors are appropriate.

When a person in your care behaves in a harmful way, report his actions to your supervising nurse. Be as specific as you can. For example, if you say, "Mr. Lightfoot was a pain in the neck today," or "Mr. Lightfoot is so messy," you are communicating only your judgments rather than facts.

A more useful way to report the behavior would be, "At 9:00 A.M., when I was helping Mr. Lightfoot shave, he suddenly grabbed the razor out of my hand and threw it on the floor, barely missing my foot, and said he wanted me to go away and leave him alone."

You may have many feelings to sort out after someone behaves in an inappropriate way. If you keep your feelings bottled up inside, they can create stress and cause you to act in inappropriate ways with other people. To help you deal with the feelings that you have with difficult situations, try some of the following suggestions.

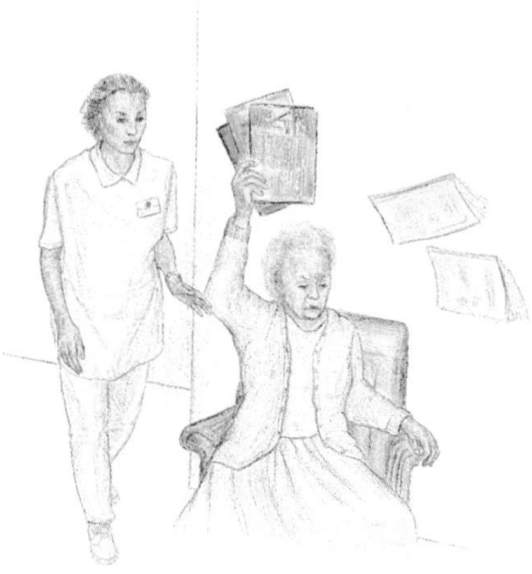

Try not to take inappropriate behaviors personally.   A person who is sick or hurt often directs inappropriate behaviors toward the people she sees most often, even if she is really upset with something or someone else. If you try not to take her behaviors personally, it will be easier for you to handle the situation (Figure 5-12).

Breathe deeply.   Take deep breaths and count to 10 or 20. Keep taking deep breaths until you feel that you are calm and in control.

Leave the room.   If you are afraid you may say or do something that is not appropriate in your role as a nurse assistant, leave the room, providing that the person is safe. If you can, go on with your duties. If you are too upset to work effectively, you may need a few minutes to yourself.

Take a break.   Ask your supervising nurse for permission to take a break so that you can take a brisk walk, get a drink of water, or breathe in fresh air.

Talk to someone.   Tell your supervising nurse or someone else you trust about your feelings. When you are talking, always respect the privacy of the person you are talking about, even if she did not treat you with respect.

Develop a plan.   Work with other members of the health care team to develop a plan of response to the person's inappropriate behaviors.

Figure 5-12
It is not unusual for someone who is sick or in pain to feel frustrated, angry, or afraid. Although your natural response to inappropriate behavior may be anger, you must try to understand the cause of the person's behavior. Try saying, "You seem to be very upset about something. Would you like to talk about it?"

You might be able to influence her behavior and also help prevent a co-worker from being faced with a similar situation.

Talk with the person.   Let her know that you are unhappy with her behavior, but that you still care about her.

Communicating with Families

When you communicate well with the person in your care, you learn a great deal about her. She is your primary source of personal information. You also can learn more about her from her family members, who are important to her and to you. By asking them questions, you can learn more about her food likes and dislikes, clothing preferences, and family and cultural traditions that may affect her care. They can tell you about the work she has done and the hobbies she enjoys. In this way, you are involving the family as part of the health care team.

In our society, the word family means many things. Traditionally, family has been defined as a mother, a father, and children. Family usually implies a connection by blood, but today many people consider it to mean much more than that. What does family mean to you? Who are the people in your family?

When we are young, we can experience family in one of the following ways:

❖ **Biological.** We are related biologically, or by blood, to both parents.
❖ **Step.** We are related biologically to one parent who has remarried, which gives us a step-parent.
❖ **Foster.** We are not living with either of our biological parents, but another family is taking care of us temporarily in their home.
❖ **Adoptive.** We are not living with either of our biological parents, but another family has made us a part of their family permanently. Or we are living with one biological parent, and that parent's spouse adopts us.
❖ **Institutional.** We are not living with either of our biological parents or in another traditional family setting. We are living in a place with other children who do not have parents or traditional families. This place is often called an orphanage.

Family is important in our world and to each of us as individuals because it helps us meet our needs. Early in our lives it is family that meets these needs. As we grow and mature, we may begin to consider friends and organizations in the community as part of our family. We call this larger circle our relationship system. Thus, a larger family group or relationship system helps us meet our needs. For many individuals, this family also includes a partner, such as a husband, wife, or significant other. Throughout our lives, the circle that we call family may continue to change as significant people come and go in our lives.

The family can be an important member of the health care team. Because families are different, some want to be participating members of the team, and others do not. You can encourage families and help them feel more comfortable by getting to know them, learning about their family history, talking with them, and listening to them (Figure 5-13).

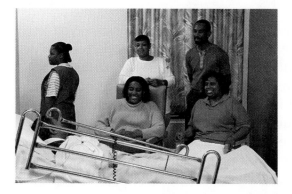

Figure 5-13
You can learn family members' names and find out when they like to visit. Then you can let them know that you are expecting them by planning your caregiving around their visits, bringing extra chairs to make them comfortable, and providing privacy for them.

You also can learn a great deal about the person in your care by observing how her family members relate to one another. At the same time, you must stay on the outside of their family circle and avoid making judgments, expressing opinions, or taking sides when there are disagreements, because these actions may add to stress or unresolved family problems.

Family members also may want to learn things about the person from you. For example, Mrs. Ryan's family may want to know how well she is eating, sleeping, and getting along with other people. Families want to know if their loved ones are getting better or worse. Be sure to answer questions about her activities of daily living. If a family's question needs a medical answer, refer the family to the doctor or nurse.

Use your communication skills to help family members. Listen to them and inform your supervising nurse if someone in the family has questions about the condition of the person in your care, or if someone has a complaint.

Families can feel reassured by your skilled caregiving, but they also may feel resentful or guilty because they can no longer provide care for their loved one or because she became ill or her condition got worse when they were taking care of her.

Family members generally want to continue to be involved with caregiving. They may continue this involvement by trying to make sure their loved one receives the best care possible. They may ask many questions or say that things are not being done correctly. What they may mean is that things are not being done the way they would do them.

To put the family at ease, be sure to talk with them about your role in providing care for their loved one and explain why you do things in a certain way. When possible, use their caregiving suggestions, but make sure that these recommendations support the principles of care.

Box 5-1   How Families Can Help

Give the nurse assistant information:	Likes and dislikes (activities, food, colors), habits (sleeping, bathing, elimination), feelings and fears, past history (career, children, hobbies)
Play a role in caregiving:	Feeding, ambulation (walking), hair care, nail care, bathing, and backrubs
Play a role in decision making:	Care planning and levels of care, restrictions on movement, maintaining household, discharge planning, needed support services
Give emotional support:	Visiting or phoning; sending cards, letters, and photos; listening and talking; showing affection (hugging, touching)
Give financial support.	

Sometimes family members may want to help but aren't sure how to fit in with other members of the health care team. You might hear a family member say, "I just feel so helpless," or "I wish I could do something to help." When family members are frustrated because they don't know what they can do to help, you can make suggestions such as those in Box 5-1.

In a nursing home setting, encourage families and friends to participate with the resident in activities. Explain the benefits of the activity: how it provides a way for meeting new people, how it breaks up the day and makes it more interesting, and how it can be stimulating and motivating. Offer to stay with the resident and her family at a new activity to help them become comfortable in the new situation.

Communicating with People When Teaching

The people in your care need to learn about their illnesses, injuries, disabilities, or medical conditions. As a nurse assistant, you help these people learn how to **adapt** their lives so that they can stay healthy or comfortable. To help them, you must know how people learn and how to teach. When you teach, your communication skills become very important.

adapt
(uh-DAPT)   To change a behavior to adjust to a certain illness or condition.

Your Role as a Teacher

Teachers from your school days probably talked in front of their classes, wrote on chalkboards, and gave structured tests. They taught formally. But teaching is also an ongoing process that often happens informally through conversations or as one person watches another do things.

You help other members of the health care team teach people what they need to know. You may intentionally teach people new activities or new ways of doing familiar activities because it is part of the care plan. Or you may teach informally by performing your daily tasks, talking with people about their concerns, and giving them new

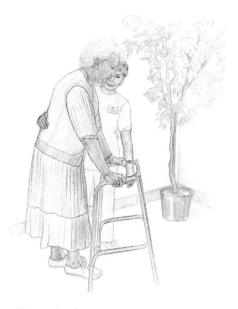

Figure 5-14
By reinforcing what the physical therapist taught, this nurse assistant helps Mrs. Garcia adapt to her condition and maintain her independence.

information so that they can make correct choices. Through all these ways you help them understand how to adapt to the changes in their lives (Figure 5-14).

You can be a good teacher by practicing your three roles: reinforcing, teaching, and observing and reporting.

Reinforcing.   Your supervising nurse may ask you to reinforce, or strengthen, the teaching that another health care worker has begun. Perhaps the physical therapist taught Mr. Wilson how to move and walk with a cane. You can reinforce these lessons by observing his use of the cane when you help him get from one place to another.

Teaching.   Your supervising nurse may ask you to teach a person how to do certain things that are within the scope of your job responsibilities. For example, she may ask you to teach someone who has a weak arm how to dress himself or how to use a special fork or spoon.

Observing and reporting.   Your supervising nurse may also ask you to observe and report on how well someone is doing, as well as on areas in which the person needs additional teaching. You may see Mr. Wilson using his cane incorrectly. You would first correct the situation if it were unsafe, and then you would report this observation to your supervising nurse.

The Learning Process

To communicate effectively through teaching, you must understand how people learn and how you can help in their learning process.

How people learn.   The adults and children that you teach, as well as their family members and friends, learn better when *they*—

❖   Can practice what they are learning.
❖   Can associate new information with their past experiences and with something they already know.
❖   Can clearly see a reason or purpose for their learning.
❖   Are treated with respect.

They also learn better when *you*—

❖   Listen to what they are saying or asking.
❖   Have patience.
❖   Give encouragement and feedback.
❖   Take time out if they are not feeling well or are upset.

How the learning process works.   Learning is an ongoing process, during which a person's knowledge, attitudes, and behaviors change. Learning is not restricted to the classroom. Every day you learn by reading, working, communicating with your friends and family, listening to the radio, and watching television. Just as you learn from other people and experiences, the people in your care learn from you.

When you were a child in school, you learned what your teacher and school chose to teach you. As an adult, you make choices about what you learn, based on what is important to you. Just as you chose to learn to become a nurse assistant, the adults in your care choose what they want to learn. What they learn and how they learn are affected by many things, including knowledge, attitudes or feelings, and experience.

❖ **Knowledge.** A person's learning is affected by what he already knows. For example, if Mr. Wilson already knew how to plan nutritious meals when he changed to a diabetic diet, he probably had an easier time learning to plan and prepare a new diet than someone who doesn't know anything about meal planning. However, he may have had a harder time learning if the information he received was different from what he already knew (Figure 5-15).

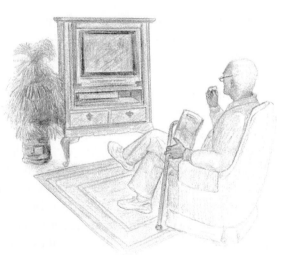

Figure 5-15
For many years, Mr. Wilson snacked on potato chips and peanuts, thinking they were good for him. He may have a hard time accepting his new diabetic diet, which eliminates or reduces these foods.

❖ **Attitudes or feelings.** The person's learning also is affected by how he feels about what he needs to know. For example, if a man believes that cooking is woman's work, he may not want to learn about nutrition and meal planning.

❖ **Experience.** The person's past experience affects how he learns. For example, if someone with high blood pressure tasted a few meals with less or no salt and liked them, it is easier to teach him how to prepare foods with less salt. On the other hand, if he didn't like the way low-salt meals tasted, he might find it harder and need more encouragement to learn how to cook with less salt.

Look at Box 5-2 to see how knowledge, experience, and attitude help Mr. Rivera switch from a safety razor to an electric razor.

By talking with Mr. Rivera, you discover his knowledge level, his attitude, and his behavior. You learn that he may need more information about his disease and its conditions, because he doesn't seem to

Box 5-2   **Changing Razors**

Mr. Rivera, the 78-year-old man in your care who had a stroke, takes medication that increases the amount of time it takes for blood to clot. Because even a small cut may bleed a long time, Mr. Rivera has to avoid any skin injury. Your supervising nurse alerted you to watch for any signs of bleeding during personal care. She also instructed you to have Mr. Rivera switch from shaving with a safety razor to shaving with an electric razor to help prevent nicking his skin. One morning, while helping Mr. Rivera shave, you have the following conversation with him.

Mr. Rivera: "I don't see why I have to use this electric razor. I've been shaving with my safety razor for years, and I never had a problem."

You could say: "I know you like the safety razor better, Mr. Rivera, but, because of the kind of medication you are taking, it is important that you don't cut yourself. The electric razor doesn't nick your skin. It is better for you to use."

Mr. Rivera: "I don't like electric razors, but I don't like bleeding either, so I guess I'd better try it."

understand how his medication affects his blood. You supply some needed information. You should report your observation to your supervising nurse so that she can provide Mr. Rivera with more information. You also find out that, even though Mr. Rivera still prefers his safety razor, he is willing to try a new behavior.

The Teaching Process

During his morning shower, you try to help Mr. Rivera transfer himself from his wheelchair to a shower chair. During the past few days, your supervising nurse and the physical therapist have been teaching him how to do the transfer. You have been told to reinforce the instructions and to encourage Mr. Rivera to do as much of the transfer by himself as possible. Mr. Rivera makes several unsuccessful attempts. After his third try he mumbles, "Oh, forget it. I'm sure my wife knows how to do this. I sure don't."

You can help Mr. Rivera learn to do the transfer if you understand the four steps of the teaching process: assessing the person's knowledge, planning what you have to teach and how to teach it, implementing your teaching plan, and evaluating the impact of your teaching.

Assessing.   Before you begin to teach, you and your supervising nurse work together to assess what the person already knows and feels about the information he needs to learn. First, your supervising nurse makes a formal assessment by looking at several different factors, including age, past education and knowledge, present health status, and illness. She takes into account that certain disease conditions have very specific learning needs. For example, she knows that Mr. Rivera has weakness and some paralysis on his right side as the result of a stroke. She knows that he needs to learn to move around by himself but also that he depends on his wife to help him.

After your supervising nurse completes the formal assessment, she tells you what she thinks the person needs to learn and how you can help. She may ask you to repeat or reinforce certain points while you provide care.

Then, every day as you provide care for the person, you continue to observe what he does or does not know and help your supervising nurse understand more about his needs. You look for any hints or clues from the person that may suggest that he needs more information. For example, Mr. Rivera may say, "I know the nurse and physical therapist showed me how to do this, but I keep forgetting. Besides, my wife knows how to do it." Some clues are not this obvious. Mr. Rivera's statement about his wife knowing how to do it may have been a message that he needs more information or that he is frustrated. You report this observation to your supervising nurse.

Planning.   When your supervising nurse knows what the person needs to learn, she usually plans what needs to be taught and how it should be done. When she tells you what to teach, first review the information and skills before planning how to present them to the person. Plan how to fit the teaching into the time that you spend providing care for the person. For example, you might plan to help Mr. Rivera learn to dress himself during his personal care times. And you might plan to bring a long-handled shoe horn so that he can put on his shoes without bending over and getting dizzy as you learned he had done before. First, you plan to teach him how to put on his pants. When he does that well, you plan to teach him how to put on his shoes. You save teaching him how to button his shirt until last because he thinks this will be the hardest task. This teaching plan becomes a guideline to make sure you communicate the information he needs.

To make sure that your plan is what your supervising nurse wants, discuss it with her and ask any questions that you may have about the procedures you will teach.

Implementing.   Once you have an assessment and a plan, implement your plan to put it into action. An important part of implementing your plan is choosing when to teach. Teach only when you have enough time, when the person is feeling well, and when his surroundings are quiet and private for learning. Otherwise, postpone or adjust your teaching plan until conditions are good enough for the person to learn.

For example, Mr. Rivera has repeated difficulty with buttoning his shirt. He makes several attempts but just can't get the button through the buttonhole. After his fourth try he says angrily, "I just can't do it! I'll never be able to do it! It's hopeless."

You could say, "I'm sure you must feel frustrated, but I'm sure you'll get it. Why don't you take a little break right now?"

By recognizing that Mr. Rivera is upset and suggesting that he wait, you are communicating your calm and patience. You may know from

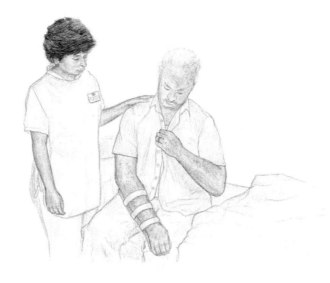

Figure 5-16
The nurse assistant notices that Mr. Rivera is becoming frustrated while trying to learn a dressing task. She will re-evaluate and modify her teaching plan for him.

your own experience that trying to do something difficult when you are frustrated is almost impossible (Figure 5-16). What Mr. Rivera really needs to do is to take a break and relax.

Evaluating.   After assessing, planning, and implementing your teaching plan, you must test, or evaluate, how effective the teaching was by observing the person and asking questions to find out how much he learned. For example, all week you and Mr. Rivera worked together on dressing. Today, when you come in to help him with his personal care, he has already eaten his breakfast and is in the process of getting dressed. You notice that he is able to put on his shirt and button it with only a little difficulty.

Evaluating shows you how effective your teaching is, if the person understands, and if you need to repeat anything. Ask the basic evaluation question: Is the person willing and able to do the task or use the information that I was teaching him? To find the answer to this question, you should ask the person to demonstrate what he learned. After you evaluate, you should give prompt, helpful, and realistic feedback on how the person is doing. You also must report your evaluation to your supervising nurse.

Reinforcing What You Teach

If people in your care are overwhelmed by the amount of information you give them, use teaching skills to help them remember what you teach and communication skills to find out what they didn't understand.

Help the receiver remember the message.   If you have a great amount of information to teach, separate the message into several parts, ask for confirmation from time to time, and give a summary of all the information when you are finished.

Encourage people to ask questions.   To find out if people understand the information, encourage them to communicate by regularly inviting questions. To let them know that others also may have the same questions, you might say, "Many people ask me questions about this." And to encourage questions, praise people when they ask, by saying, "That's a good question. I'm glad you asked!" If a person asks a question that you don't know how to answer, say that you don't know the answer and that you want to check with your supervising nurse. Write down the question, find out the answer, and then give the information to the person as soon as you can.

Learning the Language of Caregiving

One day after work, you and a co-worker go to a restaurant for dinner. As you walk into the restaurant, you hear the waitress yell back to the short-order cook, "BLT on white! Hold the mayo!" You may wonder what language she is speaking. To some people, these words may not sound like any English words they have ever heard before. But these words are restaurant "lingo" for "a bacon, lettuce, and tomato sandwich on white bread, without mayonnaise."

People who provide health care also use a special language that everyone "on the inside" knows. It helps them to communicate more effectively with one another. For example, when a nurse says that Mrs. Wang needs "ostomy" care, most people don't know what she is talking about. But the people on her health care team know that she is talking about a surgical opening in Mrs. Wang's body that needs care.

As a nurse assistant, you learn this special medical language, or terminology, so that you can communicate effectively with others on your health care team. You understand the directions that your supervising nurse gives to you, other nurse assistants understand what you need when you ask for their help, and other members of the health care team understand what you have observed and reported.

In the medical setting, it is important to be clear and **precise** in describing behavior, illness, and treatment. Medical terms are precise: They mean the same thing to the person who is hearing or reading the terms as they do to the person who is speaking or writing them.

precise
(pree-SISE)   Another term for *exact*.

How Small Words Make Large Words

Many medical words seem to be a mile long and impossible to pronounce. They really are just many small words that are hooked together. Many words in the English language have a beginning, a middle, and an end. The beginning is called a **prefix**, the middle is called the **root**, and the end is called the **suffix**. For example, an everyday word that has these three parts is *preschooler*. The prefix *pre* means *before*. The root *school* means *a place for teaching and learning*. And the suffix *er* means *a person or thing that.* . . . When you put the three meanings together, you have *a person who is before learning,* or *someone who is not old enough to be in school.* The root word can be a word that stands by itself, such as the word *school*. But prefixes and suffixes cannot stand alone. They always are

prefix
(PREE-fiks)   The first part of a word that comes before the root word and changes the meaning of the root.

root
The middle part, or base, of a word.

suffix
(SUH-fiks)   The last part of a word that comes after the root word and changes the meaning of the root.

attached to root words. *Pre* and *er* are not strong enough to stand by themselves. But, when you attach them to a root word, they are powerful enough to change the meaning of the word.

Most words do not have all three parts. A word may have a prefix and a root, such as *replace,* which has the prefix *re* (again or back) and the root *place* (put or position). For example, "After the floor dries, the man replaces the furniture." Together, the prefix and the root mean *put back.*

Or a word may have a root and a suffix, such as *alcoholic,* which has the root *alcohol* (an intoxicating liquor) and the suffix *ic* (having to do with). The root and the suffix together mean *having to do with alcohol.* For example, "Only one bowl of punch was alcoholic. The other one was just fruit juice. So the recovering alcoholic took his drink from the nonalcoholic punch bowl."

Box 5-3 contains some familiar everyday English words and some medical words that give you an idea of how roots, prefixes, and suffixes are combined to form longer words with specific meanings.

In addition, words created from prefixes, roots, and suffixes may leave out, change, or add certain letters so that they conform to rules of spelling and pronunciation. That is what happened with the last word in Box 5-3, *physiology.* The prefix is *physio-,* but the *o* was cut out when it was combined with *ology,* so the word is not *physioology,* but *physiology.* This change also happens with the word *ejaculate,* which is combined from the prefix *ex* (out or out of) and the root *jaculor* (throw) to make the word that means *to discharge suddenly and briefly.*

Using Medical Terminology

As a nurse assistant, you do not have to memorize all the possible combinations of medical words. But you must know the meanings of prefixes, roots, and suffixes and how to combine them to understand the longer words. Box 5-4 contains words that relate to the heart.

From this list, you can see how knowing just one word gives you a clue for understanding many other words. When you know the meaning of the different parts of a word, you can identify each piece and then figure out what the whole word means. A list of word parts appears in Appendix B, Glossary of Word Elements.

Using Medical Abbreviations

Remember at the beginning of this section how the waitress yelled back to the cook for a *BLT?* BLT is an **abbreviation** for **b**acon, **l**ettuce, and **t**omato. BLT is made up of the first letters of the three things that are on the sandwich. An abbreviation that we often use is *USA.* USA is an abbreviation for the **U**nited **S**tates of **A**merica. USA is made up of the first letters of the three most important words in the phrase.

In the language of medicine, members of the health care team use abbreviations to save time and space. For example, when a doctor surgically removes the tonsils and adenoids of a patient, he performs a *tonsillectomy and adenoidectomy.* But, when he records informa-

abbreviation
(uh-bree-vee-AY-shun)   A shortened version of a word. An abbreviation is often made up of the first letters of several words.

Box 5-3   **Forming Words**

Prefix	Root	Suffix	Word	Meaning
re- (again or back)	-use (to put into action or service)	-able (that can be)	reusable	that can be used again

Example: The blanket and spread may be reusable linens.

Prefix	Root	Suffix	Word	Meaning
ab- (away; from; away from)	-use	-er (a person or thing that)	abuser	a person who uses or treats someone or something in a way that is different from the acceptable way

Example: The abuser is often someone the victim knows.

ab-	-norm (standard; pattern)	-al (pertaining to)	abnormal	not as it should be; not in the usual pattern

Example: The person's bowel elimination pattern has become abnormal.

ab-	-norm	-ality (the condition of being)		a condition in which things are not as they should be

Example: The test on the specimen shows if there is an abnormality.

co- (with)	-operate (work)		cooperate	to work together with someone

Example: When people on the team cooperate, the work is more easily done.

	tracheo- (tube that carries air to the lungs; windpipe)	-tomy (cutting into)	tracheotomy	surgical operation of cutting into the trachea

Example: A nurse assistant must provide special care to someone who has had a tracheotomy.

	ana- (living)	-tomy	anatomy	study of a living body based on dissection or cutting open

Example: When you study anatomy, you learn about the separate parts of the body.

	physio- (of the body)	-ology (a science or knowledge of)	physiology	science of the normal function of a living body or its parts

Example: We must know about the kidneys, heart, lungs, and blood vessels to understand blood physiology.

tion about the procedure, he writes "T and A." Likewise, on a person's chart you may see that he had a "CBC," which is the abbreviation for *complete **b**lood **c**ount.*

Not all abbreviations stand for the first letters of the words in a phrase. For example, *no.* stands for *number,* and *fld.* stands for *fluid.* Some abbreviations used in medical settings do not seem to relate to

Box 5-4   Forming Medical Words

"Cardio" is a root word that means "heart." If you add different prefixes and suffixes to "cardio," you get a variety of terms to use when communicating about the heart. For example:

Prefix	Root	Suffix	Word	Meaning
	cardio-	-ology	cardiology	science of heart function and disease
	cardio-	-ologist	cardiologist	specialist who studies and treats heart disease
	cardio-	-vascular	cardiovascular	having to do with the heart and blood vessels
	cardio-	-pulmonary	cardiopulmonary	having to do with the heart and lungs
myo-	-cardium		myocardium	heart muscle

the words they stand for. For example, *q* stands for *every, qd* stands for *every day,* and *q2b* stands for *every 2 hours.* You must memorize abbreviations like these, because they may not look like the words they represent. If you are not sure about an abbreviation, look it up before you use it.

As a nurse assistant, you use these abbreviations in your daily work, but you must use only the abbreviations that everyone else in your health care setting uses. A table of abbreviations appears in Appendix C, Glossary of Abbreviations, at the back of the textbook. It includes the abbreviations most commonly used in most health care settings.

Communicating About the People in Your Care

When you use medical terminology, you communicate about the person in your care with other caregivers on that person's health care team. Every day, health care workers must pass information from one group of caregivers to another so that all caregivers can provide coordinated, high-quality care. For example, the caregivers who work at night must give information to the people who provide care during the day. They must write down the information so that it is not forgotten.

Or your supervising nurse may give you a lot of information about a new person in your care: "Mr. Chalmers was admitted from the emergency room last night complaining of chest pain and shortness of breath. He has no known allergies. He is on bed rest but can get out of bed to use the bathroom. He can have nothing by mouth now, but after blood is drawn for the lab he can have fluids as desired. He can have nothing by mouth after midnight tonight. He is on oxygen at 2 liters and is on intake and output. Today he is scheduled for a complete blood count, a 6 A.M. fasting blood sugar, an electrocardiogram, and urinalysis. Get a urine specimen. Take his vital signs four times a day. Mr. Chalmers has an order for pain medication every three hours as needed and a sleeping pill at bedtime if he needs it."

To make sure you remembered everything she said, you would take notes, using the abbreviations you learned, while listening to her report: "Mr. Chalmers was adm. from E.R. last noc c/o chest pain and S.O.B.; NKA. Bedrest c BRP, N.P.O. til lab draws blood; then fld. ad lib; N.P.O. after midnight; O$_2$ at 2 L; I&O; CBC, 6 A.M. FBS, EKG, U/A (get spec.) today; VS q.i.d; pain medication q3h, prn; sleeping pill q.h.s., prn."

Communicating in Three Documents

Your supervising nurse must have written records of the care a person receives. Because you are responsible for contributing information and observations to one or all of these documents—the care plan, the flow sheet, and nursing notes—and because you have to read and use the forms, you must be familiar with all three of them.

Care plan.   Each day, the first documentation tool you use is a care plan. Care plans often are kept in a card file, and each person receiving care has a separate card in the file. A nurse obtains information from the doctor's orders and writes it on the care plan. Like other documentation tools, care plans may be kept on a computer. In place of a card, each person has a computer printout. You read the care plan every day to obtain information for providing care. The following list includes some of the information you may find in each person's care plan:

❖   The person's name, age, religion, and date of admission
❖   Diagnosis
❖   Diet
❖   Activity level
❖   Special procedures and dates
❖   Treatments, such as dressing care, intravenous therapy, respiratory therapy, and intake and output recordings
❖   Special equipment, such as an air mattress, a Foley catheter, and traction devices

Flow sheet.   Caregivers use a **flow sheet** to keep track of a person's changes over a period of time (Figure 5-17). The flow sheet often is kept in a person's room or at his bedside for immediate recording. Documentation on a flow sheet also may include vital signs, intake and output recordings, weight, measurements, treatments, and procedures. For example, Grace Smyth's flow sheet shows that on her first day in the hospital, she ate 100 percent of her diet at breakfast, 80 percent at lunch, and 80 percent at dinner. Figure 5-18 shows an example of a typical flow sheet.

flow sheet
A form used to record health care information and track changes in a person's condition over a period of time.

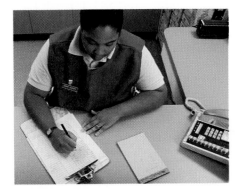

Figure 5-17
Other caregivers rely on information that you record.

Activities of Daily Living (ADL) Flow Chart

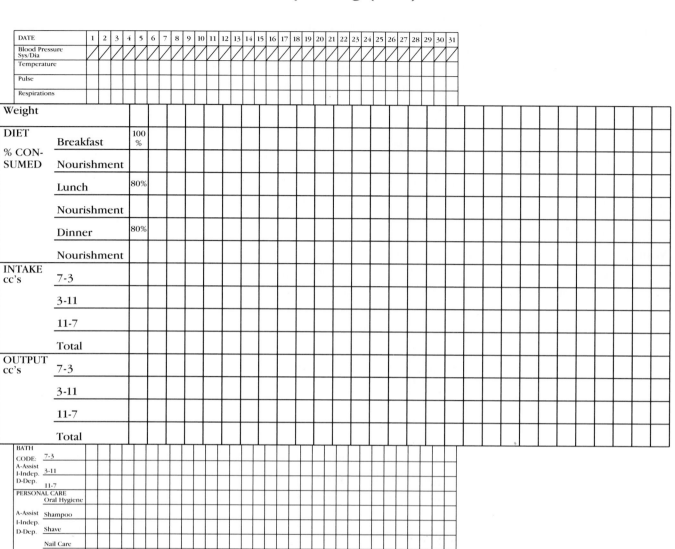

A

		1	2	3	4	5	6	7	8	9	10	11	12	13	14	15	16	17	18	19	20	21	22	23	24	25	26	27	28	29	30	31
DATE		1	2	3	4	5	6	7	8	9	10	11	12	13	14	15	16	17	18	19	20	21	22	23	24	25	26	27	28	29	30	31
Blood Pressure Sys/Dia																																
Temperature																																
Pulse																																
Respirations																																

Weight																
DIET **% CON-SUMED**	Breakfast	100%														
	Nourishment															
	Lunch	80%														
	Nourishment															
	Dinner	80%														
	Nourishment															
INTAKE cc's	7-3															
	3-11															
	11-7															
	Total															
OUTPUT cc's	7-3															
	3-11															
	11-7															
	Total															

BATH CODE: A-Assist I-Indep. D-Dep.	7-3																		
	3-11																		
	11-7																		
PERSONAL CARE A-Assist I-Indep. D-Dep.	Oral Hygiene																		
	Shampoo																		
	Shave																		
	Nail Care																		
	Skin Care																		
Diabetic Urine Test	AC																		
	AC																		
	AC																		
	MS																		
BEDRAILS UP Y - Yes N - No	7-3																		
	3-11																		
	11-7																		

LAST NAME	FIRST NAME	INITIAL	ATTENDING PHYSICIAN	ROOM NO.	PATIENT NO.
Lightfoot	Steven	P.	Dr. Connor	120	416028

Figure 5-18

A and **B**, A flow sheet is one of the three documents health care workers use to record information about a person in their care.

DATE		1	2	3	4	5	6	7	8	9	10	11	12	13	14	15	16	17	18	19	20	21	22	23	24	25	26	27	28	29	30	31
UP IN CHAIR	7-3																															
A-Assist																																
I-Indep.	3-11																															
D-Dep.	11-7																															
ROM EXERCISES	7-3																															
A-Active																																
P-Passive	3-11																															
POSITION CHANGED	7-3																															
A-Assist																																
I-Indep.	3-11																															
D-Dep.	11-7																															
BLADDER ACTION	7-3																															
C-Continent																																
I-Incontinent	3-11																															
Foley 0 × 0	11-7																															
BOWEL ACTION	7-3																															
C-Continent																																
I-Incontinent	3-11																															
0 × 0	11-7																															
CONSISTENCY	7-3																															
L-Liquid																																
S-Soft formed	3-11																															
H-Hard formed	11-7																															
PERI CARE	7-3																															
A-Assist																																
I-Indep.	3-11																															
D-Dep.	11-7																															
OTHER																																
Nursing Assistant's Initials	A.M.																															
	P.M.																															
	NOC.																															

B

Nurse Aids Signature and Initials: _____

LAST NAME	FIRST NAME	INITIAL	ATTENDING PHYSICIAN	ROOM NO.	PATIENT NO.
Lightfoot	Steven	P.	Dr. Connor	120	416028

Nursing notes. Members of the health care team read another form of communication called **nursing notes**. The supervising nurse writes nursing notes in the medical chart to record the person's condition, the care provided to her, and significant events that took place during the shift or visit. You contribute information to your supervising nurse, which she writes into the nursing notes.

Observing

As a nurse assistant, one of your biggest jobs is to be the eyes, ears, nose, and fingertips for the rest of the health care team. You spend much time with the people in your care, and you have to communicate when something changes. To communicate changes, you must observe carefully with your senses, and you must report these observations to your supervising nurse.

Table 5-5 contains examples of how to use your senses of sight, sound, smell, and touch to learn about a person's condition.

Reporting Your Observations

When you use your senses to observe the people in your care, you must know which observations are important to report, what is the best way to report the observation, and when is a good time to report it.

What to report. As you make observations, assess the person's condition and decide what information to pass on to other members of the health care team. A rule of thumb to use when deciding what information to report is, "When in doubt, report." It is best to tell your supervising nurse and let her determine if something needs to be done.

When deciding what to report to your supervising nurse, focus on the word "change." Report observations that indicate changes in:

❖ Mood, mental awareness, and independence level
❖ Vital signs
❖ Elimination
❖ Skin condition and color
❖ Appetite (Figure 5-19)
❖ Sleep habits

Figure 5-19
You don't know why Mrs. Ryan ate very little of her last two meals, but you know that, because she usually has a good appetite, you must report this observation to your supervising nurse.

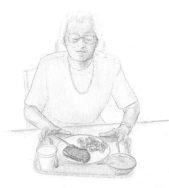

Table 5-5   **Using Your Senses to Observe**

Sense	Common Observations
Sight	*You See* . . . that the person's skin looks pale or red. open areas on the person's skin. sores in the person's mouth. that the person's hand shakes or that the person is too weak to hold a glass. that the person limps or cannot stand alone. that the person's urine, stool, or sputum has an unusual color. that the person's emesis (vomit) has an unusual color. that the person is not eating or is having trouble eating. that the person squints or bumps into things and people. that the person's usual facial expression has changed (for example, he smiles less often). that the person sleeps a lot or does not make eye contact. that the person's breathing is different, labored, or slow, or the person gasps for breath. that a part of the person's body looks different or abnormal to you (for example, one limb is larger than the other). that there is blood or other leakage coming from some part of the person's body or medical device, such as a drain or IV.
Sound	*You Hear* . . . the person coughing. the person making a noise when breathing the person complaining of a change in his condition (for example, pain, numbness, or swelling). the person crying. no response from the person when you talk to him. that the person does not speak clearly.
Smell	*You Smell* . . . that the person's breath has an unusual odor. that the person's emesis (vomit) has an unusual odor. an unusual odor in the person's urine or stool. that the person's dressing or wound has an odor.
Touch	*You Feel* . . . that the person's pulse is strong. that the person's pulse is weak. that the person's skin is warm, cool, or moist. a lump under the person's skin.

Table 5-6   **Fact and Opinion**

Fact	Opinion
The person is not putting his full weight on his left foot.	The person walks funny.
She is crying.	She must miss her dog.
He weighs 250 pounds.	He is overweight.
The person has a dry cough.	I'll bet he smoked a cigarette.
She did not eat any of her dinner.	She must be sneaking candy.

How to report.   After you decide what needs to be reported, the next step is to communicate. Give your information and assessment to others by telling or writing what you observed. Your observations of a person's condition contribute important information to the care plan. For the information to be helpful to those who use it, it must include as many accurate details as possible.

Be objective by reporting clear, accurate information and by paying attention to the facts and not to your personal opinions. Table 5-6 contains examples of differences between facts and opinions.

The following examples demonstrate helpful ways of reporting information and other ways that are less helpful:

Example 1. After Mrs. Garcia broke her hip, she used a wheelchair to get around in the hospital. Her physical therapist worked with her to improve her strength so that she could stand up. The care plan said that you should help her stand three times a day. You knew that she usually stood for 2 or 3 minutes each afternoon. One day, using your arm for support, Mrs. Garcia stood for 5 minutes.
Helpful: "Mrs. Garcia stood for 5 minutes this afternoon. She leaned on my arm."
Less helpful: "Mrs. Garcia stood for longer than usual."

Example 2. Following his stroke, Mr. Rivera has been working with an occupational therapist to relearn how to shave himself using an electric razor. When he started therapy last week, he had a hard time holding the razor and making his hand move the right way. He got frustrated and asked you to finish the job. Today you notice that he shaved his whole face.
Helpful: "Mr. Rivera has made progress with his shaving skills. He is able to shave his whole face."
Less helpful: "Mr. Rivera is doing better holding the razor."

When to report.   Two regular times for reporting are when you begin to provide care for a person and when you complete it. In some settings, especially hospitals, there is a meeting called *report*. During report, you *receive* information about each person in your care from your supervising nurse. At the end of your caregiving, you *give* a report and share information about what you observed and what you did for each person in your care.

Also, report to your supervising nurse right away whenever you think it is necessary. Use the guidelines in this chapter, information throughout this book, and the six principles of care to guide you as you decide what to report and when to report it.

Information Review

Circle the correct answers and fill in the blanks.

1. The five elements of communication are
    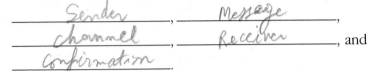
    _____Sender_____, _____Message_____,
    _____channel_____, _____Receiver_____, and
    _____Confirmation_____.

2. When you communicate a message to someone, what should you do after you deliver it? You should—
    a. Expect the person to do what you told him.
    b. Ask for confirmation that the message was understood.
    c. Communicate the next message.
    d. Look for written communication.

3. When entering the room of a person who is blind you should—
    a. Walk up quietly and touch the person on the back.
    b. Knock on the door, wait for a response, and introduce yourself.
    c. Knock on the door and go in.
    d. Talk in a low voice.

4. What two channels of communication could you use to communicate with someone who is deaf?
    a. Nonverbal and written
    b. Verbal and confirmation
    c. The sender and receiver
    d. Written and verbal

5. Several days ago you taught Mr. Rivera to shave with an electric razor instead of a safety razor. He needs to use an electric razor for medical reasons. Today he gets his electric razor out without making the usual comments about how he dislikes shaving this way. You want this behavior to continue. What should you do? You should—
    a. Ignore the situation because he has already changed his behavior.
    b. Tell him you're surprised that he didn't complain today.
    c. Tell him he probably will be able to go back to his old razor in a few months.
    d. Give his shoulder a squeeze and tell him that he is doing a great job.

6. Mrs. Morgan's daughter always asks you what you are doing and tells you how she provided care for her mother when Mrs. Morgan was at home. The daughter often goes to the nurses' station to ask questions or complain about her mother's care. What could you say to help the daughter feel more comfortable? You could—

   a. Ask Mrs. Morgan to tell her daughter that she likes the care you provide.

   b. Tell the daughter that her mother likes the care she is receiving.

   c. Tell the daughter that what you are doing is the right and only way to provide care.

   d. Tell the daughter what you are doing and why you are doing it, and ask her to help with her mother's care.

7. Before you teach Mrs. Ryan about her skin care, what must you learn from her first?

   a. Nothing; just teach her what she needs to know

   b. What she knows and how she takes care of her skin

   c. How she takes care of her hair

   d. What her favorite brand of soap is

8. You see a new medical word and are not sure what it means. There is no dictionary available. How do you try to figure out its meaning?

   a. Look at the different parts of the word, especially the root, to see if you know the meaning of any of the word's parts

   b. Look at the suffix to see what the word means

   c. Say the word out loud

   d. Ignore it

9. Three documents that health care workers use to communicate about the people in their care are the

   _____ Care plan _____

   _____ Flow sheet _____, _____ nursing notes _____, and

   _____

10. When deciding what to report to your supervising nurse, you should focus on—

    a. Any change in a person's behavior or condition.

    b. The person's appearance.

    c. What the person does from moment to moment.

    d. Whom the person talks with during the day.

Questions to Ask Yourself

1. Mrs. Alvarez is getting better after suffering a stroke but wants you to do everything for her. How can you encourage her to start taking care of herself again, and how can you reinforce her efforts?

2. What subjects would you find difficult to discuss with a person in your care? How would you respond if someone started to talk with you about these subjects?

3. How would you feel if a person in your care cursed and threw a glass at you? How would you respond to that person? How would you handle your feelings?

4. Mr. Chin's adult son doesn't visit his father at the nursing home very often. You know that the father would like to see his son more often. What could you do?

5. Mrs. Cohen's two daughters argue loudly in their mother's room about the kind of care each one thinks her mother should be receiving. Their voices get louder and louder, and you see that Mrs. Cohen is getting more and more upset. What could you do to ease the situation?

6. Mr. Dutta believes that a special ointment from a "healer" can cure his open sore, and he uses it, even though his doctor instructed him not to. What should you do?

7. While you help Mr. Rivera transfer himself from the bed to the wheelchair, he says that your directions don't match the way he learned to do it. What should you do?

8. You notice that Mrs. Roth's daughter often brings a box of chocolate candy when she comes to visit her mother. Both you and Mrs. Roth know that candy is not permitted on her diet, but she eats it anyway because she says she doesn't want to hurt her daughter's feelings. What should you do?

9. Mrs. Wang normally greets you with a smile and pleasant conversation. Today she doesn't. Also, she seems to be sleepy and says she isn't hungry. You remember that she had many visitors yesterday, but you also know that several people in the unit have colds. What additional observations could you make to help your supervising nurse or the doctor assess her condition? How do you record/report your observations?

6

Keeping People Safe

Goals

After reading this chapter, you will have the information to—

Explain why safety is the most important principle of care.

Use good body mechanics to help others and protect yourself.

Maintain equipment and use it safely.

Practice fire safety.

Help people cope with natural disasters, such as earthquakes, hurricanes, and tornadoes.

Provide first aid for people who are choking or who have suffered falls, fainting, seizures, bleeding, shock, or burns.

Keep the home environment safe for people in your care.

Keep children safe from hazards in their own environments.

After practicing the corresponding skill in the skills book, you will be able to—

Provide first aid for a conscious choking adult or child using abdominal thrusts.

Provide first aid for a conscious choking adult using chest thrusts.

The primary nurse has already begun talking with Amber Clark when you arrive to help create a home health care plan. You learn that both she and her 15-month-old son, Dominic, were in a car crash last week and have just come home from the hospital. Ms. Clark has a fractured collarbone, which limits her mobility. Both she and Dominic have concussions.

Because of the limitations caused by the broken collarbone, Ms. Clark is unable to lift Dominic. This disability makes it difficult for her to provide daily care, such as feeding and diapering, for her son.

Her injury also makes it difficult for her to move quickly to get Dominic out of harm's way. As you talk with the primary nurse and Ms. Clark, you watch Dominic as he moves around the tiny apartment. You notice that he runs around, falls easily, and looks with curiosity into every corner. He laughs at his own antics and charges into each new adventure without any signs of fear. The more you watch him, the more you become concerned about his safety.

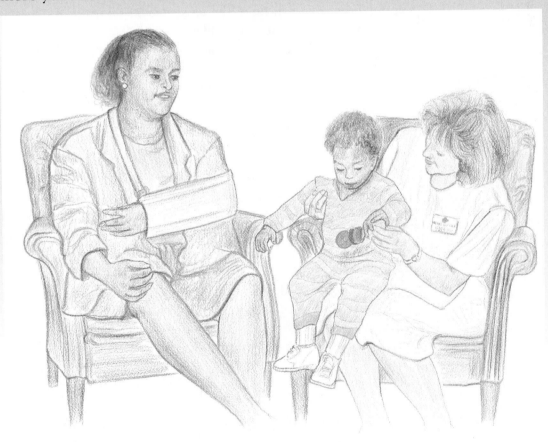

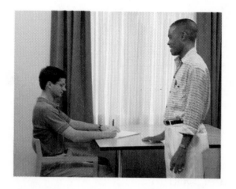

Figure 6-1
You may have to remind yourself several times a day to stand or sit correctly.

alignment
(uh-LINE-ment) Correct positioning to keep the spine straight and to avoid any twisting, straining, pressure, or discomfort.

abdominal
(ab-DOM-in-uhl) Pertaining to the abdomen, the part of the body between the ribs and the groin.

Setting the Stage for Safety

Safety is the most important principle of care because it is the foundation of everything else you do. If you're not safe, you cannot meet the needs of the people in your care. If people are not safe, they will not benefit from the care you provide them.

Practicing the other principles of care without practicing safety is like setting a table that has a wobbly leg. No matter how clean your dishes and utensils are, or how nutritious your dinner is, you can't eat the meal if the table tilts and your dinner is in your lap.

The key to safety is prevention, or trying to keep things from going wrong by considering the things that *can* go wrong and taking steps to avoid them.

Using Good Body Mechanics

As you read over Ms. Clark's care plan, Dominic continues to move about the apartment. Suddenly he falls down on the floor and begins to cry. You walk over to him, stoop down next to him, and pick him up in your arms. You hold him close as you return to the sofa and carefully put him in Ms. Clark's lap.

As a nurse assistant, you lift and move things all day long and often rush as you carry out your responsibilities. These factors—lifting, moving, and rushing—can lead to back injuries over time. Every time you twist your body quickly or in a way it is not meant to twist, you increase the chances of injuring your back. You may think that you hurt your back when you bend down to pick up a pencil, but the injury may be the result of repeated abuse from using bad body mechanics.

Using good body mechanics is one way to prevent injuries. You practice good body mechanics if you keep your back straight when you sit or if you bend your knees when you lift. You can sit, stand, and lift in certain ways that improve your body **alignment** (Figure 6-1).

If you ever have driven a car that is out of alignment, you know that it's hard to steer, the tires wear down unevenly, and it's unsafe. Human bodies that are out of alignment have similar problems. Body parts get pulled out of shape, which leads to discomfort and injury.

Sitting.   Follow these tips for improving alignment when sitting:

❖ To distribute your weight evenly and lessen strain on your lower back, sit with your knees slightly higher than your hips. Keep your back straight, your **abdominal** muscles tightened, and your shoulders straight and centered above your hips (Figure 6-2).

❖ To turn while sitting, turn your entire body, not just your chest and shoulders.

❖ To select a chair that is right for you, sit down with your back against the back of the chair. The chair is the correct height and depth for your body if two thirds of your thigh length is on the seat and your feet comfortably reach the floor. If the chair is not the right size, select a different chair, or use devices such as firm pillows and foot props to adjust the size.

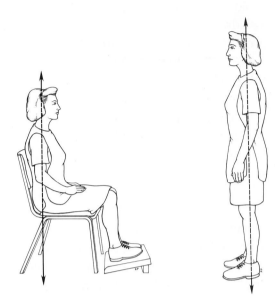

Figure 6-2
Good Body Alignment While Sitting.

Figure 6-3
Good Body Alignment While Standing.

Standing.   You can use good body mechanics to improve your alignment when you stand (Figure 6-3) by following these steps:

1. Relax your knees so that they do not lock.
2. Put your weight evenly on both legs and stand with your feet shoulder width apart.
3. To reduce pressure on your lower back, stand up straight with your stomach muscles tightened and buttocks tucked under, your head up, and your chin level.
4. Align your upper body by keeping your shoulders right over your hips.
5. To turn your body, start with your feet and let your upper body follow, rather than turning from the waist.

Lifting.   You can use good body mechanics to improve your alignment when you lift by following these steps:

1. Before lifting, place your feet about 12 inches apart, with one foot slightly in front of the other. This position provides a broad base of support that makes it hard for you to lose your balance or to be knocked down.
2. Before lifting, make sure the person or object you lift is close to you so that you don't have to lean over or reach.
3. While lifting, keep the person or object close to your body.
4. While lifting, keep your upper body erect and bend only your knees.
5. Lift smoothly without jerking.
6. To turn, lift first, pivot with your feet, and turn smoothly, making sure not to twist your body when your arms are loaded.

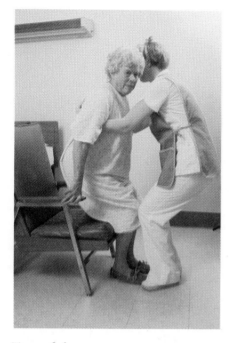

Figure 6-4

When helping someone sit, you must practice good body mechanics to protect the person's safety and yours.

hazard
(HAZ-erd)   Something that is very dangerous.

obstruction
(ob-STRUK-shun)   Something that blocks.

By using good body mechanics, you keep yourself safe and are better able to provide safety for others.

You can help the people in your care use good body mechanics to avoid injuries and be more comfortable. One way to help them is by assisting them with proper alignment. You can help people maintain proper alignment when they lie in bed, sit in a chair, stand (Figure 6-4), use a walker, or walk.

A person who spends most of the time in bed or in a chair may slump to one side from time to time. Help the person stay comfortable and avoid injury by reminding or helping him to stay aligned. You can use pillows, rolled towels, or other devices to support the person. You will read more about these techniques in Chapter 9, Positioning and Transferring People.

Promoting Safety for Others

Providing a safe environment is the responsibility of all health care team members, and preventing injuries is the best safety measure. By using common sense and your knowledge of the person in your care, you can think about things that might go wrong and take steps to prevent them from happening. If a person in your care is physically weak, unfamiliar with the surroundings, or confused or unsteady, you know that this person is more likely to fall or injure himself, so you take steps to prevent such a fall or injury. For example, Mr. Lightfoot's legs are unsteady when he gets up quickly from his chair. One day he anxiously waits for a phone call. As the time of his expected call nears, you suggest that he sit by the phone.

You can use common sense and knowledge about potential **hazards** to prevent things from going wrong. To spot potential hazards, look around a room each time you enter it. If you see a safety threat, correct it right away.

To help ensure the safety of the people in your care, as well as your own safety, remember these tips:

❖ Make sure doorways and floors are free from **obstruction**.
❖ Wipe up spills immediately, following infection control procedures when necessary.
❖ Walk. Don't run.
❖ Store all medicines and cleaning materials in locked cabinets and closets.
❖ Turn hot water on last and off first.
❖ Check the temperature of water coming out of faucets to be sure it is correct for performing a procedure. For general purposes, the temperature of hot tap water should be at or below 120 degrees Fahrenheit. If water seems too hot, report this concern immediately to your supervising nurse.
❖ Check food temperature to make sure it is not too hot. If food is steaming or a plate is too hot to touch, wait until the food stops steaming or the plate has cooled a little before serving the meal.
❖ Check handrails and grab bars to make sure that they are tightly fastened.

- ❖ Encourage people to use handrails and grab bars in the shower, bathroom, and hallways.
- ❖ If a person wears eyeglasses, make sure they are clean.
- ❖ If a person uses a hearing aid, make sure it works and encourage the person to use it when he needs to.
- ❖ Put the call signal within easy reach. Answer calls for help promptly (within 3 to 5 minutes), but respond immediately if you suspect that there is an emergency or that the person may be in pain, may be having trouble breathing, needs help going to the bathroom, or may be frightened. Someone needing to go to the bathroom may tire of waiting for you and try to get there alone, risking a fall.
- ❖ Handle people gently, especially children and the elderly. Their skin may be fragile and may injure easily.
- ❖ Unless a person objects, make sure a night-light is on at bedtime.
- ❖ Make sure people are familiar with their surroundings.
- ❖ Report any **incident** to your supervising nurse, even if no injury occurs.

incident
(IN-suh-dent)   Anything unusual that happens and has the potential to cause harm.

If an injury or incident happens, you are legally responsible for reporting it. When you report an incident, you must gather the important information and give it to your supervising nurse. The information you gather goes into an incident report, which is a written description of what happened.

Observing and reporting incidents accurately are important parts of your job. Immediately report any incident involving you or another person to your supervising nurse, because your memory of what happened is likely to be fresh and accurate right after it happens. If questions about the incident come up later, the incident report often is the only source of information. A complete incident report contains answers to the following questions:

- ❖ When did the incident happen? (time, date)
- ❖ Where did the incident happen?
- ❖ What caused the incident? (For example, was water on the floor?)
- ❖ Who was the person involved in the incident?
- ❖ Was the person injured? If so, describe the injury.
- ❖ Was the person confused before or after the incident?
- ❖ Was the person alone?
- ❖ Were there witnesses to the incident? If so, who?
- ❖ Who gave assistance or first aid?
- ❖ What kind of assistance or first aid was given?
- ❖ Did a doctor treat the person?

Include other information that would be a useful part of the record or that is required in your employer's incident report.

Using Equipment Safely

As a nurse assistant, you use many pieces of equipment that make your job easier and the people in your care safer. But, because most equipment has moving parts, you can cause serious injuries if you do not use it properly.

Before using any piece of equipment, be sure you understand how it works. Read the product manual and follow instructions exactly. (If no manual is available, you may find instructions on a sticker or label attached to the equipment.) Before using the equipment with the person in your care, practice the correct procedure for using it by yourself. If you are not completely confident about using the equipment, ask your supervising nurse for help rather than risking any danger to yourself or the person in your care.

Maintaining Personal Equipment

Regularly check personal equipment to make sure that it is working as it should (Figure 6-5). Anything that is broken, even something as simple as a comb, is a safety problem.

The person in your care may use a personal safety device, such as a cane or walker. To increase the safety of such devices, inspect them from time to time to make sure that the rubber tips on a cane or walker have not become worn and that the frame on a walker is tight.

Locking Side Rails

People in your care sometimes need side rails on their beds. Only a doctor can order side rails that run the full length of a person's bed. Make sure you understand how to use them, because the many different types all operate a little differently. If you are unsure about how to use the type you have, ask for help. After raising or lowering side rails, test them to make sure they lock securely. If a side rail does not lock properly, stay with the person and summon help.

If there is a strong chance that a person in home health care might fall out of bed and there is no way to prevent a fall, use a low bed or put a mattress on the floor as a last resort. When you leave the bedside of a person who is in a mechanical bed, always leave the bed in the lowest postion.

Using Brakes

The brakes provided on equipment that has wheels—beds, wheelchairs, shower chairs, and carts—prevent the equipment from rolling. Imagine how unsafe and difficult it would be to help someone into a wheelchair that kept moving.

Before using a piece of equipment that has wheels, try out the brakes. Make sure you know how they work and that they work properly. If they do not work properly, do not use the equipment. Report the equipment problem to your supervising nurse.

Before helping a person into or out of a wheelchair, lock the brakes and make sure the chair is secure. Also, before stepping away

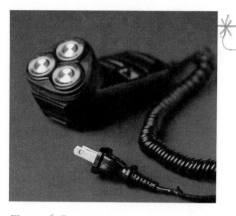

Figure 6-5

Small appliances can be hazardous if they don't work properly or if the cords are in bad condition.

Table 6-1   **Using Equipment Safely**

Always	Never	Why?
Dry your hands thoroughly before handling electrical equipment.	Pull electrical equipment out of water.	The electrical current in the water could kill you.
Plug electrical equipment into an outlet near the place where you will be using it.	Use extension cords, except in an emergency.	The cord could trip someone, or it could overload a circuit and cause a power outage or fire.
Follow the manufacturer's directions for using electrical equipment.	Use equipment unless you have been trained to use it and feel sure of yourself.	If you use equipment incorrectly, you may injure yourself or a person in your care.
Use equipment that is clean and in good repair.	Use defective or broken equipment, and <u>never</u> permit the person in your care to use personal equipment that could present a hazard.	Using broken or defective equipment could cause serious injury to you or a person in your care.
Ensure that each person in your care has his own razor, toothbrush, hairbrush, and other personal equipment.	Share personal equipment among people.	Keeping personal equipment personal maintains infection control.
Store equipment in closets or in other out-of-the-way areas.	Store equipment in halls or other areas where people walk.	Equipment that is improperly stored obstructs free movement.

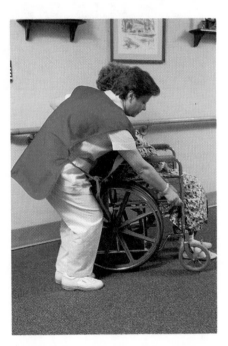

from a person who is in a wheelchair, make sure both wheelchair brakes are locked securely (Figure 6-6).

Following Safety Tips

Read the additional tips for using equipment safely in Table 6-1.

Practicing Fire Safety

Fire safety is an important concern for everyone because fires rarely affect just one person. Practicing fire safety makes sense for you, but also for the people in your care. They may be at greater risk from fire than most people because they are more likely to have limitations in mobility, hearing, vision, or understanding, which interfere with their ability to successfully react to a fire. These limitations also make cigarette smoking especially dangerous for them.

Figure 6-6
Remember to lock the brakes on both wheels of the wheelchair.

impaired
A condition in which something is diminished or weakened.

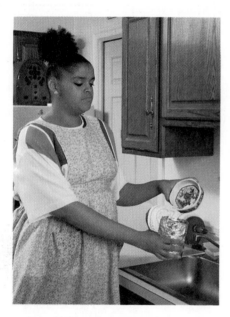

Figure 6-7
Empty ashtrays into approved containers. Before discarding the contents of an ashtray, thoroughly wet them.

Preventing and Preparing for Fires

Although you may make your best effort to prevent fires, sometimes they can occur for reasons beyond your control, and you must be prepared. To prevent fires, be careful about cigarettes, know where fire alarms and extinguishers are located and how to use them, look for and remove fire hazards, be careful around oxygen, and know whom to call in case of fire.

Be careful about cigarettes.   Cigarettes and other smoking materials are a major cause of fires, but you can help prevent fires by following these tips:

❖ Supervise the people in your care whenever they smoke.
❖ Follow your employer's rules about smoking. Permit smoking only in designated areas.
❖ Remove smoking materials from the reach of any person who has **impaired** thinking.
❖ If you provide care for people who smoke, make sure they smoke only in appropriate places and safely extinguish their cigarettes (Figure 6-7).
❖ Never permit smoking around a person who is using oxygen.

Know where fire alarms and extinguishers are located and how to use them.   Whether you work in a hospital, in a nursing home, or in a person's home, fire alarms or smoke detectors should be installed and in working order to warn of fires. Fire extinguishers should be available to cope with fires if they occur. Take advantage of these devices by following these rules:

❖ Know the location of fire alarms and fire extinguishers, and know how to use them.
❖ Know the location of fire doors, and keep them free from obstruction.
❖ In a private home, look for smoke detectors on each level and on the ceiling outside of each sleeping area. Test their batteries to make sure they work. Also, look for a fire extinguisher. If you think that the home needs improvement in fire safety, discuss this concern with your employer.
❖ Know the fire escape routes. Hospitals and nursing homes generally post fire escape routes for each room or area (Figure 6-8).

Figure 6-8
Know fire escape routes ahead of time so that you can proceed immediately. You may have only seconds to escape.

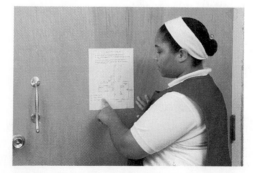

If you work in a private home, plan two fire escape routes from each room that you and your client spend time in. Never use an elevator to escape from a fire.

Look for and remove fire hazards.   Use your eyes and your common sense to remove things that could start fires or prevent escape from a fire. Follow these tips:

- Remove or report clutter promptly, because clutter on floors, in hallways, and in front of doors is a safety hazard, a fire hazard, and an escape hazard.
- Know how to unlock windows.
- Be aware of any open flames, such as those in gas water heaters, furnaces, and stoves. Keep flammable materials, such as paints or clothing, away from electric stoves and warming appliances, such as coffee makers, because they have coils that stay hot and that can become dangerous. Don't store flammable materials, such as cleaning products and newspapers, near furnaces and hot water heaters. Keep curtains, dish towels, or pot holders away from a kitchen stove burner, because fabrics can ignite.
- Look for electrical hazards, such as frayed cords and overloaded outlets. Remove or report them, as appropriate.

Be careful around oxygen.   Because oxygen is highly flammable, you must take special precautions if a person in your care uses it. Follow these oxygen safety guidelines.

- Never remove or shut off oxygen during its administration.
- Never adjust the flow of oxygen.
- Post "No Smoking" signs in a room where oxygen is in use, and do not permit anyone to smoke in the room.
- Make sure that no candles, gas heaters, or other items with open flames are in the room.
- Do not use electrical appliances that could create sparks, such as hair dryers and electric razors, while oxygen is in use. (Battery-operated appliances generally are safe to use, but you and your supervising nurse should check each item for safety before using it.)
- Use a room humidifier to decrease static electricity.
- Use clothing and bedding made of cotton rather than a synthetic fiber.
- If the oxygen tank is portable, make sure it is secure on a floor stand.
- Make sure that the person in your care, as well as others who come in contact with him, understands and follows these oxygen safety guidelines.

Know whom to call in case of fire.   Your employer's fire emergency plan may direct you to signal a fire by pulling a fire alarm or sending some other signal. Although the plan may designate a specific person to summon the fire department, you still must know the telephone number to call. In some communities you call Emergency Medical

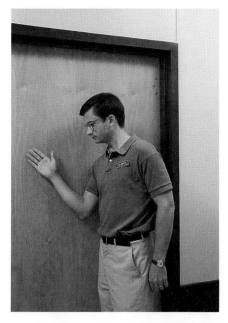

Figure 6-9
A door feels hot if there is a fire on the other side.

Services (EMS), usually by dialing 911. In other communities you call a separate telephone number. Look in the front of the phone book to see which number to call in your community, and write down the number in a permanent place near the phone.

Following a Plan When a Fire Occurs

If a fire breaks out when you are working, follow the fire emergency plan set by your employer. In addition to guidelines for whom to call and how to call them, it should include information about when and how to evacuate the people in the building, and any special measures to take to prevent a fire from spreading. These guidelines usually are practiced in periodic fire drills.

Use the following precautions and attempt to alert any other people in the building:

❖ Touch a door with the back of your hand before you open it (Figure 6-9). If it is hot, do not open it. Leave the room another way. If the door is cool, stand to one side and open it slowly. If you observe heavy smoke on the other side, close the door.
❖ Stay low. Smoke rises, and it is easier to breathe when you are closer to the floor.
❖ Use stairs, not an elevator.
❖ If your clothing or that of another person ignites (catches fire), *stop*, *drop* (to the ground), *roll* over and over (to extinguish the flames), and *cool* (use water to cool the burn site).

Coping with Natural Disasters

When a natural disaster happens, many people are injured in a short period of time. The types of natural disasters that occasionally occur where you live may differ from those that occur in other parts of the United States. For your own safety, you should know what types of disasters occur in your area (Figure 6-10).

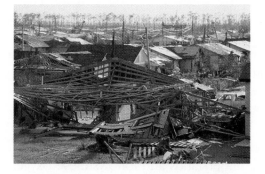

Figure 6-10
Because natural disasters such as hurricanes are not always predictable, you should learn ahead of time what your employer expects you to do so that you can act quickly and efficiently.

disaster plan
(di-ZAHS-ter) A set of safety procedures to follow in case a natural disaster occurs.

Your employer's **disaster plan** or emergency plan explains your role in the event of a natural disaster. No matter what your role, always remain calm in the event of a disaster. Because people and their visitors may become frightened and confused, you play a critical role and can calmly explain what is happening and reassure them that you will help them move to a safe area. When helping to move a person who cannot walk, use a wheelchair or a bed. After people are moved to a safe place, make sure a staff member remains with them to keep them from wandering into dangerous areas. The presence of a staff member is especially important for people who have impaired vision or hearing or who are confused.

Earthquakes

An earthquake occurs when the earth moves, shakes, or rolls. This activity in the earth may cause buildings to shake, windows to shatter, and objects to fly around. It also can cause fires to start and can generate large ocean waves. Earthquakes can occur in most states, and they may occur at any time without warning.

    If an earthquake occurs, follow these safety tips:

- ❖ Stay calm.
- ❖ If you are inside a building, stay inside. Protect yourself, especially your head, from falling or flying objects. Take cover under a large, heavy object, such as a desk or table.
- ❖ If you are outside, stay outside. Move away from buildings, trees, and overhead wires.

    After the earthquake, follow these safety tips:

- ❖ Check for injuries. Never try to move seriously injured people unless they are in danger of further injury.
- ❖ Be prepared for aftershocks (smaller quakes after the first tremor).
- ❖ Use your flashlight to inspect for damage. *Do not use* appliances, other electrical equipment, or services requiring electricity, gas, water, or sewage disposal if these systems may be damaged. If you smell gas or see a broken line, shut off the main valve or inform the person responsible. Don't try to turn utilities back on.
- ❖ Listen to the radio or television for information about the emergency.
- ❖ Watch for fallen power lines.
- ❖ Clean up spilled medicines, drugs, flammable liquids, and other materials.
- ❖ Never smoke. Earthquakes can create gas leaks, and an open flame from a match or cigarette lighter can cause an explosion.
- ❖ Use the telephone only in a life-threatening emergency.

Hurricanes

A hurricane occurs when the winds of a large tropical storm increase to 74 miles per hour or more. A hurricane brings heavy rain, coastal and inland flooding, and sometimes tornadoes. Hurricanes strike the U.S. coast from Texas to Maine, as well as Puerto Rico and the U.S.

Virgin Islands. Hurricane season lasts from June through November, with August and September being the peak months.

A hurricane watch means a hurricane is possible in your area. If a hurricane watch is issued in your area, follow these safety tips:

❖ Listen for weather reports on the radio or television. In a hospital or nursing home, know which personnel are assigned to listen to the reports.

❖ Make sure you have access to a supply of fresh water.

❖ Have a flashlight with fresh batteries available.

❖ Follow your supervising nurse's instructions, which may include evacuation preparations, such as asking people to stay out of bed or moving bedridden people into chairs. Make sure a staff member stays with people after they have been moved to safety. You also may have to check outdoor areas and remove or secure loose objects and prepare to board up windows.

A hurricane warning means a hurricane is approaching your area. If a hurricane warning is issued in your area, follow these safety tips:

❖ If an evacuation order is issued, follow your employer's emergency procedures to safely evacuate the people in your care.

❖ If you are not told to evacuate, keep people away from windows.

❖ Move people into interior rooms.

❖ If some people cannot easily get out of bed, move them in their beds into the hallways or push their beds against the wall. Make sure a staff member stays with them.

❖ Close the doors to rooms and close fire doors (Figure 6-11).

❖ Make sure doorways to halls, fire doors, and exits are not blocked.

❖ Cover people with blankets or bedspreads to protect them from flying glass in case windows break.

❖ Monitor weather conditions carefully.

Tornadoes

A tornado is a spinning, funnel-shaped windstorm that moves along the ground. Tornadoes have winds up to 200 miles per hour and can develop from severe thunderstorms and sometimes hurricanes. Tornadoes have occurred in every state of the United States. Primary tornado season is March through August, but tornadoes can happen at any time of year.

A tornado watch means that a tornado is possible in your area. If a tornado watch is announced, follow these safety tips:

❖ Listen for weather reports on the radio or television. In a hospital or nursing home, know which personnel are assigned to listen to the report.

❖ Be alert to weather conditions, blowing debris, and the sound of an approaching tornado. A tornado often sounds like a freight train. Inform other staff members if you see or hear anything.

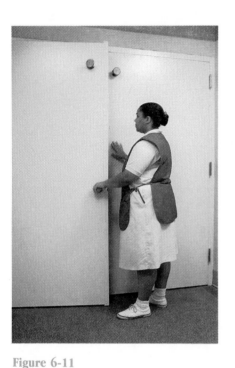

Figure 6-11

Closing doors during most natural disasters can help protect people from flying debris.

❖   Have a flashlight with fresh batteries available.
❖   Follow your supervising nurse's instructions, which may include
    evacuation preparations, such as asking people to stay out of bed
    or moving bedridden people into chairs. Make sure a staff mem-
    ber stays with the people after they have been moved to safety.
    You also may have to check outdoor areas and remove or se-
    cure loose objects.

A tornado warning means that a tornado has been spotted or is
about to strike in your area. Sometimes tornadoes strike so rapidly
that you may not get a warning. If a tornado warning is announced
or you think a tornado is near, follow these safety tips:

❖   Sound alarms.
❖   Move people from any large rooms and away from windows.
❖   Move people into interior hallways near exits or into closets or
    bathrooms.
❖   If some people cannot easily get out of bed, move them in their
    beds into the hallways or push their beds against the wall.
❖   Close the doors to rooms and close fire doors.
❖   Make sure doorways to halls, fire doors, and exits are not
    blocked.
❖   Cover people with blankets or bedspreads to protect them from
    flying glass in case windows break.
❖   Monitor weather conditions carefully.

When you are prepared for a disaster, you are able to act calmly
and help the people who depend on you. You also must be prepared
to cope with emergencies.

Providing First Aid

You've read about how to keep yourself safe, how to use equipment
safely, and how to practice fire safety. You've also looked at how you
can cope with natural disasters. As a nurse assistant you also have to
cope when specific emergencies occur.

When an emergency occurs, the worst thing you can do is nothing.
The decision to get involved, however, can be a hard one to make.
In this section, you will read basic information about a few medical
emergencies and how you can respond to them. To expand your
knowledge of how to respond to emergencies, you can take an
American Red Cross First Aid Course.

When an emergency happens, you may feel confused. However,
you can train yourself to stay calm and think before you act. Ask
yourself, "What is the best help I can give?" You can provide proper
help if you know the following three basic steps, which you can take
in any emergency:

1. *Check* the scene and the person.
2. *Call* 9-1-1 or your local emergency number.
3. *Care* for the person.

Before you can help the person, you must make sure the scene or the area is safe for you and any bystanders. To gather information for determining such safety, look over the scene and take the following actions:

❖ Look for anything that might make the scene unsafe. For example, does the person have any electrical wires in his hand? Is it safe to touch him? **Don't put yourself in danger.**

❖ Try to find out what happened. Look for clues.

❖ Look carefully for more than one injured person.

❖ Do not move a seriously injured person unless there is immediate danger, such as fire, flood, or poisonous gas.

❖ If the person is lying on the floor or ground, is silent, and is not moving, find out if he is conscious or unconscious. Look for other signals of injury that are life-threatening or may become life-threatening, such as no breathing or breathing with difficulty, no pulse (read about measuring pulse rate in Chapter 8, Measuring Life Signs), and severe bleeding. As you check the person, use your senses of seeing, smelling, and hearing.

Know your local emergency number. It may be 9-1-1, 0 (zero) for operator, a local seven-digit number, or a special response number where you work (Figure 6-12). Post your emergency number by the phone at home and work.

Calling for help is often the most important action you can take to help an injured person. If you are the only person on the scene, stay with the person and shout for help. If no one responds to your shout, get to a telephone as quickly as possible and then return to the person. If you are working in a nursing home and the injured person is unconscious, call your supervising nurse, as well as your local emergency number. If the person is faint, drowsy, confused, dizzy, or drifts in and out of consciousness, notify your supervising nurse.

After you have checked the scene and the person, you may need to provide care. Always provide care for life-threatening emergencies before providing care for those that are not life-threatening. Help the person rest comfortably, keep him from getting chilled or overheated, and reassure him by talking to him.

If the person is conscious and able to talk, ask him what happened. Ask him if he hurts anywhere and, if he has pain, ask him where it is located and what it is like—for example, burning, aching, sharp, stinging. Ask him when the pain started and how bad it is. Be calm and patient. Speak normally and simply.

When responding to an emergency, remember the emergency action steps: check, call, and care. These steps guide your actions in an emergency and ensure your safety and the safety of others.

First Aid for Choking (Airway Obstruction)

Choking is one form of airway obstruction that occurs when an object blocks a person's airway. A person who is choking may quickly stop breathing and lose consciousness.

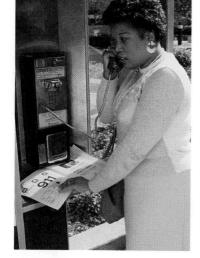

Figure 6-12
Local emergency phone numbers are easily found.

Common causes of choking.   About 3,000 people (80 percent of these are elderly) will choke to death this year. Choking occurs when a person—

❖   Tries to swallow large pieces of food that are poorly chewed.
❖   Drinks alcohol before or during eating. (Alcohol dulls the nerves that help a person swallow.)
❖   Wears dentures. (Dentures make it difficult to sense the size of food when chewing and swallowing.)
❖   Talks excitedly or laughs while eating, or eats too fast.
❖   Walks, plays, or runs with objects in his mouth.

Learn from your employer what is expected of you should a person begin to choke, especially when you are alone with the person.

Signs and symptoms of choking.   The key to saving a person's life is being able to recognize when someone is choking. Two types of obstructions that you must know about are "partial airway obstruction" and "complete airway obstruction." You also must be able to recognize the differences between them and know which first aid procedure to perform.

❖   **Partial airway obstruction.** When a person has a partial airway obstruction, the care you provide depends on whether the person has good or poor air exchange. Air exchange is the movement of air in and out of the lungs.
        With good air exchange. When a person has a partial airway obstruction with good air exchange, he can cough forcefully. He also may wheeze between breaths. If he is able to cough forcefully on his own, do not interfere with his attempts to cough up the object that is blocking his airway. Stay with the person and encourage him to continue coughing.
        With poor air exchange. When a person has a partial airway obstruction with poor air exchange, he will have a weak, ineffective cough and may make a high-pitched noise while breathing. The obstruction may begin with poor air exchange, or it may begin with good air exchange and turn into an obstruction with poor air exchange. Respond to partial airway obstruction with poor air exchange as if it were complete airway obstruction.
❖   **Complete airway obstruction.** When a person has a complete obstruction of the airway, he will not be able to cough, speak, or breathe. He may clutch at his throat with one or both hands. This is the universal distress signal for choking. You must act right away to clear his airway.

Abdominal thrusts for a conscious person.   Yesterday evening, after a tiring day at work, you decided to have dinner at a small, local restaurant. You were eating your dinner when you heard a woman begin to yell, "Oh, help! Somebody help!" You looked in the direction of her voice and saw the woman slapping the back of a middle-aged

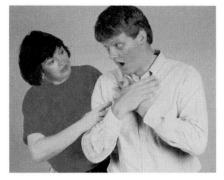

Figure 6-13
A person who is choking often clutches his throat.

man, who had both hands at his throat and was gasping for air (Figure 6-13). You quickly walked over to the man, helped him to stand up, and positioned yourself behind him. You then wrapped your arms around his waist, made a fist with one hand (Figure 6-14), grasped that fist with your other hand, and pressed your fist into his abdomen with a quick upward thrust (Figure 6-15). Three times you thrust your fist into his stomach. On the third thrust, a piece of chicken flew out of the man's mouth and onto the floor. Perspiring and shaken, the man slumped onto the chair where he had been sitting. "Thank you so much," the woman said. "How can I ever thank you enough?"

Figure 6-14
As you start to give abdominal thrusts, place the thumb side of your fist against the middle of the person's abdomen.

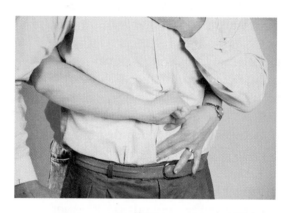

Figure 6-15
Grasp your fist with your other hand and give quick upward thrusts into the abdomen.

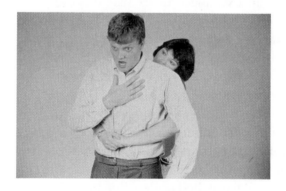

In this situation it was important to get the man to his feet so that you could perform abdominal thrusts. It is also important to know that hitting a person on the back when he is choking can make matters worse and can lodge the object farther into his windpipe.

To provide first aid for choking (airway obstruction) in a conscious adult or child, follow the step-by-step procedures that are explained in Skill 1, Option 1, in the skills book.

Chest thrusts for a conscious person. Today at lunch, you are providing care for Mr. Rivera who had a stroke, which resulted in right-side paralysis. He sits in his wheelchair while you help him eat. Suddenly, he begins to choke. First, you call for help. Because he is sitting, you perform chest thrusts rather than abdominal thrusts to loosen the food that is blocking his airway. Use chest thrusts any time you are not able to get your arms around the waist of a choking person to deliver effective abdominal thrusts. Also use chest thrusts for a person who is overweight (obese) or a woman who is in her last stages of pregnancy. You may perform chest thrusts if the person is sitting in a wheelchair, sitting in a chair, or standing.

To perform chest thrusts for a conscious person, follow the step-by-step procedure that is explained in Skill 1, Option 2, in the skills book.

Chest thrusts for an unconscious person.   If the object on which the person is choking is not quickly coughed up by your attempts to help, the person may become unconscious. You will probably have some warning that this is about to happen. The person may begin to fall forward or back toward you. Should this occur, lower the person to the floor and once more call for help. Stay with the person until help arrives.

The procedure for performing chest thrusts for an unconscious person is not part of this nurse assistant training material. To learn the steps of this procedure, you may take an American Red Cross First Aid or **Cardiopulmonary Resuscitation** (CPR) course.

First Aid for Falls

Falls happen often. As with fires and other potentially dangerous situations, prevention is the best safety measure. You can aid in the prevention of falls. For example, if the person in your care has difficulty walking or needs assistance when walking, encourage him to call you for help. If you are willing to help and let the person know that you are concerned for his safety, he will feel better about calling for your assistance, and you may prevent serious injuries that often result from falls.

When helping a person walk, or when helping a person move to a different location, prevent a potential fall by making sure no obstacles are in the way.

If a person begins to fall, catch him, if possible. Keep your feet apart, back straight, and knees slightly bent. Put your arms around his waist or underarms, keep him close to your body and, bending your knees, lower yourself and the person slowly to the floor. Call for help. (For more information about proper body mechanics, read Chapter 9.)

If a person does fall, do not leave him. Call for help. Do not move him until directed by your supervising nurse. Help the fallen person to be comfortable. Reassure him (Figure 6-16). Be prepared to give necessary information to your supervising nurse for the incident report.

If you walk into a room and see that a person has fallen, look around. Survey the scene. Look at the person. Does the person respond? Is the person's airway open? Is the person breathing? Does he have a pulse? Call for help.

cardiopulmonary resuscitation (kar-dee-oh-PULL-mon-air-ee/ree-sus-suh-TAY-shun)   Also known as CPR, a series of manual or mechanical procedures used to restore circulation and breathing after the heart and respiration have stopped.

If the person is responsive, ask him what happened (Figure 6-16). Does he feel any pain? Where is the pain? How bad is it? Check the person's vital signs. (Read Chapter 8.) Assist your supervising nurse during a head-to-toe exam. Help make the person comfortable.

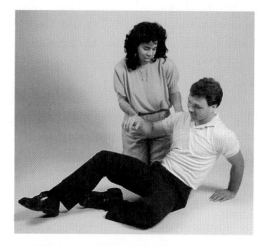

Figure 6-16
Reassure the person who has fallen and avoid moving him if possible.

First Aid for Fainting

syncope
(SING-kuh-pee)   A temporary loss of consciousness caused by a lack of blood flowing to the brain. It may occur because of fatigue, fear, pain, or blood loss.

Fainting, also known as **syncope**, is a safety or emergency problem that you may have to manage. If a person shows signs of fainting, such as paleness and cool, moist skin, move the person from an upright position to a flat, horizontal position. In this position, normal blood circulation to the brain often resumes, and the person who has fainted usually regains consciousness within a minute.

If you see someone fainting, catch him, if possible. Help him to the floor, as in the section on first aid for falls. Call for help. Raise his legs about 8 inches, loosen any tight clothing, and observe any changes in his position.

First Aid for Seizures

epilepsy
(EP-uh-lep-see)   An ongoing condition of the brain marked by changes in the level of consciousness and/or abnormal muscle or sensory activity.

You may need to provide care for a person who has a seizure. A seizure occurs when injury, disease, fever, or infection interferes with the normal functions of the brain and the electrical activity of the brain becomes irregular. This irregularity can cause a loss of body control. One medical cause of seizures is a condition known as **epilepsy**.

Before the seizure occurs, the person may have an aura, which is an unusual sensation or feeling, such as a visual hallucination; a strange sound, taste, or smell; or an urgent need to get to safety.

Seizures may range from mild blackouts that others may mistake as daydreaming, to uncontrolled muscular contractions, also called convulsions, that may last for several minutes. Infants and young children are at risk for seizures brought on by high fever.

Your job is to make the person who is having a seizure as safe as possible. Call for help. Do not try to stop the seizure. Do not attempt to restrain the person. Protect the person from injury. If there is fluid in his mouth, turn him on one side so that the fluid drains from his mouth. Do not try to place anything between his teeth. Stay with the person until help arrives and reassure and comfort him. After the seizure, he will be tired and want to rest.

First Aid for Bleeding

When you see someone bleeding, call for help. The signs of severe external bleeding include blood spurting from a wound and blood that won't stop after you have taken reasonable measures to control it.

Each type of blood vessel bleeds differently. (Read about the circulatory system in Chapter 8.) When a person bleeds from an **artery**, the blood flows rapidly from the wound and in large amounts, and the color of the blood is bright red. This type of bleeding is life-threatening and is harder to control than bleeding from a vein. When a person bleeds from a **vein**, the blood flows from the wound at a steady rate, without spurting, and the color of the blood is dark red or maroon. When a person bleeds from the **capillaries**, the blood oozes slowly from the wound, the color is lighter than blood flowing from the veins, and bleeding stops easily.

Direct pressure. You can control external bleeding by applying direct pressure with your hand on the wound. Elevate the wound above the person's heart level, unless you suspect a broken bone. Put on gloves if they are nearby. Press firmly against the wound with a clean cloth or bandage. If the person who is bleeding is able, have him apply the pressure to the wound.

Pressure bandage. If a wound on the arm or leg does not stop with direct pressure or elevation, apply additional dressings over any dressing that is already on the wound. Secure a self-adhesive roller bandage over the dressing. Continue wrapping the bandage snugly around the limb. Use overlapping turns to cover dressings completely and secure them in place. Tie off the bandage. Check to be sure that the bandage is not too tight by feeling the radial (wrist) or pedal (foot) pulse, which should not be slowed or absent. Also look at fingers or toes to ensure that their color is not bluish. (For more information about the pulse and circulation, read Chapter 8.)

Pressure points. If bleeding continues after applying a pressure bandage, your supervising nurse may apply pressure at a pressure point, with your assistance. While maintaining direct pressure on the elevated wound, locate the pressure point at the **brachial artery** (if the wound is on the arm) or **femoral artery** (if the wound is on the leg), and apply pressure over the appropriate artery.

First Aid for Shock

Every blood-loss injury is accompanied by some degree of shock and should be treated promptly. Shock is the condition that occurs when

artery
(ARE-ter-ee) Any of the branching blood vessels that carries oxygen-rich blood from the heart to all parts of the body.

vein
(vayn) Any of the blood vessels that carries blood from all parts of the body to the heart.

capillaries
(KAP-uh-ler-ees) Any of the small blood vessels with a slender, hairlike opening that attaches the end of an artery to the beginning of a vein.

brachial artery
(BRAY-kee-uhl) An artery in the arm at the inside bend of the elbow.

femoral artery
(FEM-er-uhl) An artery at the groin where the thigh meets the hip.

the flow of blood returning to the heart is inadequate for normal function, resulting in a lack of oxygen to all body organs and tissues. This lack of oxygen starts a series of responses that produce specific signals of shock. If a person is in shock,—

❖ He will be restless and irritable.
❖ His pulse will be weak and rapid.
❖ His breathing rate will increase and be shallow.
❖ His skin will be pale or bluish, cool or moist.
❖ He will have excessive thirst.
❖ He will experience nausea and vomiting.
❖ He will be drowsy and lose consciousness.

Call for help. Monitor the person's breathing for any developing problems. Position him according to the injury. Maintain normal body temperature. Reassure the person and stay with him.

First Aid for Burns

A person in your care may experience burns if his body is exposed to fire, steam, hot liquids, certain chemicals, electricity, the sun, or other forms of radiation. Burns first destroy the first layer of the person's skin. (For more information about the skin, read about the integumentary system in Chapter 9.) If the burn progresses, it injures or destroys the second layer of his skin. Because burns may break the skin, they can cause infection, loss of fluid, and loss of temperature control. Burns can damage underlying body tissue. Burns also can damage the person's respiratory system and eyes.

In general, people over age 60 have thinner skin, and children under age 5 have less-developed skin. As a result, people in these age groups may burn more severely.

Degrees of burns.   Depending on the severity of the burn, it may be classified as superficial (first degree), partial-thickness (second-degree), or full-thickness (third degree).

A superficial burn involves only the top layer of skin. The skin is red and dry, the burn is usually painful, and the burned area may swell.

epidermis
(ep-uh-DER-mis)   The outer protective layer of skin.

dermis
The sensitive layer of skin beneath the epidermis.

A partial-thickness burn involves both the **epidermis** and the **dermis**. The burn looks red or mottled, has blisters, and is usually painful. The area often swells and may look a little wet from the loss of fluid through the damaged skin layers.

A full-thickness burn destroys both layers of skin, as well as any or all underlying structures—fat, muscle, bones, and nerves. This burn can be extremely painful or, if the nerve endings in the skin are destroyed, it can be relatively painless. It may look white or charred (black), or it may look like a partial-thickness burn. Because the burn is open and the body loses fluid, the person is at risk for going into shock or getting an infection.

Box 6-1   **Dos and Don'ts of Burn Care**

Dos

Cool a burn by flushing it with cool water.

Cover the burn with a dry, sterile dressing.

Take steps to minimize shock.

Don'ts

Don't apply ice directly to partial-thickness or full-thickness burns.

Don't touch the burn with anything except sterile or clean dressings.

Don't remove pieces of cloth that stick to a burned area.

Don't try to clean a full-thickness burn.

Don't break blisters.

Don't use any kind of grease or ointment on severe burns.

Dos and don'ts of burn care.   When providing care for someone who has a burn, observe the advice in Box 6-1.

If you are working in home health care, read the following section with specific information about safety in the home. If you choose not to read the next section, please turn to the end of the chapter to read "Information Review" and "Questions to Ask Yourself."

Safety in Home Health Care

When you are a caregiver in someone's home, you must pay special attention to the most important principle of care—safety—so that both you and the client are in a safe environment. When you ensure safety in a person's home, you lower the chances of the person being injured. This increased level of safety may mean that the person is able stay at home, which promotes his independence, another important principle of care.

Traveling Safely

In addition to promoting safety in your client's home, you must be concerned about your safety when traveling to and from your home. You may travel at night or provide care for people who live in areas you don't know or believe are not safe. Follow the tips below to ensure your safe travel, as well as your timely arrival:

❖   When driving, plan your route. Get clear directions, and mark the route on a map, rather than guess about where you are going. Use main roads whenever possible, especially if you are unfamiliar with the area or must drive at night.

❖ Drive and travel defensively. Make sure your car is in good working condition. Drive with caution and with the doors locked. If your car breaks down, raise the hood, return to the car, lock the doors, and wait for the police. If a stranger offers assistance, keep the doors locked, remain in your car, and ask the person to telephone the police for help.

❖ When using public transportation, such as a bus or train, phone the transportation information number to find out about the best route. Schedules vary according to the time of day and the day of the week.

❖ When walking, walk smart. Carry a whistle or some kind of alarm. Walk in the center of the sidewalk, away from doorways, alleys, and shrubbery. Walk purposefully and pay attention to your surroundings. Have your keys ready to open your car or house door as soon as you get there.

❖ If something looks wrong—a door is open, or a window is broken—when you arrive at your client's home, do not go in. Call the police from a safe place. ***Do not enter the house until help arrives.***

❖ If you go to your client's door and no one responds to your knock, try to find out if he is inside by checking to see if the door is locked, by looking in the window, or by phoning him from a safe place. Follow your agency's policy for specific procedures. These procedures may include calling your supervising nurse, calling the person's emergency contact person, or calling the police.

Practicing Good Home Security

When you first arrived at the Clark's home to help create their health care plan, 15-month-old Dominic had been actively running through the apartment until he fell down and began to cry. You picked him up and put him in his mother's lap. Now he has stopped crying about his fall and scoots down from her lap. He heads for the outside door, reaches up and, to everyone's surprise, opens the door and walks into the apartment hallway.

Practicing good security measures is a good idea for both you and your client. Follow these safety tips to protect your client, and to protect yourself in your own home:

❖ Keep all outside doors locked at all times. No neighborhood is so safe that you can afford to overlook this simple advice.

❖ Keep the windows locked. This security measure is especially necessary for windows at ground level, where an intruder could easily enter. If you open windows in a room for ventilation, try to stay in that room.

❖ Don't let strangers into the house. Use a peephole or window to see who is at the door before deciding whether to open it. If you don't know the person at the door who insists on being admitted, call the police and your supervising nurse.

❖ Check the identity of visitors, such as medical workers and repair people, before letting them in the house (Figure 6-17). You may feel embarrassed by asking them to drop their identification through the mail slot, but your priority is protecting your safety and the safety of the person in your care.

Looking for Potential Hazards in the Home

When you enter a client's home, do a **safety survey** by looking around for potential hazards. First, look for unsafe conditions, such as anything that could cause falls, burns, poisoning, or other injuries.

Get to know the person's house. Find the smoke detectors and fire extinguishers and be sure they work correctly. Locate the fuse box or circuit breakers, and know how to replace a fuse and turn the electrical power off and on. Check any special equipment your client needs in the home, such as safety gates for a small child or safety rails for a person who is unsteady, to make sure that it is safe and works well. Make sure a list of emergency numbers is next to each telephone with ambulance, fire, and police numbers, as well as other important numbers.

If you can correct a hazard right away, do so. Otherwise, make a list of things that have to be done. To help you do this, copy and use the safety checklist that appears as Appendix D at the end of this book. Use your judgment and your employer's procedures to decide whether to correct the hazard yourself or to ask the client, the client's family, or your employer to arrange for necessary action.

Safety concerns for the home.   Because no two homes are alike, no list can include everything in every home that could cause a problem. As a home health aide, think about the most common ways people are injured in their homes, and then check for potential hazards. Table 6-2 lists potential hazards and tells you what to look for and what to do when you identify them.

Safety concerns for the person in your care.   Some people in your care may cause special safety concerns, such as the following:

❖ **Providing safe care for the person whose thinking is impaired.** To keep a thinking-impaired person safe, lock away poisonous items, such as cleaning products, medications, and alcoholic beverages, as well as dangerous items, such as knives or guns. Take steps so that you will know if the person attempts to leave the house. You may have to remove control knobs from the stove to prevent the person from using it.

❖ **Providing safe care for an infant or child.** To keep an infant or child safe, make sure no choking or suffocation hazards, such as window blind cords, plastic bags, or small pieces from toys, are present. An infant's crib is safe if no pillows are in it and if the slats are no more than 2⅔ inches apart. All unused electrical outlets should have safety covers. Poisonous items, such as

safety survey
(SUR-vay)   Examination of a home to make sure it contains no safety hazards.

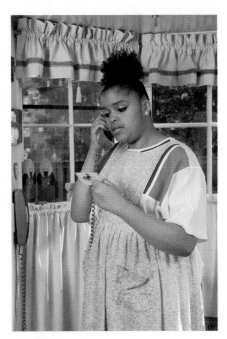

Figure 6-17
One way to verify the identity of a repair person is to call his or her employer.

Table 6-2 **Checking for Potential Hazards**

Potential Hazard	What to Look for	What to Do
Fire hazards	Fire extinguishers, smoke detectors, flammable objects (such as cleaners and paints), space heaters	Check to see if extinguishers and detectors are there and if they work properly. Check to see if flammable objects are stored safely. Make sure space heaters are being used safely. Watch for frayed cords and notify the client and family if you find any.
Tripping or falling hazards	Throw rugs, untacked carpeting, extension cords, boxes, low pieces of furniture	Walk through the home and look for anything that could cause someone to trip or fall.
Medication	Labels, expiration dates	Check to see that all medication containers have legible labels. If the expiration date on a label has passed, report this information to your supervising nurse. Make sure medication is stored away from extreme heat, light, cold, or moisture. Avoid storing medication on windowsills or on the stove.
Lighting	Lights, night-lights	Make sure there is enough lighting so that the person can get around the house without difficulty and that night-lights are placed where they are needed.
Doors and windows	Locks, escape routes	Check to see that doors and windows have good locks and that the locks are used to keep the home safe from intruders. Make sure that doors and windows are not blocked and that they can be unlocked in an emergency.
Stairs	Carpeting, handrails, gates	Look at indoor and outdoor stairways to make sure they are free of cracks and sagging, loose carpeting. If there are handrails, make sure they are tight. If young children are in the house, check for safety gates at the top and bottom of each stairway.
Bathroom	Water temperature, nonskid surfaces, handrails, cleaning products, floor, appliances	Make sure the hot water is a safe temperature (120 degrees or less). Check the tub or shower for nonskid surfaces. Check next to the tub or shower and the toilet for handrails. Make sure the person has a call signal nearby. Make sure cleaning products are safely stored. Check for anything that could shatter—glass bottles or drinking glasses. Make sure the floor is in good condition—no loose tiles, no damp spots. Make sure small appliances such as radios, electric toothbrushes or razors, and hair dryers are either battery operated or kept unplugged when not in use.

cleaning products, medications, and alcoholic beverages, should be kept well out of the reach of children, and the telephone number of the local Poison Control Center should be included in the list of emergency numbers by every phone. Make sure dangerous items, such as knives or guns, are locked away.

Small children must never be left alone, even for a second, near a body of water, such as a bathtub or swimming pool. You may have to take special steps to ensure that unattended children can't get to water. Make sure that safety latches are on cabinet doors and that an appropriate safety seat is in the car. Safety gates should be placed at both the top and the bottom of each stairway.

NOTE: Accordion-style gates should never be used to contain a child, because the child's head and neck may become wedged between the slats.

Table 6-2   Checking for Potential Hazards—(cont'd)

Potential Hazard	What to Look for	What to Do
Kitchen	Fabrics, cleaning products, appliances, floor, cleanliness	Make sure curtains, towels, cleaning products, and other flammable items are kept away from the stove. Check to see if small appliances, such as toasters and electric frying pans, are in good condition—no frayed cords or other evidence of electrical hazard. Make sure the oven is not being used to heat the house. Make sure that the floor is clean and free of debris and that there are no loose tiles. Make sure the room is clean and sanitary.
Bedroom	Safety hazards, bed height, medications, call signal	Check to see if an electric blanket or space heater is being used safely. Make sure all safety procedures are being followed if oxygen is used. Check a humidifier to make sure it is on a solid surface. Check for slippers or other items on the floor that are tripping hazards. Check the bedside table for clutter. Make sure the bed is the right height for the person and not so high or low that the person has difficulty getting in or out of it. Make sure that medications are properly stored. Make sure a call signal is available if the person needs one.

Note: Change the place where the person stores medication only with the person's permission. Look for potential errors that may result from the way medications are stored (too many in one place, similar names or colors together). Extra medicine should be stored in a closet that has a light switch inside. That way, a person can clearly see the medicine she is reaching for and may not grab the wrong one by mistake. Keep daily medication in a highly visible place, such as the top of a dresser or nightstand. If children or confused people are in the house, make sure medication is stored out of their reach. When discarding medications that have expired or are no longer needed, check with your supervising nurse for your agency's policy. A common practice is to flush them down the toilet, but first it is important to document what medication you are discarding, why, and how much you are discarding. Never throw medications in the wastebasket. A child or a confused person may pick them up and swallow them.

❖ **Providing safe care for a person who has physical limitations.** If a person in your care has impaired vision or difficulty walking, you must be especially careful that he has secure footing wherever he goes and extra lighting, if necessary (Figure 6-18). Don't move furniture and other items without first telling the person, since it's important for his surroundings to be familiar to him.

   If the person's hearing is impaired, he might not be able to hear a smoke detector's signal. Smoke detectors with lights work well for hearing-impaired people.

   Finally, think about any special features of the home that are a safety concern. If you provide care for someone in an upper floor of an apartment building, make sure that the person cannot fall from a balcony or open window. If a person's house has a swimming pool, make sure the person cannot fall into it. Outdoor steps or walkways may become slippery when it rains, and radiators or heat registers may become very hot. Think about anything unusual in the home that may cause harm, and then think about what you can do to lessen the danger by correcting the hazard or taking steps to keep the person away from it.

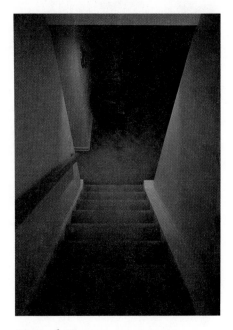

Figure 6-18
A poorly lit stairway is a safety hazard, especially for someone with impaired vision.

Following a Plan When a Fire Occurs

In a private home, conduct your own fire drill from time to time. If a fire does break out, take the following important measures to ensure your own safety and the safety of the person in your care:

❖ Stay calm.

❖ If it is safe or possible to do so, close doors to contain the fire.

❖ If it is safe to go to the person in your care, help him evacuate the home. Attempt to alert any other people in the home. Follow the precautions listed previously in the section on practicing fire safety.

❖ After you leave the building, call the fire emergency number (9-1-1 or the local fire department) from a neighboring building or pay phone. State whether any person is trapped in the home and stay on the line until the dispatcher hangs up. Stay close to the scene until the fire department arrives. Let them know whether anyone is trapped in the home and exactly where the person is.

❖ If you cannot get out of a room, first close the door and block out as much smoke as possible by stuffing material such as wet towels around the door. Put something easy to spot in the window to alert fire fighters that you are there.

❖ Follow your employer's procedures for reporting the fire to the employer and others, such as family members.

Practicing Infant Safety

An infant thrives in an environment where she feels safe and loved. You respond to her need for love by hugging and holding her close. You respond to her cries, which tell you that something is wrong, by determining if she is hungry, thirsty, uncomfortable, or in pain. You respond to her need for safety by observing the following special safe practices:

❖ When holding an infant, be sure to use two hands. Support her head and neck, pick her up with smooth movements, and don't wear jewelry that may scratch her (Figure 6-19).

❖ Keep your nails clean and short. Long fingernails can be a hazard.

❖ Keep infants away from drafts, air conditioners, and fans.

❖ Never turn your attention away from an infant on a sofa, changing table, high chair, bed, or other place from which she could fall without first making sure she is secure. Always use safety straps in high chairs, because infants move quickly and manage to find ways to get out. Make sure the straps fit snugly but are not too tight.

❖ Don't use pillows around infants. You may have seen people make "walls" with pillows to keep a baby from falling off a bed.

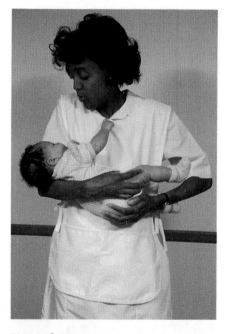

Figure 6-19
Holding a baby correctly not only keeps her safe physically but also helps her build trust by making her feel secure.

This is dangerous because the baby could roll over, put her face into a pillow, and **suffocate**.

❖   Always keep small objects away from infants because they can choke on them.

❖   Lay a baby on her side after feeding. An infant who is laid on her back may spit up and choke. Change the baby's position as you would for anyone who is in bed most of the time.

suffocate
(SUF-uh-kate)   To die from a lack of oxygen.

Information Review

Circle the correct answers and fill in the blanks.

1.   The most important principle of care is—
    a.   Independence.
    b.   Communication.
    c.   Dignity.
    d.   Safety.

2.   By practicing good body mechanics, you can avoid a
    _____Back_____ injury.

3.   Before using any equipment, you should—
    a.   Check to make sure it is working properly.
    b.   Unplug it.
    c.   File an incident report.
    d.   Stand up straight.

4.   What would you do if a fire alarm sounded while you were at work?
    a.   Leave the building and go home
    b.   Ask another nurse assistant what was happening
    c.   Follow your employer's policies for fire alarms
    d.   Ignore the fire alarm, because it is probably only a fire drill

5.   If your clothing ignites in a fire, you should—
    a.   Run, cover, and cool.
    b.   Stop, drop, roll, and cool.
    c.   Call EMS.
    d.   Blanket, bathe, and bandage.

6.   One of the first things to do when a natural disaster strikes is to—
    a.   Unplug appliances.
    b.   Call the weather bureau.
    c.   Close all the doors.
    d.   Gather fire extinguishers.

7.   In any emergency, take three basic steps:
    _____check_____ the scene and the person,
    _____Call_____ 9-1-1 or your local emergency number, and provide _____Care_____ for the person.

8.   Two types of airway obstruction are
    _____Partial_____ and _____Complete_____.

9. Sign(s) of fainting, or syncope, are—
   a. Flushed skin and perspiration.
   b. Excessive thirst.
   c. Pale coloring and cool, moist skin.
   d. Muscle spasms.

10. When a person bleeds from an ___artery___, blood flows rapidly and in large amounts. When a person bleeds from a ___vein___, blood flows at a steady rate, without spurting.

Home Health Care

1. If you find safety hazards in a client's home, you should—
   a. Correct *all* safety hazards immediately.
   b. Correct the two biggest hazards found in your safety survey.
   c. Make a list of all safety hazards and correct those you can do immediately. Discuss the remaining hazards with your supervising nurse.
   d. Tell the client to correct the hazards before your next visit.

2. You are providing care in a home where children and confused people are present. Where is the best place to store medication?
   a. In a high bathroom cabinet
   b. On a window sill
   c. In a corner of a kitchen counter
   d. In a locked box in a well-lit hall closet

3. Using a ___pillow___ around a baby is dangerous because the baby could put his face in it and suffocate.

Questions to Ask Yourself

1. A chair, a plant stand, a small table, and some boxes are on the floor directly in front of the window. You want to water several plants on the sill. What should you do to protect your back?

2. You need to pick up a heavy suitcase and place it on the edge of a waist-high table. What should you pay particular attention to as you move?

3. Mrs. Kennedy has poor vision and uses a walker. What special measures would you take to make sure her room is safe?

4. Ms. Bernstein gets into a wheelchair before you notice that the brake on the left wheel doesn't work. What should you do?

5. You notice that Mr. Brown's electric razor keeps shutting off by itself. Mr. Brown taps on it to get it started again. What should you do?

6. You enter Mr. Lee's room and see flames shooting out of the trash can, creating a great deal of smoke. Both Mr. Lee and his roommate are coughing and calling for help. Neither person can walk by himself. What things should you do and in what order?

7. You enter the room of Mrs. Bateman, who is on oxygen. Her visitor is smoking. What should you do?

8. Your 82-year-old client is unsteady when she walks, but she refuses to have handrails installed. She says they are ugly and leave holes in the wall. You believe that she is in real danger of falling. What should you say?

9. You are providing care for 30-year-old Emilio Sanchez, who is recovering from leg injuries he sustained in a car crash. You notice that his electric razor and hair dryer are kept plugged in on a shelf over the bathroom sink and that the railing on the steps is loose. What should you do?

10. Your client looks forward to frequent visits from his daughter and small grandchildren. But you are always nervous when they are there because they usually sit on the deck, which leads to the backyard swimming pool. How would you discuss your concerns?

11. A small child is playing in the living room. You enter the room and see marbles on the floor and the child lying very still in the middle of the floor. You call to him and he doesn't answer. What do you do next?

12. Mrs. Chue asks to be taken for a ride in her wheelchair. As you park the wheelchair next to her bed and put down the side rails, you hear the person in the next room calling for assistance. You tell Mrs. Chue you'll be right back. While you are gone, she decides she feels good enough to get into her wheelchair by herself. When she gets up and tries to grab the wheelchair, it rolls back and Mrs. Chue falls to the floor. You return to the room and find Mrs. Chue lying on the floor. She moans and indicates that her left foot hurts. You tell Mrs. Chue not to move, call for assistance, and stay with her until help arrives. What information would you give your supervising nurse to complete an incident report? What safety measures could have prevented this incident?

7

Controlling the Spread of Germs

Goals

After reading this chapter, you will have the information to—

Apply general infection control measures to control the spread of germs.

Clean, disinfect, and sterilize objects.

Use universal precautions when necessary.

Use isolation procedures when necessary.

Explain isolation procedures to someone in isolation.

After practicing the corresponding skills in the skills book, you will be able to—

Wash your hands to control the spread of germs.

Put on and take off protective clothing.

Open and close a trash bag and double bag contaminated trash and laundry.

During morning report at Metropolitan Hospital Center, your supervising nurse tells you about your new patient, Louise Wang, an 83-year-old woman who was admitted through the Emergency Room from Morningside Nursing Home last night. Because she was diagnosed with highly contagious staph pneumonia, she is in isolation in room 117. Last year, she had part of her intestines removed because of colon cancer and has a colostomy. That means that you will have to provide care for the surgical opening in her abdomen that allows feces from her intestines to empty into a bag rather than through her rectum. In addition to colostomy care, she needs help with a complete bed bath and with transferring from the bed to the chair, as she is very weak. Your supervising nurse also tells you that Mrs. Wang is originally from China, but speaks and understands English very well.

You decide to visit Mrs. Wang immediately because you think she might be afraid. Before going into her room, you wash your hands and put on a gown, mask, and gloves. Outside her room, you notice the sign posted on her closed door. The sign requests visitors to report to the nurses' station.

You knock gently, then a little louder when you hear no response. When you finally hear a faint "come in," you open the door to see the back of a small, gray-haired woman lying in bed. You walk toward the bed, gently calling Mrs. Wang's name and telling her who you are. When she turns toward you and sees your masked face, her eyes open wide before she turns back to face the wall.

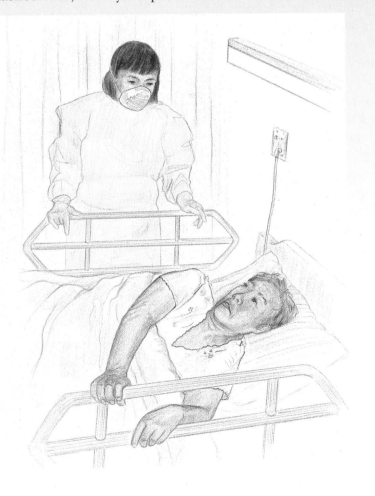

Germs and Infection

Louise Wang is in a room by herself because she has staphylococcus pneumonia, also called staph pneumonia, a disease that other people could catch from her. Colds and flus also are diseases that people can get from one another. Have you ever caught a cold or flu from someone? You can lessen your chances of getting sick and avoid passing on an illness to someone else by learning about germs, how they can cause illness, and how you can help control their spread.

Germs is the word that most people use to describe tiny living things that are too small to see but are all around us and can cause disease. Scientists call them **microorganisms**. Microorganisms, such as bacteria, viruses, yeasts, and molds, can be seen only with a microscope. Some microorganisms are harmful to humans and some are not. Harmful microorganisms that cause disease are called **pathogens**.

Sometimes pathogens move from place to place and may spread disease from one person to another. These diseases are called **infectious**. **Infection** is a general term for a disease caused by bacteria, viruses, or other germs that enter and infect the body in a variety of ways.

You use different precautions and take certain actions to control the spread of germs that cause different infectious diseases. This practice is called **infection control**, which is one of the six principles of care. You probably already use some of these precautions in your daily life without thinking much about them. If you cough or sneeze, for example, do you cover your mouth or turn your head to control the spread of germs? If someone you know has a cold or flu, do you try to keep your distance from that person so that you won't catch her germs (Figure 7-1)? Do you always wash your hands after using the bathroom? If you do these things, you already are controlling the spread of infection .

Practicing infection control is especially important when providing care for older people, because they have a harder time protecting themselves from infection. In addition, after an older person gets an infection, it is more difficult to eliminate it from her body.

When you work in any health care setting, you help control the spread of infection if you understand what is meant by clean and what is meant by dirty. Clean items or surfaces are considered to be free of dirt and pathogens, or disease-causing germs. Dirty items or surfaces are considered to be **contaminated** because they contain dirt or pathogens. An unused item is considered to be clean until it comes in contact with a person or his environment (Figure 7-2). It is then considered to be dirty and cannot be reused for another person.

In a hospital or nursing home, the clean utility room has clean, unused supplies, such as linens and dressings. The dirty utility room has trash containers and reusable supplies that must be cleaned or laundered. When you provide care for a person in her home, you can help the family understand the difference between clean and

microorganisms
(my-crow-OR-guh-niz-ums) Tiny living things that can be seen only through the magnification of a microscope.

pathogen
(PATH-o-jen) A harmful germ or microorganism that causes disease.

infectious
(in-FEK-shus) Spreading or capable of spreading rapidly. Infectious germs are also described as communicable and contagious.

infection
(in-FEK-shun) A harmful condition caused by the growth of germs in the body.

infection control
Action taken to control the spread of germs. Infection control is one of the six principles of care.

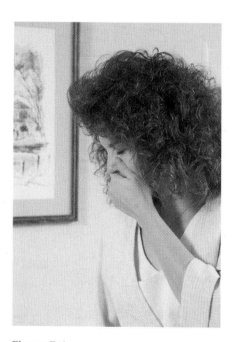

Figure 7-1
You probably already practice some common methods of infection control.

contaminated
(kun-TAM-in-ay-tid) Containing dirt or disease-causing germs.

dirty work areas. Together, you might decide to keep one part of the kitchen as clean, where food can be prepared and supplies stored, and a different part as dirty, where trash and used items can be put for disposal.

How to Recognize an Infection

In addition to practicing the everyday control of spreading germs, you must know how to recognize infection. For example, germs live and multiply on and in your body. They grow rapidly wherever they have warm temperatures, moisture, darkness, and food. Think of an area of your body that is dark and moist. That is a place where germs live, grow, and multiply fast. That is a place where an infection might occur.

Although some germs are useful and necessary in certain areas of the body, these same germs may cause disease if they spread to another part of the body. For example, certain bacteria in the stomach and intestines help to digest food. But, if these same bacteria are present in the kidney or bladder, they can cause an infection.

An infection occurs when pathogens grow inside the body, and almost any part of the body can become infected. You can recognize a possible infection in a person's body by certain **symptoms**. The symptoms are not always the same, because they vary according to the kind of germ and the place in the body where the infection is occurring. Box 7-1 contains some of the common symptoms that help you recognize an infection.

If you observe that someone in your care has one or more of the symptoms in Box 7-1, report it to your supervising nurse, just as you report any changes that you observe with your senses. (Read Table

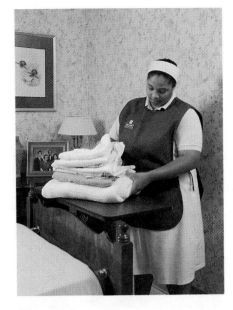

Figure 7-2
Always place clean items on a clean surface.

symptom
Any change that you observe in a person's body or in the way it functions that may indicate an infection.

Box 7-1   **Common Symptoms for Recognizing an Infection**

High body temperature	Vomiting
Red or draining eyes	Diarrhea
Stuffy nose	Cloudy or smelly urine
Coughing	Joint pain
Headache	Muscle ache
Sore throat	Skin rash
Flushed face	Sores
Loss of appetite	Redness around a wound or incision
Nausea	Drainage from a wound or incision
Stomach pain	Swelling

5-5 in Chapter 5 again.) By recognizing infections early, you increase the chances of treating them and preventing their spread to others. Although it is important to know the symptoms of possible infection, you must always practice infection control, even when you do not observe any symptoms.

How Germs Spread

To control the spread of germs, you need to know how germs move from one place to another. Germs are most commonly spread through direct and indirect contact.

Direct contact. If you are not protected by gloves while you provide care for Mrs. Wang's colostomy, you can get bacteria directly from her feces onto your hands. These germs will spread to you through direct contact. Direct contact means that germs spread from one living thing to another living thing—from Mrs. Wang to you, for example. If you kiss a person who has a cold, you can catch the cold. The germs will spread by direct contact (Figure 7-3). Infections also can occur by direct contact if you touch drainage from a person's infected wound or if someone coughs or sneezes directly on you.

Indirect contact. If Mrs. Wang drinks from a glass, some of the pathogens that caused her illness are transferred to the glass. Then, if you handle the glass, you can get these same germs on your hands. If you then touch the inside of your nose or mouth, or if you have a crack in your skin, you can develop the infection. The germs will spread by indirect contact.

Indirect contact means that germs are spread by way of an object. Usually this situation occurs when an infected person touches something and then someone else touches that same object (Figure 7-4). For example, if you have a cold and blow your nose into a tissue, and someone else picks up the tissue to throw it away, he can get your cold by indirect contact. The germs will spread from your nose secretions to the tissue to his hand. You can get other infections by indirect contact if you—

❖ Eat contaminated food such as a custard that has been left out of the refrigerator overnight.
❖ Use contaminated water or drink it.
❖ Handle dirty equipment.
❖ Handle soiled linens.
❖ Handle dressings that are contaminated with wound drainage.

How to Control the Spread of Germs

When you understand what germs are and how they spread, you can use precautions to keep them from spreading. In addition, if you are always ready to recognize potential infection and take positive actions, such as washing your hands, you can control the spread of germs and infection every day.

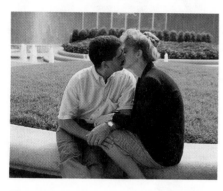

Figure 7-3
Kissing someone who has a cold is a common way of getting an infection by direct contact.

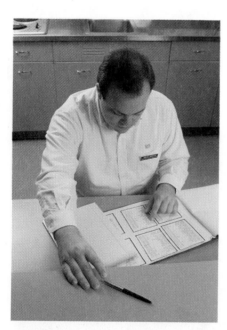

Figure 7-4
Sharing items can spread germs, because commonly borrowed items, like pens, often are contaminated with harmful microorganisms.

Taking precautions every day.   You can control the spread of germs 24 hours a day by taking the following actions:

❖ **Wash your hands.** Read the next section on handwashing to know the appropriate times for washing your hands (Figure 7-5).

❖ **Use an antimicrobial soap.** If possible, use **antimicrobial** soap from a liquid soap dispenser, rather than from a bar that is used by others.

❖ **Eat well.** Select a well-balanced diet to stay healthy.

❖ **Discuss any illnesses.** Before doing any personal care, discuss any illness you may have with your supervising nurse.

❖ **Clean.** Keep yourself, the person in your care, and the person's space clean. You can remove dirt and some germs from an object if you clean the object with soap and water. Or you can **disinfect** the object to remove disease-causing germs by soaking it in a **disinfectant** solution. To destroy all germs, **sterilize** the object by treating it with gas, liquid, dry heat, or pressurized steam. A special department of the hospital or nursing home, often called Central Supply, usually sterilizes objects. In a person's home, you can sterilize durable objects by boiling them in water for 20 minutes.

❖ **Keep dirty linens away from your uniform.**

❖ **Hold dirty or contaminated items still.** Avoid spreading germs from items, such as dirty linens, thermometers, or clothing, when you move them.

❖ **Bag dirty linens.** Place dirty linens in a laundry bag in a person's room before you carry the bag to the laundry hamper outside the room (Figure 7-6). Place wet and soiled linens in a plastic or leakproof laundry bag .

❖ **Clean, dry, and store utensils.** Follow your employer's policy for cleaning, drying, and storing utensils after you use them.

❖ **Ensure single use of personal equipment.** Make sure only one person uses personal items such as bedpans, urinals, washbasins, emesis basins, toothbrushes, toothpaste, lotion, and soap.

❖ **Cover bedpans and urinals.** To contain fluids when carrying them from one place to another, always cover bedpans and urinals.

❖ **Recognize and report symptoms of infection.** Be on the lookout for any symptoms of infection and report any symptoms immediately to your supervising nurse.

❖ **Prepare food carefully.** When preparing food for yourself or for another person—
  Wash your hands first.
  Rinse off the tops of cans before opening them.
  Wash fruits and vegetables before using them.
  Cook food properly; cook chicken and pork thoroughly.
  Clean dishes and utensils after each use.
    When using cutting boards to prepare chicken, pork, or other meats, wash them thoroughly with hot soapy water immediately

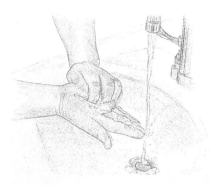

Figure 7-5
Handwashing is the most important method for reducing the spread of infection.

antimicrobial
(an-ti-my-CROW-bee-uhl)   Capable of killing or slowing the growth of pathogens.

disinfect
(dis-in-FEKT)   To remove disease-causing germs.

disinfectant
(dis-in-FEK-tunt)   A substance that destroys disease-causing germs.

sterilize
(STAIR-uh-lize)   To destroy all germs.

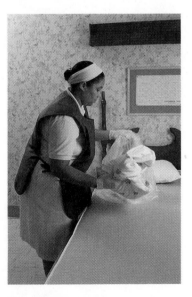

Figure 7-6
Bagging dirty linens where they are used is an effective way to control the spread of germs.

after use. Use separate cutting boards for cutting meat and for cutting vegetables that are not going to be cooked.

❖ **Serve meals immediately.** After food arrives from the dietary department of a hospital or nursing home, or as soon as you prepare food in a client's home, serve it immediately.

❖ **Store foods carefully.** Make sure people do not store food in their rooms, unless the food is nonperishable and is stored in a tightly sealed container. For example, if Mrs. Wang does not finish her lunch but wants to keep a cup of chocolate pudding to eat later, explain to her that unrefrigerated food can grow bacteria that could make her ill if she eats it several hours later. Tell her that if she is hungry later in the day, you will bring her a fresh serving of pudding.

Washing your hands. Washing your hands is the most important thing you can do to control the spread of germs. As a nurse assistant, you wash your hands in a special way so that they are free of germs. The specific procedure for handwashing is explained step by step in Skill 2 in the skills book.

As you practice the handwashing procedure, remember these tips about infection control:

❖ Keep your fingernails trimmed short and use a nailbrush or orangewood stick to remove any dirt underneath them (Figure 7-7).

❖ Don't wear rings to work, except for a simple wedding band. The tiny spaces in jewelry provide a good place for breeding germs, which may spread from one person to another.

❖ Because you must wash your wrists along with your hands, push your watch above your wrist, put it in your pocket, or pin it to your uniform.

❖ If you must use your hand to twist on the faucet, use a clean paper towel to turn it on so that you don't have direct contact with germs on the faucet.

❖ If antimicrobial soap is not available from a dispenser, rinse the bar of soap before and after you use it.

❖ Rub your hands together briskly to loosen and remove dirt and germs.

❖ Wash for at least 10 seconds and longer if your hands are contaminated with body fluids.

❖ Use a paper towel to turn off the faucet.

❖ Dry your hands thoroughly to keep them from chapping.

Look at Box 7-2 to make sure you are using every possible opportunity to keep your hands clean.

Sometimes you may think that handwashing is a "pain in the neck" when you have so much else to do. But the one time you say, "I'll skip it. I'm too busy," may be the time you infect yourself or someone else with germs from another person.

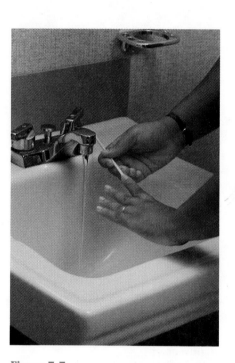

Figure 7-7
By paying careful attention to nail care and wearing only simple jewelry, this nurse assistant helps control the spread of germs.

Box 7-2   **When to Wash Your Hands**

> ### As a Nurse Assistant, You Should Wash Your Hands—
> As you are coming on duty.
> Before and after contact with a person in your care.
> After using the bathroom.
> After coughing, sneezing, or blowing your nose.
> Before handling food.
> After smoking.
> Before handling clean linens.
> After handling dirty linens.
> Before going home.
> Any other time you think it may be important.

Universal Precautions and Isolation Procedures

Health care workers control the spread of germs by always practicing universal precautions and following **isolation procedures** when they are necessary.

Practicing Universal Precautions

As a nurse assistant, you come in contact with many different substances that are produced by and released from a person's body, such as blood, vomitus, tears, semen, vaginal secretions, saliva, urine, feces, and sweat. These substances are called **body fluids**. If a person has an infection, these body fluids can contain pathogens. Some serious pathogens, such as **human immunodeficiency virus** (**HIV**) and those that cause **hepatitis**, may be spread when a person comes in contact with an infected person's body fluids, especially blood.

HIV, which is carried in the blood and some other body fluids, causes **acquired immune deficiency syndrome** (AIDS). AIDS can spread in two ways: by sexual contact with an infected person or by contact with the infected person's blood. (For more information on AIDS, read Chapter 17, Providing Care for People Who Have AIDS.)

Another virus, called **HBV**, causes one form of hepatitis—hepatitis B—that also is carried in the blood and other body fluids. As with HIV, HBV can spread by sexual contact or by contact with an infected person's blood. HBV also can spread by contact with an infected person's saliva.

Blood must be present in other body fluids that may not otherwise be a source of infection. But, because there is no way of seeing the blood in some body fluids, you should consider all body fluids to be infectious.

You must practice universal precautions whenever you might come into contact with any body fluids, such as when assisting with a

isolation procedures
(pro-SEE-dyurs)   Practices used to separate a person from others and prevent the spread of infection.

body fluids
Liquid substances produced by the body.

human immunodeficiency virus
(im-you-no-duh-FISH-uhn-see)   The microscopic organism that causes AIDS.

HIV
An abbreviation for **h**uman **i**mmunodeficiency **v**irus.

hepatitis
(heh-puh-TY-tis)   A disease or condition marked by an inflammation of the liver.

acquired immune deficiency syndrome
(uh-KWY-erd/im-MYOUN/duh-FISH-uhn-see/SIN-drum)   A condition caused by the human immunodeficiency virus that results in a breakdown of the body's defense systems.

HBV
An abbreviation for **h**epatitis **B** **v**irus.

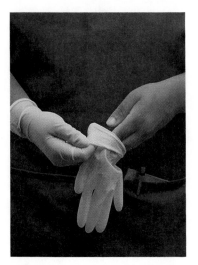

Figure 7-8
Wearing disposable gloves is an important part of infection control and an important universal precaution.

Box 7-3   **Ten Universal Precautions**

1. Wear latex gloves.
2. Wash your hands and other skin surfaces immediately and thoroughly if contaminated with body fluids or if you have handled potentially contaminated articles.
3. Wear protective clothing, such as a gown and a mask, when required.
4. Handle sharp instruments carefully.
5. Wear gloves if you have open cuts or oozing sores.
6. Clean up blood or body fluid spills promptly.
7. Handle linens carefully.
8. Bag contaminated articles carefully.
9. Put waste in a leakproof, air-tight container.
10. Keep resuscitation masks or bags on hand in a hospital or nursing home setting.

medical procedure or when providing personal care (Figure 7-8). Even if you think the person in your care is not infected, you must follow the ten universal precautions. Box 7-3 contains a list of the universal precautions you must follow when you might come into contact with body fluids. Read about the precautions in the following paragraphs, memorize them, and make them a way of life as you work as nurse assistant.

Wear latex gloves.   Wear latex gloves when—

❖ You touch blood.
❖ You touch semen and vaginal secretions.
❖ You touch **mucous membranes**.
❖ You touch any body fluids that may or may not contain visible blood.
❖ The person in your care has broken skin or you have broken skin on your hands.
❖ You must handle items on surfaces soiled with blood or other body fluids.

mucous membrane
(MYOU-kus)   A thin layer of body tissue that lines body passages and cavities that communicate directly or indirectly with the outside, such as the inside of the mouth, nose, eyes, vagina, and rectum.

Change gloves and wash your hands after each contact with a person.

Example: You wear latex gloves when you provide oral hygiene care, perineal care, or care for someone who has open sores on his skin or a draining wound. You also wear latex gloves when you touch a contaminated dressing.

Wash your hands and other skin surfaces.   Wash your hands and other skin surfaces immediately and thoroughly—

❖ If you are contaminated with blood or other body fluids.
❖ If you have handled potentially contaminated articles.
❖ After removing gloves.
❖ Before putting on new gloves.

Example: Amber Clark pulls off her bloody wound dressing and places it on the table next to the sofa. When you arrive at her apartment to provide home health care, you unintentionally pick up the dressing along with some pieces of paper. You are not wearing gloves. After disposing of the dressing in a leakproof, airtight container, you must wash your hands right away with antimicrobial soap.

Wear protective clothing.   Wear protective clothing, such as—

❖   A gown or apron when your clothing might become soiled with body fluids or excretions.
❖   A mask and protective eyewear if you think blood or other body fluids might splash into your mouth, nose, or eyes (Figure 7-9).

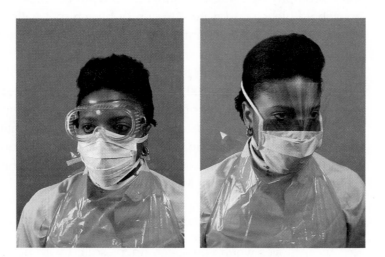

Figure 7-9
Use protective equipment whenever you are likely to be exposed to blood or other body fluids.

Example: The nurse asks for your help to position a person onto his side. The person has a large, open, draining wound that needs cleaning. The nurse explains to you that a great deal of solution will be used to clean the wound and it is likely to splash. You must put on a gown to protect your clothing and a mask and protective eyewear to protect your mouth, eyes, and nose.

Handle sharp instruments carefully.   To avoid wounds from sharp instruments contaminated with blood or body fluids—

❖   Immediately dispose of sharp items (such as razors) without recapping them, because you may cut or injure yourself if you try to recap a sharp instrument.
❖   Put all sharp items in a **sharps container**.

Example: Stephen Lightfoot has just finished shaving with a disposable safety razor. It is your responsibility to dispose of used items and clean the surrounding area. You immediately put the razor in the container marked "sharps."

sharps container
A sturdy box with a tight-fitting lid that cannot be punctured by sharp objects such as needles or razors. Use of a sharps container protects health care workers from injury and exposure to contaminated items.

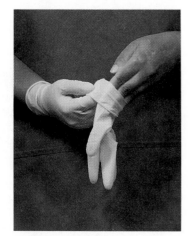

Figure 7-10
Frequent handwashing can lead to dryness, irritation, and breaks in the skin. Until your hands heal, wear gloves when providing care.

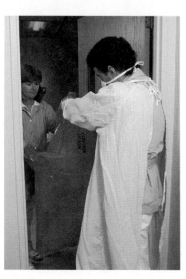

Figure 7-11
Placing a second bag over a bag containing contaminated items is called double bagging. This procedure works well with two people, but the person outside the room does not have to be gowned, masked, or gloved as the person on the inside does.

speculum
(SPEK-you-lum)   An instrument used to examine a body passage or cavity.

Wear gloves when you have cuts or sores.   Wear gloves when giving care if YOU have an open cut or oozing sore. Make sure you—

❖ Wear gloves when giving direct care and handling equipment.
❖ Examine yourself daily, because scratches, cuts, and breaks in the skin often occur without your knowledge (Figure 7-10).
❖ Discuss precautions with your supervising nurse before assisting with care.

   Example: This morning, while slicing fruit, you cut your finger. You apply a bandage and go to work. You must wear gloves when you give care today and every day until the cut is completely healed.

Clean up blood or body fluids promptly.   Clean up blood or body fluid spills promptly by using a freshly mixed disinfectant solution, such as household bleach and water (¼ cup of bleach to 1 gallon of water), or any other approved disinfectant. Mix a fresh solution of bleach daily.
   Example: After drawing Mrs. Wang's blood for some lab tests, the lab technician drops the vial of blood on the floor. The stopper falls off the vial, spilling blood onto the floor. He carefully picks up the stopper and vial and disposes of them in the sharps container, as they have become contaminated. He uses a bleach solution to clean the floor. He removes his continimated gloves, washes his hands, and regloves before redrawing Mrs. Wang's blood.

Handle linens carefully.   Handle linens carefully and be sure to—

❖ Wear gloves when you touch linens soiled with body fluids.
❖ Keep linens as still as possible to prevent contaminating yourself or putting germs into the air.
❖ Bag all soiled linens where they were used. Do not sort or rinse them in areas where you provide care.
❖ Put wet linens into leakproof bags, carry linens in these bags, and never put soiled linens on the floor.

   Example: Before changing Mrs. Wang's linens, you notice wet, blood-tinged drainage on the pillow case and bottom sheet. Wear gloves while making her bed, and bag the dirty linens in a plastic bag as soon as you remove them from the bed.

Bag contaminated articles carefully.   Bag contaminated articles carefully and be sure to—

❖ Put articles, such as thermometers and **speculums**, that have been contaminated with germs or body fluids into a puncture-proof bag.
❖ Put a second bag over the first bag if the first bag may have been contaminated (Figure 7-11).

Example: The doctor has used a special piece of equipment to examine Mrs. Wang. After the examination, the equipment is contaminated with body fluids. The nurse asks you to first wash and then soak the equipment in a disinfectant solution before bagging it and informing Central Supply that it needs sterilizing.

Put waste in a leakproof, air-tight container.   Put waste in an air-tight container that—

❖ Does not leak and may be thoroughly cleaned.
❖ Has a tight-fitting cover (unless it can be maintained in a sanitary condition without a cover).

Example: You place waste from Josie Miller's bedside in a plastic trash bag that you tie and discard in a larger, air-tight, covered container. In the hospital, the container may be the trash bin in the dirty utility room. In the home setting, this container may be the garbage can.

Keep resuscitation masks or bags on hand.   In a hospital or nursing home, know where resuscitation masks or bags are kept, as you may have to get them in a hurry. When a person stops breathing and needs rescue breathing or CPR, the nurse or doctor will give oxygen to the person by applying a mask or bag over the person's mouth and nose (Figure 7-12).

Example: A nurse calls an emergency on the floor where you work. Your job is to assist with getting the equipment that is needed. You are told to get the resuscitation mask. You must know what it is, where it is, and why it is used.

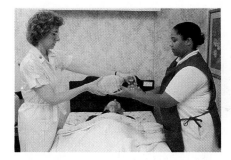

Figure 7-12
You can help the doctor or nurse give effective CPR by quickly getting the resuscitation bag.

Following Isolation Procedures

You know from your supervising nurse's report that Mrs. Wang is in respiratory isolation because her staph pneumonia is contagious. In addition to following the general principles of infection control and universal precautions when you provide care for Mrs. Wang, you focus on the isolation procedures you must follow to protect yourself and others from her contagious disease. Before serving her breakfast, you check the supply table outside her private room to make sure everything you need is there: masks, gloves, a container for soiled linens, plastic bags, and a container for contaminated trash. You also check to make sure her breakfast is served on disposable plates, with disposable utensils, and you remind yourself to close her door after you enter her room.

If someone is placed apart from other people, we say that person is in isolation. If you had chicken pox as a child, you may remember that your mother kept you in your room and didn't let your playmates visit (Figure 7-13). She may have used paper plates and plastic utensils that she could throw away after you used them. By doing these things, your mother practiced methods of isolation at home. A

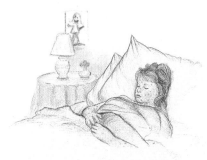

Figure 7-13
A child who has a contagious disease may have to stay in her own room to keep others from catching the disease.

person may be isolated from other people if she has a contagious disease. Examples of contagious diseases that often are cared for at home are measles, chicken pox, hepatitis, tuberculosis, conjunctivitis, infected sores, and some kinds of diarrhea. What are some other contagious diseases that you or your family members may have had?

When a doctor suspects or confirms that a person has a contagious disease, you must take additional precautions and follow additional procedures to control the spread of the disease to other people. The health care worker who writes the orders for the person's care decides which of several isolation categories to specify. He bases his decision on two things: the type of germ that causes the person to have a contagious disease and how that type of germ spreads. Sometimes a doctor orders reverse isolation procedures to protect a person who may easily get an infection from microorganisms carried by health care workers or other people. A person who is already sick may be isolated to prevent her from developing an additional infection. When a person is placed in isolation in the hospital or nursing home, a sign is posted outside the room. Box 7-4 contains the kind of information that may be posted outside an isolation room.

Box 7-4   **Isolation Sign**

Visitors—Report to Nurses' Station Before Entering Room	
1. Private room indicated?	_____ No
	_____ Yes
2. Masks indicated?	_____ No
	_____ Yes, for those close to patient
	_____ Yes, for all persons entering room
3. Gowns indicated?	_____ No
	_____ Yes, if soiling is likely
	_____ Yes, for all persons entering room
4. Gloves indicated?	_____ No
	_____ Yes, for touching infective material
	_____ Yes, for all persons entering room
5. Special precautions indicated for handling food?	_____ No
	_____ Yes

6. Hands must be washed after touching the patient or potentially contaminated articles and before taking care of another patient.

7. Articles contaminated with _____ should be discarded or bagged
                                       infective material(s)
   and labeled before being sent for decontamination and reprocessing.

From Charette S et al: *Infection control manual,* Ft Smith, Ark, 1991, Beverly Enterprises.

When a person is in isolation, you must—

❖ Make sure the person knows why she is isolated.

❖ Check on her often and listen to her concerns. Try to understand her feelings and help provide care for her needs. Stress to her that isolation helps speed her recovery and prevents others from getting sick.

❖ Make sure that visitors (if permitted) follow the nurse's instructions.

❖ Keep clean items separate from dirty items.

❖ Know your employer's specific procedures for isolation.

Contagious diseases can be sorted into categories that then determine the type of isolation that is used. Six isolation categories are explained below.

1. *Strict isolation* prevents the spread of highly contagious diseases by direct contact with the infected person or any contaminated items, *as well as* any germs that may be in the air of the infected person's room.

2. *Respiratory isolation* prevents the spread of contagious diseases that may be spread by **airborne germs**.

3. *Contact isolation* is used to prevent the spread of contagious diseases by close or direct contact.

4. *Protective or reverse isolation* is used when a person's body is unable to fight off the germs carried by other people.

5. *Enteric precautions* are used when urine or stool is infected.

6. *Drainage/secretion precautions* are used when a person has a minor infection that is draining and that can be contained within a dressing. They also are used when a person has a minor infection such as conjunctivitis (pink eye).

airborne germs
Germs that are carried in the air by breathing, coughing, or sneezing.

Table 7-1 compares the similarities and differences in the procedures and equipment used in each isolation category. To practice universal precautions and isolation procedures for controlling the spread of germs, you must know what equipment to use and how to use it properly.

Equipment for Practicing Universal Precautions and Isolation Procedures

When practicing universal precautions and following isolation procedures, you must know how to use required equipment: gowns, masks, eyewear, golves, and plastic bags. When putting on protective clothing, follow the specific procedures that are explained step by step in Skill 3 in the skills book.

Gowns.   Wear a gown when required by universal precautions and isolation procedures to provide a barrier against germs. A gown is worn only one time by one person and then is placed in a laundry hamper or is thrown away. Because a damp or wet gown is a breeding place for germs and will not protect you, wear only a gown that

Table 7-1   Isolation Procedures and Categories

Procedure	Strict Isolation	Respiratory Isolation	Contact Isolation	Protective or Reverse Isolation	Enteric Precautions	Drainage/ Secretion Precautions
Keep door to private room— closed	Yes	Yes	Yes	Yes	Only if person can't be trusted to wash his or her hands	No
Wash hands when entering and leaving the room	Yes	Yes	Yes	Yes	Yes	Yes
Wear gown	Yes	Only if specific tasks require its use	Yes (when in contact with a wound)	Yes	Yes (if you may get soiled)	Yes (when touching soiled material)
Wear mask	Yes	Yes	Yes (for close or direct patient contact)	No	Yes	No
Wear gloves	Yes	Only if specific tasks require their use	Yes (when in contact with a wound)	Yes	Yes (when touching soiled material)	Yes (when touching soiled material)
Bag linens and contaminated articles	Yes	Yes	Yes	Only if linens are contami- nated	Yes	Yes
Disinfect or throw away articles from the room after use	Yes	No	No	No	No	No

NOTE: Wear protective eyewear when the possibility exists for blood or other body fluids to splash into your eyes, such as when suctioning during a tracheotomy.

is dry. Follow your employer's procedures for wearing gowns that are appropriate to the type of anticipated exposure.

Masks.   Wear a mask to keep from inhaling infectious germs into your lungs. Use a mask only once. Change your mask if it becomes moist, because a moist mask makes it easy for bacteria to enter your mouth and nose. Also change the mask after you have worn it for 20 minutes, because it will be moist from exhaled breath.

Protective eyewear.   Wear protective eyewear to keep splashes of body fluids from contacting the mucous membranes of your eyes. Protective eyewear is either reusable or disposable.

Gloves.   Wear only latex or vinyl gloves when you practice universal precautions. *Never* wash or disinfect these gloves for reuse. Always discard them. Do not use gloves that are peeling, cracked, or discolored or that have punctures, tears, or evidence of deterioration. In the home, you may decontaminate and reuse general-purpose utility gloves worn for housekeeping and laundry.

Use vinyl gloves when handling oil, because oil causes latex gloves to weaken and tear. Use latex gloves when handling alcohol, because alcohol weakens vinyl gloves. Do not wear gloves as a "second skin" throughout the day. Put them on and remove them as needed.

Plastic bags.   Use leakproof plastic trash bags to provide protection from wet items. When closing a used trash bag, touch only the outside of the bag. When a bag contains items contaminated with body fluids, label it as contaminated or put it in a red bag. When handling plastic trash bags, follow the specific procedure that is explained step by step in Skill 4 in the skills book.

Responding to the Person's Needs

As you enter Mrs. Wang's room, she turns her face away and covers her eyes so that you can't see her tears. "Good morning, Mrs. Wang," you say and then introduce yourself. You explain that you will be taking care of her today. When you suggest that she seems upset and offer to help her, Mrs. Wang shakes her head and looks out the window. You suggest that it must be hard to be cooped up in her room by herself on such a nice day.

"At the nursing home I like to sit on the sun porch with my roommate Agnes," she replies.

You suggest that she must feel very lonely in her isolation room and offer to tell her why she has a private room and why you are wearing a mask. She looks at you and smiles sadly.

Even though you must practice infection control, you have to be sensitive to Mrs. Wang's needs. How would you feel if the door to your room had to be closed all the time for isolation? Perhaps you would feel as if no one wanted to be near you or that no one liked you. How would you feel if the people providing personal care for you wore gloves? How would you feel if they were completely covered with gowns, masks, and gloves (Figure 7-14)?

Try to imagine what it would be like to be in isolation. How do you think you would feel? Lonely? Angry? Depressed? Maybe embarrassed or afraid? You can be more sensitive to the person's needs if you try to imagine what it would be like to be in her situation.

In this chapter you read about germs and how they spread. You also read about universal precautions and isolation procedures and know when to follow these practices to protect yourself and others. In addition, you now know what equipment you need and how to use it. You understand the important role you play in controlling the spread of germs and in meeting the needs of the people in your care, not just physically, but emotionally as well.

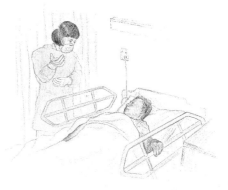

Figure 7-14
By explaining why you are wearing a gown, mask, and gloves, you can help a person in your care get used to seeing you in protective clothing.

Information Review

Circle the correct answers and fill in the blanks.

1. The two most common ways that germs are spread are by
   _____*indirect*_____ and _____*direct*_____ contact.

2. Three ways for removing germs from a contaminated object are
   _____*cleaning*_____, _____*disinfecting*_____, and
   _____*sterilizing*_____.

3. When you take dirty linens to the laundry hamper you should—
   a. Shake them first.
   b. Hold them away from your uniform.
   c. Take only one sheet at a time to prevent contamination.
   d. Save steps by tossing them into the laundry hamper from a short distance.

4. What is the most important thing you can do to control the spread of germs?
   a. Bag all contaminated linens
   b. Wash your hands
   c. Always cover bedpans and urinals when carrying them from place to place
   d. Eat a well-balanced diet and stay healthy

5. You should practice universal precautions—
   a. When you provide care for any person.
   b. Only when you provide care for people infected with HIV or HBV.
   c. Only when a person is in isolation.
   d. Only when you need to wash your hands.

6. What is one time when you must wear latex gloves?
   a. When you give someone a backrub
   b. When you cough or sneeze
   c. When you serve meal trays
   d. When you touch blood or other body fluids

7. When handling sharp items, dispose of them in a
   _____*sharps*_____ _____*container*_____.

8. If you have a cut or open sore on your hand, what must you do to protect yourself from infection?
   a. Avoid providing care for people with infections
   b. Stay away from work until the wound heals
   c. Wear gloves while providing care
   d. Handle only clean items

9. Which of the following is a reason to place someone in isolation?
    a. The person has many infected dressings.
    b. The person had surgery.
    c. The person has germs.
    d. The person wants the privacy of a single room.
10. Four items of protective equipment that you may wear when practicing universal precautions and isolation procedures are
    _____mask_____, _____gloves_____,
    _____gown_____, and _____eyewear_____.

Questions to Ask Yourself

1. How can you control the spread of infection when you provide care for a person with an open wound?

2. How can you spread infection if you have a cold?

3. In the past, how have you spread germs through direct and indirect contact? Think of three ways.

4. What will you do in the future to avoid spreading germs by direct and indirect contact? Think of three ways.

5. You are providing care for an 8-year-old child who is in isolation because he has chicken pox. How would you explain to him why he can't leave his room and go to the playroom? What could you do to relieve his boredom?

6. You are changing the linens in Mrs. Wang's isolation room when you realize that you brought only one sheet instead of two. How would you handle this problem? What would you do first?

7. How can you help Mrs. Wang get the information she needs about isolation and infection control? How can you help her with her feelings of loneliness?

8. When you arrive at Amber Clark's apartment at 9:00 A.M. to provide home health care, you discover the remains of the previous night's casserole sitting on the kitchen counter. What should you do?

9. When you put on gloves to help Mr. Wilson with mouth care, he eyes the gloves and says, "I don't have AIDS, you know. Why are you wearing those things?" How should you respond?

10. Emma Jones, who works as a nurse assistant, became engaged over the weekend. She wants to wear her new engagement ring to work on Monday so that she can show it off. What does she need to consider when deciding whether to wear the ring?

8

Measuring Life Signs

Goals

After reading this chapter you will have the information to—

Discuss the importance of measuring vital signs.

Know when and how to measure vital signs.

Help improve a person's cardiovascular and respiratory function.

After practicing the corresponding skills in the skills book, you will be able to—

Read, clean, and shake down a glass thermometer.

Take and record a person's oral, rectal, and axillary temperature with a glass thermometer.

Use an eletronic thermometer.

Count and record a person's radial pulse and respirations.

Take and record a person's blood pressure.

When you arrive on duty today at Morningside Nursing Home, you learn that you will provide care for Agnes Ryan. You have provided care for Mrs. Ryan before and know that, although she is 90 years old and has arthritis, she is an active, interesting woman. She stays out of bed much of the day, talking with staff and other residents.

Today, however, you discover Mrs. Ryan in bed, coughing a dry, hacking cough. When she tries to talk to you, she coughs even more. Between coughs she manages to tell you that she aches all over. Her face looks flushed, and when you touch her she feels warm and dry.

When you report these changes in Mrs. Ryan to your supervising nurse, she tells you to take her vital signs. You try to take her temperature orally, but she cannot keep the thermometer in her mouth because of the cough. Her vital signs are not what they normally are: Her temperature is 103.6 degrees Fahrenheit rectally, her pulse is 110 and thready, and her respirations are 26 and shallow. Her blood pressure is 134/94, which is higher than it usually is. You report the vital signs to your supervising nurse, who goes to Mrs. Ryan's room to do a further assessment. She says that she will phone Mrs. Ryan's doctor.

Before leaving Mrs. Ryan's room to call the doctor, your supervising nurse tells you to make sure that she rests in bed and drinks plenty of fluids. A short time later, while you are giving Mrs. Ryan some juice, your supervising nurse returns with some medicine for the fever. Shortly after Mrs. Ryan takes the medicine, her doctor arrives, examines her, and orders a liquid medicine for the cough and antibiotic capsules to prevent an infection.

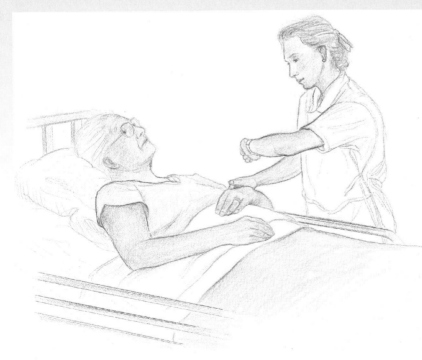

Later in the day, your supervising nurse commends you for being alert in your observations and taking accurate vital signs. She tells you that, because Mrs. Ryan received medicine for her symptoms quickly, she will be more comfortable. In addition, she says, the antibiotic prevents pneumonia, which can be life-threatening for older people.

Using Vital Signs to Measure Body Function

When you walked into Mrs. Ryan's room, you knew that things were not as they usually were. You heard Mrs. Ryan coughing, you saw that her face was flushed as she lay in her bed, and you felt that her skin was warm to the touch. You used your senses to observe that something was wrong with Mrs. Ryan.

These observations alerted you and your supervising nurse to check further. For example, you measured her body temperature to determine if she had a fever. You also measured her pulse rate to know how fast or slow her heart was beating, her respiration rate to determine how fast or slow she was breathing, and her blood pressure to see how much pressure her blood was putting on the walls of her arteries.

vital
Necessary for life.

Temperature, pulse, respiration, and blood pressure all are **vital** indicators of life. In the medical world, the measures of a person's temperature, pulse, respiration, and blood pressure are called vital signs. Vital signs give you information about how the person's body is functioning.

In this chapter, you will learn how to measure a person's vital signs. Health care workers use their own language for talking about vital signs. They talk about a person's TPR, which stands for **t**emperature, **p**ulse, and **r**espiration, and BP, which stands for **b**lood **p**ressure. When you take someone's TPR and BP, you record the numbers as "readings." The nurse and doctor use the TPR and BP readings to decide what treatment or medication the person may need. The importance of these readings to the person's care makes it essential that you measure these signs accurately, record them correctly, and report any changes in them to your supervising nurse.

When to Measure Vital Signs

Two times that you always measure a person's vital signs are: (1) when the person is admitted to a hospital or nursing home or when she first starts receiving care in her home, and (2) when you observe a change in someone's usual condition. When a person first starts receiving care, your supervising nurse may ask you to take her vital signs frequently, because it is one way to tell how her body is functioning. These frequent readings let the doctor know the usual vital sign numbers for that person. After the doctor knows a person's usual numbers, he may order the vital signs to be taken on a less frequent, but regular, basis. The frequency varies from one person to another. For example, someone who has a heart problem needs to have her vital signs measured more often than a person who has no heart problem or other major illness.

If you observe and report a change in a person's condition, your supervising nurse may ask you to take her vital signs more frequently. The changes you observe may be physical or behavioral. When you saw that Mrs. Ryan was flushed and felt that she was warm to the touch, you observed a physical change (Figure 8-1). When you observed that Mrs. Ryan, who is usually active and sociable, was tired

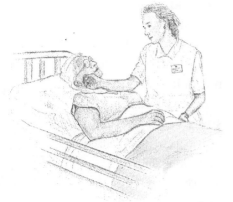

Figure 8-1

Use the back of your hand to determine if a person's skin feels warm to the touch, because the back of your hand is more sensitive than the palm.

Glass ther	Oral	Rectal	Auxill
O – 5-8 min	surger oral	surgery	tip in the middle
A – 10 min	oxygen	heart attack	
R – 3 min	nose feeding	diarrea	
		R. blockge	

Radial pulse   eye level
Apical pulse   breastbone

and stayed in bed, you observed a behavioral change. When your supervising nurse asked you to take vital signs, your observations were verified: Mrs. Ryan's body temperature was high, she had a **thready pulse**, her respirations were **shallow**, and her blood pressure was high.

Responding to the Person's Needs When Taking Vital Signs

Measuring vital signs is part of providing regular care. If you work in a hospital or nursing home, you may be asked to take the vital signs of everyone who needs to have them taken at that time, or you may take just one person's vital signs. If you provide care in a client's home, you take the vital signs of just one person at a time.

Some employers may refer to taking vital signs as "routine vital signs." The word "routine" refers to *which signs* you measure—not to *how* you measure them. You always observe the six principles of care when you take a person's vital signs. For example, you remember to provide privacy for a person while you are measuring her vital signs.

You also have to be sensitive to how a person feels about having her vital signs measured. One person may be afraid of or upset about having her temperature, pulse, or blood pressure taken. Another may worry because she believes it means she is sick. Sometimes a person in your care may be tired and may not want to be bothered. Or a person may be embarrassed because you must take a **rectal** temperature through the **anal** opening.

As you take a person's vital signs, be sure to do these three things: (1) Reassure her that the procedures are important to her care, (2) ensure her dignity and privacy, especially when taking a rectal temperature, and (3) most important, perform the skills accurately.

Measuring a Person's Body Temperature

Body temperature indicates the amount of heat in a person's body. The human body keeps its temperature fairly constant by responding to heat and cold. If the body gets hot, it sweats to get rid of some of the heat, or it breathes more air in and out of the lungs. When the body gets cold, it shivers to create heat from muscle activity.

Normal Range of Body Temperature

Body temperature can vary slightly from one person to another and among age groups (Figure 8-2). A person's normal body temperature usually changes slightly during the day. Generally, it is lower in the morning after sleeping, when body functions have slowed down, and higher in the afternoon after activity. A person's body temperature may rise when her emotions increase and may fall when she feels depressed. It also may increase or decrease with the temperature of the air.

What is a normal body temperature? No single temperature is normal for everyone, because body temperature changes in response to

thready pulse
A condition in which the force of the pulse is very weak.

shallow
Not deep.

rectal
(REK-tuhl)   Of or referring to the lower portion of the large intestine just inside the anal opening.

anal
(A-nuhl)   Of or relating to the opening at the end of the rectum through which feces pass.

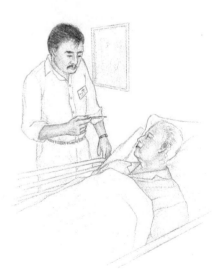

Figure 8-2
Body temperature usually is higher in newborns and lower in the elderly.

Table 8-1 Normal Range of Body Temperatures for Three Methods of Measurement

Method	Normal Range (° F)	Average (° F)
Axillary	96.6 to 98.6	97.6
Oral	97.6 to 99.6	98.6
Rectal	98.6 to 100.6	99.6

many things. Instead, a range of numbers describes what is normal for most people. You have to know the normal range of body temperatures, because you must report temperatures above or below the normal range to your supervising nurse. If a person has a temperature reading above the normal range, illness has caused a fever.

You will learn to measure temperature in four different ways. When you place an instrument called a thermometer in a person's mouth, you are taking an *oral temperature*. When you place the thermometer under a person's arm, you are taking an *axillary temperature*. (The underarm is called the axilla.) When you insert the thermometer in a person's rectum, you are taking a *rectal temperature*. When you place a probe in a person's ear, you are taking a *tympanic temperature*. (The eardrum is called the tympanic membrane.) The normal range of temperatures is different for each of the first three methods of taking body temperature, and the tympanic method can reflect either the oral or the rectal range.

A thermometer measures temperature in units called "degrees." Degrees can be measured on two different scales: Fahrenheit or Celsius. On the Fahrenheit scale, the freezing point of water is 32 degrees, and the average, normal human body temperature is 98.6 degrees. On the Celsius scale, the freezing point of water is 0 degrees, and the average normal human body temperature is 37 degrees. In this book, temperatures are measured on the Fahrenheit scale. Fahrenheit is abbreviated as "F." Table 8-1 shows the normal range of body temperatures for each of the first three methods of measuring body temperatures. A recent study suggests a slightly different range of normal adult temperatures and average temperature.* At this time, however, the temperatures in Table 8-1 are still the accepted ones. The average body temperature varies quite a bit, depending on which method you use to measure it. For example, compared to the average oral temperature of 98.6 degrees Farhenheit, the average axillary temperature is 1 degree lower and the average rectal temperature is 1 degree higher.

*Mackowiak MD et al: A critical appraisal of 98.6° F, the upper limit of the normal body temperature, and other legacies of Carl Reinhold August Wunderlich, *JAMA* 268:1578, 1992.

Types of Thermometers

To take a person's temperature, use one of three types of thermometers: glass, electronic, or tympanic.

Glass thermometer.   A glass thermometer is made of clear glass with a hollow shaft in the middle, which contains mercury. Mercury travels from a bulb at one end of the thermometer through the shaft toward the other end, called the stem. When taking someone's temperature, insert the bulb end of the thermometer into the person's mouth, under her arm, or into her rectum. The bulb warms from body heat, and the mercury moves further up the shaft toward the stem. Because it takes time for the mercury to warm to the same temperature as its surroundings, it is important not to remove the thermometer too soon, or the reading will not be accurate.

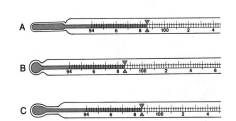

Figure 8-3

Three types of glass thermometers are **A,** oral, **B,** rectal, and **C,** security.

Three types of glass thermometers are oral, rectal, and security (Figure 8-3). They differ in the shapes of their mercury bulbs. The oral glass thermometer, which you use for taking only oral temperatures, has a long, slender bulb. The rectal and security thermometers have rounder, stubbier bulbs. You should use the rectal thermometer for taking only rectal temperatures, but you can use the security thermometer for taking oral, rectal, or axillary temperatures.

Although you can use the security thermometer for all three methods of taking body temperature, once you use a thermometer to take a rectal temperature, you should never use it to take an oral or axillary temperature. To avoid confusion, the thermometer manufacturer often colors the ends of thermometers in red if they are going to be used for taking rectal temperatures. (To remember this clue, think "Red for Rectal.")

As you read earlier, glass thermometers are marked in either degrees Fahrenheit (F) or degrees Celsius (C). The shaft of a glass thermometer is marked with a series of long and short lines extending from 94 to 108 degrees Fahrenheit or from 34 to 43 degrees Celsius. On a Fahrenheit thermometer, each long line on the thermometer represents 1 degree, and each of the four shorter lines between the long lines represents 0.2 degree. On a Celsius thermometer, each long line represents 1 degree, but each shorter line in between represents 0.1 degree. See Skill 5 in the skills book and look again at Figure 8-3 to see the lines on the thermometers.

Electronic thermometer.   The electronic thermometer is a small, battery-operated machine that looks something like a calculator. It is connected to a probe that resembles a thermometer, but it has no mercury. A person's body temperature is calculated electronically inside the machine. The machine beeps when the person's temperature has been registered, and the number of the temperature appears on a small digital screen.

You can use an electronic thermometer to take a temperature by any method (Figure 8-4). It measures a person's body temperature in 2 to 60 seconds. The probe of the thermometer has a disposable

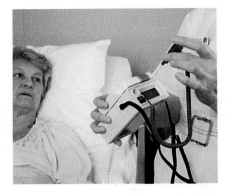

Figure 8-4

An electronic thermometer can be used to measure oral, rectal, or axillary body temperature.

cover, which you throw away after taking the person's temperature. Probes on electronic thermometers also may be colored red for the rectal method and blue for the oral and axillary methods.

Tympanic thermometer.   The tympanic thermometer, which is becoming more widely used, measures heat waves given off by the eardrum. This type of thermometer has a specially designed probe that you place in the person's ear to measure the heat waves and translate them into a temperature reading, which is displayed on a digital screen. The tympanic thermometer is accurate and fast (Figure 8-5).

Cleaning a Glass Thermometer

Glass thermometers are fragile and can break easily, so they must be stored in holders. In some health care settings, glass thermometers are all stored together in one container. In most homes, thermometers are stored in individual holders at the bedside or in the bathroom. A holder protects a thermometer from breaking, but it also provides a place for germs to grow. Because of this possibility of infection, you must wash a glass thermometer with soap and water twice: before you use it—to remove any germs that may have grown while it was stored in the holder, and after you use it—to remove secretions that may harbor germs. Use cold water, because hot water can cause the mercury to shoot through the shaft and break the glass. Use soap and water rather than alcohol to clean a thermometer. When cleaning a glass thermometer, follow the specific procedure that is explained step by step in Skill 5 in the skills book.

Taking a Person's Temperature with a Glass Thermometer

When taking a person's oral temperature, make sure that she has not had recent mouth surgery and does not have a mouth disease. Also make sure that she is not receiving oxygen and is not having trouble breathing, is not confused or unconscious, and is not paralyzed on one side of her body or face. Do not take an oral temperature if she is breathing through her mouth or if she has a tube in her nose. Do not take a child's oral temperature if she is under the age of 5. Also delay taking the person's temperature by 15 minutes if she has eaten, smoked, or had anything to drink within the past 15 minutes.

To take an accurate oral temperature using a glass thermometer, you must understand how the thermometer works and what conditions can affect the reading.

Before using the thermometer, make sure that it is in perfect condition and is not chipped, cracked, or broken. Make sure the mercury is mostly contained in the bulb, rather than in the shaft of the thermometer. To move the mercury into the bulb, "shake down" the thermometer with a flick of your wrist until the mercury column is below 94 degrees.

After placing the bulb of the thermometer in the person's mouth, allow at least 5 minutes for the mercury to register the person's internal body temperature. If you take the oral temperature of an adult

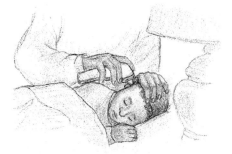

Figure 8-5
The use of the tympanic thermometer does not require the removal of clothing, which makes it less frightening to children than the rectal or axillary methods.

in your care, you usually do not have to hold the thermometer in place. You can make use of the waiting time by measuring and recording other vital signs. (If you take a rectal or axillary temperature and have to hold the thermometer in place, you won't be able to record other signs at the same time.) When taking a person's oral temperature with a glass thermometer, follow the specific procedure that is explained step by step in Skill 6 in the skills book. Generally, the oral method is the preferred way to measure a person's body temperature, because it is the easiest method and requires little preparation. Taken correctly, it is an accurate reflection of the body's internal temperature.

The rectal method for measuring a person's body temperature also accurately reflects internal body temperature, but it requires more preparation and can be embarrassing for adults and frightening for children. Take a person's rectal temperature when an oral temperature would be inaccurate or might cause injury. When taking a person's rectal temperature with a glass thermometer, always use a rectal thermometer that is in perfect condition. Make sure that the person does not have diarrhea or a blocked rectum. Make sure that she has not recently had a heart attack or rectal surgery or injury or that she does not have hemorrhoids. Allow at least 3 minutes for the temperature to register. Follow the specific procedure that is explained step by step in Skill 7 in the skills book.

The axillary method is the least accurate way to measure a person's body temperature. This method requires you to keep the thermometer in place for 10 minutes. Take an axillary temperature only if the person cannot tolerate either an oral or a rectal thermometer. Make sure the person is sitting or lying down during the procedure and not walking around with the thermometer under her arm. Use only a glass thermometer that is in perfect condition. When taking a person's axillary temperature with a glass thermometer, follow the specific procedure that is explained step by step in Skill 8 in the skills book.

Sometimes certain situations require you to take special precautions when measuring a person's body temperature. Read Table 8-2 on p. 178 to learn how to respond to these situations.

Taking a Person's Temperature with an Electronic Thermometer

Electronic thermometers are quick and easy to use. You do not have to clean the electronic unit or shake it down as you provide care from one person to another. You insert the probe of the thermometer, which has a disposable cover, into the mouth, rectum, or axilla of a person in your care. The unit beeps to indicate when the internal body temperature has registered and displays this number on a small digital screen. After you discard the probe cover, the thermometer is ready for reuse.

Some electronic thermometers operate on nonrechargeable batteries, and others periodically have to be plugged into recharging devices so that they are always ready to use. Because most health care

Table 8-2   Precautions for Using a Glass Thermometer

Situation	Problem	Solution
Chipped, cracked, or broken glass on thermometer	Can cut mouth, lips, rectum, or axilla	Check thermometer before use and discard if chipped, cracked, or broken
Broken thermometer	Mercury is a poison that can injure the person who touches or swallows it	Check thermometer before use; follow employer's guidelines for cleaning up a broken thermometer
Person just drank hot or cold fluid or smoked a cigarette	Temperature of fluid or cigarette smoke influences temperature of mouth	Wait 15 minutes before taking oral temperature or use another method if permissible
Person has had recent mouth surgery or has mouth disease	Thermometer may cause injury	Take temperature using rectal, axillary, or tympanic method
Confused person	May bite down on thermometer and may injure herself	Take temperature using rectal, axillary, or tympanic method
Unconscious person or person paralyzed on one side of body	May not be able to keep mouth closed, resulting in inaccurate temperature reading	Take temperature using rectal, axillary, or tympanic method
Person has trouble breathing or breathes through mouth, or person has tube in nose and cannot keep mouth closed	Cannot get accurate temperature reading	Take temperature using rectal, axillary, or tympanic method
Person receiving oxygen experiences cooling of the body tissues around the mouth	Cannot get accurate temperature reading	Take temperature using rectal, axillary, or tympanic method
Person has a blocked rectum, hemorrhoids, or has had recent rectal surgery	Rectal thermometer can cause injury	Take temperature using oral, axillary, or tympanic method
Person has had a heart attack	Rectal thermometer may stimulate the urge to strain and may increase the workload of the heart	Take temperature using oral, axillary, or tympanic method
Person is embarrassed about having rectal temperature taken	May be uncooperative	Explain the reason for taking rectal temperature to encourage cooperation
Person perspires under the arms	Moisture can affect the temperature reading	Dry the axilla with a tissue

facilities have a minimum number of electronic thermometers, it is important that each caregiver replaces the equipment immediately after use so that it is available for others to use.

An electronic thermometer is often used for many people, so you must practice good infection control procedures. Remember not to put the thermometer down on dirty surfaces. If the thermometer has a cord, place it around your neck so that the only part that contacts the person or his surroundings is the probe cover.

Periodically, some electronic thermometers may have to be recalibrated, or readjusted. If you suspect that a thermometer is not giving an accurate body temperature reading (for example, every person's temperature that you take is exactly the same), let your supervising nurse know so that the machine can be repaired. When taking a person's temperature with an electronic thermometer, follow the specific procedure that is explained step by step in Skill 9 in the skills book.

Taking a Child's Temperature

For children under 5 years of age, take a rectal, axillary, or tympanic temperature. The rectal or tympanic methods are preferred, because they provide the most reliable measurement of temperature. However, if a child is very upset or uncooperative and a tympanic thermometer is not available, it is safer to take an axillary temperature rather than a rectal one. As with adults, do not take a rectal temperature if a child has diarrhea or has had rectal surgery.

To take an infant's rectal temperature, position the baby on her back. Hold her ankles up with one hand and bend her knees to expose the anus (Figure 8-6). With the other hand gently insert only the bulb of the lubricated thermometer into the rectum and hold it in place for 3 minutes. Always hold onto the thermometer while it is in the rectum.

To take a child's rectal temperature, have the child lie on his side with his knees flexed, or have him lie on his stomach. A child may be more likely to cooperate if he is held across his parent's lap while you take his rectal temperature (Figure 8-7). Be sure to insert the bulb gently, insert only the bulb, and hold the thermometer in place while the child's temperature is registering.

For children over the age of 5 years, take an oral temperature. However, use a security thermometer, rather than an oral thermometer, because it is easier for a child to hold in his mouth. Always stay with a child who has a thermometer in his mouth to make sure that he remains still— lying down or seated— so that he doesn't break the thermometer or injure himself.

The normal temperature for a child is the same as it is for an adult, although a child's temperature may change very rapidly. Young children especially can run very high temperatures. If you work in a hospital, be sure to report any temperature changes immediately. In a home setting, refer to the chart in Table 8-3 to help you decide when and to whom to report temperature changes.

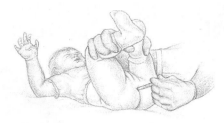

Figure 8-6
Hold an infant's ankles to keep her from kicking when you take her temperature.

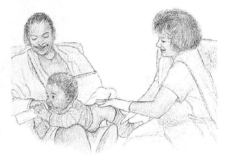

Figure 8-7
The security of being held by a parent often calms a child and helps him cooperate.

Table 8-3   **When to Report a Child's Temperature Change in a Home Setting**

Report to Your Supervising Nurse Immediately When the Child Is. . . .	And the Axillary Temperature Is*. . . .	Or the Rectal Temperature Is. . . .
Under 4 months old	99° F or higher	101° F or higher
Over 4 months old	103° F or higher	105° F or higher

*When the axillary temperature is this high, take a rectal temperature, if possible, to confirm the reading. Report the high temperature immediately to your supervising nurse, or, if she is not available, report it to someone else in authority who can take immediate action or direct you to monitor the child's condition.

BodyBasics

Carotid artery

Jugular vein

Brachial artery

Superior vena cava

Pulmonary artery

Heart

Aorta

Inferior vena cava

Radial artery

Femoral artery and vein

BodyBasics

❖   The Cardiovascular System   ❖

Life depends on a heart that pumps blood. Using blood vessels as its vehicle, blood travels throughout the body, making its first stop at the lungs to pick up oxygen for delivery to every cell. During the blood's return trip to the heart, the liver and kidneys filter out harmful and useless waste.

The heart, made mostly of thick muscle, is about the size of a man's fist and weighs about 12 ounces. It is divided into four compartments, called chambers, which are separated by small valves that act like miniature swinging doors that keep blood flowing in one direction. Several blood vessels supply the heart with blood.

Blood vessels called arteries carry blood away from the heart. The largest artery, the aorta, has strong, elastic walls that won't tear under the high pressure of the blood as it is pumped from the heart. Arteries that carry blood to the internal organs and arms and legs are smaller, and smaller still are the arterioles that carry blood to individual cells. Blood vessels called veins carry blood on its return

trip to the heart. Veins are thinner than arteries because they carry blood under less pressure.

Blood is made of cells and plasma, the fluid that carries the cells. Red cells carry oxygen, white cells fight infection, and platelets help clot the blood.

How the Cardiovascular System Ages

As people grow older, their veins and arteries lose some of their elasticity, so blood pressure may rise and circulation may decrease. Poor eating habits, little exercise, and a family history of heart disease increase an older person's chance of having a heart attack.

Fascinating Fact

Our bodies have 10,000,000,000 (10 billion) tiny blood vessels called capillaries that connect arteries and veins. They are so small that red blood cells, visible only through a microscope, have to squeeze through them in single file.

Measuring a Person's Pulse

When your supervising nurse asked you to check Mrs. Ryan's vital signs, one of the signs you checked was her pulse. The pulse indicates how the cardiovascular system is working. (See Body Basics, The Cardiovascular System.) Each time the heart beats, it pushes blood through tiny tubes called arteries that carry blood throughout the body. The heartbeat creates a wave, which you can feel if you put your fingers over certain places on the body. In between beats, the heart rests. Then it beats again, causing another wave that you can feel. The wave that you can feel is called the pulse.

The pulse provides information about how a person's heart is working, and this information helps the doctor plan her care. Because this information is so important, you must be able to describe what the pulse feels like.

You can compare a pulse that comes at regular intervals to the ticking of a clock. You can describe this pulse as having a regular rhythm. If the interval between pulses is uneven, describe the rhythm as being *irregular*. If the force of the pulse is easy to feel, describe it as a *full* or *strong pulse*. If the force of the pulse seems to push up against your fingertips, describe it as a *bounding pulse*. If the force

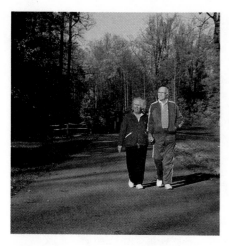

Figure 8-8
Even a slight amount of exercise can make a person's heart beat faster. If you know a person has been exercising, wait 5 to 10 minutes before taking his or her pulse.

stethoscope
(STETH-o-skope)   An instrument used to listen to body sounds.

of the pulse is very weak and you can barely feel it, describe it as a *thready pulse*. When you use these words to describe how the person's pulse feels, you give the doctor information about the person's heart.

When you count the number of times you feel a person's pulse beat in a minute, you know the rate at which the person's heart is beating. This number is called the heart rate, or pulse rate. Many things can cause the pulse rate to speed up or slow down (Figure 8-8). Think of a time when you felt like your heart was beating very fast. Perhaps you were scared or had just run up a flight of stairs. Maybe you were excited, upset, or angry, which caused your heart to beat faster. Other conditions that may speed up your pulse rate are pain, fever, or significant blood loss. Mrs. Ryan had pain and fever with the flu, and her heart rate was faster than normal. Just as some things can speed up pulse rate, other things, such as sleep, certain drugs, and depression, can slow it down.

Because so many things can affect the pulse rate, it is important to count the pulse when the person is sitting quietly. The average rate for an adult is between 60 and 84 beats per minute, although athletes have slower-than-average rates that may even fall below 60 beats per minute. The average rate for a 6-year-old child is between 70 and 110 beats per minute, and it is even higher for infants.

You can feel the pulse in several places on a person's body. Table 8-4 describes the seven common places where you can feel the pulse.

Most of the time you measure a person's radial pulse on the wrist, and, except for the apical pulse at the top of the heart, you use the same procedure regardless of which pulse area you use. To measure an apical pulse, you use a **stethoscope** because you cannot feel an apical pulse with your fingers. (Read about the stethoscope later in this chapter in the section on measuring a person's blood pressure.) Because you usually take all vital signs at the same time, you can

Table 8-4   **Where to Feel the Pulse**

Pulse Area	Location
1. Apical	At the top of the heart, just under the left breast
2. Brachial	At the inside bend of the elbow
3. Carotid	On the neck on the side of the Adam's apple
4. Femoral	At the groin where the thigh meets the hip
5. Pedal	On the top of the foot
6. Radial	On the inside of the wrist at the base of the thumb
7. Temporal	At the side of the forehead above the outer corner of the eye

count a person's pulse while you are waiting for her oral temperature to register. You may notice that, when a person's temperature
rises, her pulse rate also rises. This condition occurs because, for
each degree Fahrenheit that body temperature rises, the heart beats 8
to 10 beats faster per minute.

Counting and Recording a Person's Radial Pulse

When you are getting ready to take a person's pulse, approach her in
a calm, unhurried manner so that she does not become upset or agitated and her heart rate does not increase. Make sure that she is in a
comfortable, relaxed position. If she has just come back from a stren-
uous physical therapy session, or has just had a painful procedure
done, remember that these experiences will increase her heart rate.
If possible, you should come back a little later after she has had time
to relax.

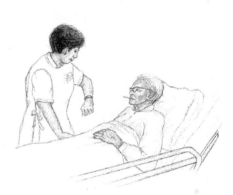

Figure 8-9
Usually you take the person's pulse
along with her oral temperature.

When you are first learning to take a radial pulse, it is easy to push
too hard on the wrist and flatten the artery so that you don't feel anything. Remember to press lightly against the wrist, with your fingers
over the radial pulse (Figure 8-9), and count the number of beats per
minute, using a watch with a second hand. Until you become comfortable with counting the pulse rate, start timing the pulse when the
second hand is on the "12" so that you don't lose track of when you
started counting. Never use your thumb to feel a person's pulse, because your thumb has its own pulse and you may count *your* pulse
rate instead of the person's pulse rate. Count the pulses for 1 full
minute. Note the pulse rhythm and force so that you can describe
them accurately. Write down the pulse rate immediately, noting any
irregularities in the rhythm and any changes in the force that you
feel.

Report any irregularities in rhythm and any pulse rate that is below 60 beats per minute or above 100 beats per minute to your supervising nurse. Irregular rhythms and very slow or very fast rates
may indicate a medical problem. Earlier, when you measured Mrs.
Ryan's vital signs, her pulse was faster than usual because of her pain
and fever. When taking a person's radial pulse, always keep the person's arm close to her body and not in the air. Follow the specific
procedure that is explained step by step in Skill 10 in the skills book.

Taking an Apical Pulse

When measuring the pulse of some adults and younger children
whose arteries are small and whose heartbeats are fast, you must take
an apical pulse. You use a stethoscope to count the apical pulse by
listening to it rather than feeling it. With a stethoscope, you are listening to the heart beat, which should reflect the same beats per
minute as those felt at other pulse points. Count the beats for 1 full
minute, and record the number of beats as the apical pulse rate. To
take an apical pulse, follow the procedure that is explained step by
step in Skill 10 in the skills book.

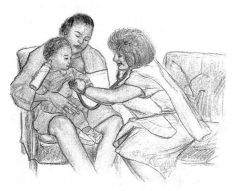

Figure 8-10
Being held by a parent may calm a child, allowing you to get a more accurate pulse reading.

Taking a Child's Pulse

A small child typically is afraid of an unfamiliar person, especially a nurse assistant approaching with strange-looking equipment. It is difficult to take a child's pulse rate if he is crying or upset. Try to enlist the child's cooperation and encourage the parent to hold the child (Figure 8-10). To help the child relax, let him play with another stethoscope or play a listening game. Because activity can affect the reading, report what the child was doing when you took his pulse.

The average pulse rates for children of different age ranges appear in Table 8-5.

Table 8-5   **Pulse Rates in Children**

Age	Pulse Rate (beats per minute)
Newborn to 1 year	140 to 170
1 to 2 years	80 to 160
2 to 6 years	80 to 130
6 to 14 years	70 to 110
14 to 18 years	60 to 100

Counting and Recording a Person's Respirations

Respiration, the process of breathing, consists of two parts: inspiration and expiration. Taking breath in is called *inspiration,* and letting breath out is called *expiration.* One rise (inspiration) and fall (expiration) of the chest equals one respiration. (See Body Basics, The Respiratory System, on p. 186.)

How do you know if a person's breathing is normal? A person with normal respiration breathes quietly and easily. Her breathing seems effortless and regular. If you watch her chest, you see both sides of her chest rise and fall equally.

How do you know if a person's breathing is **abnormal**? Difficult, erratic, or noisy breathing is considered abnormal. Abnormal breathing indicates that the person is experiencing some medical problem. You may observe that a person is breathing abnormally if—

❖ She sounds like she has a rattle or wetness in her chest.
❖ Her breathing is uneven.
❖ She has **dyspnea**.
❖ Her lips look blue or gray and the base of her fingernails looks blue. (Either of these conditions, called **cyanosis**, develops when a person doesn't get enough oxygen. Oxygen-rich blood is bright red, while blood that is low in oxygen is darker and looks blue through the skin.)

abnormal
(ab-NOR-muhl)   Not normal or regular.

dyspnea
(disp-NEE-uh)   The condition of having difficulty in breathing.

cyanosis
(si-uh-NO-sis)   The condition of having a blue or gray color, due to lack of oxygen in the blood.

If you observe any of these abnormal signs, report them immediately to your supervising nurse.

Many things affect the way a person breathes. A person who slouches may not breathe deeply, because her lungs don't have room to expand. Another person with lung or heart problems may have difficulty breathing when he is lying flat. To breathe comfortably, he may need to sit up, have his bed elevated, or use several pillows (Figure 8-11).

The same things that make a person's heart beat faster also make her breathe faster, such as exercise, anger, fear, pain, excitement, fever, and significant blood loss. Likewise, the same things that slow down her heart rate can also slow down her breathing, such as rest, depression, and certain drugs.

Sometimes, especially after exercise, a person's body may need to take in more air. Her chest rises more to create more space for air to enter. This condition is called deep breathing. If the chest rises and falls very little, as it does during sleep, this type of breathing is called shallow.

Because a person can make herself breathe faster or slower just by deciding to do so, you must count her respirations without her being aware of what you are doing. Usually, you count a person's respirations when you take her oral temperature and before or after taking her pulse. If you count her pulse first and continue to keep your fingers on her wrist, she may not be aware that you are counting her respirations. Count the person's respirations for 1 full minute, counting one rise and one fall of the chest for each respiration (Figure 8-12). When counting and recording a person's respirations, follow the specific procedure that is explained step by step in Skill 11 in the skills book.

Counting an Adult's Respirations

A normal healthy adult breathes 14 to 20 times a minute. Because loud noises or pain can affect the reading, note if either of these situations occurred while you were counting. Earlier, when you counted Mrs. Ryan's respirations, they were fast and shallow due to her pain and fever.

Counting a Child's Respirations

For an accurate reading, count a child's respirations while she is quiet or asleep. If you also plan to take a temperature or blood pressure reading, count the respirations first in case the child becomes upset and starts to cry. Respiration rates in children are higher than in adults (Table 8-6) and may be irregular. Report if the child has an abnormal rate or any difficulty breathing.

Taking and Recording a Person's Blood Pressure

Blood pressure measures the pressure of the circulating blood on the walls of the arteries. Each time the heart beats, it pumps blood

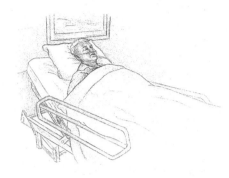

Figure 8-11
Because Mr. Lightfoot has difficulty breathing, the head of his bed is elevated to help him breathe more easily.

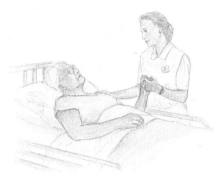

Figure 8-12
Mrs. Ryan's respirations are fast and shallow due to her pain and fever.

BodyBasics

❖ The Respiratory System ❖

The human body depends on oxygen to live. Without it, the heart couldn't beat, the stomach couldn't digest food, and hair wouldn't grow. Air containing oxygen enters the body through the respiratory system.

When a person inhales, air enters the body through the mouth and nose. It swirls through the sinuses, the hollow spaces in the skull, and then makes its way through the trachea, or windpipe, the thick tube that leads from the throat to the lungs. On its trip to the lungs, tiny hairs called cilia warm and clean the air.

This warmed air continues along the trachea, which splits into two slightly smaller tubes called bronchi, which enter the right and left lungs. The bronchi divide again and again like branches of a tree, becoming smaller and smaller tubes that end in little air spaces called alveoli.

Each lung has millions of alveoli that conduct the real business of respiration, the exchange of life-giving oxygen and body waste called carbon dioxide. Blood flows past the alveoli and picks up oxygen from the air in the lungs. Then, the alveoli take the body's wastes from the blood, which the person blows out by exhaling air through the same path as the air that was inhaled.

How the Respiratory System Ages

As people age, their lungs become less elastic, and their rib cage muscles may become weak, resulting in shallow breathing and a greater chance of developing pneumonia or other lung infections.

Fascinating Fact

We each have 300,000,000 (300 million) alveoli, a number that is greater than the number of people in the United States. If one person's alveoli were opened up and spread out flat, they would cover an area equal to about eight room-size carpets.

Table 8-6 Respiration Rates in Children

Age	Normal Rate (times per minute)
Newborn to 1 year	35
1 to 2 years	30
2 to 6 years	20 to 25
6 to 10 years	19 to 21
10 to 16 years	17 to 19
16 to 18 years	16 to 18
Adult	16 to 20

BodyBasics

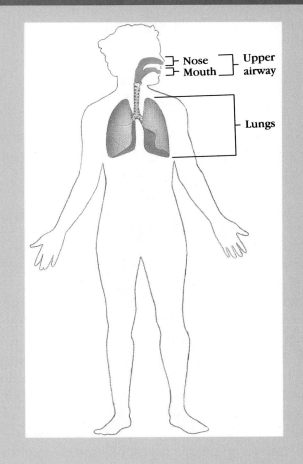

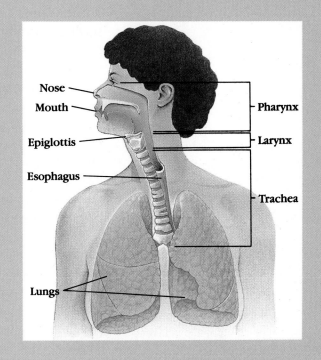

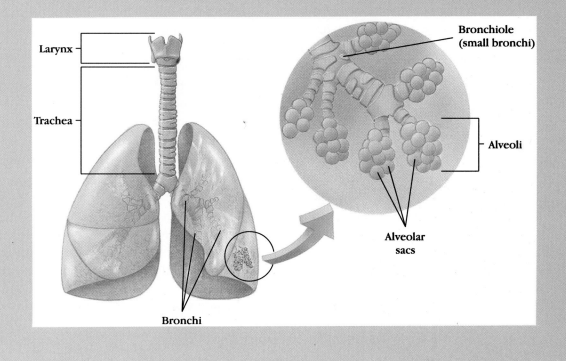

through the heart and lungs and into the arteries. The pressure of the blood against the walls of the arteries when the heart pumps is called the systolic pressure. The pressure of the blood against the walls when the heart relaxes is called the diastolic pressure. A blood pressure reading consists of these two numbers, which are written like fractions. The larger systolic reading goes on the top, and the smaller diastolic reading goes on the bottom. For example, in the number 120/80, 120 is the systolic pressure, and 80 is the diastolic pressure. The systolic pressure is always higher.

To understand blood pressure, imagine the heart as a pump and the arteries as a hose connected to the pump. When you turn on the pump, water is pushed through the hose. When you turn off the pump, water continues to go through the hose for a time, but the pressure inside the hose decreases. The water eventually stops flowing, unless the pump is turned on again. The heart is like the pump—pumping and resting, pumping and resting—as it pushes blood through the arteries.

What would happen if some sand got into the water hose? The sand would make it more difficult for the water to flow through the hose. The sand causes the pressure inside the hose to increase, because the pressure in a tube increases as the size of the opening of a tube decreases. Think about what happens when you put your finger partially over the end of a hose while the water is running through it (Figure 8-13). The opening that the water goes through gets smaller, and the water spurts out farther and harder.

The same thing happens to the arteries in the body if they get clogged up with a fatty substance called cholesterol. The cholesterol buildup makes the openings of the arteries smaller. When the heart pumps blood into the arteries, the pressure inside the arteries increases because the opening is smaller. Fatty, cholesterol-rich foods can clog arteries, and people with clogged arteries may have high blood pressure.

Some other factors that influence the increase or decrease in blood pressure appear in Table 8-7. In addition, men frequently have higher blood pressure than women, and some ethnic groups tend to have higher blood pressures than others. Children whose parents had or have high blood pressure are more likely to develop high blood pressure. For all people, blood pressure varies throughout the day and is usually lowest in the morning when they first get up.

What is a normal blood pressure reading for an adult? Each person has a blood pressure range that is normal or usual for her. A systolic reading that ranges between 90 and 139 is considered normal, and a diastolic reading that ranges between 60 and 89 is considered normal. Blood pressure in children is generally lower than in adults, and blood pressure tends to increase with age because the arteries become narrower and more rigid.

Equipment for Measuring Blood Pressure

You use two pieces of equipment when measuring a person's blood pressure. First, you place a **sphygmomanometer**, consisting of a

pumps blood

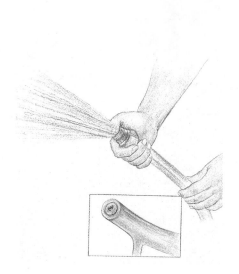

Figure 8-13
There is more pressure in a clogged artery, just as there is more pressure in the hose when you put your thumb over the end of it.

sphygmomanometer
(sfig-mo-ma-NOM-eh-ter) An instrument used to measure blood pressure.

Table 8-7   **Factors That Influence Blood Pressure**

Influencing Factor	Increase(s) Blood Pressure	Decrease(s) Blood Pressure
Arteries clogged with cholesterol	X	
Eating salty foods	X	
Eating fatty foods	X	
Eating healthy foods		X
Alcohol consumption	X	
Being overweight	X	
Lack of exercise	X	
Regular exercise		X
Physical stress	X	X
Smoking	X	
Emotional stress	X	X
Some kidney diseases	X	
Medications	X	X

cuff and a **manometer**, on the person's arm (Figure 8-14). Then you listen to the sounds of her pulse with a stethoscope.

Using a stethoscope.   The stethoscope consists of two pieces of tubing that are connected at one end to a flat disk called a **diaphragm**. The earpieces, which are connected to the other end of the tubing, fit into your ears, and the diaphragm is placed on the person's brachial pulse (refer again to Table 8-4) for measuring blood pressure. The diaphragm amplifies the sound of the pulse, or makes it louder, so that you can hear it better.

Before taking a person's blood pressure, check the tubing and diaphragm for cracks and holes that could make it difficult to hear and could cause you to make an error in the blood pressure reading. To prevent the spread of infection, use alcohol to clean the diaphragm after each contact with a person. If you use a stethoscope that is used by other caregivers and is used on a regular basis, clean the earpieces with alcohol before putting them in your ears. When using a stethoscope to measure a person's blood pressure, follow the specific procedure that is explained step by step in Skill 12 in the skills book.

Using a blood pressure cuff.   The cuff of the sphygmomanometer is placed on the person's bare arm. Do not put it on the side that is weak from a stroke or that is the same side as where a woman has had a breast surgically removed (mastectomy). The cuff is made of

cuff
The inflatable band of a sphygmomanometer that wraps around the arm.

manometer
(ma-NOM-eh-ter)   The gauge on a sphygmomanometer that measures systolic and diastolic blood pressure.

diaphragm
(DYE-uh-fram)   The thin, usually plastic, disk of a stethoscope that is placed on the skin to magnify body sounds.

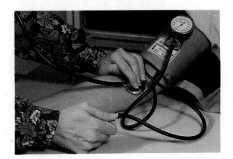

Figure 8-14
Properly using blood pressure equipment takes practice.

bladder
A pouch that holds air inside the cuff of a sphygmomanometer.

valve
A device that controls the flow of air in an instrument such as a sphygmomanometer or fluid in an organ such as the heart.

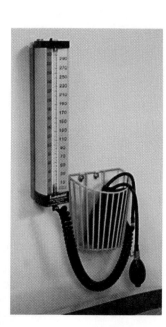

Figure 8-15
A Mercury Manometer

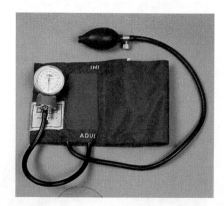

Figure 8-16
An Aneroid Manometer

palpate
To examine by touching or feeling.

fabric and comes in several sizes. It has a rubber **bladder** inside, which is connected at the end to a hose with a rubber ball, called a bulb. A **valve** in the bulb opens and closes to control the flow of air into the bladder. The valve is controlled by a screw. If you turn the screw to the left, it opens the valve and lets the air escape from the bladder. If you turn the screw to the right, it closes the valve so that when you pump air into the bladder with the bulb, the valve keeps the air inside the bladder, making the cuff tight.

When you pump air into the cuff, the bladder pressure increases until it is strong enough to stop the blood flow through the brachial artery. At this point, you don't hear anything through the stethoscope. As you turn the valve to release pressure on the brachial artery, the cuff pressure eventually matches and then drops below the systolic blood pressure. When the cuff pressure reaches this point, you begin to hear the pulse sounds. As the cuff pressure drops to equal the diastolic pressure in the artery, the sounds that you hear change or fade away.

Understanding the manometer.   The gauge that measures systolic and diastolic pressure is called a manometer. The numbers on the gauge show the pressure in millimeters. The larger the number, the greater the pressure. Three types of manometers that you may read are mercury, aneroid, and electronic.

The mercury manometer shows the pressure readings on an upright gauge with a straight column of numbers (Figure 8-15). The mercury moves up the column from zero to the higher numbers as you inflate the cuff. The numbers show the pressure in millimeters of mercury (mm Hg).

The aneroid manometer shows the pressure readings on a round dial with an arrow that points to the numbers (Figure 8-16). Although there is no mercury column, the numbers on the dial are equal to millimeters of mercury (mm Hg). The arrow moves from zero to the higher numbers as you inflate the cuff.

The electronic manometer eliminates the need for using a stethoscope and listening for the pulse sounds, because it takes the blood pressure readings for you and displays them on a digital screen like the one on an electronic thermometer.

Taking a Person's Blood Pressure

When you take an adult's blood pressure, do it in two steps. First, obtain an estimate of the systolic pressure. Wrap the cuff around the person's arm. **Palpate** the radial pulse. Squeeze the rubber ball to inflate the cuff until you can no longer feel the pulse. The number at which you no longer feel the pulse is the *estimated* systolic pressure. Now that you have an idea of the systolic pressure, let the air out of the cuff quickly to make the person more comfortable.

In the second step, to obtain an accurate reading, locate the brachial pulse and place the diaphragm of the stethoscope over that pulse. Inflate the cuff 30 points beyond your estimated systolic pressure. Then slowly deflate the cuff as you **auscultate** or listen for the pulse sound to begin. The number on the gauge at the point where you begin to hear the pulse sound is the systolic reading. As you continue to deflate the cuff, the pulse sound changes or stops. The number on the gauge at the point where you hear the pulse sound stop is the diastolic reading for an adult.

As you use the equipment, you will learn to adjust the valve so that air is released slowly from the bladder. When you deflate the cuff slowly, it makes a quieter sound, which makes it easier to decide exactly when you hear the pulse sounds appear and disappear. Remember both numbers so that you can record the readings accurately.

Sometimes you may not hear clearly or you may not be sure of what you heard. If you do not hear the pulse clearly, let all the air out of the cuff. Wait 1 minute before you try again. This pause allows time for the blood vessels to relax. Never try to take a person's blood pressure more than twice on one arm because repeated **compressions** of the arteries may give an incorrect reading.

To use the electronic manometer, place the cuff on the person's arm as you do when using the mercury and aneroid manometers. Some machines inflate the cuff automatically, while others require you to inflate the cuff manually with a bulb. When the cuff deflates automatically, the blood pressure reading and usually the pulse appear on the digital screen.

When taking a person's blood pressure, observe the precautions listed in Table 8-8 on p. 192 and follow the specific procedure that is explained step by step in Skill 12 in the skills book.

Taking a Child's Blood Pressure

When you take a child's blood pressure, use the right size cuff. A cuff that is too large gives a reading that is too low. A cuff that is too small gives a reading that is too high. Try to get the child to cooperate during the procedure by using words and concepts that the child understands (Figure 8-17). For example, you may tell the child that the cuff is going to give his arm a "big hug" when you squeeze the black ball. Often it helps if the child sits on his parent's lap.

Table 8-9 on p. 192 lists the range of normal or usual blood pressure readings in children. As a group, younger children generally have lower blood pressures than older children do.

auscultate
(OS-kuhl-tate)   To listen for sounds produced by the body's organs.

compression
(kum-PRESH-un)   The act of pressing or squeezing together.

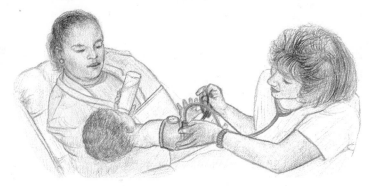

Figure 8-17
You can use an object, such as a toy or bottle, to distract a child and gain cooperation while taking blood pressure.

Table 8-8   Precautions for Taking a Person's Blood Pressure

Precaution	Reason
Place the cuff on the person's bare arm.	Clothing increases the size of the arm and may give an incorrect reading. When the diaphragm is placed on clothing, it creates noises that make it difficult to hear pulse sounds.
Select the correct cuff size: adult-size for most adults, extra-large for some adults, and child-size for small people.	Using the correct size results in an accurate reading.
Wrap the cuff smoothly and snugly.	A smooth wrap gives an accurate reading.
Position the cuff correctly, with the center of the bladder over the brachial artery.	Correct positioning gives an accurate reading.
Do not place the cuff on a cast.	The cuff cannot compress the cast, which results in no reading.
Do not place the cuff on an arm with an IV in place.	The pressure from the cuff could stop the flow of fluid and possibly cause the needle to clog or dislodge from the vein.
Do not place the cuff on the weak arm of a person who has had a stroke, on a person's paralyzed arm, or on the arm on the side of a woman who has had a mastectomy.	Circulation in these conditions is impaired, resulting in an inaccurate reading. Also, an inflated cuff decreases circulation in the arm and may cause some damage.

Table 8-9   Blood Pressure Readings in Children

Age of Child	Systolic Blood Pressure Diastolic Blood Pressure
Newborn to 1 year	65-91 50-56
2 to 5 years	90-95 55-56
6 to 12 years	96-107 57-66
13 to 15 years	109-114 63-67
16 to 18 years	112-121 66-70

Data from Whaley LF, Wong DW: *Nursing Care of Infants and Children,* ed 4, St Louis, 1991, Mosby.

As with all vital signs in a child, blood pressure readings can change very rapidly. Report even small changes in blood pressure to your supervising nurse. Also, be sure to note the activity of the child while you are taking the blood pressure reading so that the significance of any changes can be evaluated.

Improving Cardiovascular and Respiratory Function

When providing care to an elderly person, you can help her improve her cardiovascular and respiratory functions by observing her and monitoring her vital signs. You can remind her to do certain things and encourage her to do things in a certain way. Be patient while she does things for herself and report any concerns about her to your supervising nurse.

Helping a Person's Cardiovascular System Work Better

To help a person's cardiovascular system work better, you can—

❖ Provide more time for the person to complete tasks.
❖ Provide more time for her to rest.
❖ Encourage the person to exercise every day.
❖ Encourage her to eat healthy meals.
❖ Encourage her not to smoke.
❖ Monitor her vital signs.
❖ Observe any changes in her skin, because poor circulation can lead to pressure sores.
❖ Report right away to your supervising nurse if the person has any of the following conditions:
　　Shortness of breath
　　Change in vital signs
　　Change in skin color or injury to her skin

Helping a Person's Respiratory System Work Better

To help a person's respiratory system work better, you can—

❖ Remind the person to take deep breaths during the day, because deep breathing fills the lungs with air and helps them stay more flexible.
❖ Encourage the person to rest between activities, such as between eating and bathing.
❖ Encourage her to take time to stop, rest, and breathe deeply when walking.
❖ When the person is lying down, raise her upper body to make breathing easier.
❖ Encourage her not to smoke.
❖ Report right away to your supervising nurse if the person has any of the following conditions:
　　Shortness of breath
　　Difficulty breathing
　　Blue or gray color (cyanosis)
　　Unusual confusion (often the first sign of pneumonia)

Information Review

Circle the correct answers and fill in the blanks.

1. Temperature, pulse, blood pressure, and respirations usually
    are taken together and are referred to as—
    a. Life measurements.
    b. Vital signs.
    c. Routine measurements.
    d. Monitoring.
2. Two times when you always measure a person's vital signs are
    when the person is ____admitted____ to a hospital,
    nursing home, or home health care and when you observe a
    ____change____ in someone's usual condition.
3. The normal range for an adult's oral temperature is
    ____97.6____ to ____99.6____.
4. An elevation of body temperature is called—
    a. Cyanosis.
    b. Shallow.
    c. Compression.
    d. A fever.
5. Irregular is a term used to describe the
    ____Rhythm____ of a pulse, and thready is a term used
    to describe the ____force____ of a pulse.
6. The ____Brachial____ pulse is located inside the bend
    of the elbow and is used for measuring blood pressure.
7. The instrument used to listen to heart sounds when taking
    blood pressure or an apical pulse is called a—
    a. Stethoscope.
    b. Diaphragm.
    c. Valve.
    d. Thermometer
8. Never use your ____thumb____ to count the pulse on
    another person.
9. Difficulty with breathing is called ____dyspnea____.
10. When you count the number of times a person breathes per
    minute, you are counting her—
    a. Pulse.
    b. Temperature.
    c. Respirations.
    d. Emotional level.

Questions to Ask Yourself

1. You are taking Josie's vital signs. She is complaining of being dizzy, especially when she sits up. Her BP is 90/52. What should you do?

2. What could you do to calm a child who is afraid of having his BP taken?

3. When you go into Mrs. Clement's room to take her oral temperature, you notice a cup of hot coffee on her table. What should you consider, and what should you do?

4. Mr. Smith is smoking when you enter his room to take his temperature. What should you do?

5. You are taking an infant's temperature rectally, and the baby begins to have a bowel movement while the thermometer is in place. What should you do?

6. When you take Mr. Wilson's pulse at 8:00 A.M., the rate is 72 and the rhythm is regular. When you take it again at 9:00 A.M., it is 56 and irregular. What should you do?

7. Mrs. Miller breathes quietly when she is sitting up but begins to breathe noisily and faster as soon as you lower the head of her bed. What should you do?

8. Mr. Rivera is asleep and breathing so quietly that you have difficulty seeing his chest rise and fall. What should you do?

9. Josie keeps trying to carry on a conversation while you are trying to measure and record vital signs. How should you handle this situation? What should you say to her?

10. Baby Jerome is crying when you get ready to take his vital signs. What should you do?

9

Positioning and Transferring People

Goals

After reading this chapter, you will have the information to—

Help prevent bedsores on the people in your care by providing good skin care and changing their body positions.

Assess situations before positioning or transferring people.

Protect your safety and the safety of the people in your care when you position or transfer them.

Make people comfortable when you position and transfer them.

Work with another nurse assistant to position and transfer people.

After practicing the corresponding skills in the skills book, you will be able to—

Help move a person around in bed.

Help move a person into several different positions.

Transfer a person from a bed to a chair.

Use a mechanical lift to transfer a person from a bed to a chair.

Reposition a person in a chair.

You have been providing care for 78-year-old Victor Rivera since he was transferred from the hospital to Morningside Nursing Home several weeks ago. An earlier stroke left him paralyzed on his right side and incontinent of urine and stool. Immediately after suffering the stroke, he was unable to speak, but his speech has improved with the help of the speech therapist at the nursing home.

You are concerned that, because of his illness and poor circulation, Mr. Rivera could easily develop a bedsore if he stays in one position too long. Yet, because of his paralysis, Mr. Rivera is unable to move much by himself. So every day, according to his care plan, you help him change position at least every 2 hours. By changing his position and relieving pressure on certain parts of his body, you help provide comfort and help prevent bedsores from developing on his dry, fragile skin. When Mr. Rivera's wife comes to visit every day, she helps by gently rubbing lotion into his skin.

This morning, when you first check on Mr. Rivera, you notice that he had been positioned on his side for sleeping. But he has moved his unaffected leg, which caused the pillow that was between his knees to shift out of position, so his knees have been lying against each other. As you reposition him, you check the inner surfaces of his knees and notice a red spot on each knee. You report the condition of Mr. Rivera's skin to your supervising nurse.

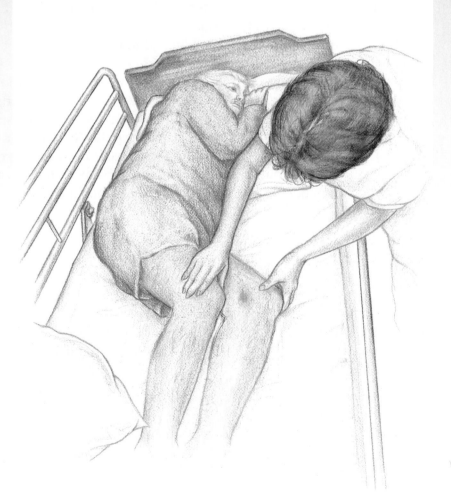

Preventing Decubitus Ulcers

Like Mr. Rivera, someone in your care may not be able to move by himself due to illness, injury, or a medical problem. A person who stays in one position for too long becomes stiff and uncomfortable and may develop a bedsore, or **decubitus ulcer**. Decubitus ulcers usually develop on pressure point areas, which include the ears, elbows, shoulder blades, hips, **coccyx**, knees, ankles, and heels. These parts of the body are bony areas that are protected by only a thin layer of fat and muscle under the skin. When a person stays in one position too long, pressure increases on certain points on his body. When he repeats certain activities, such as sliding down in the bed, friction affects other points on his body. Points of pressure or friction can decrease or cut off blood circulation to parts of the person's body. When he is unable to change position or repeats the same movements, pressure and friction continue and cells die, leaving reddened, pale, or darkened areas that can quickly become decubitus ulcers.

You may have experienced pressure in a minor way if your foot or arm ever "fell asleep" after being in the same position for too long. How did it feel? What did you do to relieve the discomfort? How would you feel if you could not move to stop the discomfort?

The big difference between what you experience if your foot or arm falls asleep and what some people in your care experience is that you can move to relieve pressure and restore circulation, and your cells can continue to function.

People who cannot move or have limited movement also have problems with friction, which causes the skin layers to tear apart. The injured skin then breaks down, which results in sores. People who are extremely overweight may develop such sores when body parts rub together in areas such as the buttocks and thighs, under folds of fat on the abdomen, and under the breasts. Even the continuous rubbing of medical tubing on a person's skin can cause decubitus ulcers. Box 9-1 shows steps you can take to protect a person's skin integrity.

Several factors put Mr. Rivera at risk for developing a decubitus ulcer. He—

❖   Has dry skin.
❖   Has been sick in bed for almost 6 weeks.
❖   Has poor circulation.
❖   Is unable to move himself without help, because he is paralyzed on one side.
❖   Has a poor appetite due to difficulty in chewing and swallowing. (Poor nutrition and poor fluid intake increase the likelihood of skin breakdown.)

When you provide care for a person who has to stay in bed, you must give frequent skin care and help change his position. You also must be on the lookout for any clues, such as the red spot on his knees, so that you can report signs of bedsores that may be develop-

---

decubitus ulcer
(duh-KYOO-bi-tuhs/UHL-ser)   The medical term for a bedsore or pressure sore, caused by pressure or friction, which cuts off circulation. A decubitus ulcer can quickly progress into a deep, infected crater.

coccyx
(COCK-siks)   The "tailbone," or end of the spine.

Box 9-1   **Protecting Skin Integrity**

To Prevent This . . .	*Do This* . . .
Direct Pressure	Change the person's position at least every 2 hours.
	Observe and report immediately any reddened, pale, or darkened areas of the skin.
	Make sure the person is in good body alignment. Use appropriate positioning devices when needed.
	Use special protective devices to relieve pressure and protect skin. Some examples of protective devices are air and water mattresses, special foam mattresses that look like egg cartons, and heel and elbow protectors.
Friction	Get help when moving the person—be sure to lift him all the way off the mattress.
	Elevate the head of the bed no more than 30 degrees (except when a person is eating, requires a procedure, or has difficulty breathing). This will keep the person from sliding down in bed.
	Use a drawsheet to move and turn the person.
	Keep equipment and devices such as tubes from getting caught under a part of the person's body.
Skin-to-Skin Contact	Check for skin changes under skin folds, especially under breasts, and under the folds of fat on people who are overweight.
	Position the person so that air circulates around his arms and legs to keep skin from touching skin.
Moisture	Wash, rinse, and dry the person's skin thoroughly.
	Check people with incontinence at least every 2 hours and keep their skin clean and dry.
	Cover a vinyl chair with a pad or sheet.
	Have the person wear moisture-absorbing clothes made from natural fabrics such as cotton.
Poor Circulation	Elevate the person's arms and legs.
	Provide mild massaging, including good back and skin care.
	Observe the person's skin frequently and report any changes to your supervising nurse.
Harmful Contact from Splints and Clothing	Pad splints and check the person's circulation often.
	Check to make sure shoes and nylon stockings fit correctly.

To Improve This . . .	*Do This* . . .
Nutrition	Encourage the person to drink an adequate amount of fluids.
	Encourage the person to eat a well-balanced diet.
	If the person has anemia, encourage him to eat foods that are rich in iron.
Sleeping Conditions	Make a tight, neat, wrinkle-free bed.
	Check the bed for items such as hair pins and barrettes and remove them.
Mobility	Move the person often.
	Help with range-of-motion exercises.

Box 9-2   **Signs and Stages of Decubitus Ulcer Development**

Stage I

An area is red, pale, or dark and does not improve after the pressure has been removed.

What to Do

1. Report this stage to your supervising nurse and discuss a plan of care with her.
2. As a preventive measure to help increase blood circulation and keep the skin moist and flexible, massage the skin around the discolored area gently in a circular motion using alcohol-free lotion.
3. Use another preventive measure to relieve pressure: Reposition the person to keep weight off areas that are red, pale, or dark in color, and make sure his body is properly aligned.
4. Continue with other preventive measures to reduce pressure and friction, such as using pillows and blankets to keep one skin surface from touching another; using special protective devices, such as air and water mattresses (alternating pressure pad mattresses that fill and empty to relieve pressure and stimulate circulation), special foam mattresses that look like egg cartons, gelatin-filled pads for chairs and wheelchairs, sheepskin to protect bony areas, and heel and elbow protectors with self-fasteners; and keeping linens under the person as wrinkle free as possible.
5. Use additional preventive measures to reduce friction when moving the person: Get help from a co-worker, use a drawsheet, and lift the person all the way off the mattress.
6. As another preventive measure to reduce friction, elevate the head of the bed no more than 30 degrees so that the person will not slide down or have pressure on the coccyx. If the bed must be elevated more than 30 degrees, such as during mealtime, slightly elevate the person's knees as well.
7. To prevent friction with people who have feeding tubes or other medical devices, keep tubes from getting caught under the person's body.

Stage II

Persistent redness and blistering lead to a breakdown of the skin's surface.

What to Do

1. Report this stage to your supervising nurse and discuss a plan of care with her.
2. Reposition the person to keep weight off this area.
3. Continue with preventive measures.

Stage III

Skin breakdown has reached the inner tissue, and an ulcer now looks like a shallow crater. There may be some drainage from the wound.*

What to Do

1. Report this stage to your supervising nurse and discuss a plan of care with her.
2. Reposition the person to keep weight off this area.
3. Continue with preventive measures.

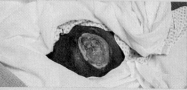

Stage IV

Skin is damaged in a deep crater that extends to the muscle or bone. Wound drainage or crust formation usually is present. The wound often becomes infected.*

What to Do

1. Report this stage to and discuss a plan of care with your supervising nurse, who will provide treatment.
2. Reposition the person to keep weight off this area.
3. Continue to provide preventive measures so that other areas of the skin stay intact.

*Stage III and Stage IV decubitus ulcers often require surgery to remove dead skin so that healing can occur.

ing. To know how to recognize each stage and what to do, look at Box 9-2.

Keep preventive measures in mind as you provide care for Mr. Rivera. To relieve pressure, help him roll over in bed. To make him more comfortable, help move his arms, legs, and body into different positions, and help him move to different areas of the bed and from the bed to a chair and back.

Whenever you change Mr. Rivera's position, be sure to relieve the pressure points he was on. For example, if he is lying on his back with the head of the bed raised, reposition him on his side. When he is on his back, his shoulder blades, coccyx, heels, and elbows are under pressure. If you position him on his side, his ear, shoulder, hip, knee, and ankle are under pressure. It would *not* be good to change Mr. Rivera's position from lying on his back with the head of the bed raised to lying on his back with the bed flat, because the pressure points he was lying on would not be relieved.

Promoting Proper Body Alignment

When you reposition Mr. Rivera, prop him up with pillows to help prevent pressure and friction and to help maintain proper body alignment. Review the Body Basics for the Integumentary, Muscular, and Skeletal Systems to learn more about how the body works so that you can understand the importance of promoting proper body alignment and comfort for Mr. Rivera.

Make sure Mr. Rivera's bones and joints are in a natural position that feels comfortable to him. Also, when you position him in bed, support his bones and joints to minimize the strain on them. For example, you could place a small towel under his calves to lift his heels away from the mattress and relieve pressure. Since muscles that **flex** joints are stronger than those that **extend** them, a paralyzed or inactive limb may tend to curl upward. For this reason, when positioning a person who has a weak or paralyzed arm, support the arm so that the wrist is higher than the elbow. Since the limb may curl upward, people who cannot move their wrists, hands, fingers, or heels often need special devices to prevent this curling (Figure 9-1).

flex
To bend.

extend
To straighten.

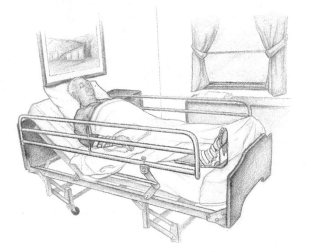

Figure 9-1
Mr. Rivera wears a splint on his right hand to keep his wrist and hand extended, rather than flexed. He wears a bootie to keep his right heel extended.

BodyBasics

❖   The Integumentary System   ❖

The human body has a covering of skin, hair, and nails called the integumentary system that protects the body from the outside world. The skin acts as a barrier to bacteria, keeps water inside the body, contains sense organs that allow people to feel, and regulates body temperature.

The skin, which is more than a simple protective sheet, is made up of several parts. The outer layer, called the epidermis, is firm and dry to the touch. Beneath the epidermis, the dermis holds glands and hair follicles. Sweat glands produce sweat to keep the body's temperature in a safe range, and oil glands make oil to keep the skin soft and flexible. Hair follicles produce the hairs that cover most of our bodies. Blood vessels in this layer provide nutrients and oxygen to all skin cells. Underneath the skin is a layer of fat that cushions, protects, and insulates the body.

How the Integumentary System Ages

As people age, their skin becomes less elastic, the amount of fat under the skin decreases, and their bodies produce less oil. As a result, their skin tends to be dry and looks wrinkled. Older people also have more skin cancers, usually caused by sun damage that adds up over a lifetime.

Fascinating Fact

The skin is the largest organ in the body. The skin of an adult weighs about 6 pounds and, if spread out flat, would cover an area 3 feet wide and 6 feet long. A piece of skin the size of a quarter contains 1 yard of blood vessels, 4 yards of nerves, 25 nerve endings, 100 sweat glands, and more than 3 million cells. The skin produces vitamin D when the body is exposed to sunlight. Vitamin D is artificially added to milk and dairy products to ensure that people, especially children, receive an adequate amount. Human bodies need vitamin D to absorb the calcium that is needed to fill up the spaces created by bone cells.

When and How to Position and Transfer

Because a person who is unable to move without help must be repositioned at least every 2 hours to avoid damage to his skin, he usually is placed on a schedule for regular turning. The schedule uses a sequence of positions (described later in this chapter and in the skills book) that allows parts of his body to be free of pressure when he is in certain positions. For example, during the first position, he may be on his back, but in the second position, he may be on his side, with no pressure on his back. A typical 12-hour rotation schedule* for a person who needs regular repositioning might look like the following:

6:00 A.M.	Left-modified side-lying position
8:00 A.M.	Semi-Fowler's position

*Rotation schedules, with 2-hour intervals for repositioning, are carried out around the clock, even while the person is sleeping.

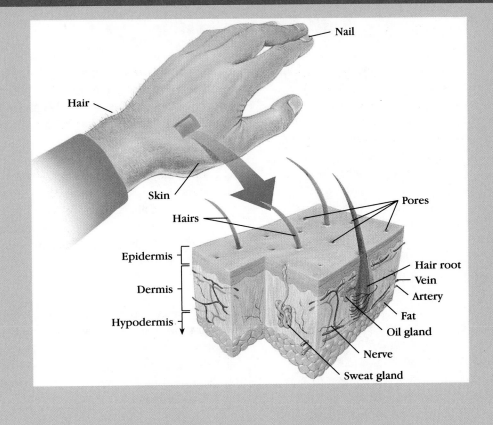

10:00 A.M.	Right-modified side-lying position†
12:00 P.M.	Supine position (raise head into semi-Fowler's position for lunch)
2:00 P.M.	Left-modified side-lying position
4:00 P.M.	Prone position‡
6:00 P.M.	Right-modified side-lying position

By paying close attention to the places where the person's body comes into contact with the bed, you ensure that he is not lying on one spot for long periods of time. You play an important role in reducing the likelihood of his developing bedsores.

Whenever you move or position a person, remember two important factors: First, assess the situation and plan what to do and how to do it; and second, carry out your plan using the good body mechanics that you read about in Chapter 6, Keeping People Safe. In addi-

---

†If this schedule were for Mr. Rivera, you would not position him on his right side, because he is paralyzed on his right side.
‡Using the prone position may require a doctor's order.

BodyBasics

❖ The Muscular System ❖

Every movement in the human body, from the blink of the eye to the beat of the heart, depends on muscles. The body has hundreds of muscles that come in all sizes, from the delicate muscles in the ear to the thick, powerful muscles in the legs.

Muscles do their work by getting shorter, or contracting, in response to electrical impulses sent through nerves. To recover from their work, they relax, or get longer. Some muscles, which are under a person's control, are attached to bones by tendons and contract with voluntary actions such as walking. Other muscles, which are not under a person's control, surround the blood vessels, digestive tract, and other body parts that work involuntarily.

Some muscles, such as those in the arms and legs, work together in contracting and relaxing teams. For example, when a person bends his arm at the elbow, muscles on one side of his arm contract, pulling on the joint and causing it to bend, while muscles on the opposite side relax. To straighten his arm, the opposite happens. These muscle pairs work together to make movement controlled and smooth. A person is able to stand straight because teams of muscles around his spine contract and relax in perfect harmony.

How the Muscle System Ages

As people age, their muscles get smaller and less elastic and lose strength. Large muscle loss in the hips and knees affects balance. More fat cells and connective tissue begin to replace muscle fibers. People can help their muscles remain strong with regular exercise and a healthy diet.

Fascinating Facts

Have you ever noticed your muscles twitching? This normal movement occurs when a single nerve sends its electrical impulse to the muscle. The impulse isn't strong enough to make the whole muscle move but is just strong enough to make a couple of muscle fibers contract.

tion, to successfully position and transfer someone without causing injury to him or yourself, give clear directions to the co-worker who is assisting you and to the person you are positioning. Before moving the person, check the bed for any tubes or personal items that may get in the way, and check the brakes to make sure they are locked. Finally, when you finish the procedure, make sure the person is comfortable, that his body is in proper alignment, and that he is supported by any necessary blankets and pillows.

The following sections list factors to consider and some questions to ask as you assess, communicate, and complete a positioning or transferring skill for a person such as Mr. Rivera.

Assess

mobility
(moe-BIL-uh-tee)   The ability to move.

Gather information about Mr. Rivera's **mobility** and independence, as well as his environment, and determine a plan of how you will help him move every 2 hours.

Mobility and independence.   Find out about Mr. Rivera's mobility and level of independence by talking with your supervising nurse and

BodyBasics

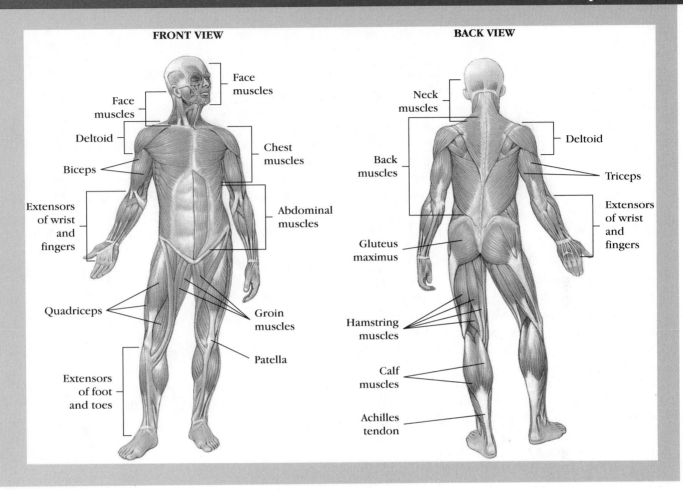

FRONT VIEW

- Face muscles
- Face muscles
- Deltoid
- Biceps
- Extensors of wrist and fingers
- Quadriceps
- Extensors of foot and toes
- Chest muscles
- Abdominal muscles
- Groin muscles
- Patella

BACK VIEW

- Neck muscles
- Back muscles
- Gluteus maximus
- Hamstring muscles
- Calf muscles
- Achilles tendon
- Deltoid
- Triceps
- Extensors of wrist and fingers

checking the care plan. Find out about Mr. Rivera's weight and muscle strength and his ability to use his arms and legs so that you know how much he can help. Ask these questions:

❖ Can he bear all his weight on one leg or both legs?
❖ Is one side stronger than the other?
❖ Can he maintain his sense of balance?
❖ Does he have visual or **perception** problems?
❖ Do visual or language problems affect his understanding of instructions or his surroundings?
❖ Does he have pain when he moves?
❖ Is he afraid of being moved?
❖ Has he ever suddenly refused to cooperate?
❖ Are his movements **predictable**?

Environment.   Ask yourself these questions about the room and equipment:

❖ How much room do you need to complete the move?
❖ What obstacles, such as tubes or personal items, are in the way?

perception
(pur-SEP-shun)   A person's awareness of his environment through his senses.

predictable
(pree-DIK-tuh-bull)   Can be known in advance.

BodyBasics

❖ The Skeletal System ❖

The skeletal system supports and protects the body. Without a skeletal system, the human body would collapse like a jellyfish. To support the body, muscles are draped over bones, made mostly of calcium, and cartilage, the firm tissue that supports and connects parts of the skeletal system. To protect vital organs inside the body, the skull surrounds the brain, the twelve ribs and breastbone (sternum) cover the heart and lungs, and the backbone (vertebral column) guards the spinal cord.

Adults have 206 bones in various sizes and shapes. The smallest bones (ossicles) inside the ear are no larger than the head of a match. The largest bone (femur) in the leg is the thick, sturdy bone between the hip and the knee. Long bones, such as those in the arms and legs, are not solid structures but have center cavities filled with red marrow, which produces red blood cells, and yellow marrow, which is mostly fat cells.

Joints, the place where neighboring bones are connected by ligaments, allow the skeleton to move. Some joints work like door hinges and others are like a ball and socket.

How the Skeletal System Ages

As people age, their bones lose calcium, become fragile, and break more easily. This is especially true for women. Female hormones keep calcium in bones, but after menopause women's bodies no longer produce these hormones. The vertebrae begin to collapse, and some women actually lose an inch or more in height and may develop a humpback. In addition, their joints become less flexible and begin to wear away, resulting in a form of arthritis. Their walking slows, and their steps may take on a shuffling gait.

Fascinating Fact

Without weight-bearing exercise, such as walking, bones tend to lose the calcium that makes them hard. They can take on a sponge-like, porous appearance and become very brittle. Because of this change, the bones of inactive people can break with only small amounts of stress on the bones.

---

drawsheet
A bed sheet about 5 feet wide that is placed under a person, across the middle third of the bed. A drawsheet is useful in positioning and transferring procedures.

❖ Where do you get a **drawsheet**? (In a home setting, make a drawsheet by folding a top sheet in half, widthwise.)
❖ What equipment do you need? (Check to see what equipment is available, and be sure you know how to use it.)
❖ What height should the bed be?
❖ How will you position yourself to avoid injury?
❖ Do the bed and wheelchair have brakes? (Be sure to lock them when necessary.)

Sometimes you may have to use special equipment, such as a mechanical lift or a metal trapeze above the bed (Figure 9-2). This equipment is designed to help with positioning and transferring when the person being moved cannot assist you with the move. You also can use it if the person is too heavy or if there is any risk to you or the person being moved. Lack of this specialized equipment, however, is not an excuse for improper positioning. If special equipment is not available and you believe it is necessary, discuss this concern with your supervising nurse.

BodyBasics

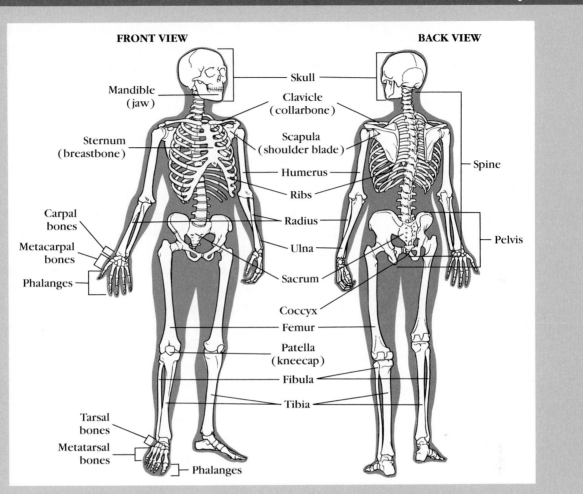

FRONT VIEW   BACK VIEW

- Skull
- Mandible (jaw)
- Clavicle (collarbone)
- Sternum (breastbone)
- Scapula (shoulder blade)
- Humerus
- Ribs
- Spine
- Carpal bones
- Radius
- Metacarpal bones
- Ulna
- Phalanges
- Sacrum
- Pelvis
- Coccyx
- Femur
- Patella (kneecap)
- Fibula
- Tibia
- Tarsal bones
- Metatarsal bones
- Phalanges

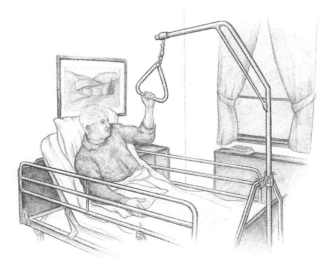

Figure 9-2
A trapeze enables people to change positions by themselves or with some assistance.

Determining a plan.   After you have the necessary information about the person and his environment, determine if you need any help to move him. To prevent injury to yourself and Mr. Rivera, you need another nurse assistant to help you with most positioning techniques. Two people can lift or move someone more easily than one person can. You must arrange with a co-worker to help you, and then remember to return the favor when he or she asks you for help.

Communicate

After you decide what to tell Mr. Rivera and the co-worker assisting you, explain each step of your plan to them.

What to communicate.   Emphasize good body mechanics to both Mr. Rivera and your co-worker as you explain each step of the plan to them. Tell Mr. Rivera what he can do to help make the move easier. Encourage him to help as much as possible and make sure he understands and agrees with your plan. Tell your co-worker exactly what his or her responsibilities are and make sure he or she understands the plan. For example, you could tell Mr. Rivera to use his unaffected arm to lock arms with you so that you can support his head while your co-worker moves his pillow or ties his nightgown.

When to communicate.   Explain the procedure before you begin. Then, as you move through the steps, explain each step as you come to it. For example, you might say to Mr. Rivera, "Now, we are going to help you roll over onto your left side." And you might say to your co-worker, "When I count to three, lift the drawsheet."

Complete

Finish the procedure and make sure Mr. Rivera is comfortable and safe. Ask yourself:

❖ Did I protect all the pressure point parts of his body?
❖ Does this new position put pressure on different bony parts of his body than the last position did?
❖ Did I support his back, arms, and legs with pillows?
❖ Did I smooth out the sheets under him to prevent his lying on uncomfortable wrinkles?
❖ Does Mr. Rivera look comfortable?

Ask Mr. Rivera if he is comfortable. Complete the procedure by checking to see if his spine is straight and his body is in proper alignment by putting up the side rails, if necessary, and by making sure the call signal is within reach of his strong hand. If a person in your care is unable to speak at all, it is important to watch his facial expressions. If he grimaces or frowns, he may be uncomfortable. If he is unable to communicate at all, you must look at his position to make sure his body is in proper alignment.

Types of Positions and Transfers

You can position people in many ways to provide safety and comfort. For example, you go to Mr. Rivera's room to prepare him for breakfast. He is lying on his left side in a **modified side-lying position**, with a rolled blanket supporting his back. He has a pillow between his knees to reduce strain on his upper hip and to prevent pressure on his knees and ankles. His paralyzed arm rests on a pillow (Figure 9-3). You ask a co-worker to help you position Mr. Rivera in a high

modified side-lying position
A position in which a person lies partially to one side with his back supported.

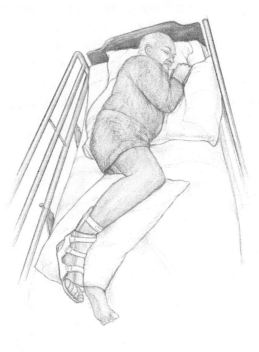

Figure 9-3
Use the modified side-lying position when you reposition a person in bed to prevent bedsores. Many people prefer to rest or sleep in this position.

Fowler's position for eating. You roll him onto his back, move him up in bed, and elevate the head of his bed so that he can sit up and eat (Figure 9-4). After breakfast, you collect Mr. Rivera's food tray and tell him it will soon be time for his personal care. He shakes his head and, with effort, tells you that he wants to rest. Although you had planned to start your day by providing personal care for Mr. Ri-

Fowler's position
A position in which a person sits up with the head of the bed elevated for support.

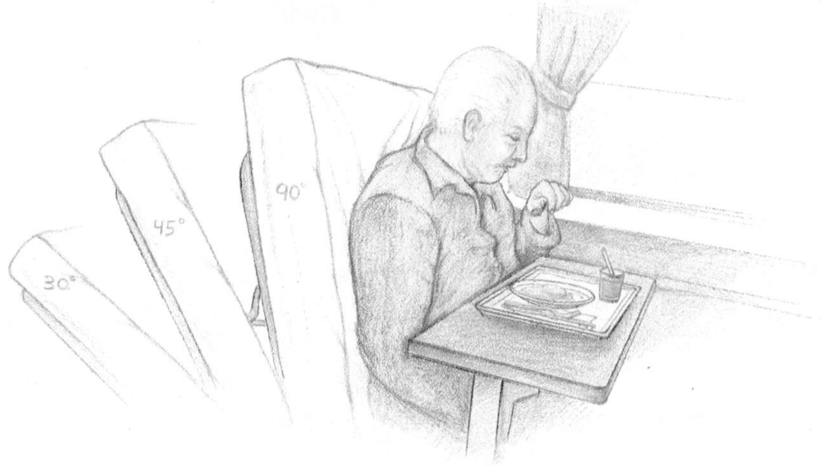

Figure 9-4
Three types of Fowler's positions are—
❖ High Fowler's position with the head of the bed elevated almost 90 degrees.
❖ Fowler's position with the head of the bed elevated about 45 degrees.
❖ Semi-Fowler's position with the head of the bed elevated about 30 degrees.

vera, you observe that he seems tired, and you adjust your schedule to meet his needs. Because he has just eaten, you encourage him to rest in the semi-upright position called the semi-Fowler's position. You lower his head and make him comfortable.

Later you return to Mr. Rivera's room to help him with his bath. To do this personal care procedure, you lower the head of the bed and put him into a **supine position** (Figure 9-5). During the bath you have to turn him onto his side to wash his back and give him a backrub (Figure 9-6). Because of his paralysis, he finds it difficult to position himself but is able to help turn with his unaffected side. After his bath, Mr. Rivera agrees that he would like to get out of bed and sit in his wheelchair. His mobility is limited because of his right-sided paralysis, but he can balance himself with assistance and can support his own weight. You ask a co-worker to help you transfer Mr. Rivera into the wheelchair using a transfer belt (Figure 9-7). Later, when you check on him, you notice that he has slumped over and slipped down in the wheelchair. You and a co-worker reposition him (Figure 9-8).

supine position
(SUE-pine) A position in which a person lies flat on his back.

Figure 9-5
Help a person into the supine position when he needs to lie flat on his back to rest or sleep. This position is also useful when helping someone with a bed bath.

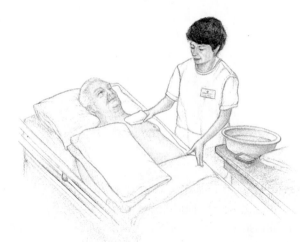

Figure 9-6
Help a person turn onto his side when he needs a complete bed bath, a backrub, or assistance getting onto a bedpan.

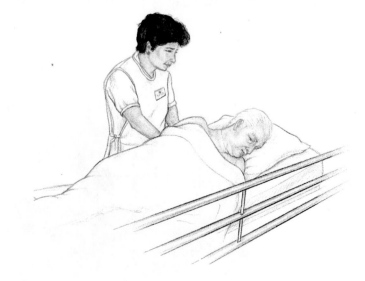

Throughout the day and night, you and other nurse assistants reposition Mr. Rivera every 2 hours. Even though it may seem inconsiderate to awaken someone to move him, it is better to interrupt his sleep than to let him sleep in the same position for more than 2 hours, which could cause pressure sores. If you are gentle and quiet, you can move him without bringing him to a full waking state.

Occasionally you assist a person into the prone position when you help him lie on his stomach. This position is useful for relieving pressure on other areas of the body, but it is not used often because many people find it uncomfortable. In many health care settings, the prone position requires a doctor's order.

When positioning or transferring someone, follow the specific procedures that are explained step by step in Skills 13 through 20 in the skills book. You must perform these skills well, because, as a nurse assistant, you have the important job of positioning and transferring people in your care. You provide for their safety and comfort by understanding the importance of using good body mechanics to protect

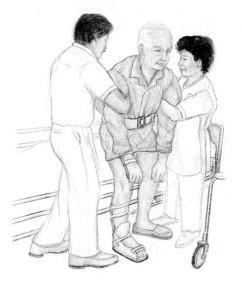

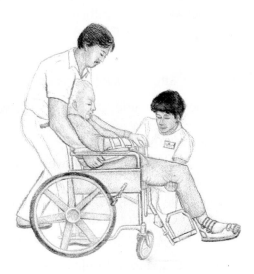

Figure 9-7

If a person can support himself, you can help him transfer from the bed to a chair or wheelchair without a transfer belt. If he needs help to maintain his balance, you must use a transfer belt. If he needs more than minimal support, use a transfer belt and the assistance of a co-worker. If the person cannot help you with the move, or if he is overweight, you and a co-worker can use a mechanical lift to make the transfer.

Figure 9-8

Help a person reposition in a chair when he has slouched down and cannot move back up without assistance.

yourself and others and by putting people in proper body alignment to prevent pressure sores and injury. You apply your skills to the people in your care in a personalized manner, taking into consideration their needs and their ability to help you. You also recognize the importance of teamwork when you ask a co-worker for help or help another co-worker in positioning and transferring people.

Transporting a Person in a Wheelchair

If you work in a hospital or nursing home, you may have to transport people from one part of the facility to another. Sometimes you will transport the person on a stretcher. (Read about transporting a person on a stretcher in Chapter 20, Providing Care for People Having Surgery.) The other way to safely transport a person is in a wheelchair. Follow these important tips:

❖ Always walk on the right side of the hall.
❖ When going down wheelchair ramps, turn the chair around and walk down backwards, with the person facing uphill. This backward positioning decreases the risk of tipping the chair and injuring the person.
❖ To avoid bumping into other people, use caution when walking past doorways and around corners or when entering hallway intersections.
❖ To enter an elevator, turn the chair around and enter the elevator backwards. Once inside, turn the chair around again and exit the elevator backwards. This backward positioning prevents the small wheels on the front of the chair from jamming in the space between the elevator and the floor.
❖ Always lock the brakes when the wheelchair is stopped and when the person remains in the wheelchair for a period of time.
❖ Always check with your supervising nurse before leaving a person unattended in a wheelchair.

If you plan to work in home health care, please read the next section. Otherwise, read "Information Review" and "Questions to Ask Yourself" at the end of the chapter.

Positioning and Transferring in the Home Health Setting

As a home health aide, you may not have another person present to help position or transfer a client. In addition, the client may be in a stationary bed that cannot be raised or lowered. The bed may have a head or foot that cannot be lowered, requiring you to use adaptive equipment.

If the head of a person's bed cannot be elevated, try some alternative ways to create a backrest that raises the person's head and shoulders to a 30- to 60-degree angle, such as—

❖ Stacking up several pillows up against the headboard or wall.
❖ Turning a straight-backed chair upside down against the headboard or wall.

❖ Inserting a foam wedge pillow between the person's back and the headboard or wall.

❖ Placing a padded board between the person's back and the headboard or wall.

❖ Using a pillow armrest.

❖ Making a backrest from a cardboard box that has four flaps (Figure 9-9). To make this backrest, follow these steps:

   1. Cut down the front side of the box at the corners. Let the front side fall forward and lie flat.

   2. Score (cut partially through) the two sides of the box diagonally from corner to corner on the inside. Bend the sides inward along the scored lines.

   3. Bring the cover flap of the back of the carton forward and place it over the folded sides.

   4. Bring the front flap up and over the folded sides and cover the back flap.

   5. Fold the excess cardboard over the back of the box and tape or tie securely.

Each home situation presents unique challenges for positioning and transferring clients. To ensure that you don't injure yourself or the client, you must apply the same principles of safety and good body mechanics that you learned in Chapter 6. If you have any concerns about safety, tell your supervising nurse.

When you provide care for a client who is able to assist and who is predictable, it may be safe for one person to position or transfer him. Assess the situation, using the questions in the earlier section of this chapter. If it seems to be a safe situation, follow the specific one-person procedures that are explained step by step in Skill 13 in the skills book. Otherwise, explain your assessment to your supervisor so that she can provide additional help or train family members to help you.

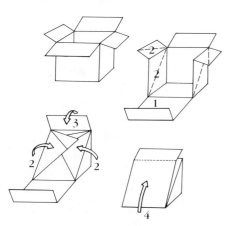

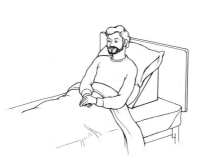

Figure 9-9
Make a backrest from a cardboard box.

Information Review

Circle the correct answers and fill in the blanks.

1. Decubitus ulcers or ___bedsores___ can easily develop on pressure points of the body because these areas are protected only by thin layers of ___fat___ and ___muscle___ under the skin.

2. On which areas can pressure sores develop?
    a. Eyes, ears, nose, and throat
    b. Ears, elbows, and ankles
    c. Heels and wrists
    d. Coccyx and buttocks

3. What is the *first* sign of a decubitus ulcer?
    a. A reddened area on the skin
    b. A fever
    c. An open sore
    d. Bleeding

4. To avoid damaging the skin of a person who is unable to move without help, you should reposition him—
    a. When you can fit him into your schedule.
    b. Every 4 hours.
    c. At least every 2 hours.
    d. When you come to work and before you go home.

5. When planning to move a person, you first assess. Some of the things you must know are—
    a. The person's height.
    b. How much time you have to move the person.
    c. How recently the person ate.
    d. The person's mobility, level of independence, and ability to help.

6. A ___drawsheet___ is placed under a person to help with positioning and turning him.

7. It is important that you ___explain___ your plan to the person so that he understands what you are going to do and how he can ___help___.

8. When you help a person sit up in bed with the head of the bed raised, that person is in a ___Fowler's___ position.

9. Supine position means the person is flat on his ___back___.

10. Always lock the ___brakes___ on a wheelchair when the chair is stopped and the person is remaining in the chair for a period of time.

Questions to Ask Yourself

1. Mr. Rivera has been sitting in a Fowler's position and watching television for the past 2 hours. When you come to help him change position, he wants to lie on his back and sleep. What should you do? ✓

2. Why is it important to change Mr. Rivera's position so often? How often should his position be changed? *2 hrs*

3. Why could Mr. Rivera could easily develop pressure sores or decubitus ulcers? Give three reasons. *poor circulation, dry skin & poor diet*

4. What do you consider before getting Mr. Rivera out of bed and into the wheelchair? Which type of transfer method should you use?

5. What important things should you think about to protect yourself from injury when positioning and transferring Mr. Rivera? *ask for help*

6. You are wheeling Mrs. Paulson down the hallway in a wheelchair. Because she has a cast on her right leg, you have raised the leg supports of the wheelchair so that her leg is supported out in front of her. You are approaching an intersecting hallway. What would you do to ensure her safety as you enter the intersection? *slow down & look carefully*

7. Mr. Eller, who is paralyzed on his right side, is sitting in a chair next to his bed. Every time you look into his room, he has slumped over to his weaker side. What could you do to position him properly and maintain his alignment?

8. Mrs. Hillman, who weighs 200 pounds, begins to stand up from the chair where she is sitting. Knowing that she often gets dizzy without warning, you offer to help her, but she insists that she is able to stand up by herself. What safety precautions should you take to prevent potential injury? How many people are needed to move her safely?

9. Mrs. Romano is sitting in the chair in her room while her niece is visiting. When Mrs. Romano says she wants to get back into her bed, her niece says that she will help her. You offer to help, but the niece says she can do it by herself. What should you do? *no*

10

Assisting People with Personal Care

Goals

After reading this chapter, you will have the information to—

Be better prepared to provide each person with thoughtful, individualized care that respects the private nature of personal care.

Know how to incorporate the six principles of care when assisting adults and children with personal care.

After practicing the corresponding skills in the skills book, you will be able to—

Assist with good mouth care, including mouth care for someone who has dentures, as well as for someone who is unconscious.

Help people bathe and shampoo in bed, in the shower, and in the tub.

Assist with good grooming care by helping someone brush and comb his hair, shave, clean and trim his fingernails, and clean his feet and toenails.

Help a person with dressing and undressing.

Assist a home health care client with medications.

Three mornings each week, you go to George Brady's home to help provide personal care. Mr. Brady is 68 years old and is terminally ill with cancer. His wife tries to help with his care but has arthritis and isn't strong enough to perform many of the tasks. When you first started helping Mr. Brady 2 months ago, he was able to get out of bed to take a tub bath. But, now, as his cancer has progressed and he has become weaker, you have to give him a bed bath. On the days when you do not come to his house, Mrs. Brady gives him a partial bed bath.

As you enter his room with Mrs. Brady, she says, "Look, Honey, your nurse assistant is here to help you with your bath and to shampoo your hair."

Mr. Brady looks your way, smiles, and lifts his hand in a weak wave. "G'morning," he says.

After you explain to Mr. Brady how you will be helping him with his personal care, you gather supplies and close the door to his room. First you help him brush and floss his teeth. Mr. Brady is able to shave his face, using an electric razor, so you wash his face and then stand by to help if he needs assistance. You help Mr. Brady undress for his bath, take care to keep him warm during the bath, and pay special attention to his skin. After the bath, you shampoo, condition, and towel dry his hair. During the bath, you have him soak his hands so that you can clean and trim his fingernails. You also have him soak his feet in a basin of water so that you can clean his toenails.

Now that Mr. Brady is bathed, you help him into the bedroom chair so that he can get dressed in a warm sweat suit and rest for a few minutes while you comb his hair and make his bed.

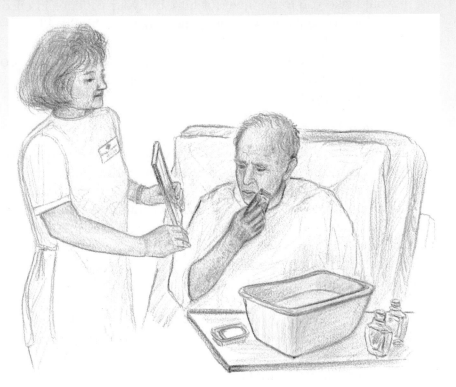

Focusing on Personal Care

Personal care includes positioning and transferring people, which you read about in Chapter 9; healthful eating, which you will read about in Chapter 12; and elimination, which you will read about in Chapter 13. It also includes mouth care, bathing, shampooing, grooming, and dressing and undressing, which you will read about in this chapter.

Assisting with Personal Care

To assist with personal care in a sensitive manner, put yourself in the place of the people in your care. Imagine what it would feel like to have a stranger brush your teeth, bathe you, comb your hair, and dress you.

Every day you make choices about what to wear, when to get up, how to style your hair, and many other personal decisions. These actions and decisions say something about you and your personal needs, self-image, and independence. The people in your care need to make these same decisions for themselves, but they may need your help to carry out the actions. You must respect the way people want their personal care done, because they each must maintain their own personal needs, self-image, and independence.

Remember to think about what the people in your care need to feel good, how much they can do for themselves, and how you can help them feel good about themselves. For example, even though Mr. Brady is very weak, he still wants to brush his teeth, shave, and help dress himself. It takes him longer to do each of these tasks than it would take you to do them for him. But your patience in encouraging him to do these tasks independently helps him feel better about himself.

Because it is so important to respect a person's needs and promote a good self-image and independence, assisting with personal care involves making many decisions.

When to Help with Personal Care

As nurse assistants, you and your co-workers make sure the people in your care are clean, safe, and comfortable throughout the day and night. In the morning, you help a person prepare for breakfast by helping him go to the bathroom or use another method to eliminate. You also help him wash his face and hands and brush his teeth. You offer him fresh drinking water and assist with any other care that makes him comfortable. After breakfast, you usually help the person bathe and dress. During the day, you take care of any other personal care needs that arise.

At night, you help a person prepare for bed by helping him undress, use the bathroom, wash his face and hands, and brush his teeth. You also make sure his bed linens are smooth and wrinkle free, offer him fresh drinking water, and assist with any other care that makes him comfortable (Figure 10-1).

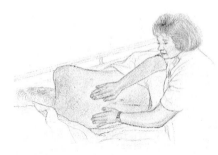

Figure 10-1
A backrub is relaxing and helps promote sleep.

Assisting with Mouth Care

When you get up in the morning, how does your mouth feel? What do your teeth feel like after you eat a meal? Part of your responsibility in assisting with personal care is to help provide mouth and teeth care, also called oral hygiene. This important part of daily care includes care of the mouth, teeth, gums, tongue, lips, and soft parts of the inside of the mouth, such as the cheeks and the roof. A person in your care may want to take care of his own mouth, as Mr. Brady did.

Encourage the people in your care to be independent, but make sure they all receive proper mouth care. Assist them as much as necessary, which may involve helping some people brush and floss their teeth, helping others clean their dentures, or providing special mouth care for **unconscious** people. Remember to use universal precautions, especially wearing latex gloves, when you assist with mouth care.

unconscious
(un-KON-shus)   A state of mind in which a person does not respond to the world around him.

Why Help with Mouth Care?

A clean mouth and clean teeth help prevent mouth odors and infection. An unclean mouth and unbrushed teeth can cause a person to be uncomfortable, to lose his appetite, to drink less fluid, and to be less healthy overall. It also may keep him from wanting to talk or be with other people.

If a person does not brush his teeth, **plaque** builds up on the gums. Eating sugars and starches causes the bacteria in plaque to grow. These bacteria, in turn, produce acids, which destroy the outer surface of the tooth, leading to tooth decay. If plaque is not removed by brushing the teeth, it hardens into tartar, which only a dentist can remove. If tartar is not removed, it can cause gum irritation, infection, and possibly tooth loss.

Good mouth care is important for people of all ages, but it is especially important for the elderly. Table 10-1 on p. 220 contains examples of dental conditions that affect the elderly.

plaque
(PLAK)   A sticky, colorless layer of bacteria that forms constantly on the teeth.

fluoridated
(FLOOR-uh-day-ted)   Containing fluoride, a chemical that helps decrease tooth decay. Toothpaste and drinking water often are fluoridated.

How to Help with Mouth Care

When assisting with mouth care, always wear latex gloves. Use a toothbrush that has soft bristles with rounded ends to remove plaque and food particles from the teeth and to stimulate circulation in the gums, which helps keep them healthy. Generally you should use **fluoridated** toothpaste when you clean a person's teeth. Fluoride is important for keeping teeth strong and healthy, but too much fluoride can cause teeth to discolor. In a few areas of the United States, the water supply contains a high percentage of fluoride, and dentists recommend using toothpaste that does not contain fluoride.

To finish cleaning the teeth, use dental floss to remove plaque and food particles from between the teeth (Figure 10-2). Waxed dental floss slides between the teeth more easily than unwaxed dental floss does, and it makes the procedure more comfortable for a person who has sensitive gums. Flossing, like brushing, also stimulates the gums.

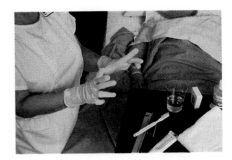

Figure 10-2
Tools for mouth care.

Table 10-1   **Dental Conditions Affecting Elderly People**

Sign of Change	Reason
Plaque builds up faster.	Decreased saliva production
Teeth appear slightly darker.	Changes in bonelike tissue under tooth enamel
Mouth is drier.	Decreased saliva production; medications, especially for high blood pressure
Teeth are more susceptible to decay.	Drier mouth; other conditions or diseases that may decrease the ability to effectively brush and floss the teeth
Dentures become uncomfortable.	Drier mouth
Gums may bleed easily.	Gum disease
Pus forms between gums and teeth.	Gum disease
Denture fit changes.	Gum disease
Bad breath persists.	Insufficient or improper brushing or flossing; gum disease

Use mouth sponges to remove mucus and secretions from the gums, tongue, and palate of people who are unconscious or who wear dentures. Mouth sponges are soft enough to clean the tender tissues of the mouth without injuring them.

Brushing and flossing.   Like Mr. Brady, the people in your care should brush their teeth twice a day and floss once a day. Rinse the teeth with diluted mouthwash before and after brushing, and use a soft-bristle toothbrush to clean all surfaces of the teeth. Brushing the upper teeth first, and then the lower teeth, controls the amount of saliva produced. After brushing the teeth, brush the tongue to control bacteria, which cause mouth odor.

Toothbrushes lose their effectiveness when the bristles become worn, bent, or frayed. To maintain good mouth care, replace toothbrushes when they show signs of wear, or at least every 6 months.

If you are going to floss, check with your supervising nurse or the care plan to make sure that a person's teeth can be flossed. Some people taking certain medications may bleed excessively if their teeth are flossed. To keep a person's gums from bleeding when you floss, insert floss without pressing against the gums. Whenever you brush or floss, observe changes in the person's mouth and report any swollen, red, or tender gums, as well as bleeding, white patches, or pain.

When helping someone brush and floss his teeth, follow the specific procedure that is explained step by step in Skill 21 in the skills book.

Denture care.   When you provide care to one of your other clients, 73-year-old Dorothy Roth, you assist with a different kind of dental care, because she wears dentures, also called false teeth. Mrs. Roth can clean her own dentures but needs help.

People in your care may wear complete (full-mouth) dentures, which replace all of their teeth, or partial dentures, which replace only a portion of their teeth. Wearing dentures decreases gum shrinkage after teeth have been removed and maintains the shape of the mouth. It also improves a person's speech and makes it easier for her to eat. In addition, wearing dentures improves a person's self-image. If people in your care wear dentures, remind them to remove the devices for at least 8 hours each day to rest their gums.

Handle dentures carefully so that they do not chip or break (Figure 10-3). Be sure to label each person's dentures and denture cup to keep them from being misplaced or lost. Read the information in Box 10-1 on labeling dentures to learn how to do this.

After removing dentures, brush and floss the person's natural teeth if she has any. Wash the dentures with cold water, because hot water may change the shape of the dentures. When storing the dentures in the denture cup, cover them with water, not denture cleaner, because the cleaner may weaken the metal parts of the dentures. Observe changes in the person's mouth and report any swollen, red, or tender gums, as well as bleeding, white patches, sores or pus between gums and natural teeth, and ill-fitting or broken dentures.

When you help someone take care of her dentures, follow the specific procedure that is explained step by step in Skill 22 in the skills book.

Providing Mouth Care for an Unconscious Person

You may be responsible for providing care to a person like 25-year-old Tamara Frazier, who is unconscious as the result of a car crash.

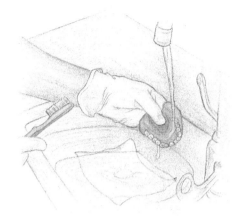

Figure 10-3
When removing dentures from the mouth, grip them firmly, as they become slippery when coated with mucus or saliva. When cleaning dentures, hold them over a padded surface in case they slip from your hands.

Box 10-1   **How to Label Dentures**

Professional dentists and dental employees can mark dentures permanently. If dentists or dental employees aren't available, you can mark them with surface-marking techniques that are not as durable as permanent denture labeling but that help to avoid losing or misplacing dentures. Often hospitals and nursing homes have denture-labeling kits that contain all necessary supplies. If a kit is not available, use the following method.

1. Thoroughly clean and dry the dentures.
2. Use an abrasive pad to roughen the area on the lingual (tongue) side of the denture.
3. Use an extra-fine felt-tip pen* to print the wearer's name, initials, or Social Security number in the roughened area of the dentures.
4. Allow markings to dry and then coat them with two layers of clear, acrylic resin.† Ask a local dentist for the product available in your area.

From *Techniques for denture identification,* Chicago, 1984, The American Dental Association Council on Prosthetic Services and Dental Laboratory Relations.
*"Sharpie" pens by Sanford Corporation have been tested for toxicity and, according to research reports, are not toxic if used in small quantities inside the mouth.
†Clear fingernail polish should *not* be used as a coating, because it has not been tested for toxicity or durability.

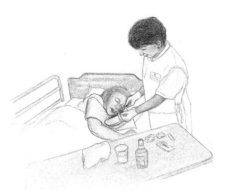

Figure 10-4
Reposition an unconscious person and provide mouth care for her every 2 hours during the day and night.

aspirate
(AS-puh-rate)   To breathe in.

An unconscious person cannot swallow adequately and does not have normal mouth movements that keep the mouth clean and moist. Mucus and other mouth secretions, which tend to coat the teeth of a person who is unconscious, must be removed regularly. You must provide mouth care for an unconscious person every 2 hours throughout the day and night because her mouth can become very dry (Figure 10-4).

An unconscious person may not respond to you, but she may be able to hear you. People who regain consciousness sometimes remember and talk about the frustration of hearing what was going on but not being able to move or talk while they were unconscious. Therefore, as you provide care, always talk to an unconscious person and tell her what you are doing.

Because of her decreased ability to swallow, it is essential that you position an unconscious person's head so that she won't **aspirate** any fluids into her lungs. Put the head of her bed as flat as possible and turn her on her side so that fluids will run out of her mouth instead of going down her throat, which could cause her to choke. Observe changes in the person's mouth and report any swollen, red, or tender gums, as well as bleeding, white patches, or sores.

When you provide mouth care for an unconscious person, follow the specific procedure that is explained step by step in Skill 23 in the skills book.

When to Help with Mouth Care

As a nurse assistant, help the person with mouth care—

❖ Every morning.
❖ Every evening.
❖ After the person eats a meal (as often as possible).
❖ Every 2 hours, if the person is unconscious.
❖ After the person vomits.

Assisting with Bathing and Shampooing

Have you ever had to be bathed by another person? If so, how did you feel? Was the person who bathed you sensitive to your feelings? Have you ever bathed another person? Do you have any fears about bathing another person?

Part of your responsibility in assisting with personal care is to help people with bathing. Helping a person with bathing is important because it gives you an opportunity to observe physical and emotional changes in the person. When you help someone bathe, observe his skin for redness, open sores, or bruises (see Body Basics, The Integumentary System, in Chapter 9), as well as any signs of physical abuse (see Chapter 3, Protecting People's Rights). During bathing, you may notice changes in the person's mood, which may be a clue that something is wrong.

What does it feel like to have someone else wash your hair? What does it feel like to have someone gently rub, or massage, your head, or scalp? How do you feel after your clean hair is dried and styled? Many people enjoy having someone else wash their hair.

Helping a person shampoo his hair also is an important part of your responsibility in assisting with personal care. Shampooing helps clean the scalp, stimulate circulation, and improve the person's self-image. The ideal way to shampoo someone's hair is in the shower or tub, although the same procedures can be used for shampooing at the sink.

Many people like to have their hair washed in a beauty shop. You can encourage a nursing home resident to arrange for an appointment with the hairdresser.

When you help a person with bathing or shampooing, you often have to consider whether he bathes and shampoos in the bed, the shower, or the tub. If he bathes in the bed, will you shampoo his hair while he is in the bed, or will you transfer him to a stretcher and wash his hair over a sink? If the person bathes in the shower or tub, can he get there by walking, or will you need to push him in the wheelchair? If the person bathes in the tub, will you have to use a mechanical lift?

The person in your care also has needs and preferences that influence your decision-making. Does he prefer the tub or the shower? Does he like to use soap on his face? When he is not shampooing in the shower, does he like to wear a shower cap? How often does he like to shampoo? Does he like to use conditioner after shampooing?

Why Help Bathe and Shampoo?

Bathing does a lot for a person: It refreshes and relaxes him, eliminates body odor, removes dirt and dead skin cells, and stimulates movement and blood flow, or circulation, through the body (Figure 10-5). In addition, washing with soap and water reduces oily secretions, which provide a place for odor-producing bacteria to grow. When a person shampoos, he removes dirt, oil, and bacteria from the hair and also prevents **dandruff**.

dandruff
(DAN-druff)   Flaking skin from the scalp.

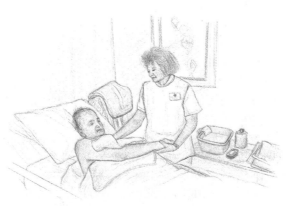

Figure 10-5
When helping someone bathe, you may need only to wash his back, or you may need to do a complete bed bath, as you did for Mr. Brady.

How to Help with Bathing and Shampooing

When you help a person bathe and shampoo her hair, you must observe the principles of care. As always, safety is the most important

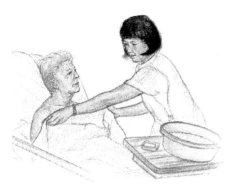

Figure 10-6
When helping someone bathe, be sure that you know and respect her personal and cultural feelings about modesty.

perineal care
(per-uh-NEE-uhl)   A nursing procedure in which a person's body is cleaned from the genitals to the anus.

principle. Because bathrooms, showers, and tubs can be dangerous places, make sure that showers and tubs have nonskid mats and surfaces and that grab bars are tightly fastened to the wall. To prevent burns, check the temperature of shower or bath water by touching the inside of your wrist to the water. Your fingers are less sensitive than the inside of your wrist, and by using them you could underestimate the water temperature. Ensure the person's safety by remaining with her while she is in the shower or tub.

Protect your own safety by using proper body mechanics. When bathing a person who is in bed, protect your back by helping the person move to the side of the bed where you are working. Make sure the bed is in the highest possible position. If the bed doesn't elevate, wash one side of the person at a time to avoid bending and reaching.

To provide dignity and privacy during bathtime and to keep the person warm, keep her covered as much as possible (Figure 10-6). Practice proper infection control measures by wearing disposable gloves when providing **perineal care**. When assisting a woman with perineal care, bathe her from front to back (the genitals to the anus). Cleaning in this direction avoids contaminating the urethral opening with bacteria from the anal area. (Review the drawing of the reproductive system in Chapter 4, Understanding People.) When helping a man with perineal care, wash from the urethral opening outward to prevent infection. For both women and men, use a different part of the washcloth for each stroke to prevent the spread of germs.

Bathing and shampooing in bed.   A complete bed bath involves bathing all parts of a person's body while she is in bed, as well as giving a backrub. A partial bed bath involves bathing only these parts of the body: face, hands, axillae, perineal area, back, and buttocks. When assisting with a complete bed bath, help the person maintain her independence by discussing with her how she can help. A person may be able to help only by washing her face, but any amount of self-care is good. If the person has more ability, you may suggest that she do her own perineal care. In this case, hand her the washcloth and provide privacy for her, after making sure she is safe.

When shampooing the hair of someone who is in bed, place a waterproof sheet under the person's head to keep the bottom sheet from getting wet. Or position the person on a stretcher with side rails and wash her hair at the sink (Figure 10-7).

Many people enjoy a backrub after a bath. After washing and drying a person's back, put lotion on your hands and rub them together to warm the lotion. Rub the lotion into the person's skin, using circular motions, to relax her and stimulate circulation.

When you help a person with a complete bed bath, follow the specific procedure that is explained step by step in Skill 24 in the skills book.

Showering and shampooing.   Many people enjoy bathing and shampooing in the shower. Before helping someone shower, reserve the

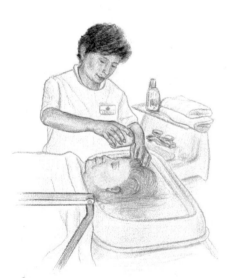

Figure 10-7
When you use this method for shampooing, water from the shampoo tray flows directly into the sink, avoiding any possibility of getting the bedding wet.

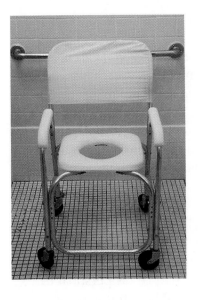

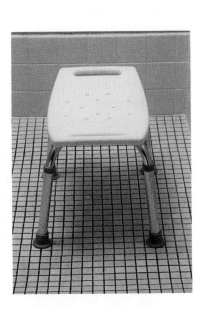

Figure 10-8
A shower chair is a waterproof chair on wheels. It is used to move a person into and out of the shower.

Figure 10-9
A shower seat is a removable chair or bench that enables a person to sit while showering.

shower, if necessary, and determine if you need any special equipment. Assess the person to decide if he is steady on his feet or if he needs to use a shower chair or shower seat (Figures 10-8 and 10-9).

Determine the best way to get the person to the shower room or bathroom: by walking or by riding in a wheelchair or shower chair. Accompany him to the shower room or bathroom to ensure his safety.

When you help a person with bathing and shampooing in the shower, follow the specific procedure that is explained step by step in Skill 25 in the skills book.

Tub bathing and shampooing.   Today at the nursing home, you help Mr. Wilson with a tub bath after his evening meal. He always enjoys a bath before he goes to bed. He says he sleeps better after a nice, warm bath.

Before helping someone with a tub bath, reserve the tub room, if necessary. Assess the person to determine if he can get into and out of the tub by himself or if you have to help him with a mechanical lift (Figure 10-10). The information in Box 10-2 helps you make this decision.

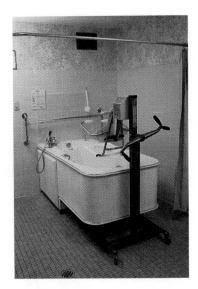

Figure 10-10
If you use a mechanical lift to help a person into the bathtub, be sure to get special instructions, and practice before using the lift.

Box 10-2   **When Can a Person Safely Get into and out of the Tub Without a Lift?**

To help a person into the bathtub without the use of a lift, the person should—
   ◆   Be predictable.
   ◆   Be able to reliably bear all or most of his own weight.
   ◆   Be able to stand on one foot and lift the other foot over the edge of the tub with a minimum of assistance.
   ◆   Be able to lower his body onto the tub seat or into the tub.

Determine the best way to get the person to the tub room or bath-room: by walking or by riding in a wheelchair or shower chair. Accompany him to the tub room or bathroom so that you can prevent a possible fall. When you fill the bathtub, check the water temperature with a bath thermometer to make sure that the temperature is not over 105 degrees Fahrenheit. Shut off the hot water first to prevent hot water in the faucet from dripping on the person's skin.

When you help a person with bathing and shampooing in the tub, follow the specific procedure that is explained step by step in Skill 26 in the skills book.

When to Help with Bathing and Shampooing

Set up regular bathing times based on the person's independence level, his preference for when to bathe, and your employer's policy on bathing. Assist him with shampooing as part of his personal care, following whatever schedule he would like, although it is recommended that a person wash his hair at least once or twice each week.

Assisting with Grooming

Why is grooming important to you? What does your hairstyle say about you? What does your beard or mustache say about who you are? How are your fingernails an expression of who you are? Does the way you look affect how you feel about yourself? A clean, well-groomed appearance improves your sense of well-being and makes you feel better about yourself.

Part of your responsibility in assisting with personal care is to help people with grooming. This important part of personal care includes brushing and combing the hair, shaving or grooming the beard, cleaning and trimming the fingernails, and cleaning the feet and toes. Some people in your care may want to do their own grooming, as Mr. Brady did when he used his electric shaver. Team up with the person by helping him with the tasks he cannot do and encouraging him to do the ones that he is capable of doing. For example, Mr. Brady could shave but was not able to clean his nails, so you helped him with that task. If someone in your care is unable to groom himself, you must provide the care for him.

You must know what kind of grooming each person in your care needs. Think about how you would feel if a stranger had to do your grooming. What if someone styled your hair in pigtails? Or what if someone shaved off your mustache? Or how would you feel if someone hastily applied the wrong color of lipstick to your mouth? How would you feel if your parent or grandparent was treated in this way?

If you can relate personally to these situations, you understand why each person must be treated as an individual. If you can imagine what it would feel like to depend on someone else to help you with your grooming, these feelings will help you provide better care to others.

Why Help with Grooming?

In addition to improving the person's self-esteem, grooming can help prevent painful tangles in the hair and possible injuries from jagged or long nails. Good foot care is an essential part of grooming, because the feet have a large number of sweat glands that remove wastes from the body. Foot care is especially important for anyone who has poor circulation in the legs and feet and for elderly people who may not be mobile enough to care for their own feet.

How to Help with Grooming

Generally people like to groom themselves. If physical limitations prevent this, you may have to help with grooming or encourage the use of adaptive devices (Figure 10-11).

To make good use of personal care time, combine tasks. For example, while a person in your care soaks his hands for nail care, use this time to brush and comb his hair. If a man in your care wears a beard or mustache, periodically wash it during bathtime to remove accumulated oil and food residue. Follow the person's desire for grooming. For example, he may want to use a special soap on his beard or mustache.

Brushing and combing hair.   The way a person wears her hair generally reflects how she feels about herself. The amount of time she spends on her hairstyle on a given day may reflect how she feels that day. You must consider the person's feelings along with variations in hair types and styles when you help brush, comb, and style someone's hair (Figure 10-12).

Remember to brush hair gently so that you do not pull it out. Some medications and medical treatments cause hair to be brittle or fall out. To prevent hair from breaking and to detangle the ends, start brushing from the ends of the hair, working toward the scalp, and work in small sections.

If a person's hair is tangled, use a comb with widely spaced, blunt teeth so that you don't hurt the person's scalp. Work slowly and in small sections so that you don't break the hair. In extreme cases, wet the hair and apply conditioner before combing and then wash and rinse the hair after you have removed all the tangles.

People of African descent may have very curly hair and dry scalps. If the person prefers, use oils, creams, or lotions when assisting with hair care to make the hair easier to comb and to moisturize the scalp. Generally, apply these creams to the scalp after shampooing and massage them into the scalp and hair. For people who have coarse hair, it may be easier to comb the hair when it is wet, after shampooing. Some people with very curly hair may find it easier to keep their hair tangle-free if it is braided. Check with the person to make sure that she wants her hair braided. If she does, be careful not to braid the hair too tightly, because hair tends to draw tighter as it dries and may pull too tightly on her scalp.

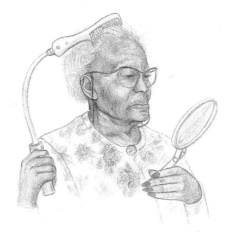

Figure 10-11
A person who has difficulty raising her arms can use a long-handled comb to comb her hair.

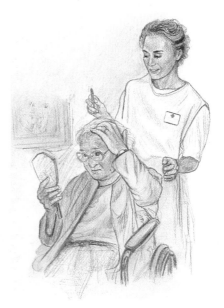

Figure 10-12
Like Mrs. Ryan, most people want to decide how to style their hair.

As you groom a person's hair, encourage her to look in the mirror. Report to your supervising nurse any unusual conditions, such as sores on the person's scalp, unusual flaking or dandruff, excessive hair loss, or tangles that can't be removed.

When you help a person with brushing and combing, follow the specific procedure that is explained step by step in Skill 27 in the skills book.

Shaving with a safety razor. Many men prefer to shave with a safety razor instead of an electric razor. Safety razors may either be disposable or have standard handles that hold replaceable blades. Whenever you handle a razor blade, you must take special precautions to avoid nicking or cutting yourself and the person in your care.

Because certain medical disorders and some medications can cause excessive bleeding if a person is cut, always ask your supervising nurse if a person should be shaved with a safety razor. Before helping a man shave, inspect his skin for moles, birthmarks, or sores. Shave carefully around these areas to avoid scraping or cutting, which could cause bleeding. Encourage the person to use shaving cream, because it softens the skin and helps the razor glide over the skin. Also, encourage him to use after-shave lotion, because the alcohol in after-shave helps keep germs from growing and acts as an **antiseptic** on **abrasions**. Men who have very curly beards may prefer not to shave, but to use **depilatory cream** or powder to remove facial hair.

After helping a man shave, report any red areas, sores, nicks, or cuts on his skin to your supervising nurse. To avoid cutting yourself or the person in your care, place the used razor in a sharps container or, if it is reusable, place the blade end down in a container, but don't recap it (Figure 10-13). Make sure each razor is used by only one person, because blood particles may be left on the blade, which could spread infection from one person to another.

When you help a person shave with a safety razor, follow the specific procedure that is explained step by step in Skill 28 in the skills book.

Shaving with an electric razor. Mr. Brady insists on doing his own shaving with the new cordless electric razor that Mrs. Brady bought him for his recent birthday. "You know how I grumbled when the wife bought this contraption for me?" Mr. Brady says. "Well, even though it doesn't shave close like my old safety razor, I'm really getting to like it—mainly because I can sit here in bed and shave all by myself."

Like Mr. Brady, some people use electric razors for convenience. Other people may have to use them for medical reasons. Use electric razors instead of safety razors on all people with blood-clotting disorders and on people taking medication that changes how fast the blood clots. For safety, check the condition of the razor to make sure that the screen has no holes and the cord isn't frayed.

antiseptic
(an-tuh-SEP-tik)   A substance that stops the growth of germs.

abrasion
(uh-BRAY-zhun)   A tiny cut or scrape.

depilatory cream
(duh-PILL-uh-tor-ee)   A lotion that dissolves hair and removes it from the surface of the skin.

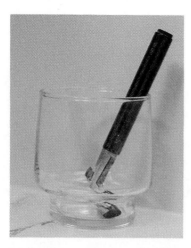

Figure 10-13
To avoid cutting yourself, never recap a sharp object. If the object is reusable, store it safely to prevent other people from injuring themselves.

Use an electric razor only in a room where no one receives oxygen, because the combination of the electric razor and the oxygen could set off a spark and start a fire. A battery-operated or rechargeable razor may be safe to use in a room with oxygen, but you must clear such use with your supervising nurse.

To keep the razor in good working order, take it apart and clean it when finished. As when shaving with the safety razor, report any red areas, sores, nicks, or cuts on the person's face to your supervising nurse.

When you help a person shave with an electric razor, follow the specific procedure that is explained step by step in Skill 29 in the skills book.

Cleaning and trimming fingernails.   Helping to wash someone's hands is part of daily personal care, and assisting with care for the fingernails is done as needed. When helping to care for someone's fingernails, have the person soak his hands in warm water for 5 minutes to soften the nails and make them easier to trim. The soaking may be done as part of the bath. Push the **cuticles** back gently with a washcloth to help prevent hangnails. Help keep a person's nails trimmed and smooth to prevent injury to his skin.

cuticles
(KYU-tuh-kuhls)   The skin at the base of the fingernails and toenails.

NOTE: Use caution when trimming the nails of a person who has diabetes, poor circulation, paralysis (on the paralyzed side), or decreased sensation in the hand.

Report to your supervising nurse any changes in the person's hands, such as reddened or discolored areas, sores, hangnails, or badly torn nails.

When you help a person clean and trim his fingernails, follow the specific procedure that is explained step by step in Skill 30 in the skills book.

Helping with foot care and cleaning toenails.   To assist with foot care, help the person out of bed and into a chair, if possible, as this position allows him to place his feet directly into a washbasin of water. If the person cannot get out of bed, help him to lie flat or position him in a semi-Fowler's position, place the washbasin on a towel near his foot, flex his knee, and place his foot into the basin. Help the person soak his foot for at least 5 minutes to loosen dirt under the nails and make them easier to clean. After helping a person clean his toenails, dry his feet and toes thoroughly. Then massage lotion into his feet (Figure 10-14). After assisting with foot care, report to your supervising nurse any changes in the person's feet, such as reddened or discolored areas, sores, breaks in the skin between the toes, injuries to the feet, toenails that need trimming, and ill-fitting shoes and socks.

NOTE: Although you may assist a person with general foot and toenail care, it is generally a doctor or nurse who cuts a person's toenails because of the chance of injury that may come from cutting nails too short or cutting the skin around the nails. Using orange sticks to clean under the toenails may also cause injury. Do not use

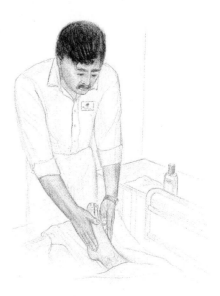

Figure 10-14
When assisting with foot care, gently massage the feet with lotion, working from the toes to the ankles. Do not massage the legs, as this could dislodge blood clots, if any are present.

them if the person has diabetes, poor circulation in the feet, paralysis of the legs, or decreased sensation in the feet.

When you help a person with foot care and cleaning his toenails, follow the specific procedure that is explained step by step in Skill 31 in the skills book.

When to Help with Grooming

Help a person with grooming—

❖ As part of regular care.
❖ When the person asks.
❖ When your supervising nurse asks.

Assisting with Undressing and Dressing

How important are clothes to you? What does it feel like when you wear your favorite clothes or when you wear something you don't like? Deciding what to wear is part of who you are. It is part of your self-image. Getting dressed every day helps you maintain your sense of identity. Making choices about what to wear encourages you to maintain control over your independence.

Every day when you get up and decide what to wear, you consider the weather, where you are going, who you will be with, and how you feel that day. Can you imagine if someone else made the decision for you? Suppose he or she selected clothing that was wrinkled, too big or small, or mismatched? What would that do to your self-image?

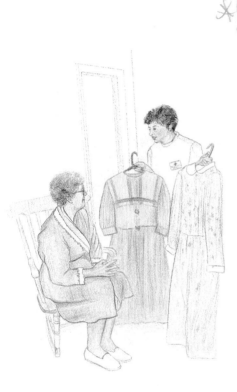

Figure 10-15
For someone like Mrs. McDay, who has a hard time making decisions and selecting clothing, you can offer two appropriate choices and say, "Which one would you like to wear today?"

The person in your care also likes to decide what to wear. Even though you may think it easier to pick out the clothes for her, she needs to decide what outfit to wear each day. How can you help someone decide what to wear? Even if the person has difficulty making decisions, you can offer two selections (Figure 10-15).

When helping someone select clothing, consider—

❖ The person's preference.
❖ The person's physical capabilities.
❖ Changing conditions, such as the time of day, scheduled activities, and the weather.

Why Help with Undressing and Dressing?

Dressing properly is important to help a person maintain dignity, stay warm, and prevent his body from being exposed. Wearing shoes also helps to protect the feet from possible injury.

Undressing is also important. Over a period of time, a person's clothing absorbs perspiration, a waste product from the body, which needs to be washed out of the clothes.

How to Help with Undressing and Dressing

Today, you encourage Mr. Brady to wear a nice, warm sweat suit. He sits in the bedroom chair to get dressed while you make his bed. Mr.

Brady takes a long time to fasten his sweat suit jacket, but you make the bed and talk with him as he completes the task. By providing time for Mr. Brady to finish snapping his jacket, you encourage his independence.

When helping someone get dressed, provide for his safety by making sure he sits down when putting on or taking off clothing. Sitting down eliminates the risk of the person standing on one foot, possibly losing his balance, and falling. Make sure the person is dressed appropriately for the weather and situation. Provide privacy and warmth by keeping the person covered as much as possible while undressing and dressing. For example, when helping a woman, adjust the bath blanket so that it covers her shoulders and upper body and remove her gown from underneath the bath blanket so that she is not exposed. When helping a man, cover him with a bath blanket before removing his pants.

To save time and energy, arrange the clothes in the order in which you help the person put them on. If the person has an **IV**, make sure that the sleeves of the clothing are large enough for the IV or bottle to fit through. Put the bag or bottle and tubing through the sleeve first, and then put the arm in the sleeve. If the person has a weak or paralyzed side, remove the clothing from the unaffected side first, but put on clothing from the affected side first.

When you help a person get undressed and dressed, follow the specific procedures that are explained step by step in Skills 32 and 33 in the skills book.

IV
(eye-VEE)   An abbreviation for **intravenous**. An IV is a type of medical equipment that supplies medicine and other liquids to a person intravenously, or through a needle inserted into his vein.

When to Help with Undressing and Dressing

Help a person undress and dress—

- ❖   Every morning.
- ❖   Every evening.
- ❖   Before and after the person takes a shower or bath.
- ❖   Whenever the person's clothes are soiled.

Providing Personal Care for Children

When you go to the home of Amber Clark and her 15-month-old son Dominic, you provide care for both the mother and her son. Ms. Clark broke her collarbone in a car collision and is unable to lift her son and provide his personal care. The care that you provide for this child is similar to the personal care that you provide for his mother, but because he is small and at a different stage in his development, you have to do some things differently.

Providing Mouth Care for a Child

Today, when you visit the Clarks, Ms. Clark says that Dominic has been very fussy. She thinks he is cutting more teeth, but she can't hold him to examine his mouth. You hold Dominic on your lap and look into his mouth. His gums are red and swollen, and you can see

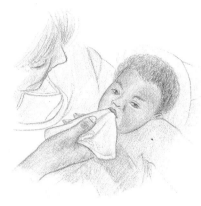

Figure 10-16
Good mouth care is important for children because it keeps teeth and gums healthy and promotes the development of healthy permanent teeth.

the white teeth just under the gum. This condition is a clue that you must be very gentle on that area of his mouth when you clean his teeth.

Many children have six to eight teeth by the time they are 1 year old. If a child's gums are not too tender from teething, use a moist cloth or gauze square wrapped around your finger to gently clean the teeth (Figure 10-16). If the child is over 1 year of age, use a very soft toothbrush dipped in water. Hold the child on your lap to provide comfort and security.

Babies around 1 year of age frequently go to bed with a bottle. If the baby drinks milk or juice from the bottle, the residue from these liquids can lead to early tooth decay. Because Ms. Clark usually puts Dominic to bed with a bottle of milk, you encourage her to substitute water for the milk at bedtime.

Children usually like to try brushing their own teeth, and it is important to encourage their independence by letting them do so. They usually are not able to clean their teeth effectively until the age of 6 to 10 years. Before then, an adult should brush the child's teeth, and the child should be encouraged to brush his own teeth either before or after the parent's brushing. He should brush for 3 minutes. Use an egg timer to let the child know when the 3 minutes have passed and to make brushing a fun time for him. Children should brush their teeth two to three times a day, making sure to brush just before bedtime.

You can brush a child's teeth when the child is in bed as you would an adult's teeth. You also can position yourself behind a child who is either seated or standing. Use one hand to cup the child's chin and the other to hold the toothbrush.

Check with your supervising nurse about whether it is advisable to use fluoridated toothpaste and mouth rinses in your geographic area. In many places, dentists recommend the use of fluoride toothpaste and, for children over 6 years, the daily use of a fluoride mouth rinse to reduce the possibility of tooth decay.

When you provide care for a child who is NPO (not eating or drinking by mouth), brush his teeth twice each day with a soft toothbrush dipped in water. Because some medicines are heavily sweetened to improve their taste, children should brush their teeth or rinse their mouths with water after taking these medicines. A child should also brush his teeth after vomiting to remove gastric juices, which can wear away tooth enamel. If using the toothbrush causes an ill child to gag, have him rinse his mouth with water and spit it out.

Children with physical impairments may have to use toothbrushes that have been specially adapted with larger or curved handles or self-adhesive fabric fasteners, which make them easier to hold. Electric toothbrushes also may be useful.

Bathing and Shampooing a Child

Dominic squeals with delight when you begin to run water into the tub for his bath. He loves bathtime. You gather together the plastic water toys and put them in the tub. After checking the tub water for the correct temperature, you turn the hot water off first, then the cold. You close the bathroom door before undressing Dominic so that he will stay warm. While Dominic plays in the tub, you sit on the toilet lid and watch him as he splashes about. After a few minutes, you kneel next to the tub and start to wash him.

Bathing a child.   When helping children bathe, it is important for you to know the age and developmental stage of each child and also his capabilities so that you can safely and appropriately provide care. Generally, older and adolescent children are very concerned about privacy, and younger children enjoy playing at bathtime.

Safety is the most important thing to keep in mind while bathing children. Never leave a child alone in water. Check the water carefully to make sure that it is between 100 and 105 degrees Fahrenheit (or just warm on the inside of your wrist). Fill the tub no more than one-third full and instruct the child, if it is appropriate, not to turn the hot water faucet by himself. To prevent falls, make sure nonskid mats are in the tub. Also helpful are safety rails or specially designed seats to support the child who cannot sit by himself. Do not use bath oils in the tub, because they make the tub and the child slippery and hard to hold onto.

If you have to help a child into a tub, be sure to use good body mechanics. If the child is small, bend your knees to squat and lower the child into the tub. Avoid bending over from the waist (Figure 10-17). A large tub may be awkward, uncomfortable, and unsafe for bathing a small infant. In a home setting, you may use an infant tub on a table top as an alternative (Figure 10-18). To hold an infant, place one arm under his neck and back and hold onto the arm on the side farther away from your body. This position gives you a firm grip on the infant and helps to make him feel more secure. Use your other hand to support the buttocks. Gradually lower the child into the water so that he has a chance to become accustomed to the water temperature and so that he isn't startled by the water.

Use one hand to wash an infant or small child who cannot sit without support, while holding and supporting him with your other hand. Wash from top to bottom, rinsing each part as you go so that the child does not become too slippery to hold onto. Also, as with adults, soap is very drying to the skin and may cause vaginal irritation in some little girls. Use soap sparingly and do not let it soak in the bath water. To keep the child warm, wrap him in a towel as soon as you remove him from the tub. Then help him get dressed.

Toddlers generally enjoy playing with unbreakable cups and toys in the bath. Provide time for play if possible, but do not leave the child alone. Older children and adolescents may have strong feelings about privacy and, as you would with adults, you should make every effort to give them privacy as long as you can do so safely.

Use the same basic procedure that you would use to bathe an adult in bed when you give a bed bath to an older child or adolescent or help him with a tub bath or shower.

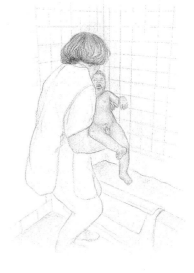

Figure 10-17
Be sure to hold a child close to your body as you lower him into the bathtub.

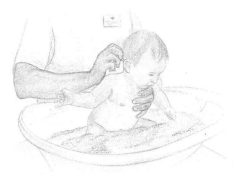

Figure 10-18
Place a specially designed infant tub on a surface that allows you to bathe a child without bending over and straining your back.

Shampooing a child's hair.   If the child is healthy, shampoo his hair once or twice a week. Adolescents may wish to shampoo their hair more frequently, because the scalp produces more oil at this stage of development. Shampooing can be done during the bath or separately.

Shampoo an infant's hair by applying baby shampoo to the scalp with one hand, while you support him as you did when you lowered him into the tub. Tip him back so that water and shampoo do not run into his eyes. Rinse out the shampoo by using the washcloth or an unbreakable cup to pour water over his head.

If a child is confined to his bed, wash his hair in the bed, using the same procedure you use for an adult. Encourage the child to help by holding a washcloth or towel over his eyes. Wrap the child's head in a towel immediately after the last rinse and follow instructions from your supervising nurse about using a blow dryer to dry his hair.

Providing perineal care for infants and children.   For children who wear diapers, it is important to clean the perineal area thoroughly (review Body Basics, The Reproduction System, in Chapter 4) to remove secretions and all traces of urine and feces from the skin. Be sure to observe the condition of the skin as you clean the area and to report all redness or skin irritation. Put on disposable gloves when you provide perineal care.

If a male child has been circumcised, clean the tip of his penis using strokes moving outward from the urethra. Use only a minimal amount of soap, and rinse thoroughly. If the child is uncircumcised, gently retract the foreskin until you feel resistance (the foreskin usually cannot be retracted fully until about the age of 4) and, using a clean section of the washcloth or a clean, moist cotton ball, clean around the head of the penis, moving from the urethra outward. Rinse in the same pattern and dry well. Be sure to return the foreskin to its original position, because leaving the foreskin retracted may interfere with circulation in the head of the penis. After washing and rinsing the penis, clean the scrotum and then the anal area.

When providing perineal care for a female child, wash any skin folds in the groin first. Then, using a separate section of the washcloth or clean cotton balls for each wipe, separate and clean the labia and then the urethral areas, moving from front to back. Use soap sparingly and rinse thoroughly. After washing and rinsing the labia and urethral areas, clean the anal area. Be sure to remove all secretions, because they can cause skin irritation. Observe the skin for any abrasions or changes in skin color. Report any concerns to your supervising nurse.

Combing a Child's Hair

Dominic hates hair-combing as much as he loves bathing. Today, you use a new approach to try to get him to sit still so that you can comb his hair. You brought along a blunt-toothed comb with a short handle and an unbreakable hand mirror. You put Dominic on your lap and hand him the new comb and mirror. Dominic begins to "comb" his hair and look at himself in the mirror. While he plays this game, you are able to comb his hair without having Dominic fuss and squirm.

Periodically comb a child's hair to remove tangles and prevent them from becoming extensive. Some children love to have their hair combed, while others don't want to be bothered. As the child gets older, combing is an important part of building good grooming habits and promoting healthy self-esteem.

To remove a stubborn tangle from a child's hair, first wet the hair and then apply conditioner to the tangle, which makes the hair shafts slippery. Applying conditioner often enables you to remove the tangle painlessly by combing. Start combing at the ends of the hair and work your way toward the scalp. Rinse the conditioner out of that section of hair or give the child a total shampoo.

Dressing a Child

Because Dominic is such as active child, you always sit with him on the floor when you dress him. He has a special floor blanket that you spread out before placing his clothes on top of the blanket. Then you and Dominic sit together on the blanket while you dress him. To help distract him and to keep him busy while you dress him, you also put two or three small toys on the blanket to hand to Dominic in case he gets bored and tries to wriggle out of your hands.

Dressing a young child on a clean blanket spread on the floor is very safe, because the child cannot roll off, fall, or get hurt. With a less active child, you can bring your supplies to the cribside or dressing table and work safely there. Because a child can move very quickly, never leave him unattended and always keep at least one hand on him if he is on a high surface. Infants and children can be very active, and at times you may think that you are trying to dress a moving target. Because of their activity, it is essential that you gather all your supplies and have them within arm's reach, yet out of reach of little fingers. Older children can be dressed in bed or while seated in a chair.

Stretchy knits or loose-fitting clothes are easier to put on than tight-fitting garments. One-piece garments for infants are convenient and easy to fasten and refasten during diaper changes. Pants for infants and toddlers may have snaps or other closures that make diaper changing easier.

Putting on a knit shirt or undershirt.   Gather up the shirt into a circle at the neck and pull it down over the child's head. Then thread your own fingers through the sleeve. Grasp the child's hand and guide it through the sleeve. Repeat the process with the other sleeve (Figure 10-19).

Putting on a one-piece sleeper.   Place the infant on his back. Gather up the leg of the sleeper that has no snaps and put it on his foot and

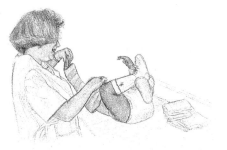

Figure 10-19
When dressing a child, gently pull his hands through the sleeves rather than pushing them through. This keeps the child's fingers from getting caught in the sleeves.

leg. Repeat with the other leg of the sleeper. Bring the sleeper up over the infant's torso. Insert his arm into one sleeve as described above and then into the other sleeve and finish fastening the garment. If you dress an older child while he sits in a chair, put the one-piece sleeper on his feet, and then have him stand as you pull the garment up and put his arms through the sleeves.

Putting on pants.   Place the infant on his back. Put your hand through the garment leg, starting at the bottom, and then grasp the infant's foot and guide his foot and leg through the garment leg. Repeat the process for the other leg. Finish by pulling the waist up over the diaper. Have an older child sit while you put his feet into the garment legs and then have him stand while you pull the pants up to his waist.

Putting on socks.   Gather the sock up and place it over the child's toes. Pull it over his heel and leg. Smooth out wrinkles before putting on shoes.

Putting on shoes.   Open the laces and fasteners of the shoe and pull out the tongue. Place the child's foot into the shoe, replace the tongue, and fasten snugly but not too tightly. Be aware of how the shoe fits, and report ill-fitting shoes to your supervising nurse.

To learn about assisting with medications in a home health setting, please read the next section. Otherwise, read "Information Review" and "Questions to Ask Yourself" at the end of this chapter.

Assisting with Medications in the Home Health Setting

One additional responsibility in personal care that a home health aide has is assisting with medications. Only doctors and licensed nurses may actually give medications to people. It is illegal for you, as a home health aide, to give any medication to a person in your care, including **over-the-counter medicines**, as well as **prescription medicines**. The law defining who can give medication protects both you and the person in your care. Giving medication is a big responsibility. If a person is given the wrong medication, he could be injured, and the person who gave him the medication could be held responsible for the injury.

In the home health setting, however, you can help the person who must take medication by reminding him to take it. You can bring the medicine container to the person and you can open it. You *cannot* pour out the medicine or remove it from the container in any way. Your supervising nurse may set up a schedule and instructions, such as the time, the **route**, and the amount.

For the safety of your client who takes medication, learn the following five rights (Figure 10-20) of administration:

You also can assist the person by steadying his hand to keep liquid medicine from spilling.

over-the-counter medicines
Medications, such as aspirin, cold remedies, laxatives, ointments, and eyedrops, that anyone can buy without a doctor's prescription.

prescription medicines
Medications that can be sold only by the order of a doctor.

route
(ROUT) When referring to medications, this is the way the medication should be taken: for example, taken by mouth, applied as an ointment, or given as a rectal suppository.

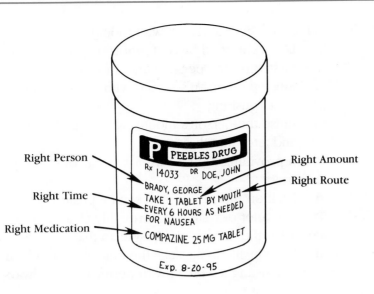

Figure 10-20
Be sure to check the five "rights" and the medication expiration date when assisting with medication in home health care.

When assisting a client with medications, follow the procedure that is explained step by step in Skill 34 in the skills book.

If a person asks you to fix some special kind of tea or home remedy, check with your supervising nurse first. Also, notify your supervising nurse if your client—

❖   Is not taking medication as prescribed.
❖   Is taking more or less than the prescribed amount.
❖   Is taking medicine other than what his doctor prescribed, including over-the-counter medicine.
❖   Is taking medication at times other than those ordered.
❖   Has **side effects** after taking medications.
❖   Says the medication doesn't seem to be working.
❖   Has any questions concerning medications.

Also, let your supervising nurse know—

❖   If a medication container is missing a label or if the label is hard to read.
❖   When you notice or your client tells you that he has just a few pills left from a prescription.
❖   If a medication has expired, because the strength of the medication cannot be guaranteed after the expiration date. (The expiration date is printed on the container label.)
❖   If you suspect that anyone in the household is misusing any type of medicine.

side effect
An action, other than the intended action, caused by a drug. Usually this action is an undesired effect.

Information Review

Circle the correct answers and fill in the blanks.

1.   When you provide care, you must respect each person's need to maintain his own—
   a.   Toothbrush, razor, and wardrobe.
   b.   Personal needs, self-image, and independence.
   c.   Grooming.
   d.   Toenails.

2. When you help a person with mouth care,—
   a. Use a stiff toothbrush to thoroughly clean his teeth.
   b. First rinse the person's mouth with plain water.
   c. Rinse the person's mouth with full-strength mouthwash after brushing.
   d. Rinse the person's mouth with diluted mouthwash before and after mouth care.

3. When providing mouth care for an unconscious person, it is important to—
   a. Position the person in a supine position.
   b. Use a lot of water to thoroughly clean the person's mouth.
   c. Turn the person on his side so that he does not aspirate.
   d. Remain silent, because the person cannot hear you talk.

4. When assisting a woman with perineal care, always wipe from _____Front_____ to _____back_____, using a clean part of the washcloth for each stroke.

5. Use a bath blanket when giving a person a complete bed bath to keep him from getting ___cold, chilled___ and to show respect for the person's ___dignity___ and ___privacy___.

6. When helping a person get ready for a shower or tub bath, determine the best way to get him to the shower room, tub room, or bathroom by—
   a. Reserving the shower or tub room.
   b. Using a safety belt.
   c. Using a mechanical lift.
   d. Walking or by riding in a wheelchair or shower chair.

7. When you finish using a disposable safety razor to shave someone,—
   a. Recap the razor. Put it in the person's drawer.
   b. Do not recap the razor. Put it in the person's drawer.
   c. Do not recap the razor. Put it in the "sharps" container.
   d. Do not recap the razor. Put it in a plastic bag and put the bag in a trash can.

8. The person you provide care for has a weak right arm. To help him put on a shirt, you put his ___weak, right arm___ arm into the sleeve first.

9. ___Safety___ is the most important thing to keep in mind when bathing children.

10. The five rights of medication administration are?

right __person__, right __route__,
right __medication__, right __~~does~~ amount__,
and right __time__.

Questions to Ask Yourself

1. Mrs. Jaskowitz is right-handed, but due to her stroke, she is not able to use her right hand to grip the toothbrush. How would you help Mrs. Jaskowitz brush her teeth?

2. Mr. Randal is unconscious. What would you talk about while you provide mouth care for him?

3. What would you look for on a person's skin during bathtime? What would you report to your supervising nurse?

4. You are bathing Mrs. Feld when Mr. Lloyd, a confused gentleman from down the hall, walks into the room. He tries to enter the privacy curtain, but cannot seem to find the opening immediately. What would you do?

5. You walk by Mrs. Kitzmiller's room while a new nurse assistant is styling her hair. You have assisted Mrs. Kitzmiller before, and you know she likes to wear her hair in a bun. The new nurse assistant is putting it in pigtails. What would you do?

6. Because of a problem with his leg, Mr. Wingard has been having bed baths without a shampoo for 10 days. He only likes to wash his hair in the shower. Today your supervising nurse has asked you to make sure his hair is washed. How would you do this?

7. Mrs. Lanver wants to help dress herself, but she is very slow. What can you do to increase her independence and maintain her dignity?

8. A 2-year-old child cries and screams every time you try to give him a bath. How could you keep him both calm and clean?

9. A 7-year-old child who is confined to a wheelchair selects a striped shirt and plaid pants to wear. You suggest a solid-color shirt to match the plaid pants or a solid-color pair of pants to match the striped shirt. But the child insists on the outfit she chose. After you finish dressing the child in the stripes and plaids, her mother comes into the room and yells at you for putting a mismatched outfit on her child. What would you do?

10. Mrs. Roth takes one pill from each pill bottle every day. One day, you notice that the one bottle is almost empty, while the other still has about 10 pills. Mrs. Roth says she takes two pills every day. You wonder if she has been taking two pills from the same bottle. What would you do?

11

Providing Care for the Person's Place

Goals

After reading this chapter, you will have the information to—

Respect a person's belongings while maintaining her place.

Operate and maintain different types of beds.

Use and maintain different types of equipment for a bed.

Demonstrate principles of infection control in maintaining a client's living area.

Assist with a client's cleaning and laundering.

After practicing the corresponding skills in the skills book, you will be able to—

Make an unoccupied and an occupied bed.

Change crib linens.

Agnes Ryan shares a room with Louise Wang at Morningside Nursing Home. Mrs. Ryan's part of this room has become home to her. A quilted wallhanging, which she made many years ago, hangs on the wall next to her bed. Every day she straightens one of her quilts, which is folded at the foot of her bed. She keeps a little stack of books, a pad of paper and pen, and her reading glasses on her nightstand, along with an arrangement of silk flowers and a lamp. She likes to keep these things arranged in a particular way so that she knows just where they are.

Mrs. Ryan also enjoys the family photos that are arranged on her half of the double dresser that she shares with Mrs. Wang. She likes to keep the pictures in a certain order so that she can tell visitors her favorite stories about her loved ones without having to search for the pictures.

One day, a new nurse assistant, who had never assisted with Mrs. Ryan's care, moved things around as she was providing morning care. Mrs. Ryan became very upset when she discovered all her things had been moved from her nightstand. She yelled at the new nurse assistant and told her not to touch her things again. She then told her to leave the room and not to come back. She wanted someone else to provide care for her—someone who would respect her home. The new nurse assistant was surprised at how upset Mrs. Ryan became. "It's not like I took anything," she said to her supervising nurse. Then her supervising nurse talked with her to help her understand the importance of respecting each resident's home space and personal belongings.

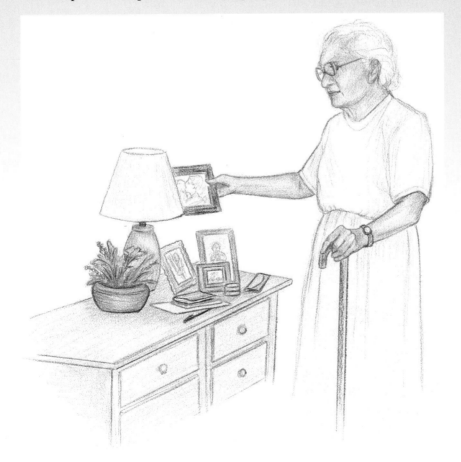

What Is a Person's Place?

Think about the word "home." What do you picture in your mind when you think of home? Do you think of a favorite, comfortable chair where you sit down after a long, hard day? Do you picture a special gift that someone gave to you? Does "home" trigger thoughts about family pictures on the wall?

What do you feel when you hear the word "home?" Do you feel that home should be a place where you feel safe and where you belong?...a place where you would want to find comfort, love, and security?

environment
(en-VY-run-ment)   The surroundings in which a person lives.

Home is your personal space. It is where you reside. As a nurse assistant, one way that you you help with a person's care is by maintaining her **environment**, or her place. One person's place may be the hospital, where her "home space" is usually part of a room. Another person's place may be a nursing home, where she receives care in her room and in shared areas, such as a dayroom. Still another person's place may be her own home, where she receives home health care.

Has someone ever come into your home and picked up or moved your things so that you couldn't find them? How did you feel? Did you feel as if that person came into your space where he or she didn't belong?

All your personal belongings are special. They say something about who you are. They often hold special meaning and may remind you of a certain place, person, or time.

A person in your care is sensitive about who touches her belongings or comes into her personal space. You must be sensitive to that person's needs by showing that you care and that you respect her belongings and her immediate surroundings. You show your sensitivity by always—

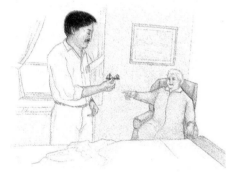

Figure 11-1
If you find glasses or other personal items in the bed while you are making it, ask the owner where you should put them.

❖ Asking the person if there is something special that she would like, such as two pillows instead of one.
❖ Telling the person you would like to move something and asking where to place it (Figure 11-1).
❖ Telling the person you would like to make or change her bed.

As a home health aide, you work in different kinds of homes. Many older people and people with disabilities may live in small apartments, or sometimes in one room. You may work with families in a poor area of a city or in a rural area. Space and materials may be limited. In some areas, you may find outdoor toilets. It is important for you to be able to "make do" with the materials that are available in the home.

Whether home is a person's own home, a nursing home, or a hospital, you help maintain that place so that it is special and personal. You help each person by maintaining a place that is safe, loving, and secure. In addition, you provide care for each person's place by keeping belongings tidy, making and changing beds, and practicing infection control so that the home space is clean and odor free.

Bedmaking

Bedmaking may seem like a very routine task. At home, you may make your bed every day. Or you may hardly ever make your bed. You may change your sheets once a week. Or you may change your sheets every few days. No matter what the routine for bedmaking is in your own home, the way you do it and when you do it are important to you. A clean, fresh bed is important to almost everyone. It is especially important to someone who spends most of her time in bed.

As a nurse assistant, you help with each person's care by making and changing beds according to each person's needs and according to the requirements of your employer.

Types of Beds

People in your care may be in different types of beds, depending on where they are receiving care and what their particular needs are. You should not operate any special bed unless you have—

❖ Received instructions on how to operate the bed properly.
❖ Practiced operating the bed.

Gatch-frame bed.   A gatch-frame bed has joints at places that allow the head and/or foot of the bed to be raised. A simple gatch-frame bed operates manually. You raise either the head piece or the foot piece and then adjust a horizontal bar (which lies across the bed), securing the bar into notches on the frame of the bed. You can adjust the bed to several different heights, depending on which notches you use.

Other manual gatch-frame beds have cranks that you turn to raise the head or foot portion of the bed. With some gatch-frame beds, you can raise or lower the entire bed, while others are stationary.

Electric bed.   An electric bed has head and foot sections that you can raise and lower electrically. Because the control panel normally is located within the person's reach, she usually can operate the bed without your assistance.

Specialty beds.   Some facilities have the following specialty beds that licensed nurses generally operate:

❖ **Stryker frame.** This special bed is used when it is necessary to change a person's position from prone to supine or supine to prone without moving her in the bed. To accomplish this repositioning, the person is secured into the bed, sandwiched between two frames, and gently "flipped" over (Figure 11-2).
❖ **Clinitron.** This bed has a mattress that is filled with a sandy material that supports and conforms to the shape of the person's body. Warm air circulates through the mattress to provide an

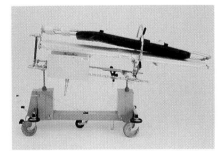

Figure 11-2
A person whose spinal column is injured may be placed on a Stryker frame to heal.

even temperature. It is used for people who have severe bed-sores or burns.

Special Equipment for Beds

People who need increased comfort in a standard bed can use special equipment, such as foam mattress pads and alternating pressure pads.

Foam mattress pad.   A foam mattress pad increases comfort and reduces the risk of developing pressure sores. Often it is contoured, resembles an egg carton, and is called an EGGCRATE mattress (Figure 11-3). It is placed on top of the standard mattress, and the bottom sheet is tucked in loosely around it. A person may need more than one foam pad on the mattress to aid in the treatment of pressure sores. To put a foam mattress pad on a bed:

❖ Transfer the person from the bed to a chair, if possible. If the person is unable to be placed in a chair, use the procedure for making an occupied bed to position the pad. When making an occupied bed, follow the procedure that is explained step by step in Skill 36 in the skills book.

❖ Strip the linens from the bed.

❖ Place the foam mattress pad on the bed with the wavy side up.

❖ Place the bottom sheet over the foam mattress pad.

❖ **Miter** the corners by following the procedure for making an unoccupied bed that is explained step by step in Skill 35 in the skills book. Tuck the sheet in loosely, so that it does not reduce the cushioning effect of the pad. If one sheet is not large enough to cover both the mattress and the pad, use two sheets. Use one to cover and tuck in around the mattress, and then lay the foam mattress pad over the sheet. Use the other sheet to cover and tuck in around the foam mattress pad.

❖ Put on a drawsheet and tuck it in loosely (Figure 11-4). Also use the drawsheet to move and position the person. Do not use the foam mattress pad as a lifting sheet, because it is not strong enough to support the weight of a person and may tear.

Alternating pressure pad (air mattress).   An alternating pressure pad, which is placed on top of the standard mattress, has channels that are connected to a pump that alternately fills and empties the channels with air. The pad is useful in preventing pressure sores and stimulating circulation.

Before using the pad, read the manufacturer's instructions for operation and safety practices. Follow these instructions, as well as general rules of electrical safety. To use the pad:

❖ Transfer the person from the bed to a chair, if possible. If the person is unable to be placed in a chair, use the procedure for making an occupied bed (Skill 36 in the skills book) to position the pad.

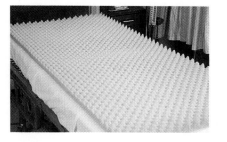

Figure 11-3
An EGGCRATE mattress (shown here on top of sheets) is used by a person who has pressure sores or has the potential to develop them.

miter
(MY-ter)   To square off the corners of bed linens by neatly tucking them under each other.

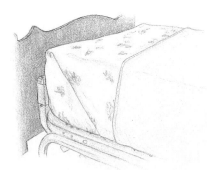

Figure 11-4
The sheet and drawsheet are loosely tucked so that the EGGCRATE mattress does not flatten, and the corners of the sheet are mitered so that they will not come untucked.

❖   Strip the linens from the bed.

❖   Unfold the alternating pressure pad on the bed with the inlet tubes facing up at the foot of the bed.

❖   Hang the air pump on the bedframe, or place it on the floor on a clean surface.

❖   Check the tubing to make sure it has no kinks, holes, or cracks.

❖   Attach the tubing to the air pump connectors.

❖   After following the instructions on the pump to determine the proper start-up pressure setting, plug the pump into an electrical outlet and turn on the motor. Make sure the cord is out of the way so that no one trips over it.

❖   After several minutes, check the filling and emptying of the channels.

❖   Cover the alternating pressure pad with a large sheet tucked loosely under the mattress, rather than mitered, to avoid pinching the tubing. Also, limit the layering of linens, as the thickness reduces the effectiveness of the pad. You may use a drawsheet to help with positioning and transferring.

❖   Check the effectiveness of the pad by placing your hand under the person's thigh. If you can feel the bottom of the pad when the channel is inflated, increase the pressure of the pump. Check periodically to make sure the mattress is functioning.

❖   To avoid puncturing the pad, do not use pins to attach anything to it.

❖   When changing linens, check to see that the alternating pressure pad is clean and dry. If it is not, clean it, using the manufacturer's method of cleaning.

Bed cradle.   A bed cradle is a framework that keeps the top **bed linens** from rubbing against and putting pressure on various parts of a person's body, especially the toes. The top linens are placed on the bed over the bed cradle to prevent direct contact.

bed linens
(LIN-ens)   Sheets, pillow cases, mattress covers, blankets, and bedspreads.

When to Make a Bed

As a nurse assistant, you provide care for many people who spend much of the day out of bed. However, you also provide care for some people who are unable to get out of bed. The frequency with which you change bed linens depends on how much time the person spends in bed, and it also depends on your employer's policies. One universal rule to follow: Change all linens immediately if they are wet or contaminated because they can cause skin irritation that can lead to sores.

In a hospital or nursing home, change the bed linens according to the policies of your employer. For people who are able to get out of bed, you may change the linens every day, as nurse assistants in most hospitals do, or only on days when people shower. For those people who cannot get out of bed, change the linens every day.

For people receiving home health care, change linens according to your employer's policy or at least once a week—more often if the person spends most of her time in bed.

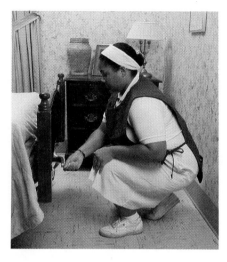

Figure 11-5
Remember to use good body mechanics when you adjust a bed with a hand crank.

Generally, most facilities and health care agencies change beds in the morning after bathing, grooming, and dressing are completed. But the time of day for changing beds also varies according to the needs of the person in your care.

How to Make a Bed

Bedmaking in a health care setting is probably different from the way you perform this task at home. First, you probably make many more beds at work than you do at home, which places extra strain on your back muscles. For this reason, you must protect your back by conserving your energy and using good body mechanics (Figure 11-5). Second, you must take special infection control measures when making beds in a health care setting.

When making beds in a health care setting, save time and energy by stacking bed linens in the order in which you use them, so that the bottom sheet or the mattress pad is on the top. Also, save time by folding reusable linens, such as blankets and spreads, and putting them over a clean place, such as the back of a chair, until you are ready to put them back on the bed.

Save more time and energy by making one side of the bed at a time. When you work from one side of the bed, you also use better body mechanics, because you don't reach across the bed. Keep from twisting your upper body by standing in front of the section of linen that you are tucking under the mattress. When making an unoccupied bed, work with the bed in a flat position and at a comfortable height so that you don't injure your back (Figure 11-6). When making an occupied bed, put the bed only as flat as the person can tolerate, because some conditions and diseases make it hard for a person to tolerate lying flat. In a home setting, the bed may be low, and you may not be able to raise it. In such situations, you may have to squat or kneel, keeping your upper body erect, to make the bed.

When you gather supplies for bedmaking, take only the linens you need into the person's room. In a hospital or nursing home, once linens have been taken into a person's room, they cannot be used for another person, and they have to be laundered, even if they weren't used. This regulation maintains infection control. Other ways you can practice this principle of care are by keeping linens away from your uniform, washing your hands before handling clean linens, keeping clean and dirty linens from touching the floor, not shaking linens, rolling dirty linens tightly and bagging them immediately after taking them off the bed, and washing your hands after handling soiled linens.

Before removing dirty bed linens, respect the person's property by checking the linens for personal items, such as eyeglasses, dentures, or hearing aids, that the person may have left in the bed. These items are expensive to replace if they are lost or broken.

Make sure you know how to use the types of linens in the place where you work, because linens vary from one health care setting to another and from one individual to another. Sheets may be flat or

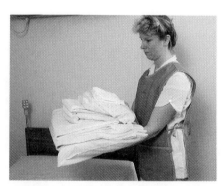

Figure 11-6
Raising the bed to the highest position and stacking bed linens correctly save you energy and time and protect your back.

fitted, washable or disposable. Bed linens may also include mattress pads or covers.

Put the person first when you are making her bed, and after you have finished making her bed, make sure that she is comfortable and safe before you leave her room.

Making an unoccupied bed.

Earlier in the morning, you assisted Josie Miller with her shower, grooming, and dressing. When you left her room to help someone else, she was sitting in the chair reading a letter she received yesterday from her daughter who lives in England. She has told you before how much she misses her daughter.

Now, as you get ready to return to her room to change her bed linens, you think about how sad Josie might feel. You plan to take advantage of this time to talk with her and listen to her concerns. You hope this special care that you provide as you make her bed helps her feel better.

Bedmaking is an opportunity for you to spend some time in conversation with the person in your care. In addition to providing a clean, comfortable bed for her, you can use this time to show her that you think she is an important and special person.

When making an unoccupied bed, follow the specific procedure that is explained step by step in Skill 35 in the skills book.

Making an occupied bed.

Because Tamara Frazier is in a coma, she is always in her bed when you change her bed linens. Although she doesn't respond to what you say to her, you always talk to her while you make her bed. You tell her what you plan to do, and you talk about the weather, what's happening in the news, and what's happening in the nursing home. You talk about the people who come to visit her, and sometimes you even tell her about your life outside the nursing home.

When making an occupied bed, changing the bottom sheet and drawsheet is your biggest challenge. To make Ms. Frazier's bed, first position her on her side and loosen the dirty bottom sheet and drawsheet. Then roll the dirty sheets against her back and lay a clean bottom sheet on the mattress. Fan-fold the part of the clean bottom sheet that goes on the side of the bed where Ms. Frazier is now lying and place it next to the dirty sheets rolled against her back. Tuck in the clean bottom sheet. Do the same with the drawsheet. Next, roll Ms. Frazier over the rolled dirty sheets and the fan-folded clean sheets and position her on the "clean" side of the bed. Remove the dirty sheets from the bed and pull the clean bottom sheet over the mattress and tuck it in. Do the same with the drawsheet.

As you make Ms. Frazier's bed, keep the principle of safety in your mind by—

- ❖ Keeping the side rail up on the side where you are not working.
- ❖ Rolling Ms. Frazier toward you, never away from you, to avoid injury to yourself and her.

❖ Staying with her and never leaving her alone until you have completed the procedure.

Even though Ms. Frazier is in a coma, you respect her dignity by providing the same kind of privacy that you would provide to a conscious person while making the bed. You keep her covered with the top sheet, unless it is wet or contaminated, and then you cover her with a bath blanket. Before removing the dirty top sheet or bath blanket, you cover her with the clean top sheet (Figure 11-7).

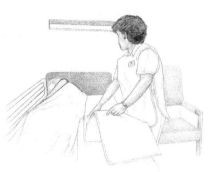

Figure 11-7
The nurse assistant is not sure if Ms. Frazier can hear or understand her, but she is careful to maintain the resident's dignity and privacy. She also talks to Ms. Frazier while she provides care.

To make Ms. Frazier comfortable, you complete the bed by making a toe pleat, which prevents pressure from the tight corners of the linens on her feet.

When making an occupied bed, follow the specific procedure that is explained step by step in Skill 36 in the skills book.

To read about bedmaking, cleaning, and laundering in a home setting, please read the next sections. Otherwise, read "Information Review" and "Questions to Ask Yourself" at the end of this chapter.

Changing crib linens.   When you provide home health care for Mary Hill and her 3-month-old daughter Melissa, you always change the linens on the baby's crib. After you finish giving Melissa her bath, you place her in the playpen in her room so that you can keep an eye on her while you change the bottom sheet and baby blanket in her crib. As you work, you talk to Melissa, and she smiles up at you from the playpen.

When you first started visiting the Hill's, you noticed that Mrs. Hill had a small pillow in Melissa's crib. You explained to her that it was not safe because the baby could suffocate in the pillow. Mrs. Hill was glad that you told her and asked you to remove the pillow from the crib and store it in the closet in Melissa's room.

When changing the linens on a crib, follow the procedure that is explained step by step in Skill 37 in the skills book.

Maintaining a Bed in a Home Setting

In a home setting, in addition to changing the linens on a person's bed, you must maintain the bed so that the mattress remains firm and free from dust that might cause allergies. To maintain the person's bed,—

❖ Brush or vacuum the bed weekly to get rid of dust and dust mites.

❖ Turn the mattress at least once a month so that the person does not sleep on the same place, which would cause uneven wearing of the mattress.

❖ Make sure the air pump works, if she uses an air mattress.

When making a bed in a home setting, it is especially important to remember to use good body mechanics, since the bed may not raise or lower. Protect your back by squatting instead of bending over and by moving around the bed instead of reaching across it.

Some people in a home setting may sleep on water beds. One type of water bed, called a soft-sided water bed, uses standard bed linens. Another type, which consists of a water-filled bladder inside a wooden frame, often requires the following special linens:

❖ Mattress pad with elastic bands that fit over the corners of the mattress

❖ Sheets with triangular corners and with the top and bottom sheets sewn together at the foot end

To put these special sheets on a water bed:

❖ Place the linens on the bed so that the bottom sheet is against the mattress and the top sheet is facing up. The corner pockets will then be on the side facing the mattress.

❖ To fit the corner of the sheet over the mattress, grab the corner of the sheet with one hand and turn the pocket inside out over your hand. With your hand inside the sheet pocket, lift the mattress and turn the pocket over the corner of the mattress with your other hand (Figure 11-8). When you let go of the mattress, the weight of the water fills the corner and keeps the pocket in place. Repeat the process for each corner.

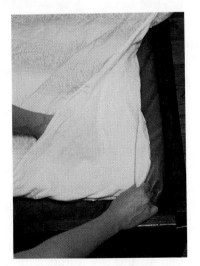

Figure 11-8
A water bed is easy to change with specially made bed linens.

❖ Tuck the sides of the sheets between the mattress and the bedframe.

❖ Use a drawsheet by pulling it taut and tucking it in the sides between the mattress and the bedframe.

❖ Tuck blankets and spreads on the bottom and sides, or simply spread them over the top of the bed, depending on the client's wishes.

❖ Check the water bed thermostat to make sure it is set at the temperature that the client prefers. The range of comfort for most people is 75 to 95 degrees Fahrenheit.

❖ Special conditioners must be added periodically to the water to keep it free from harmful bacteria. Check with the client to determine when you have to add the conditioner.

❖ The water bed is adequately filled if the mattress is level with the bedframe and not heaping over it. Yet, the person should not be able to feel the bottom of the bed when she is lying on it.

When providing care for a client who sleeps on a water bed, you must—

❖ Keep all sharp objects away from the bed.

❖ Make sure the temperature is comfortable and check the thermostat daily.

Cleaning and Laundering in a Client's Home

When you provide health care to someone at home, your primary responsibility is providing personal care according to the client's plan of treatment (Figure 11-9). Light housekeeping chores may play

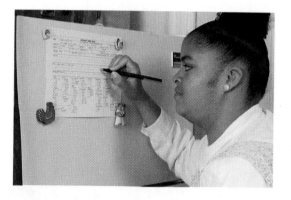

Figure 11-9
A client's care plan is often posted in the house so that everybody knows his or her responsibilities. If you are asked to do large jobs that are not listed on the care plan, check with your supervisor first.

a role in that plan. The amount of cleaning you do depends on the availability of family members, and the amount of time you spend in the home, and the requirements of the client's care plan. You may have to keep the bedroom, bathroom, and kitchen clean, as these three areas are important to the client and the care you provide for her. You also may have to do the client's personal laundry and wash her linens.

Maintaining a clean living environment helps promote the client's dignity and discourages the occurrence and spread of diseases such as colds, flu, and diarrhea. Pests, such as roaches, rats, mice, lice, and fleas, cannot thrive in a clean home. As a home health aide, you also must be concerned about a client's safety. The prevention of falls is a key factor.

Your duties as a home health aide differ from those of a house-keeper. You focus your cleaning on eliminating germs, controlling infections, and keeping the house free of safety hazards. You also may have to teach family members proper techniques to clean the household in this manner.

The home health agency that you work for has infection control policies and procedures for client care, housecleaning, and launder-ing. It is important that you understand and practice these policies and procedures. The specific cleaning and laundry duties that you are responsible for are in the care plan prepared by your supervisor or the home health care team.

Before beginning each day, you must organize your time and thoughts. You have only a limited amount of time to spend with each client. Although your primary responsibility is helping the client with basic personal care, you have to think about the areas of the client's home you must address after you provide this care.

When taking care of a client in her home, you must always re-member that, just like you, she may feel very strongly about her home and the things in it. Discuss your cleaning duties with your supervising nurse and client so that you know how much you should do, as well as what the client wants and needs to have done for her. The way that you do things may be different from the way the client does things. If you must do things a certain way to maintain safety or infection control, you may have to explain why. Or you may have to alter the procedure if the client asks you to handle things differently, providing you would not be violating a basic principle of care.

You also have to think about how the client and her family mem-bers might feel because they cannot take care of her needs. Some family members might feel insecure because someone else is doing their job. Or they may ask you to do tasks outside your responsibil-ity. The care plan is your guide. If you think a large job needs to be done or a family member asks you to do something that is not in the care plan, you must discuss it with your supervising nurse, the client, or the client's family before doing it.

Cleaning to Prevent the Spread of Germs

To prevent the spread of germs and disease, always wash your hands before beginning and after completing home maintenance tasks. You may have to carry your own soap, paper towels, and disposable hand wipes for handwashing. If there is no running water, use your hand wipes. Always observe the principles of infection control.

Also, observe universal precautions and infection control proce-dures, such as wearing gloves if you come into contact with body fluids such as blood, urine, or feces. For example, you must put on disposable gloves when handling contaminated laundry or cleaning up vomit. Throw away the disposable gloves in a covered trash can or a plastic trash bag and wash your hands when you have finished the task. If necessary, put on new gloves for the next job.

In Chapter 7, Controlling the Spread of Germs, you read about the following three levels of cleaning:

1. Cleaning: To get rid of visible dirt
2. Disinfecting: To remove harmful organisms
3. Sterilizing: To eliminate all organisms

In your job as a home health aide, you must use cleaning products safely. You also have to know when to use various cleaning agents, including the four basic kinds of household cleaning products:

1. All-purpose cleaning agents for general cleaning of many kinds of surfaces, such as countertops, walls, floors, and baseboards
2. Soaps and detergents for bathing, laundering, and washing dishes
3. Cleansers for scouring areas that are hard to clean
4. Specialty cleaners for specific tasks and surfaces, such as cleaning glass or ovens

Some cleaners also contain disinfectants. If you have to disinfect, but the cleaners you have don't kill germs, use a bleach solution. Household bleach is an inexpensive and effective chemical disinfectant for cleaning. At the beginning of each visit, prepare the solution by mixing ¼ cup of bleach with 1 gallon of water.

Because full-strength bleach has a very strong odor and is harsh on the skin, always mix it with water. Put the water in a bucket or other container first and then pour the bleach into it. Mix bleach only with water, since mixing it with anything else, especially any product containing ammonia, could make a dangerous gas. Also, make a fresh solution of bleach and water each day, because the disinfecting power of bleach goes away if the solution sits too long.

Before using the bleach solution, test a small area to make sure the solution does not affect the color of the surface, and then wash it off. Use the bleach solution to clean the bathroom, floors, and counters. Also use it as a disinfectant on a surface that has already been cleaned of visible dirt. To protect your skin, wear disposable or household gloves.

Be sure to store all cleaning products in a safe place (Figure 11-10). (Read this information again in Chapter 6, Keeping People Safe.)

Sterilization is a process that kills all germs. Boiling an item for 20 minutes is a sterilization process that kills most harmful germs. For example, you may have to sterilize baby bottles in the home. Glass bottles may be boiled, but check with the client before boiling plastic bottles. You will learn more about sterilizing baby bottles in Chapter 21, Providing Care for Mothers and Newborns.

Cleaning the Home

Today is one of your longer visits with Mrs. Roth, so you plan to help her with some additional cleaning and laundry. On your shorter visits, you help her wash and get dressed, change her bed and bath linens, and prepare her lunch. You frequently put a load of Mrs. Roth's dirty clothing or linens into the washer and dryer and usually have time to clean the toilet, sink, and tub. In addition, you clean the kitchen counters, wash the dishes that Mrs. Roth used, and dispose of

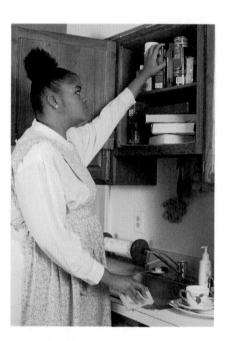

Figure 11-10
Because some cleaning products are dangerous if swallowed or used improperly, make sure all cleaning products are stored in a safe place. If children or confused people are in the home, use a high shelf or a locked cabinet.

trash. Today you also have time to launder the dirty kitchen linens and do some light dusting and floor cleaning.

Dusting.   If required, dust a client's home about once a week. If the client has an allergy, you may have to dust every day.

Cleaning floors and rugs.   Depending on the client's needs, you may have to sweep, vacuum, or wash floors and sweep or vacuum rugs in her living area. Check with the client or other family members before you wash a floor. Once you have permission, wash the floor with a cloth or mop dampened with hot, sudsy water; bleach solution; or clear water. Dry the floor with a dry mop or cloth, because wet floors may be slippery and can cause falls. Wash your hands after cleaning the floors or rugs.

Disposing of trash.   You must dispose of any trash you create while providing care for your client. You also may dispose of household trash and possibly teach family members proper techniques for trash disposal. Periodically, you may have to wash trash cans with hot, soapy water when they are dirty and rinse them with a bleach solution. Washing reduces germs and odors that grow in trash containers, as well as insects and rodents that may live and breed there. To avoid spreading any germs from handling trash, be sure to wash your hands when you finish disposing of it. In addition, observe the following procedures for different types of trash:

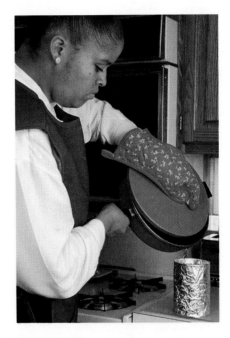

Figure 11-11
If you must dispose of grease while it is still hot, be sure to use a heat-proof container, such as a metal food can. Allow the container to cool before putting it in the trash.

❖   **Food.** To throw away food, drain off liquid, wrap the food, and put it in a paper- or plastic-lined pail. If your client has a garbage disposal, put only soft foods in it. Never put hard or stringy foods in the garbage disposal, as they may damage it.

❖   **Grease.** Pour cooled grease into a disposable container, never into the sink drain or garbage disposal (Figure 11-11). Put a lid on the container before disposing of it with the garbage.

❖   **Cans and bottles.** Rinse cans and bottles to destroy odors that might attract insects, rats, or other pests. Put appropriate cans and bottles in containers for recycling, and dispose of the others with the trash.

❖   **Contaminated and wet items.** Use plastic bags for contaminated and wet items such as used tissues, sanitary napkins, disposable underpads, adult briefs, or dressings. Double-bag and tie these items before throwing them into a plastic trash bag or covered container. Always wear disposable gloves when handling these items, and dispose of gloves properly in a plastic trash bag or covered container.

Doing the Laundry

Part of the care you may have to provide for your client is cleaning and maintaining her linens and clothing. If your client has urinary or bowel **incontinence**, you may have to do laundry several times a day. To clean contaminated linens,—

incontinence
(in-KON-ti-nense)   The inability to control the release of urine or feces.

❖ Immediately remove contaminated linens from the bed.

❖ Flush solid waste down the toilet.

❖ Put the contaminated linens in a plastic bag and take them to the washing machine or to a commercial laundry.

Because you may come in contact with body fluids on contaminated laundry, you must observe infection control procedures by keeping dirty linens away from your own clothing and wearing a gown and disposable gloves when handling linens soiled with body fluids.

When washing a client's linens or clothing, check with her or an appropriate family member about the way she prefers to have her laundry done. You may have to check clothing labels to determine how to wash certain items. For example, clothing labels may direct you to use a particular water temperature, to wash dark clothes separately, or to dry at a particular heat level.

Before washing clothes, sort them by—

❖ Color (separate dark colors and light colors).

❖ Type of fabric.

❖ Durability (separate sturdy items and delicate items).

❖ Amount of dirt (separate very dirty items and moderately dirty items).

❖ Size or weight.

While you are sorting, empty pockets, close zippers and hooks, and pretreat stains.

Select the kind of detergent and bleach that is best for the kind of fabric. For example, use light-duty detergent for delicate fabrics, such as silk, lingerie, and hosiery. Select heavy-duty detergent for sturdier items. Some detergents are "all purpose," and you can use them for all laundry. Add the detergent to the wash water before putting in the clothes.

Be sure to check the labels on each piece of clothing so that you know whether it should be dried in a dryer or on a clothesline. Whether you dry clothes and other items in a dryer or on a clothesline, be sure the clothes are completely dry before you put them away.

Place clean laundry and linens on a clean surface for folding. If you put them somewhere dirty, such as on the floor, you must wash them again.

Taking Safety Precautions

Falls and other incidents can happen in the home. Your safety and that of the client and her family are very important. Part of your job of maintaining the home is identifying and eliminating safety hazards. You can practice safety by observing the precautions that you read in Chapter 6.

Information Review

Circle the correct answers and fill in the blanks.

Bedmaking

1. To show respect for a person when you make her bed,—
   a. Make the bed when it is convenient for you to do so, no matter what the person is doing.
   b. Tell the person you would like to move something and ask her where to place it.
   c. Throw away any personal items left in the bed without asking the person first.
   d. Rearrange items on the overbed table and nightstand as you would like them.

2. Foam mattress pads are—
   a. Placed between the drawsheet and the bottom sheet.
   b. Used to lift and turn a person in the bed.
   c. Used to prevent bedsores.
   d. Tightly covered with a sheet.

3. All of the following are true about bedmaking in a home health care setting except—
   a. Making one side of the bed at a time.
   b. Storing many linens in the person's room so that you don't have to go back and forth to get them.
   c. Washing your hands before handling clean linens.
   d. Holding dirty linens away from your uniform.

4. When you make an unoccupied bed,—
   a. The person sits in a chair outside the room.
   b. Don't talk, so you can finish the task quickly.
   c. Use this time to talk and listen to the person.
   d. The person sits on the side of the bed where you are not working.

5. The biggest challenge in making an occupied bed is changing

   the _____ _____ and

   the _____.

Cleaning and Laundry

1. When a client asks you to do a cleaning task, you should—
   a. Do it even if it isn't part of the care plan.
   b. Never do it if it isn't part of the care plan.
   c. Ask your supervising nurse for instructions about whether to do the task.
   d. Ask a family member to do the task.

2. Removing harmful organisms is called—
    a. Cleaning.
    b. Washing.
    c. Sterilizing.
    d. Disinfecting.
3. When mixing a bleach solution for disinfecting, the proper ratio of bleach to water is—
    a. 1 cup of bleach to 10 cups of water.
    b. ¼ cup of bleach to 1 gallon of water.
    c. 6 cups of bleach to 1 gallon of water.
    d. ½ cup of bleach to 1 gallon of water.
4. To control the spread of germs, always wash

    _____ _____ after disposing of trash.
5. To clean contaminated linens, remove them from the bed, flush solid waste down the toilet, and place the contaminated

    linens in a _____ _____.

Questions to Ask Yourself

1. Mrs. McDay keeps a large, framed picture of her daughter on her nightstand. While making her bed, you find it necessary to move the picture to avoid knocking it over. What must you remember to do before leaving the room?

2. Mrs. Taylor has just been admitted to your floor in the hospital. She wants you to remove the linens from her bed and remake it with the pink, flowered linens she brought from home. What should you say to her?

3. Mrs. Ross cannot get out of bed, and you have to change her bed linens. You know that her delicate skin is particularly vulnerable to irritation and bedsores. What can you do to protect her skin and maintain her comfort?

4. While Mr. Gilbert showers, you change his bed linens. As you lift a pillow, his reading glasses slip from the pillowcase and fall to the floor, unharmed. What should you do to retrieve them?

5. In the clean utility room, you pick up a supply of bed linens to change Tamara Frazier's bed and stack them in the order that you will use them. In Ms. Frazier's room, you begin to remove the top sheet and realize that she has been incontinent of feces and her nightgown and bed are soiled. What should you do?

Home Health Care

1. Mrs. Feld, one of your home health care clients, sleeps on a water bed. Since you know that the bed does not raise or lower, how can you protect your back when changing the bed linens?

2. Your client says she wants you to clean the bathroom with a particular cleaner that is not a disinfectant. What can you do to keep her happy and maintain infection control?

3. You are dusting items in Mr. Phelps' bedroom. Mrs. Phelps looks into the room and smiles at you. "While you're at it," she says, "could you vacuum the drapes?" You know that this task is not on Mr. Phelps' care plan. What should you do?

4. Mrs. Garcia asks you to cook her a hamburger for lunch. After serving her the hamburger, you return to the kitchen to clean up. What should you do with the hamburger grease left in the frying pan?

5. As you sort dirty laundry in the Jones' household, you come across one of Mrs. Jones' pretty dresses. You don't know what kind of fabric the dress is made of. How do you launder it?

12

Healthful Eating

Goals

After reading this chapter, you will have the information to—

Explain how social customs, religious practices, and family background shape attitudes about food.

Describe the nutrients in food.

Describe the five major food groups.

Explain how seven kinds of special diets help people who have special dietary needs.

Explain why it is important to make mealtime pleasant.

Explain why and how to measure the amount people eat and drink.

Explain how to help people in home health care with nutrition.

Explain how to help children with nutritional needs.

After practicing the corresponding skills in the skills book, you will be able to—

Help people eat.

Measure and record a person's height and weight.

Victor Rivera's wife comes to the nursing home every day around 2:00 o'clock in the afternoon and stays until after Mr. Rivera has finished eating his dinner. When Mr. Rivera first came to Morningside Nursing Home from the hospital, where he had received treatment for a stroke that left his right side paralyzed, Mrs. Rivera asked how she might help with her husband's care. You taught Mrs. Rivera how to help her husband at mealtimes, and now she comes every day to make dinnertime a special part of the day.

During the day, you help Mr. Rivera eat his breakfast and lunch. In the nursing home's dining room, filled with light and fresh flowers, he sits at a table with Mr. O'Reilly, who also has had a stroke. Mr. O'Reilly receives help from family members who are frequent guests in the dining room. During lunch, the two men talk about the day, the weather, and local news. They have become good friends, and they look forward to having mealtimes together.

Mr. Rivera is trying to learn to eat with his left hand and finds mealtime a major challenge. His shaky left arm has been getting stronger, but he often becomes tired after feeding himself the first few bites. Today at lunch you encourage him to eat all of his mashed potatoes by himself, using the new large-handled spoon the occupational therapist taught him how to use. When he finishes, he sighs heavily and slouches back in his wheelchair. "I knew you could do it, Mr. Rivera," you say, and help him with the rest of his meal.

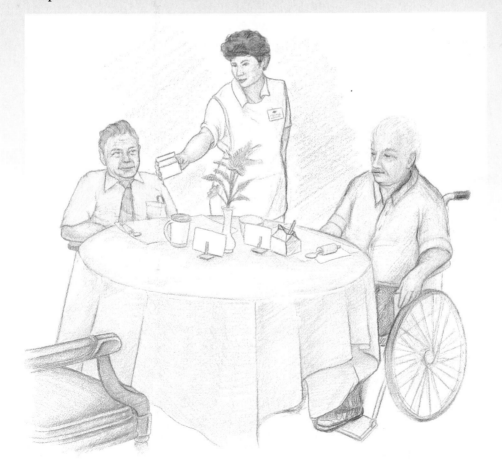

Attitudes About Food

As a nurse assistant, it is important for you to know about food and nutrition. If you eat the recommended foods, you may be healthier and better able to enjoy your life and work. The same is true for the people in your care. The right foods can help people stay healthy. They also can play a big part in helping people who are sick or injured get better.

Yet, people differ in what they eat, when they eat, and how they prepare food. Each person has certain likes and dislikes. One person may not like green beans, while another may not like chocolate. What you like to eat may seem strange to someone who grew up in a different place or who has a different religion.

Your food choices, likes, and dislikes have been influenced by where you come from and who you are. Social customs, religious practices, and the availability of ingredients all play a part in what you choose to eat. They shape your attitudes about food, attitudes that may last a lifetime. For example, one person who grew up in a Southeast Asian culture may eat rice every day with a variety of cooked vegetables, fish, eggs, and meat. He may season his foods with strong flavors such as garlic, chilies, ginger, and fresh coriander. These foods may remain part of his **diet** even if he moves far from his native country. But another person who grew up in the same culture may learn to enjoy other kinds of foods, such as pizza and tacos.

Do not depend on what you know about the person's culture or religious preferences to give you clues about what he may like to eat, because individual preferences differ. The best way to find out what someone likes to eat is to ask him (Figure 12-1).

The Basics of Nutrition

You may have heard an old saying, "You are what you eat," meaning that what you eat is reflected in your health. This saying is only partly true. Heredity, environment, and lifestyle also play a part in how healthy you are. Eating properly helps maintain overall good health, and following good nutritional habits can improve poor health.

Diet Is What You Eat

You may hear someone who is trying to lose weight say he is on a "diet." In this book, the word "diet" means all the food and liquid a person consumes. A person may choose to eat an unbalanced diet of ice cream, cookies, cake, fudge, and broccoli. Another person may choose meat, potatoes, vegetables, and fruit. Someone who is ill may need just liquids, such as broth, gelatin, and fruit juice. All these selections of food are diets.

Selecting the Major Nutrients

It is important to know what foods are in a person's diet and what **nutrients** are in those foods. Foods contain some or all of the following major nutrients:

diet
(DYE-it)   The foods and liquids that a person usually consumes.

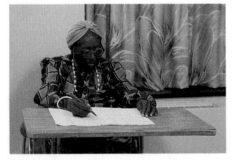

Figure 12-1
Offer the people in your care a choice of what to eat. Health care facilities in different regions of the country may offer regional foods. Many hospitals encourage patients to select meals from a menu. When preparing food in a client's home, ask him what he likes to eat.

nutrient
(NEW-tre-ent)   A substance that the body needs to grow, maintain itself, and stay healthy.

❖   Carbohydrates 6-11 servings
❖   Protein
❖   Fat
❖   Minerals
❖   Vitamins
❖   Water

To get all the necessary nutrients, a person needs to eat a variety of foods. No single food or group of foods supplies all the nutrients you need. Carbohydrates, protein, and fat supply energy for the body. The amount of energy that a food has is measured in **calories**. Have you ever looked at the label on a package of food to check the number of calories? If you eat more calories than your body uses for energy, the leftover calories are stored in your body as fat. In addition to identifying the number of calories, many food labels also identify the amounts of carbohydrate, protein, and fat that are in a serving of that food item.

Look at Table 12-1 to learn what each nutrient does, and in which foods it is found.

calorie
(KAL-uh-ree)   A unit of heat or energy produced when the body uses food.

Selecting from the Five Major Food Groups

Scientists organize similar foods together in groups. They often disagree about the number of food groups, and you may have heard

Table 12-1   **Major Nutrients**

Nutrient	What It Does	Where It Is Found
Carbohydrate	Supplies energy that is easy for the body to use; adds bulk (fiber) to the diet and helps eliminate waste material	Grains such as wheat and rice Vegetables such as potatoes, dried beans and peas, corn, squash, broccoli, and spinach Fruit such as apples, bananas, and oranges Sugars such as honey and syrup
Protein	Builds body tissue, regulates water balance, and fights disease	Milk, cheese, yogurt, meat, poultry, fish, eggs *Dried beans and nuts, seeds, grains, and peanut butter
Fat	Provides a concentrated source of energy for the body to store	Nuts, seeds, peanut butter, whole milk, yogurt, cheese, meat, fish, poultry, eggs, olives, and avocados Vegetable cooking oils, margarine, butter, mayonnaise, and salad dressing
Minerals	Regulate many body functions; build and renew bones, teeth, blood, and tissue	In all foods, but types of minerals and their amounts vary
Vitamins	Break down other nutrients into smaller parts so that the body can use them	In all foods, but types of vitamins and their amounts vary
Water	Keeps substances in solution in body tissue and regulates body temperature, circulation, and excretion	A major component of vegetables and fruits

*Incomplete proteins—must be eaten in combination wtih certain other foods to provide complete proteins when the person does not eat animal products.

that there are four, five, six, or even seven food groups. Scientists recommend the amounts you need to eat from each food group to help you select your daily meals. The five major food groups (Figure 12-2) used in this book are:

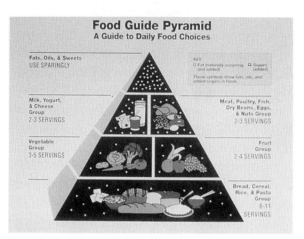

1. Grain
2. Vegetables
3. Fruit
4. Meat
5. Milk

Figure 12-2
Five Major Food Groups

diabetes
(dye-uh-BEE-tez)   A disease in which the pancreas does not secrete enough insulin and the body is not able to use all the carbohydrates, resulting in a high concentration of glucose in the blood.

oral thrush
A fungus infection that produces sore patches in the mouth.

Some other foods, such as fats, concentrated sweets, and alcohol, fall into a group identified as "fats." The amount you need to eat from each food group depends on a number of factors—your age, how healthy you are, how active you are, and whether you are male or female. If you eat too much, your body stores the extra calories as fat. Having too much body fat affects your appearance, as well as your overall health.

The nutritional needs of an ill or injured person vary, depending on what type of illness or injury he has. For example, when a person has **diabetes**, his diet often limits the number of calories he should consume, as well as the amount of sugar and fat. Or when a person has a burn or open sore and the body needs to repair tissue, his diet contains more protein and total calories for healing. A person with HIV infection or AIDS has a varied diet, depending on his health status. The focus of his nutrition should be individualized.* A great majority of those diagnosed with AIDS have difficulty swallowing and must have tube feedings at some time due to **oral thrush** or other sores in the mouth or throat.

Because very active people need more calories for energy, they need to eat more food, especially carbohydrates, which provide energy that is easy for the body to use. Men tend to need more calories than women do.

To help people know how much from each food group to eat, doctors and nutritionists make recommendations for the average person. Some guidelines for the recommended amount from each food group appear in the following paragraphs and in Figure 12-2.

*Weaver K: Reversible malnutrition in AIDS *Am J Nurs* 91(8):24-31, September 1991.

What is the right amount of grain?   You read that carbohydrates supply the body with easy energy, which is what the body needs to do its work. The body's work occurs even when people are sleeping or unconscious. A healthy person needs more carbohydrates than anything else in his diet. Because grains supply the type of carbohydrate that is used most efficiently by the body, a healthy person should eat more foods from the grain group than from any other food group. Bread, rice, pasta, and cereal are examples of foods in the grain group (Figure 12-3).

Depending on how active he is, a healthy adult should eat from 6 to 11 servings of grain each day. The size of a serving depends on what kind of grain he is eating. For example, one slice of bread is one serving, as is ½ cup of cooked cereal, rice, or pasta. When he eats a sandwich made with two slices of bread for lunch, he is having two servings of grain. What else could he eat at breakfast and dinner to get the rest of the grain he needs for 1 day?

What is the right amount of vegetables?   Vegetables also contain large amounts of carbohydrates, as well as vitamins (Figure 12-4). A healthy adult should eat three to five servings of vegetables each day. One serving of most cooked vegetables is ½ cup. A serving of raw, leafy, green vegetables such as spinach, lettuce, and escarole is 1 cup.

What is the right amount of fruit?   Like vegetables, fruits contain high levels of carbohydrates and vitamins (see Figure 12-4). A healthy adult should eat two to four servings of fruit each day. A serving of fruit is one medium apple, ½ cup of chopped fruit, or 3/4 cup of fruit juice.

What is the right amount of meat?   The body needs protein to build muscle and other body tissue. High levels of protein are found in foods in the meat group (Figure 12-5), which includes—

❖ Eggs.
❖ Red meat, such as beef, lamb, and pork.
❖ Poultry, such as chicken and turkey.
❖ Fish and shellfish, such as shrimp, crab, lobster, scallops, and oysters.

A healthy adult should have up to 6 ounces of meat each day. A 3-ounce serving of meat is about the size of a deck of cards.

When choosing foods from the meat group, keep in mind that these foods contain varying amounts of fat. Nutritionists recommend cutting down on the amount of fat consumed. Red meat usually contains more fat than poultry, and fish is generally lower in fat than meat. If you eat red meat, it is better to choose lean red meat and trim off all the visible fat before cooking. It also is better to take the skin off chicken and turkey before cooking, because most of the fat in poultry is in the skin.

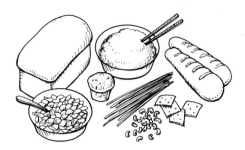

Figure 12-3
Grain Group

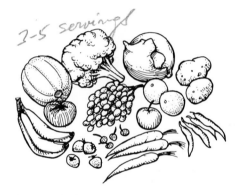

Figure 12-4
Vegetable and Fruit Groups

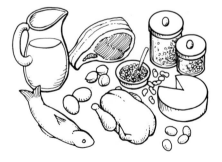

Figure 12-5
Meat and Milk Groups

9-3

What is the right amount of milk?   Like the meat group, foods in the milk group contain high levels of protein (see Figure 12-5 on p. 263). An average adult should have from two to three servings from the milk group each day. Pregnant and lactating women (those who are breast feeding) need more nutrients from the milk group and should have four or more servings each day. Children and teenagers should have from two to four servings from the milk group each day.

One serving from the milk group is 1 cup of milk, a 1-inch cube of cheese, ½ cup of cottage cheese, or 1 cup of yogurt. Foods in the milk group also can contain large amounts of fat. One way to reduce the amount of fat is to drink milk that contains 2 percent or 1 percent of milk fat instead of whole milk. Skim milk is even lower in fat than 1 percent milk. Another way to reduce fat is to eat hard, low-fat cheeses rather than soft, creamy cheeses that are high in fat and calories.

Some people do not eat meat or milk for religious, personal, medical, or cultural reasons. They can get the protein they need by eating other high-protein foods, such as whole grains, beans, and nuts, as well as extra servings of leafy green vegetables. Beans and whole grains at the same meal provide a high-quality protein.

What about fat?   Because people naturally get fats from other sources, such as meats and milk products, they should limit how much they choose to eat from this other group. Fats and oils should be the smallest part of any diet. It is better to use very little fat when cooking and to bake, roast, or boil meat instead of frying it. It also is better to use only a small amount of salad dressing and spreads, such as butter, margarine, and mayonnaise. In addition to limiting the amount of fat in their diets, people should limit their consumption of concentrated sweets, such as candy, and alcohol.

Trying to figure the right amount of nutrients to eat may seem overwhelming. But you can meet your nutritional needs by selecting a wide variety of foods from the five major food groups and eating the recommended number of servings. Table 12-2 contains some examples.

Eating for Health and Pleasure

Proper nutrition and long-term good health are closely linked. Proper nutrition means eating a wide variety of foods and choosing those that are low in fat, salt, and sugar. Eating too much of these substances can cause health problems. For example, people who eat too much **cholesterol** and **saturated fat** may develop high cholesterol levels in the blood, which can cause problems with the heart and circulatory system. Eating too much fat also has been linked to certain types of cancer. Eating too much salt can cause problems for people who have high blood pressure. Eating large amounts of sugar adds calories without adding other nutrients and contributes to tooth decay.

cholesterol
(ko-LES-ter-all)   A white, fatty substance that occurs naturally in the blood and tissues of the human body and that also is found in meat, egg yolks, liver, most dairy products, and animal fat.

saturated fat
(SAH-tyur-ay-ted)   A form of fat found in meats, cheeses, dairy products, and certain vegetable oils, such as palm and coconut oil.

Table 12-2   **What Is the Right Amount for an Adult to Eat?**

Major Food Group	Daily Servings	Examples (Size of Serving)
Grain	6 to 11	1 slice bread ½ cup cooked rice ½ cup cooked cereal ½ cup cooked pasta
Vegetables	3 to 5	½ cup cooked vegetables 1 cup raw, leafy greens
Fruit	2 to 4	1 medium apple 1 medium orange 1 medium banana 1 medium pear ½ cup chopped fruit ½ cup small berries ¾ cup fruit juice
Meat	2 (3 oz. each)	½ chicken breast 1 small, lean hamburger patty (3 oz., cooked) 3 oz. tuna 3 oz. pork (cooked)
Milk	2 to 3	1 cup milk 1-inch cube of cheese ½ cup cottage cheese 1 cup yogurt

Building good nutritional habits early in life helps keep the digestive system healthy, helps prevent **obesity**, and helps avoid the risk of long-term diseases such as cancer, heart disease, high blood pressure, **arteriosclerosis**, and diabetes in later years. (See Body Basics, The Digestive System.) When people develop health problems, they may have to change their diets.

Monitoring Special Dietary Needs

Many people require special diets because of physical disabilities or diseases. Doctors and dietitians help decide what a person should eat. For example, Mr. Rivera once enjoyed eating fried foods. But, because he had a stroke and has high blood pressure and high cholesterol, his doctor has ordered a low-fat diet that eliminates all fried foods. As a nurse assistant, you have to know what foods are in such special diets and why they are ordered. In many cases you are responsible for serving these diets, and sometimes you also must monitor how much of the food the person in your care eats. Commonly ordered **therapeutic diets** are described in the following paragraphs.

obesity
(oh-BEE-suh-tee)   Having too much body fat.

arteriosclerosis
(ar-teer-ee-oh-skluh-ROW-sis)   Hardening and thickening of the arteries.

therapeutic diet
(ther-uh-PEW-tik)   A special diet that helps a person regain his health.

BodyBasics

❖ The Digestive System ❖

Every day we eat, turn food into energy, and get rid of wastes our bodies can't use. Taking food into our bodies is called ingestion. The process of breaking food down is digestion. Sending the waste, called stool (feces) and gas (flatus), out of the body is part of elimination.

We want to eat when the brain sends a message to put food into our mouths. There, our teeth chew it and saliva mixes with it to start the digestion process. The tongue pushes food to the back of the mouth.

After we swallow, food travels down the esophagus, a muscular tube, until it reaches the stomach. There, food mixes with chemicals produced by the lining of the stomach, and the "good parts" of the food begin to separate from the "unusable parts," or waste. This process continues as partially digested food passes from the stomach and continues through the small and large intestines. Finally, waste leaves the body through the rectum and anus.

The pancreas contributes to digestion by making digestive juices called enzymes. The liver makes enzymes that break down and release sugars, starch, protein, and fat and also stores starch for later use. The gallbladder makes bile, a green liquid that helps break down fats.

How the Digestive System Ages

As we age, saliva production decreases, resulting in a dry mouth and an increase in plaque on the teeth. Intestinal muscle tone decreases, which may lead to constipation and an increase in the time it takes for food to digest. In addition, the digestive juice production decreases, which may result in vitamin and weight loss.

Fascinating Fact

The taste buds of the tongue are sensitive to four primary tastes: bitter, sweet, sour, and salt. The tongue is not equally sensitive to all tastes in every area. The back of the tongue is more sensitive to bitter, the tip of the tongue to sweet, the sides to sour, and the tip and sides to salt.

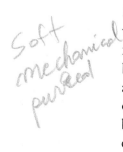

Soft, mechanical, or pureed diet. Food can be prepared in special ways to make it easier for a person to chew, swallow, and digest than food in a regular diet (Figure 12-6). In a soft diet, food such as hot breakfast cereal and mashed potatoes is prepared soft or mashed. In a mechanical diet, food such as ground meat is ground with a mechanical device. Pureed food, such as pureed vegetables and meat, is boiled to a pulp and rubbed through a sieve. Any of these three diets can meet a person's daily nutritional needs.

BodyBasics

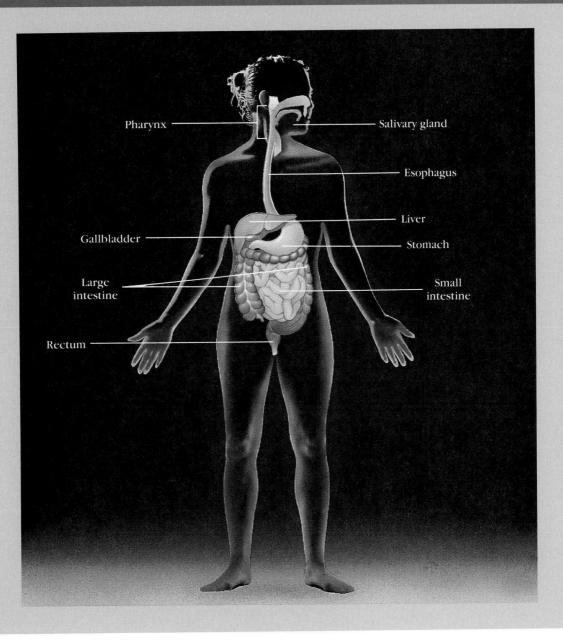

Pharynx — — Salivary gland

— Esophagus

Gallbladder —

— Liver

— Stomach

Large
intestine —

Small
intestine

Rectum —

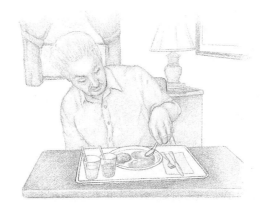

Figure 12-6
The soft foods in a mechanical diet are
ordered for someone who cannot chew
because of a stroke or other problem.
This diet is chosen over a liquid diet
because it provides complete nutrition.

Liquid diet. A doctor may order a liquid diet for a person who has digestive problems, has had recent surgery, or cannot swallow solid food. Two types of liquid diets are clear and full.

A clear-liquid diet includes liquids you can see through, such as broth; gelatin; carbonated beverages; tea; and apple, grape, and cranberry juices. A person with a short-term illness such as flu, diarrhea, or vomiting may be on a liquid diet for only 1 or 2 days to give his digestive system a rest. Because it is lacking in protein, fiber, and certain vitamins and minerals and, therefore, cannot provide adequate nutrition, a doctor must reorder this diet every 48 hours.

A full liquid diet includes fruit juices such as orange and grapefruit juice, strained soups, ice cream, milk, diluted (thinned) cooked cereal, and eggnog. A doctor orders this diet for 1 or 2 days for a person with an illness that causes digestive problems. It provides more nutrients than the clear liquid diet but still does not provide adequate nutrition. It also must be reordered by the doctor every 48 hours.

No added salt (NAS) diet. Salt and sodium may be limited for people with high blood pressure or kidney or circulatory diseases. Foods in this diet must be prepared with no added salt. The person on this diet may not use table salt, but may use a salt substitute with the doctor's approval. This diet provides adequate nutrition but limits foods that are high in salt or sodium, such as ham, bacon, cheese, regular canned soups, potato chips, lunch meat, pickles, olives, and many packaged or canned foods (Figure 12-7).

Figure 12-7
A person who eats a lot of these foods consumes a large amount of sodium. These foods are inappropriate for a no added salt (NAS) diet.

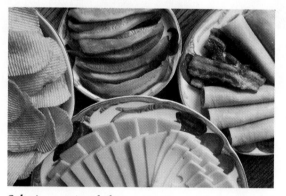

Calorie-restricted diet. A diet with 1,200, 1,500, 1,800, or 2,000 calories per day may be ordered for a person who needs to control his weight. A well-planned diet contains all the proteins, carbohydrates, and fats the person needs. The doctor or dietitian may recommend multivitamin and mineral supplements for a daily diet of 1,200 calories or fewer. For minor calorie restriction, the doctor or dietitian may order a regular no concentrated sweets (NCS) diet that eliminates only sweets, such as candy and cookies.

High-protein diet. A doctor prescribes this diet for people who do not eat enough or who need additional protein to build skin or organ tissues. A person who has been burned or has developed decubitus ulcers might be put on a high-protein diet.

Diabetic diet.   This diet, ordered for people who have diabetes, carefully defines the number of calories, as well as the amount and type of carbohydrates, protein, and fat, a person may eat (Figure 12-8).

Low-fat diet.   A doctor may order a low-fat diet for people with heart, gallbladder, or liver disease. It calls for increased protein and carbohydrates and restricted amounts of fat.

If a doctor orders one of these therapeutic diets for someone in your care, make sure the person gets only the food permitted in that diet. Eating other foods or more food than is recommended can cause health problems.

Making Mealtime Enjoyable

Because mealtime is an important part of the day, it should be as relaxing and enjoyable as possible. A person who enjoys mealtime may eat more, just as Mr. Rivera does. You can play a big part in making mealtime pleasant for the people in your care, if you observe the following general rules:

- ❖ Keep the atmosphere as cheerful and comfortable as possible and provide adequate lighting.
- ❖ For people who eat in their rooms, keep the rooms neat, clean, and free of odors.
- ❖ Allow adequate time for a person to prepare for his meal. Encourage him to go to the bathroom and wash his hands before eating.
- ❖ If needed, help the person into a comfortable, upright, sitting position, with his head up and his hips at a 90-degree angle. This position makes it easier for him to chew and swallow, as well as to manage his eating utensils.
- ❖ Serve meals promptly to make sure hot food stays hot and cold food stays cold. Some foods spoil quickly if you allow them to stand at room temperature.
- ❖ If a person is on a therapeutic diet, make sure that he gets the proper food. (Figure 12-8) If sugar, salt, or butter is not included with his meal, do not serve it without checking first with your supervising nurse.
- ❖ Identify a person's food allergies and dislikes so that these foods will not be served to him. If any of these foods are present, report this problem to your supervising nurse before serving the meal.
- ❖ Serve pureed food separately. Add seasoning, such as salt (if permitted) and pepper, to pureed food. A pureed meal does not have the appealing look of a regular diet, but a positive attitude toward the food can help a person accept it. Pureed food should have the consistency of pudding and should maintain a distinct identity from other pureed food. If you think the food needs to be thinned, check with the dietitian to determine the liquid to use. Also, check with your supervising nurse before thinning food if the person you are feeding has had a stroke or is para-

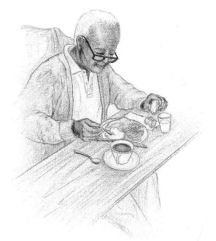

Figure 12-8

The people in your care may have medical reasons for avoiding certain foods or eating special foods. Because Jake Wilson is diabetic, the dietary department plans special meals for him that are low in sugar and fat.

lyzed on one side. Some people who have difficulty swallowing may not be able to swallow thinned, pureed food or liquid.

❖ Report any uneaten food to your supervising nurse so that a substitute may be offered. Substituting food is especially important to prevent an insulin reaction in people with diabetes who must have a specific number of calories in their diets. Ask the person why he didn't eat or if he would like something else to eat.

❖ Observe people during mealtime to determine if they need help with eating. Sometimes people leave part of a meal uneaten because they get too tired to finish. If the person does tire, you may have to help him eat more or give him a snack later.

In a nursing home, encourage residents to eat in the dining room, if possible (Figure 12-9). Assure them that they will receive as much help and direction as needed. For example, help or direct a resident to the dining room, and help him sit down. Provide protective covering for his clothing if he needs and wants it.

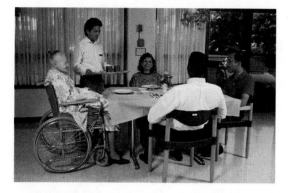

Figure 12-9
Being in the company of others and socializing are positive aspects of eating.

Helping People Eat

Some of the people in your care need assistance when they are eating, and this task may make them feel helpless. It is important for you to encourage a person to do as much as possible on his own. You may have to open a milk carton for someone whose hands are unsteady or weak. You may have to cut up meat for someone who is paralyzed on one side. You may have to steady or support the elbow of a person whose arm is weak while he feeds himself. At each meal, talk with the person about the amount of help he needs, because he may have different needs at different meals. The amount of help he needs depends in part on the kind of food served. For example, a person may be able to hold a sandwich but may not be able to cut up meat.

If you are helping someone eat, follow the specific procedure that is explained step by step in Skill 38 in the skills book. Also follow these suggestions for helping people eat:

❖ When serving a person's meal, remove the dishes from the tray and place them on the table to create a more home-like environment. Some nursing homes may serve food directly on trays with compartments for different parts of the meal.

❖ Make sure the person is positioned correctly for eating. If possible, use a dining room or kitchen chair that pulls close to the table. Make sure the person's feet are flat on the floor, and have him rest his elbows or forearms on the table if he needs support. If the person wishes, provide protection for his clothing by spreading a towel or napkin over his chest.

❖ Encourage him to hold finger foods.

❖ If you must help feed the person, ask if he has a preferred order for eating foods and preferred seasonings.

❖ If the person is going to drink hot liquids such as coffee or tea, test the temperature before serving by placing several drops on your wrist. If the liquid feels too hot on your wrist, allow it to cool slightly before serving it. Serving liquid at the correct temperature is especially important if the person drinks hot liquid through a straw, because the liquid bypasses the lips as the straw delivers liquid far back in the mouth, where it could cause serious burns to the mouth and throat.

❖ To offer a hot liquid by straw, first stir the liquid with the straw to distribute the heat evenly. Place the straw in the person's mouth. He can suck and swallow the liquid as he desires. If the person sucks too much liquid, you may have to pinch off the straw and pull it away so that he can swallow.

❖ To offer fluids by cup to a person who is not sitting up, use one hand to raise and support the person's head. Use the other hand to hold the cup while the person drinks.

❖ Offer liquids to a person only when he has no food in his mouth.

❖ Feed the person slowly. Offer a liquid first to moisten his mouth and make it easier to swallow. Then begin offering solids by filling a spoon two thirds full. Touch the spoon to the person's bottom lip so that he opens his mouth. Then touch the spoon to his tongue (Figure 12-10). This touch to the lips and tongue lets him know where the spoon is in his mouth. Allow time between bites for the person to chew and swallow. Offer liquids after several swallows of solid food, making sure the liquids are not too hot. End the meal with water to rinse the mouth.

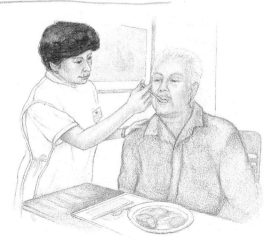

Figure 12-10
When helping someone eat, it is important to put the spoon into the person's mouth so that he will not have to move his head forward to reach for it.

❖ Name each food as you offer it.
❖ Wipe the person's mouth with a napkin, as needed.

When the person in your care has finished with a meal, remove the dishes and tidy up the table. If needed, help the person wash his hands and brush his teeth or rinse his mouth as desired.

Good nutrition is more than just eating the correct food. When helping someone eat, you can help his body work more efficiently by following the general principles related to digestion that appear in Box 12-1.

Box 12-1   **What Can You Do to Help the Digestive System Work as Well as Possible?**

1. Encourage people to drink liquids.
2. Encourage people to eat high-fiber foods, such as cereal, whole-grain bread, vegetables, and fruit.
3. Allow enough time for eating and completely chewing food before swallowing.
4. Be sensitive to a person's eating patterns. Many older people cope better with frequent small meals than with a few larger ones.
5. Remember that mealtime also serves a social need.
6. Encourage regular bowel functioning by—
   ❖ Providing privacy and time for using the toilet.
   ❖ Encouraging exercise to stimulate bowel activity.
7. Provide good mouth care.
8. Report to your supervising nurse if—
   ❖ A person's appetite changes.
   ❖ A person's bowel habits change.
   ❖ A person has signs of nausea and vomiting.

Helping a person who is blind with mealtime.   If you provide care for a blind person, remember that he can probably eat by himself if he has no other disabilities. Unless he has a special condition, the only things you have to do are—

❖ Identify the foods on the table and on the plate. Describe their locations as if the plate were the face of a clock (Figure 12-11).

Figure 12-11
You can help a person who is blind "see" his food by using the numbers on a clock face to describe the location of each item on the plate. You also can describe the location of items on the table in the same manner. For example, "The water is at 2 o'clock."

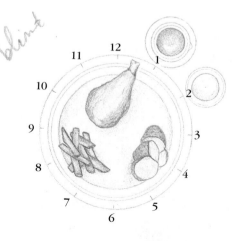

For example, if peas are on the dinner plate at the place closest
to the person, you could say, "Peas are at 6 o'clock." If potatoes
are directly across from the peas, you could say, "Potatoes are at
12 o'clock." If a glass of water is on the table near the upper
right portion of the plate, you could say, "A glass of water is at 2
o'clock."

❖   Cut up meats or anything else that needs cutting.
❖   Open containers.
❖   Describe the location of the dining utensils.
❖   During the meal, occasionally check on the person to see if he
     has overlooked some of the food and, if so, to offer assistance.

Helping someone who has difficulty swallowing.   A person who has had a
stroke that has resulted in speech difficulties may also have trouble
swallowing food. The doctor and speech therapist will make an initial
assessment of the person's ability to swallow and, if the person is
able to swallow, will order the appropriate diet. Generally, soft foods
are easier for the person to swallow than liquids, which run down
the throat. When you help feed him, observe the following guidelines:

❖   Remain with the person while he is eating.
❖   Place food toward the back of his mouth and on the unaffected
     side, because he cannot feel the food on the affected side and it
     may accumulate in his cheek.
❖   Encourage him to chew slowly and thoroughly.
❖   Eliminate distractions, such as television or many visitors, from
     the room so that the person can concentrate on eating.
❖   Encourage him to tilt his chin down as he swallows.
❖   Keep his head elevated during eating and for at least 30 minutes
     after eating.

Some people will be able to feed themselves with the help of special utensils or feeding aids, described in the next section.

Helping someone use adaptive feeding devices.   A variety of adaptive
feeding devices help a person with disabilities to gain as much independence as possible when eating. Before serving a meal, check to
see if the person uses any adaptive feeding equipment.

The most common problems people have with feeding themselves
are using utensils while trying to cope with conditions such as weak
or paralyzed limbs and poor eyesight. Information about adaptive
feeding devices and methods used to solve problems with feeding
appears in Table 12-3 on p. 274.

**Providing care for people who are fed through nasogastric and gastrostomy
tubes.**   If a person cannot swallow, has trouble swallowing, or cannot
take foods by mouth, a doctor may order a nasogastric tube or a gastrostomy tube so that the person can receive food. A doctor or nurse
inserts the nasogastric tube (NG tube) into the person's nose and

Continue 10/27/99

Table 12-3 **Adaptive Feeding Devices**

If Someone is Having Trouble With . . .	Use This Device	How to Use the Device/How the Device Helps	How to Improvise When the Device Is Not Available
1. Trying to get food on the utensil	Plate guard	Keeps food from falling off the plate as the person tries to scoop it onto the fork or spoon.	Ask the person to use his weak hand or arm to hold a piece of bread on the plate to block the food and then use his unaffected hand to push the food onto the fork or spoon.
	Scoop dish	This plate with a rounded side keeps food from falling off the plate.	
	Spork	This spoon-fork combination allows the person to either spear or scoop food onto the utensil.	
2. The plate slipping around or moving	Suction base	Place the suction base underneath the plate to hold it more securely in place.	Place a wet washcloth under the plate to increase suction and stability.
3. Grasping and holding onto utensils	Built-up utensils: Vertical or horizontal palm self-handle utensils	Slip the handle over the palm of the person's hand.	Use foam rubber or leather to build up the handles of a standard utensil or put the utensil into a bicycle handle or tennis ball.
	Utensil holder	Place the holder over the person's palm. Put the utensil inside the holder.	
	Universal cuff	Fasten the strap to the person's hand. Put the utensil handle inside the strap.	
4. Food falling off a utensil because of an arm tremor or weakness	Swivel utensil (fork or spoon)	The bowl of the fork or spoon can remain horizontal even if the person's hand shakes. It may have a built-up handle. Guide the person's hand as necessary.	Rest the person's elbow on a piece of sponge rubber on the table to lessen tremors. Guide the person's hand as necessary.
5. Using both hands and a knife to cut food	Rocker knife	A person can use one hand to cut by rocking the sharp edge over the food to cut it.	
6. Spilling liquids as he attempts to drink from a cup	Modified drinking cup	The cover and spout keep liquid from spilling.	Secure plastic wrap over the top of a cup with a rubber band and put a straw through a small opening in the top.
	Commercial straw holder	The holder keeps the straw in place.	
7. Reaching his mouth with a utensil because of limited arm movement	Extension utensil	The utensil handle is longer.	

down into his stomach. It is held in place on the face by tape. A doctor inserts the gastrostomy tube directly into the person's stomach through a surgical **incision**. The tube is clamped and held in place by **sutures** and covered with a dressing.

A nurse puts commercially prepared formula and water into the tubes, which gives the person a nutritionally adequate diet even though he cannot swallow.

When you provide care to a person who has a nasogastric or gastrostomy tube, you must observe the following important rules:

incision
(in-SIZH-un)   A cut made during surgery.

suture
(SUE-tyur)   The stitch used to join the edges of a cut or wound.

❖ Never feed the person any food or fluid by mouth. Only a nurse may feed him through the tubes or give him food or fluid by mouth.

❖ When the nurse inserts food into a nasogastric tube or a gastrostomy tube, she elevates the head of the bed at least 45 degrees to prevent aspiration. Keep the head of the bed elevated for at least 30 minutes after a nasogastric or gastrostomy tube feeding.

❖ If the person has an NG tube, clean his face around the tube by washing it gently with a washcloth moistened with warm water. Do not use cotton balls or swabs, because lint from the cotton may cause the person to sneeze (Figure 12-12). Give him mouth care at least every 2 hours to prevent his mouth and lips from becoming dry and cracked.

❖ Follow the instructions of your supervising nurse for cleaning the area around a person's gastrostomy tube. Be careful not to wet the dressing when giving the person a bath. Notify your supervising nurse if the person complains of pain or discomfort in the abdomen, nausea, or gas problems, or if you see any redness, irritation, or drainage around the tube insertion site.

❖ When providing care for a person with a nasogastric or gastrostomy tube, always position him so that he is not lying on the tube. Occasionally a person may attempt to pull out his tube. Talk with your supervising nurse about methods to use to prevent this action from happening.

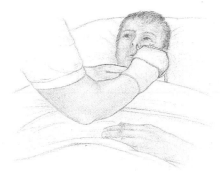

Figure 12-12
When providing care for a person who has a nasogastric tube, clean around the tube very carefully. Accidentally knocking the tube can hurt the person's nose.

Helping someone in isolation with mealtime.   Before bringing a meal tray to a person who is in isolation, first put on protective clothing as described in Chapter 7, Controlling the Spread of Germs, following the procedure that is explained step by step in Skill 3 in the skills book. Once you are in the person's room, help him into a comfortable position for eating and assist him with his meal as needed. Since a person in isolation cannot socialize with others, it is important to give him companionship if he wants it and allow him enough time to finish his meal. When the person has finished eating, dispose of any leftover food or liquid in the toilet or sink. Double-bag any reusable utensils, as well as any garbage. To avoid the spread of infection, your employer may serve meals on disposable plates, with disposable cups and utensils, to people in isolation.

Monitoring the Amount a Person Eats and Drinks

appetite
(AH-puh-tite)   The desire to eat and drink.

nauseated
(NAW-zee-ay-ted)   A feeling of sickness in the stomach.

A person's **appetite** is affected by many things. For example, he may not have a very good appetite if he is ill or **nauseated**. He may feel either very hungry or not very hungry because of medication he is taking. His appetite may change if he is worried, afraid, or sad. He may eat even when he is not hungry because he is happy, excited, bored, or lonely.

A person's appetite may be affected by the smell of food. The smell may make one person hungry, yet make another person feel nauseated. Smell also affects how food tastes. When a person can't smell food, he can't taste much. A person whose nose is stuffed up may not be hungry because he can't smell or taste the food. The next time you eat, try holding your nose to see if it makes a difference.

If the person in your care doesn't have much of an appetite or if his appetite changes suddenly, report these situations to your supervising nurse.

People with some diseases require a limited amount of calories. Others require a limited amount of fluid. For example, a person with severe congestive heart disease or kidney disease may be allowed to receive only the amount of fluid ordered by the doctor. He may not be allowed to drink or eat at all for a certain amount of time. A person who undergoes certain blood tests or procedures may be forbidden to eat or drink after midnight or for a specific number of hours before the test or procedure. To remind everyone that the person may not eat or drink, post a sign saying "NPO."

It is often important to measure and record how much the person in your care eats and drinks (intake). It is also important to measure and record how much fluid passes through his system (output). The medical abbreviation for measuring intake and output is I&O. You will learn about measuring output in Chapter 13, Elimination.

Recording the Amount of Food Eaten

It is important to record the amount of food each person eats. If someone on a special diet does not eat all his food, he may need a snack or food supplement between meals. To judge how much extra food he needs, you may be asked to record the amount of food he eats at each meal. You also may be asked to record the amount of the snack or supplement the person eats. Between-meal snacks are offered to people who have special conditions, including diabetes, poor appetite, weight loss, and decubitus ulcers. These foods may be liquid, such as milkshakes or milk, or solid, such as a sandwich.

Following are examples of different ways to estimate how much food a person eats (Figure 12-13):

❖ At lunch, you serve Mrs. Wang a cheese sandwich, tomato soup, a bowl of cherries, milk, and coffee. She eats only a few bites of the sandwich. You would record that Mrs. Wang ate 0 percent of her meal.

❖ For dinner, you serve Josie Miller a small breast of chicken, peas, broccoli, fruit cocktail, milk, and cookies. She eats all of

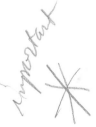

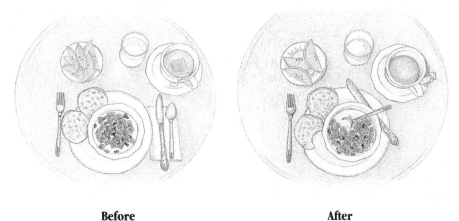

Before   **After**

Figure 12-13
How would you report how much food
the person ate?

the meat on her plate, but none of the other foods. In this case, you would record that she ate 100 percent of her meat.

❖ At dinner, Mrs. McDay sits down to a meal of mixed vegetables, potatoes, a pork chop, an apple, pudding, and coffee. She eats half of the vegetables and all of the potatoes from her plate, but none of the other foods. You would record that she ate 50 percent of the vegetables and 100 percent of the potatoes.

❖ At breakfast, you serve Mrs. Ryan one egg, two pieces of toast, orange juice, and coffee. She eats the egg and one piece of toast and drinks her coffee. You would record that Mrs. Ryan ate 100 percent of her egg, 50 percent of her toast, and 0 percent of her orange juice.

❖ Mr. Lightfoot eats all of the food that you serve him for lunch. You would record that he ate 100 percent of his meal.

Check with your supervising nurse about the proper place to record the amount of food someone eats, since the recording location varies among health care facilities. Your employer may use a form that estimates a person's appetite rather than the actual amount of food he eats. If the person's appetite is poor or his food intake is strictly controlled, your employer may use a form that looks like Figure 12-14.

The Importance of Fluid Intake

With certain illnesses, it is important to know how much fluid someone drinks and how much passes through her body. Most people must drink 6 to 8 cups (or about 1,500 to 2,000 cc or ml) of fluid each day to stay healthy or become well. A person can take fluid in liquid form, such as water, coffee, juice, milk, soup, and tea, or in solid form, such as ice cream, sherbet, or gelatin. She must consume enough fluid to replace the fluid lost each day in the form of urine, perspiration, bowel movements, and breath vapor. (When you breathe on a cold glass or mirror and it fogs up, that is fluid that you are losing from your body.)

A person must take in the same amount of fluid as her body puts out to maintain fluid balance. If a person consumes a large amount

FOOD INTAKE FORM

MEAL	TIME	FOOD SERVED	DESCRIPTION	AMOUNT EATEN
Breakfast	8:30 A.M.	Egg	Scrambled	1
		Toast	With butter	2 Slices
		Orange juice		0
		Coffee	With milk and sugar	150 cc
Snack				
Lunch				
Snack				
Dinner				

LAST NAME, FIRST NAME, INITIAL	ATTENDING PHYSICIAN	ROOM NO.	PATIENT NO.
Ryan, Agnes R.	Dr. Karlson	122-A	415778B

Figure 12-14
Food Intake Form

of fluid and doesn't lose much fluid, it could be a sign of disease. Likewise, if a person loses more fluid than she takes in, this also could be a sign of disease. When a person perspires heavily (as with a fever), vomits (as with a stomach virus), or has diarrhea (as with HIV infection/AIDS), she must replace lost fluids quickly. Sometimes a person's fluid balance may be off because she doesn't drink enough. If someone in your care is losing a lot of fluid in one of these ways or is **dehydrated**, you must tell your supervising nurse. The symptoms of dehydration include the following:

❖ Confusion
❖ Constipation
❖ Drowsiness
❖ Very dry skin or chapped lips
❖ Poor skin **turgor**

dehydrated
(de-HI-dray-ted)   Not having enough water in the body.

turgor
(TER-jer)   The ability of the skin to return to its normal shape when it is squeezed or gently pinched.

❖   Decreased urination or scanty, dark-colored urine
❖   Elevated temperature

Dehydration is a serious condition. If you suspect that someone in your care is dehydrated, tell your supervising nurse immediately.

A person in your care may become dehydrated because she does not consume enough fluid. She may be afraid she won't get to the bathroom in time. She may be sick or have a disability—such as arthritis—that makes it difficult to get up to get a drink or to hold a glass. She may be afraid that she might spill the liquid and get her bed or clothing wet. Or she may simply forget to drink fluids. You can encourage her to drink the fluid she needs by following these guidelines:

❖   Offer fluids that the person likes at the temperature she prefers. (Be sure to ask what these fluids and temperatures are.)
❖   Encourage her to drink plenty of fluids with her meal. (Drinking with a meal may not be her usual habit.)
❖   Frequently provide her with a pitcher of clean, fresh water. Encourage her to drink each time you enter the room. (Follow your employer's policy for cleaning and refilling pitchers.)
❖   Be sure the person has a clean drinking glass or cup within easy reach. Refill the glass if she can't do it. Supply a drinking straw if she needs it or a plastic container with a screw-on lid and a plastic straw if she has trouble with a glass or is afraid of spilling fluids (Figure 12-15).

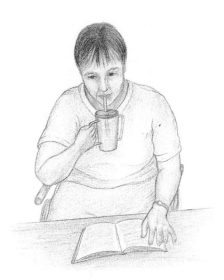

Figure 12-15
A person who is unsure of her grip and afraid of spilling liquid may feel more confident and drink more when using this type of container.

The doctor may give an order to "force fluids" for a person who is dehydrated. Forcing fluids means that the person should be urged to drink as much fluid as possible. You don't actually force the person to drink, but you encourage her to drink each time you enter the room and again on your way out. Keep a record of the amount of fluid the person does drink.

Record the amount of fluid intake and output being measured on the specified sheet of paper. One side of the sheet is for recording intake measurements, and the other side is for output. (You will read how to measure a person's output in Chapter 13.) Each time a person finishes drinking a container of liquid, mark the amount in that container on the sheet. Sometimes printed information on the container indicates how much it holds. For example, a small prepackaged milk container contains 8 ounces. In other cases, you may have to determine how much a container holds. Some facilities have lists of the amount each of their serving containers holds. If you are measuring a client's intake at home, you may have to measure how much each serving container holds. If the person does not finish the full amount in the container, estimate how much she drank and write that amount, usually in cubic centimeters (cc's), on the sheet. (See the worksheet in the skills book to practice recording fluids in cc's.) At the end of your shift, add up the amount of fluid the person drank and record the total amount on the sheet.

Measuring and Recording Weight and Height

The amount that a person eats and drinks affects her weight. It is important to keep an accurate record of a person's weight, because weight gain or loss could be related to a person's medical condition. Some people may have to be weighed every day, while others may have to be weighed only occasionally. In addition to weighing a person in your care, you must measure her height so that the doctor can evaluate the person's weight based on the normal weight range for someone of her particular height.

Because scales can vary, always weigh the person on the same scale. Also, whenever possible, weigh her at the same time of day. Have her wear as few clothes as possible, and follow your employer's guidelines about having her use the toilet before weighing.

You can use several types of scales, depending on the person's condition. When you weigh a person who can stand, use a balance scale (upright scale) or bathroom scale. If the person cannot stand, use a scale that enables you to weigh her in her wheelchair, in bed, or in a chair that resembles a mechanical lift (Figure 12-16).

When you bring a person to a balance scale to be weighed, first make sure the balance is set at zero to ensure accurate weighing. If the balance is not set at zero, ask your supervising nurse to help you change it. To learn how to use a balance scale and a bathroom scale, as well as how to measure someone's height, follow the specific procedure that is explained step by step in Skill 39 in the skills book.

To learn about helping children with nutritional needs in hospitals and home health care, as well as home health clients with nutritional needs, please read the next sections. Otherwise, turn to the end of this chapter to read "Information Review" and "Questions to Ask Yourself."

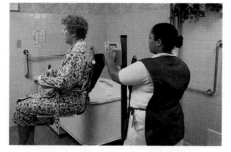

Figure 12-16
You can use this type of scale to weigh a person who cannot stand on an upright scale or a bathroom scale.

Nutrition for Children

Good nutrition often is influenced by food habits acquired in childhood. You can help children in your care establish good eating habits and wholesome attitudes toward food. These attitudes will affect their health throughout their entire lives.

Observing Appetite Characteristics in Young Children

As you provide care for children, you may observe characteristics of appetite in certain age groups. In general, healthy infants have good appetites. Children's appetites decrease toward the end of their first year and continue to decrease in their second year as growth slows down. As toddlers, children may exhibit their need for independence by choosing not to eat. Preschool children frequently eat smaller meals and may want to snack between meals. Children who are 3 or 4 years old may eat slowly but generally show an increase in appetite over the previous year. They generally eat more at one sitting than 2-year-old children. By age 6, most children have developed stable, healthy appetites. Family food preferences and behaviors strongly influence children's likes, dislikes, and eating patterns. Children generally learn to enjoy a wide variety of foods if they are exposed to them in pleasant situations.

Feeding Infants

Because infants grow and change at a rapid rate during the first year of life, you must be aware of how their feeding needs change during this time.

0 to 3 months.   Hold the infant during feedings of breast milk or formula. If the family has a history of allergies, breast feeding the baby is recommended over formula feeding. Cereal is not recommended for a child of this age, as it may be too difficult for him to digest.

4 to 5 months.   Continue feeding the infant formula or breast milk and begin baby cereal feedings. Start with 2 tablespoons of rice cereal twice daily and then introduce other single-grain cereals one at a time. Introduce multigrain cereal last. Giving the baby only one new food at a time allows him to get used to the flavor and makes it easier to determine if he is allergic to any particular type of food. (Signs of food allergy include diarrhea, rash, vomiting, and irritability.) During feedings, the baby may push most of the cereal out of his mouth due to the tongue's normal sucking action. Use the spoon to put the food back into his mouth.

   NOTE: To prevent overfeeding or choking, *never* put cereal into the baby's bottle.

6 to 8 months.   At this age, the baby may hold his own bottle of breast milk or formula, but he still should be held during bottle feedings to increase his sense of security and to meet his social needs. Introduce apple and non-citrus juices one at a time. Continue feeding the child baby cereal and begin serving him strained fruits, vegetables, and meats. Again, introduce new foods one at a time and avoid combination meals. To prepare baby food at home, steam small amounts of food over water and save the resulting cooking liquid. Place the food and vitamin-rich liquid in a blender and puree it. When using commercially prepared baby food, spoon a meal-sized portion into a bowl, and refrigerate the unused food for up to 24 hours. Feeding the infant directly from the jar introduces bacteria into the jar and contaminates the uneaten portion, which must be thrown away.

   NOTE: Do not sweeten foods with honey, because it may cause **botulism** in infants.

9 to 12 months.   Between breast or bottle feedings, begin offering the child liquids in a cup. Continue feeding the child cereal and slowly advance to chunkier toddler foods. During meals, give the child a separate spoon to encourage self-feeding skills. Introduce small finger foods such as unsugared adult cereals, cooked vegeta-

botulism
(BAH-chew-liz-um)   A severe type of food poisoning caused by bacteria found in improperly canned food and in impure honey. Untreated botulism can result in death.

bles, and fruits. Avoid giving the child nuts, raw vegetables, popcorn, grapes, and hard candy, which can easily lodge in the windpipe and cause choking. Make sure the child eats foods such as biscuits, toast, and crackers while sitting up (*never* while lying down) to reduce the possibility of choking on crumbs.

NOTE: Do not put the child to bed with a bottle of milk or fruit juice. During the night, there is ample time for the sugar in these fluids to attack the teeth and start cavities.

Feeding Children and Adolescents

When you provide care for children and adolescents, it is important to know what foods they like, how many calories they need (Table 12-4), and how you can make mealtime a pleasant part of the child's daily experience.

Table 12-4   **Daily Calorie Requirements for Children and Adolescents**

Age (Years)	Calories Required
1-3	900-1800
4-6	1300-2300
7-10	1650-3300
11-14 (boys)	2000-3700
11-14 (girls)	1500-3000
15-18 (boys)	2100-3900
15-18 (girls)	1200-3000

*From Hale E: Good nutrition for your growing child, FDA Consumer, Publication (FDA) 87-2218, Rockville, Md, 1987, US Department of Health and Human Services, p 3.

Toddler (1 to 3 years).   Begin to wean a toddler from bottle or breast feeding and offer him whole milk in a cup instead. To encourage the child to eat solid foods, limit his milk intake to 16 to 24 ounces daily. Begin serving the child table food that the rest of the family eats, keeping a watchful eye on the fat, salt, and sugar content. Avoid very spicy foods, which can be hard for a young child to digest. To prevent choking, do not give toddlers small, round, or hard foods, such as hot dogs or hard candy.

Use the child's appetite to gauge how much to serve at mealtime. Typical serving sizes for a 2- to 3-year-old child include 2 to 3 tablespoons of applesauce or cooked vegetables, ¼ of a banana or apple, ⅓ cup of orange juice, 1 to 2 ounces of meat, fish, or poultry, ½ slice of bread, ⅓ cup of cooked dry peas, beans, or lentils, and 2 to 3 tablespoons of rice or cereal. Make mealtimes fun and encourage the child to use his own cup and spoon while eating.

NOTE: Don't force a child to eat and don't use food as a reward or punishment.

Toddlers are known to be picky eaters. They commonly go on "food jags" and may eat only one food or one type of food for several days. Continue to present the child with a balanced diet by offering nutritious between-meal snacks such as cubed cheese and bread or unsalted crackers spread with peanut butter.

Preschooler (3 to 5 years). The quality of a preschooler's diet is more important than the quantity. Continue to offer a balanced diet, serving the child approximately 1 tablespoon of each food for each year of his age. You may introduce low-fat or skim milk at this time. A preschool child needs the calcium supplied by two to three 8-ounce servings of milk each day, but may not be able to drink an entire serving of milk at one time. To make sure the child gets enough calcium, serve him milk and dairy products as snacks.

Cheese cut into cubes and served with fruit or crackers makes an ideal snack, as do cheese spreads on crackers or bread. (Avoid serving cream cheese, which is full of fat and is more like butter than cheese.) Cottage cheese with fruit or plain low-fat yogurt with fruit added at home is another good snack choice. Make nutritious frozen dessert by mixing yogurt with crushed fruit in a blender and freezing the mixture in paper cups.

To increase the child's iron and protein intake, include snacks from the meat group. Cut leftover cooked meat into cubes and serve with fruit or vegetables. Make meat spreads in a food processor and spread on bread or crackers. Or offer hard-cooked eggs served with cheese. Offer sweet, high-fat, or salty foods only after meeting basic nutrition requirements. Try serving the child yogurt, raisins, and graham crackers instead of sweet desserts.

School-age child (5 to 12 years). A child grows a lot during the school-age years, and his appetite often reflects this. When serving meals, increase the portion size of each food served according to how much the child will eat, and continue to offer a balanced diet.

During the school-age years, a child's food choices and preferences are often influenced by his peers and by television commercials. Luckily, most children seem to have an avid interest in food, and this is a good time to teach them how to make healthy food choices. Encouraging a child to choose nutritious snacks such as those listed above is a good way to promote his sense of independence.

Adolescent (12 to 20 years). When serving a meal to an adolescent, plan the meal to allow for the person's need for more protein and iron, which help the body as it continues to grow and mature. Iron is especially important for adolescent girls, who begin to menstruate at this time. Adolescents who play sports need to eat more than their non-athletic peers do to keep their energy usage from affecting growth and maturity. Larger meals and between-meal snacks help supply extra calories. Young women who become pregnant also require extra calories and nutrition. To help maintain the mother's and baby's health, encourage a pregnant adolescent to have her diet professionally evaluated early in her pregnancy and to receive regular nutrition counseling.

Peers and personal body image influence food selection during adolescence. Teens who frequently eat at fast-food restaurants can maintain healthy diets if they make wise menu choices, but adolescents who experiment with dieting may seriously affect their health. Eating a balanced diet during adolescence is important for promoting good nutrition and maintaining health in the adult years.

NOTE: Government food-assistance programs are available for low-income families. If you provide care for families who are unable to provide their children with a nutritious diet, report this concern to your supervising nurse so that she or a social worker can refer them to the appropriate agency. As a nurse assistant, you may help teach nutrition and meal planning to people receiving assistance from such programs.

Promoting Healthy Food Attitudes in Children

You can help promote healthy food attitudes in children by being patient, giving positive direction and feedback, being consistent, setting a good example, and not using food as a reward.

Be patient. Young children often spill much of their food while they explore new textures and try to coordinate their bodies to handle utensils, plates, and cups. A young child learns new eating skills more easily in a relaxed atmosphere. It is important to recognize that creating messes during mealtime is a normal part of learning new skills. When helping a young child at mealtime, plan ahead for spills by minimizing their impact. Place plastic sheeting beneath the area where the child eats, and use a hand towel as a placemat. It's a good idea to keep a sponge handy. When spills occur, remain calm and encourage the child to help clean up if he is able.

Give positive direction and feedback. Teach a child to be responsible during mealtimes by helping him avoid mistakes. For example, show him where to place his cup so that he won't tip it over. Show him how to use the sponge or mop so that he can clean up his own spills. Be on the lookout for good behavior, and praise the child when he behaves well.

Be consistent. Be consistent when setting standards for eating behavior. Being very strict one day and permissive the next confuses the child and may make him anxious during mealtime.

Set a good example. Encourage adult family members to set a good example. Children learn from what they see. They often imitate family members who use good table manners and demonstrate an interest in a wide variety of foods.

Don't "use" food.   Never withhold food as a form of discipline or give it as a reward. Such practices teach a child that problems are solved by eating and may lead to eating disorders or other harmful behaviors later in life.

Controlling Obesity in Children

Several years ago, a plump child was considered healthy and cute. It was generally believed that the child would lose his baby fat as he grew and matured. Today, doctors realize that an overweight child may experience health and social problems throughout his life. Use the following guidelines to help a child build good nutritional habits and avoid obesity:

❖   Provide regularly scheduled meals and snacks to eliminate continuous eating throughout the day. Regular eating times help foster a sense of order and predictability. Encourage the child to eat slowly and to enjoy his food and, as mentioned above, encourage his parents to set a good example, because a child often will imitate a parent.

❖   Plan satisfying meals and snacks that represent a balanced and varied diet. Young children need some fat and cholesterol in their diet for proper brain development, but be careful not to serve foods that are high in fat and sugar with every meal.

❖   Do not insist that the child finish everything on his plate. Learn to adjust portion sizes according to the child's caloric requirements. A child who is rewarded for eating may overeat and associate eating with parental love and approval.

❖   Don't offer dessert as a reward for finishing the main course. A child who gulps down his dinner so that he can have dessert may believe that sweets are the best part of the meal and may eat more food than he really wants. When serving dessert, offer fruit or custard, which supplies nutrients as well as calories. Dessert isn't necessary for every meal.

❖   Monitor the child's intake of sweet beverages. Dilute sugary drinks and encourage him to drink water to satisfy his thirst. Do not serve artificial sweeteners to children, especially young children.

❖   Encourage the child to exercise by providing toys and playmates for active play. Ask the child to help with chores or activities that require body movement, such as raking leaves or mowing the lawn. Limit television watching. Often, overweight children spend more time watching television than do youngsters of average weight.

A child who becomes accustomed to overeating, eating for reasons other than hunger, and snacking on high-calorie, low-nutrient foods may continue these habits throughout life. He also may develop a physical makeup that favors fat storage and may have to struggle with excess weight his entire life. By guiding a child's nutrition during the early years, you can help establish healthful eating habits that persist into the future.

Nutrition in Home Health Care

On Monday, when you arrive to provide care for Amber Clark and her 15-month-old son Dominic, Amber looks relieved. She says that her sister did her grocery shopping for her on Saturday, but that she has been unable to prepare many dishes because of her broken collarbone.

Together, you and Ms. Clark do an inventory of the food she has in her cupboards and refrigerator and plan menus for her and Dominic. You help her choose a variety of nutritious foods for each meal. You also fix large portions of two meals that she can simply heat at mealtimes.

As a home health aide, you have an important responsibility to plan, shop for, store, prepare, and serve the most nutritious foods possible to help your client regain her health or stay healthy. You also are responsible for keeping the kitchen area clean.

Planning

To plan nutritious meals, you first must learn the eating habits, likes, and dislikes of the person in your care. You also must learn if she has religious or cultural preferences relating to food. Your supervising nurse may be able to give you some of this information, or you may have to ask the client the following questions:

❖ What do you like to eat?
❖ How do you like those foods prepared? (This question should be specific to the type of food.)
❖ Do you follow a special diet or have food preferences for health reasons?
❖ When do you like to eat? How much do you like to eat at each of those times?
❖ What kinds of snack foods do you like to eat?
❖ Is there any food you do not like? Are there foods you are allergic to?
❖ Do you have any preferences about food storage or handling?
❖ What foods do you usually buy at the grocery store when you shop? (You should ask this question of the person who usually does the shopping for the household.)

Your responsibility in meal preparation and planning varies, depending on the needs of your client (Figure 12-17). At times you may be involved in shopping for groceries. At other times you may plan and prepare meals, or you may prepare meals that have been planned by someone else. Ask the client about preferences even when she is on a special diet with limited food choices. She can make many choices within the limits of her diet. A person may ask for something her diet does not allow her to eat. For example, a per-

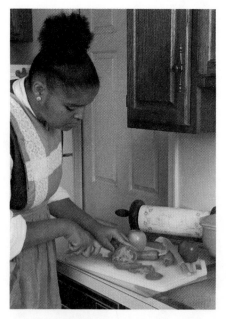

Figure 12-17
Be sure to consider your client's needs when preparing food in a home health care setting.

son on a low-salt diet may prefer pickles, which are high in salt, but you would not be able to serve them to her. You must serve only food allowed within the special diet. After your discussion with the client, plan the desirable number of meals, referring to the five major food groups for guidance in food selection.

Plan some meals that are based on leftovers. Using leftovers cuts down on the time spent preparing and enables you to buy larger quantities of items such as meat, rice, and pasta, which may save money for your client.

Shopping

For some clients, you may have to shop for groceries. Use the information you get from the client and her family to start your shopping list. Check to see what she has in the cupboards and ask her if she needs any staples, such as spices, sugar, or flour. Planning meals lets you shop for everything you need at one time. Shopping wisely saves money, too.

As a shopper, you can follow many practical, money-saving steps for both yourself and the client. For example,—

❖ Watch newspaper ads for food specials and collect money-saving food coupons. You may ask if the client shops this way.

❖ Keep an ongoing shopping list. Jot down items to be replaced as you use them, review the list with the client, and complete the list before you go shopping. Follow the list carefully as you shop.

❖ Use unit pricing. Look at Figure 12-18 to compare product prices and sizes and to help you select the most economical product.

COMPARATIVE SHOPPING

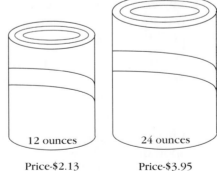

12 ounces

24 ounces

Price-$2.13
($2.84 per pound)

Price-$3.95
($2.63 per pound)

Figure 12-18
If you can efficiently use the 24-ounce can, buy it, because it costs less per pound than the 12-ounce can. However, keep in mind the client's preference for a particular brand and whether she can use the contents of the can before they spoil.

❖ Select less expensive, leaner cuts of meat. These meats may require long, slow cooking, such as braising, stewing, or overnight marinating to tenderize them.

❖ Read product labels. Label information lists ingredients and may list calories, nutrients, and number of servings per container. See Box 12-2 on p. 288 for an example of label information.

Box 12-2   **Example of Product Information on a Label**

Nutrition Information Per Serving

Serving size	9.5 oz
Servings per container	2
Calories	130
Protein	12 g
Carbohydrate	12 g
Fat	3 g
Cholesterol (5 mg/100 g)*	20 mg
Sodium	870 mg
Potassium	400 mg

Percentage of U.S. recommended daily allowances (U.S. RDA)

Protein	20	Riboflavin	6
Vitamin A	50	Niacin	30
Vitamin C	†	Calcium	4
Thiamin	4	Iron	15

Ingredients: chicken broth, carrots, chicken, tomatoes, red kidney beans, enriched macaroni product, celery, green beans, green peas, lima beans, food starch-modified, salt, dehydrated onions, hydrolyzed vegetable protein, monosodium glutamate, sugar, autolyzed yeast extract, spice, natural flavor.
*Information on cholesterol content is provided for individuals who, on the advice of a doctor, are modifying their dietary intake of cholesterol.
†Contains less than 20% of the U.S. RDA of this nutrient.

❖ Buy seasonal, fresh produce, since vegetables and fruit in season usually cost less. Whole vegetables and fruit also cost less than cut produce. For example, a whole cantaloupe costs less than a half cantaloupe that is wrapped in plastic film. Select produce that looks fresh and is not bruised or damaged. When possible, buy vegetables that are fresh or frozen, because vegetables in cans generally have a large amount of sodium or salt. If you do buy canned food, note that cut or sliced vegetables or fruit is usually less expensive than halved or whole items. (For example, sliced peaches cost less than peach halves, and cut asparagus is cheaper than asparagus spears.)

❖ Select fresh-looking packages and cans that are not dented, swollen, or bulging. Do not buy packages that are ripped or open. Damaged cans or packages may contain contaminated food.

❖ Check the expiration date when buying perishable foods that spoil quickly. Make sure you use all the food, especially milk, meats, and fish, before the "use by" date, which indicates when the food may begin to spoil.

Storing and Handling Food

Always take food home immediately after shopping. Perishable foods such as meats, dairy products, and frozen goods, or any foods that can spoil, must be stored properly and promptly. To slow the growth of harmful viruses and bacteria, observe the following basic guidelines about food storage:

❖ Purchase only what you can store.

❖ Keep the refrigerator temperature between 36 and 40 degrees Fahrenheit.

❖ Keep the freezer temperature at 0 degrees Fahrenheit.

❖ Keep the refrigerator and freezer clean and frost free. Defrost the freezer before the frost is 1 inch thick.

❖ Wrap and store perishable foods in air-tight plastic bags or plastic containers with tight-fitting lids. Store dairy products, meats, poultry, and fish in the coldest part of the refrigerator. Tightly wrap foods that are to be frozen and label the package with the contents and the date of storage.

❖ Keep dry ingredients such as flour, sugar, and pasta in tightly closed containers.

❖ Place grain items such as flour and cornmeal in the freezer for 48 hours before putting them away in the pantry. Freezing prevents insects from infesting the food, since their eggs won't hatch after being exposed to cold temperatures.

❖ Check dry storage areas for signs of insects or rodents. Do not use foods that are contaminated by pests. If necessary, ask your supervisor what to do if pests are present.

❖ Cover foods before storing them in the refrigerator.

Everyone who works in a kitchen and handles food must observe the following basic rules of sanitation and hygiene:

❖ If you suspect that food has become contaminated or has not been handled or stored properly, wrap it in plastic or aluminum foil and throw it away in a covered trash container. Too many germs in food make it unsafe to eat.

❖ Wash your hands often with soap and water when you are handling food.

❖ Clean and sanitize food preparation surfaces and utensils, especially any surfaces and utensils that come into contact with raw meats, poultry, or fish, before and after use. (Reread the sections on cleaning in Chapter 11, Providing Care for the Person's Place.)

❖ Keep hot foods hot, making sure they stay above 140 degrees Fahrenheit or higher before serving.

❖ Keep cold foods cold, storing them at temperatures of 40 degrees Fahrenheit or lower. Store appropriate foods in the refrigerator.

❖ Wash fresh vegetables and fruit carefully before using them.

❖ Discard any uneaten portion of a client's meal. The food is unsafe to use again and should not be eaten by anyone else.

❖ Keep all trash covered to prevent attracting insects and rodents.

Preparing Food

Before you start cooking, ask for a tour of the kitchen. If no one can give you a tour, take one yourself (Figure 12-19). Each person organizes her kitchen in her own way. Find out where the she keeps

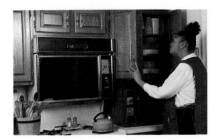

Figure 12-19
When you work as a home health aide, you may be responsible for cooking. To save time later, get acquainted with the kitchen when first visiting a new client.

pots, pans, dishes, and utensils so that you are familiar when you must cook or put away clean dishes.

Before beginning to cook, plan and organize all the food and utensils that you must have to do the job. These early steps prevent you from getting part way through the meal preparation and realizing there is something missing. If you are preparing several hot dishes, make sure that everything that needs to be served hot is completed at the same time. For example, when serving a casserole that takes 1 hour to cook and steamed vegetables that take about 10 minutes, start the casserole at 5:00 P.M. and the vegetables at 5:50 P.M. so that everything will be finished at 6:00 P.M.

Prepare foods carefully to destroy harmful germs and retain flavor and nutrients. Use the basic cooking techniques listed in the following paragraphs:

Baking. Baking is a dry-heat cooking process in the oven in which food is not exposed directly to the heat source. Bake foods, such as casseroles or breads, in oven-proof containers.

Roasting. Roasting is a dry-heat cooking process, similar to baking, that usually exposes large cuts of meat or poultry to hot air in the oven. Use an oven-proof container without a lid or cover.

Broiling and grilling. Another dry-heat cooking method is broiling. Place the food (usually meat) on a metal rack in a metal pan. Place the pan on an oven rack, and cook the food directly under the source of heat. For grilling, place the food on a rack directly over the source of heat, as in barbecuing, or place the food in a skillet or griddle on a stove burner.

Steaming. Steaming is a moist-heat cooking method that uses a burner on top of the stove. This quick, no-fat way to cook vegetables retains the maximum amount of flavor and nutrients. Place vegetables in a metal steaming rack and set it in a pot over but not in water. Cover the pot and bring the water to a boil. Check often to make sure the water hasn't boiled away.

Boiling. This moist-heat cooking method uses boiling water in a pot. Place the pot on the stove burner and bring the water to a full rolling boil. Place the food in the boiling water, cover the pot with a lid (usually), reduce the amount of heat, and cook the food until done. Periodically check to make sure the water hasn't boiled away.

Frying, stir-frying, and sautéing. Frying requires cooking foods in preheated fat or oil in a pot or skillet on the stove burner. Because the fat becomes very hot during cooking and can splatter, take extra care when putting food in or removing it from the pot. Sautéing and stir-frying require cooking thin or small pieces of food in a small amount of fat, which may be a combination of butter and vegetable oil. Foods brown and cook quickly by these methods.

Many of these techniques also may be used in a microwave oven. Follow the manufacturer's directions for proper use of the microwave oven.

To save time, prepare more than one serving of food at a time. Use the leftovers for another meal. Remember to label food containers and store warm foods in the refrigerator before they get cold. You also may want to store some of the leftovers in the freezer to save for the next week or a couple of weeks later.

You may be asked to prepare lunch for the client when you are there and to prepare something for dinner and put it in the refrigerator for her to heat later. Be sure not to serve the same thing for dinner as you did for lunch, because a person needs a variety of foods for good nutrition. If a person gets bored with what she is eating, she may not eat enough food or get the nutrients she needs.

If your client shares kitchen facilities with one or several other people, establish a schedule for when you can use the kitchen without disrupting others. Notify them that you have purchased, labeled, and stored special foods for your client. Explain the sanitary procedures you are following and ask them to use the same procedures when they use your client's plates, cups, glasses, and cooking and eating utensils.

Serving Meals

A person usually looks forward to mealtime, but food may not seem very appealing to someone who is sick. You can help make mealtime more enjoyable by using some of the following tips:

❖ Set up a mealtime schedule and stick to it so that your client doesn't get upset by any changes. However, if your client is not hungry at mealtime and wants to eat at another time, be as flexible as possible.

❖ Arrange plates and tables attractively so that food looks appealing and appetizing.

❖ Plan meals that use foods of different colors. If you planned a meal of mashed potatoes, cauliflower, and skinned breast of chicken, everything would be white. If you serve carrots instead of, or with, the cauliflower, you add some color. You might serve brown rice instead of mashed potatoes.

❖ Always use clean utensils and fresh napkins.

❖ Make sure that the client is comfortable and that she washes her hands before and after eating.

❖ Protect her clothing with a napkin or towel.

❖ Do not hurry the client while she eats.

❖ Serve hot foods hot and cold foods cold.

❖ Clear the table or remove the plate as soon as the client has finished eating.

If your client must eat in bed but doesn't have a bed table, make one from a cardboard box according to the following procedure (Figure 12-20 on p. 292):

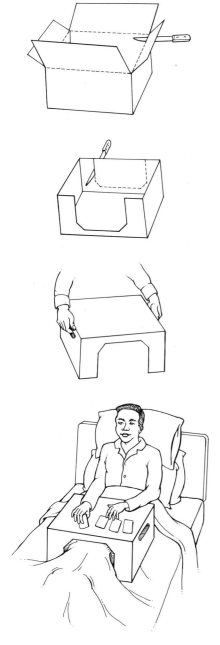

1. Cut the four flaps off a large, rectangular box.
2. Cut curved pieces out of the two longest sides of the box to create space for fitting over your client's lap. Leave at least 2 inches of cardboard at the bottom and sides to support the table.
3. Turn the box over so that the bottom faces up. Cut narrow openings near the top of each of the shorter sides so that the table can be picked up and moved.
4. To strengthen the table, cover the cut edges with tape. You also may want to cover the table with wallpaper, fabric, paint, or adhesive-backed plastic.

Before using the finished table on the bed, loosen and adjust the top bed covers so that the client can easily move her legs underneath the table.

Apply the information in this chapter to yourself, your family, and the people in your care. Make what you serve and what you eat reflect the very best you can offer. Providing proper nutrition is more than a science. It is also an art. Eating for health and pleasure is one area in which you can be both scientist and artist.

Figure 12-20
A cardboard box makes a good bed table.

Information Review

Circle the correct answers and fill in the blanks.

1. In this book, "diet" means—
   a. A way to lose weight.
   b. A list of dos and don'ts about eating.
   c. All the food and liquid a person consumes.
   d. Therapeutic.
2. A person needs more of this nutrient than all the others.
   a. Carbohydrates
   b. Protein
   c. Vitamins
   d. Fat
3. _____ Fat _____ should be the smallest part of any diet.
4. Which therapeutic diet does not provide enough nutrients to maintain good nutrition?
   a. NAS
   b. Diabetic
   c. Full liquid
   d. Pureed
5. A clear liquid diet has to be reordered by the physician every _____ 48 _____ hours.
6. A _____ high protein _____ diet is often prescribed for people who have decubitus ulcers or burns.
7. When a person has difficulty swallowing, it is easier for him to swallow _____ soft _____ foods than liquids.

8. If a person in your care is fed through a nasogastric tube, you should—
    a. Keep the person lying flat for 30 minutes after a tube feeding.
    b. Give the person water by mouth.
    c. Use cotton balls moistened with alcohol to clean around the person's mouth and nose.
    d. Keep the head of the bed elevated for 30 minutes follow- *at 45°* ing a tube feeding.

9. Which of these symptoms is *not* a sign of dehydration?
    a. Dark urine
    b. Dry skin
    c. Frequent urination
    d. Confusion

10. To promote healthy eating habits in children,—
    a. Be patient, positive, and consistent.
    b. Make them eat everything on their plates.
    c. Reward their good behavior with special treats.
    d. Tell them not to do what you do, but to do what you say.

Home Health Care

1. Handle foods properly by—
    a. Storing perishables at room temperature.
    b. Storing flour in an open container.
    c. Washing your hands with soap and water before handling food.
    d. Saving the uneaten portions of a client's food for someone else in the family to eat.

2. Food labels must indicate ___ingredients___ and may also indicate ___calories___, nutrients, and number of servings.

3. ___Steaming___ is a quick, no-fat way to cook vegetables, which retains the maximum amount of flavor and nutrients.

Questions to Ask Yourself

1. You notice that Mr. Rivera did not eat much of his breakfast or lunch. He says he feels okay and asks you not to worry. What would you do?

2. Mrs. Morgan tells you that her diabetic roommate has been stealing her cookies at lunch. You know that Mrs. Morgan's roommate cannot have cookies. What would you do?

3. Mrs. Garcia eats very little. She says she is not hungry. You suspect that she may tire easily and find it difficult to feed herself. You offer to help her eat, but she says she is too old to be fed like a baby. What would you do?

13

Elimination

Goals

After reading this chapter, you will have the information to—

Discuss daily elimination patterns and needs.

Explain special urinary needs.

Explain special bowel elimination needs.

Discuss children's elimination needs.

After practicing the corresponding skills in the skills book, you will be able to—

Help a person use the bathroom toilet, portable commode, bedpan, or urinal.

Provide perineal care for a person with a urinary catheter.

Empty a urinary drainage bag.

Apply an external catheter to a male.

Test urine for sugar and acetone.

Collect urine and stool specimens.

Give a tap water, soap solution, commercial cleansing, or oil-retention enema.

Diaper a child and collect a urine specimen from an infant.

This morning, just as you are about to help Mr. Wilson with his bath, Josie Miller presses her call signal. You make sure that Mr. Wilson is safe and comfortable and tell him that you must answer a call signal and will return as soon as possible. You then go to Josie's room, where she is trying to get to the edge of her bed. She says she needs to have a bowel movement. You think this is a bit unusual, because she already had a bowel movement just after breakfast as she normally does.

You move the portable commode to the side of her bed, put on the brake, and begin to prepare a basin of warm water when Josie says, "I don't want to use that thing today. I want to go to the bathroom and use a real toilet." You ask her if she feels well enough to walk to the bathroom or if she wants to ride to the bathroom in her wheelchair. "I'll walk," says Josie.

Although you know that she usually uses the portable commode and that you must get back to Mr. Wilson's room to help him with his bath, you tell her that you understand. You help Josie put on her bathrobe and slippers before helping her use her walker to walk to the bathroom where she can use the "real toilet." You help her onto the toilet, rearrange her bathrobe and gown, and then step outside the bathroom door, where you wait for her to finish.

After 5 minutes, you knock on the door and ask Josie if she needs help. She says she's taking care of things herself. You wait another few minutes and ask her again if she needs help. This time, you hear the frustration in her voice, and she agrees to let you come in to help her.

When you go into the bathroom, you discover that Josie has diarrhea and that she needs some assistance. You ask her permission to help her and, when she agrees, you put on gloves and clean her carefully, washing from front to back, and reassuring her.

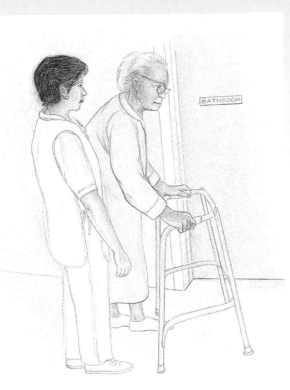

Later, after you get Josie settled back in her bed and put away the portable commode and supplies, you stop at the nurses' station to report to your supervising nurse that Josie has diarrhea. Then you return to Mr. Wilson's room, where he begins to complain about your being gone for such a long time.

Eliminating Body Waste

Every living thing eats to provide nutrients to its body. The valuable parts of the food are absorbed into the body. The wastes that are not used are **eliminated** from the body in several forms. Two of these forms of waste are **urine** and **feces**, or **stool**. Another is **perspiration**.

For most people, going to the bathroom to eliminate body wastes is a regular occurrence. It is a natural and normal process that everyone does, although the words people use to describe the process may differ. As a nurse assistant, you must use the terms that people in health care use for elimination. The correct term for the elimination of urine is **urinate**, or **void**. The correct term for the elimination of feces is **defecate**, or move the bowels. It is important for you to use these words, but in some situations it is okay to use the term preferred by the person in your care. For example, on days when Mrs. McDay is extremely confused, the only way you can get her to cooperate in using the bathroom is to use her words, "number 1" and "number 2."

Most people in our society think elimination is a personal, private matter and may be embarrassed to talk about it. Some people are brought up to think that the parts of the body used for elimination are unclean or "disgusting." They are taught not to touch those parts of the body on themselves or on other people.

As a nurse assistant, one of your responsibilities is helping the people in your care with elimination. You will learn how to provide this care with respect for their privacy and dignity. How do you feel about helping someone with her elimination needs? Feeling uncomfortable when you help a person who needs to urinate or move her bowels is normal.

How do you think people in your care feel about needing your help when they urinate or have a bowel movement? Do you think they might feel embarrassed, helpless, or angry? It's extremely important for you to be sensitive to people's feelings about needing help with a very personal function. It's also important that you always act in a positive, professional way when you help them.

Daily Elimination

A person normally eliminates 1 to 1½ quarts of urine each day. Normal urine is clear, golden yellow to amber in color and has a slight odor. In the morning, the color of urine is darker and, as the day goes on, it gets lighter. Urine changes color because a person usually takes in less fluid at night than during the day. Decreased fluid intake causes urine to be more **concentrated**, which makes the color darker. During the day, when a person drinks more fluids, the urine becomes more **diluted**, which makes the color lighter. Drinking fluids frequently helps keep urine dilute and light yellow. If urine remains concentrated for too long, it irritates the bladder and can cause an infection. (To learn how urine is produced and eliminated from the body, read Body Basics, The Urinary System.)

---

eliminate
(uh-LIM-uh-nate)   To get rid of.

urine
(YUR-in)   Liquid body waste.

feces
(FEE-seez)   Solid body waste.

stool
Another term for solid body waste, or feces.

perspiration
(pur-spi-RAY-shun)   Body waste eliminated through the skin.

urinate
(YUR-uh-nate)   To eliminate liquid waste from the body.

void
Another term for urinate.

defecate
(DEF-uh-kate)   To eliminate solid waste from the body.

concentrated
(KON-sen-tray-ted)   Containing a small percentage of water.

diluted
(di-LOO-ted)   Containing a large percentage of water.

Feces are normally brown in color, soft in texture, and formed. Because feces are about three-fourths water and one-fourth solid waste products, it is important for people to drink water to maintain regular bowel movements. The frequency with which a person has bowel movements is called his pattern of bowel elimination. This pattern varies from person to person. Some people have bowel movements every day, others every 2 to 3 days. A change in routine can disrupt a person's bowel elimination pattern. (See Body Basics, The Digestive System, in Chapter 12, Healthful Eating.)

Patterns of Elimination

An elimination pattern indicates the number of times each day a person uses the bathroom, how much time passes between voiding, and what time and how often a person usually has a bowel movement. Every person has her own normal pattern of elimination. You must learn the elimination pattern of each person in your care so that you can help maintain the pattern and recognize changes in it.

Think about your own elimination pattern. How would you feel if you had to rely on another person to take you to the bathroom at those times? How would you feel if someone tried to change your elimination pattern? For example, let's say that every day, all your life, you moved your bowels after breakfast. It would be important for the person providing care for you to know this pattern. What would happen if that person decided it was more convenient for you to have your bowel movement after lunch?

Maintaining Normal Elimination Patterns

You can help maintain a person's normal elimination pattern by learning about her pattern, answering her call signal right away, providing her privacy during elimination, giving her as much time as she needs to eliminate, being sensitive to her feelings about having to ask for assistance, having a professional attitude about elimination, and helping her urinary and digestive systems work more efficiently.

Learn about the person's elimination pattern.   To learn about the person's elimination pattern, ask her these questions:

❖ How often do you urinate?
❖ Is there anything special about your urinating habits that I
    should know?
❖ How often do you have a bowel movement?
❖ What time of day do you usually have a bowel movement?
❖ Is there anything special about your bowel movement habits that
    I should know?

If the person cannot provide the information, ask her family members or check her chart to determine a pattern.

Answer the person's call signal right away.   Because of illness, a person may not always be able to control the urge to urinate or defecate, so it is important to answer her call signal right away. As people age,

BodyBasics

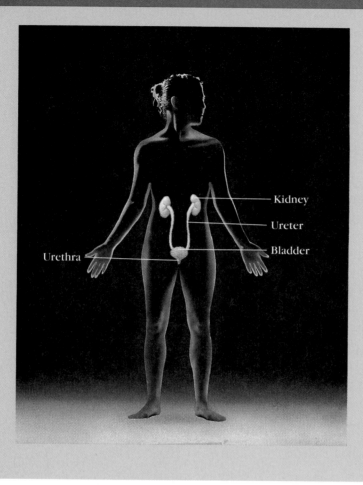

Kidney

Ureter

Bladder

Urethra

muscle tone may decrease, making it difficult to control the flow of urine. (See Body Basics, The Urinary System.)

Even for the person who has control over her elimination, it is important to answer the call signal right away, because she may need help getting out of bed or getting to the bathroom. Or, if she cannot get out of bed, she may need help using a bedpan.

When a person cannot control the release of urine or feces, this condition is called **incontinence**. The person may be truly incontinent, or she may simply have been unable to find the bathroom or get there on her own. Or, when she needed help, maybe a staff member didn't answer her call signal right away (Figure 13-1). Think about Josie and how she was trying to get out of bed when you answered her call signal. What might have happened if you had decided to ignore her call signal and give Mr. Wilson his bath first?

Provide privacy for the person during elimination.   To provide privacy, pull the curtain around the bed or close the door. Encourage the

incontinence
(in-KON-ti-nense)   The inability to control the release of urine or feces.

BodyBasics

❖ The Urinary System ❖

Every 45 minutes the body's 5 quarts of blood pass through the kidneys for purification. The kidneys are part of the urinary system, which removes wastes from the bloodstream and eliminates them as urine.

Two kidneys, bean-shaped organs about 4 inches long, are located at waist level, one on each side of the body. After removing waste materials from the blood, the kidneys mix the wastes with water and turn them into urine. The kidneys produce about 1½ quarts of urine each day.

Urine passes from the kidneys through ureters, delicate tubes connecting the kidneys to the bladder. Urine collects in the bladder until it fills to about 2½ cups. At this point, the person feels the urge to urinate, or pass urine from the body.

Urine passes from the bladder to the outside of the body through the urethra. In women, the urethra is separate from the reproductive system, with the opening located in front of the vagina. In men, both urine and semen can pass through the urethra, but never at the same time.

How the Urinary System Ages

As people age, they may have trouble with incontinence or dribbling urine. This problem occurs in men when the prostate gland enlarges, squeezing the nearby urethra, creating a need to urinate but an inability to empty the bladder completely. Incontinence can occur in women when muscles near the urethra weaken.

Fascinating Fact

Doctors first replaced a failed kidney with a working kidney in the late 1950s. Today doctors replace, or transplant, many kidneys every year. Kidneys used for transplant may be donated by a living person (preferably a family member) or by the family of someone who has died. About 80 to 90 percent of those who receive kidneys from relatives and 70 to 90 percent of those who receive kidneys from unrelated donors survive the first year.

person to eliminate in private, but let her know that you are nearby to help if she needs it. Make sure the call signal is easy for her to reach.

Give the person as much time as she needs to eliminate.   Give the person plenty of time to take care of her elimination needs. But check on her regularly so that you do not leave her stranded on the bedpan or alone in the bathroom for too long. Encourage her to remain on the toilet a few minutes after voiding to make sure her bladder is empty.

Be sensitive to a person's feelings about having to ask for assistance.   Often a person may be too embarrassed to ask for help to use the bathroom. She may feel ashamed or not in control if she cannot get to the bathroom by herself. She may be embarrassed if she needs help with perineal care.

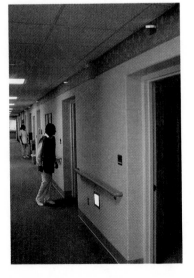

Figure 13-1

Sometimes you must make a choice about whose call signal to answer first. Be sure to answer immediately the call signals of those who have histories of incontinence.

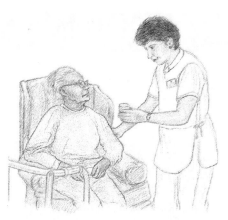

Figure 13-2
Adequate fluid intake is essential to maintaining healthy urinary and digestive systems. Because Josie has diarrhea, she needs to drink this fluid to help avoid dehydration.

Have a professional attitude about elimination.   In response to the feelings of a person in your care, approach the elimination task positively, show her respect, and make sure that your facial expressions and gestures do not show displeasure.

Help the person's urinary and digestive systems work more efficiently.   Offer the person fluids frequently during the day and encourage her to drink six to eight glasses of liquid each day to help her urinary and digestive systems work more efficiently (Figure 13-2). Also, encourage her to eat high-fiber foods, such as whole grains and fresh fruits and vegetables, and to exercise.

Helping a Person Use a Bathroom Toilet

Often when you answer a person's call signal, she needs you to help her use the bathroom toilet. If she is in bed, help her put on her bathrobe and slippers before going to the bathroom. When you help her sit on the toilet, adjust her clothing and pay attention to good body mechanics, because the bathroom may be cramped, it may be difficult to move properly, and the toilet may be low. Provide privacy for the person, but make sure she is safe before leaving her alone. While she is using the toilet, stay just outside the bathroom and check on her at least every 5 minutes to make sure that she is okay and to determine if she needs any assistance.

When helping someone use a bathroom toilet, follow the specific procedure that is explained step by step in Skill 40 in the skills book.

Maintaining a Normal Environment with an Alternative Toilet

Not everyone can use a bathroom toilet. Some people have to use an alternative toilet, such as—

❖ A portable commode, which the person sits on by the side of the bed.
❖ A bedpan, which the person sits on while in the bed.
❖ A urinal, which a man uses while in the bed or standing beside the bed.

Think about a time you may have had to eliminate somewhere other than in a bathroom. How did you feel? Did you find it easy or difficult? Think about how the person in your care might feel about using a portable commode, bedpan, or urinal.

A person who must use an alternative toilet may see elimination as a more difficult, or even distasteful, task. You can make this experience more comfortable if you make it as similar as possible to using a bathroom toilet. You can do this by—

❖ Providing privacy.
❖ Elevating the head of the bed for bedpan use. Try to have the person in a sitting position similar to sitting on the toilet.
❖ Having a man stand to use the urinal, as this position is much more comfortable. Sometimes the person cannot get out of bed.

In this case, take care to position the urinal so that the urine does not spill.

❖ Having toilet tissue nearby.

❖ Having a washcloth, soap, towel, and washbasin of water nearby so that the person can wash his hands.

Helping a person use a portable commode.   A portable commode looks like a chair with a toilet seat (Figure 13-3). Under the seat is a collection container, bedpan, or bucket (with or without a lid) that can be removed for emptying and cleaning. Some portable commodes have wheels and some do not. Sometimes they remain at the person's bedside. In other situations, you may have to bring one to the person's room for a short period of time.

Make sure the collection container is under the commode seat. Place a washbasin of warm water on the overbed table so that the person may easily wash her hands when she has finished using the commode. If the commode has wheels, lock the wheels before moving the person from the bed to the commode.

Help the person put on her bathrobe and slippers. Use good body mechanics when moving her from the bed to the chair, and adjust her clothing after you help her sit on the commode. Provide privacy for the person, but check on her every 5 minutes to make sure she is okay and to see if she needs assistance.

When helping someone use a portable commode, follow the specific procedure that is explained step by step in Skill 41 in the skills book.

Helping a person use a bedpan or urinal.   When a person cannot get out of bed to urinate or defecate, he must use a bedpan (Figure 13-4). A man may use a urinal to urinate.

Using a bedpan is not very comfortable and may feel unnatural. To help the person onto the bedpan, make the bed as flat as possible and then ask the person to bend his knees and raise his buttocks by pushing against the mattress with his feet. If he needs help, slip your hand under his lower back and lift slightly. If the person cannot help, turn him onto his side, place the bedpan firmly against his buttocks, and gently turn him onto the bedpan.

After helping the person onto the bedpan, it is important to help him into a position that best resembles sitting on a toilet. Elevate the head of the bed and ask him to bend his knees if he can. (Some people cannot bend their knees and have to keep their knees straight.) To help him off the bedpan, lower the head of the bed and have him raise his hips so that you can remove the bedpan. Or, have him turn onto his side while you remove the bedpan, taking care that the contents do not spill when he turns.

Some men find it difficult to use a urinal. A urinal is easier and more comfortable to use if the man can stand beside the bed while urinating. Because of his foot problems and the need to walk with a

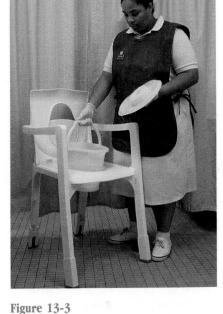

Figure 13-3
A portable commode is a good solution for a person who doesn't use a bedpan and can't get to the bathroom. To use a commode, a person must be able to sit up with little assistance.

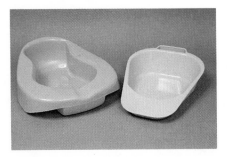

Figure 13-4
A regular bedpan is less likely to spill and is used most often. If a person cannot move enough to get on a regular bedpan (on the left), have him use a fracture pan (on the right).

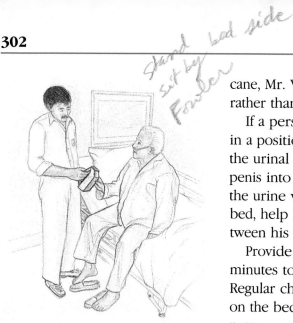

stand bad side
sit by
Fowler

Figure 13-5
If a man cannot stand at the side of the bed to use a urinal, he may prefer to sit on the side of the bed. Both of these positions are preferable to lying in bed.

diarrhea
(dye-uh-REE-uh) The frequent passage of liquid feces.

cane, Mr. Wilson prefers to use the urinal standing beside his bed, rather than walking to the bathroom.

If a person is not able to stand, help him sit on the side of the bed in a position that resembles sitting on a toilet (Figure 13-5), position the urinal comfortably between his legs, and gently help him put his penis into the urinal opening. Be sure to position the urinal so that the urine won't spill. If the person is unable to sit on the side of the bed, help him into a Fowler's position, and position the urinal between his legs.

Provide privacy for the person, but check on him at least every 5 minutes to make sure that he is okay or to see if he needs assistance. Regular checking is especially important for the person who is sitting on the bedpan or who has a urinal in place, because he can develop pressure sores.

When helping someone use a bedpan or urinal, follow the specific procedure that is explained step by step in Skill 42 in the skills book.

Measuring and Recording Fluid Output

It is important to measure a person's fluid output for two reasons: to compare it with the normal range of output and to compare it with her fluid intake (see the section on measuring fluid intake in Chapter 12) to determine the balance of fluids in her body.

To measure a person's output of fluid, use a graduate, a pitcher with measurement marks on its side. When the person finishes using a portable commode, bedpan, or urinal, pour the contents of the container into the graduate. Look at the fluid level to determine the amount to record on the intake and output (I&O) sheet. Each time a person is incontinent of stool (with **diarrhea**) or urine, make a check mark in the right place on the I&O sheet. Ask a nurse to measure or estimate the fluid output from vomit, blood, or diarrhea, if necessary. In hospitals and nursing homes, I&O sheets are totaled at the end of each shift.

Special Urinary Elimination Needs

As a nurse assistant, you play a key role in identifying potential urinary elimination problems by observing and reporting changes in a person's urinary elimination pattern. For example, if someone in your care usually voids every 2 to 3 hours and suddenly starts asking to void every ½ to 1 hour, you would report the change to your supervising nurse.

You might identify another potential problem when you observe and report that a person is not taking in enough fluid. You would suspect this problem if the amount of the person's urine decreased and the color and smell became darker and stronger.

To help you identify changes in urinary elimination patterns, look at Body Basics, The Urinary System. What are the parts of the system? What does the system do? Remembering the system, the parts of the system, and how the system works helps you understand about special urinary elimination needs.

Some people develop urinary problems due to physical conditions, changes in diet, or poor personal hygiene. Also, as people grow older, they often develop urinary problems because of changes that occur in the urinary system. Common urinary problems include urinary incontinence and urinary tract infection. Urinary incontinence is loss of control of the release of urine from the bladder, and it is not a normal process of aging. Several factors can lead to urinary incontinence:

* Damage to the brain that keeps the individual from feeling the urge to urinate
* Weakness of the muscles surrounding the opening of the bladder
* Medications
* Confusion about where to go to the bathroom
* Difficulty in moving, which makes it hard to get to the bathroom
* Not having a call signal answered immediately
* Urinary tract infection

A urinary tract infection can occur in any part of the urinary system (or urinary tract)—kidney, bladder, ureter, or urethra—and it can be painful for the person with the infection. Several of the following symptoms may indicate such an infection:

* Pain or burning sensation when urinating
* Frequent or urgent need to urinate but only a little urine is released at a time
* Cloudy, concentrated (dark yellow), and possibly foul-smelling urine
* Milky mucus shreds or blood in the urine
* Fever

If someone in your care has any of these symptoms, you should report this information to your supervising nurse.

A urinary tract infection can be caused by any of the following situations:

* Not enough fluid intake
* Incomplete emptying of the bladder
* Poor perineal care
* Poor urinary catheter care

When you respond to people who have special urinary elimination needs, you must remember that the people in your care cannot meet their own needs. They rely on you to help them and to offer support and encouragement. Give the best care possible when you provide care for a person who is incontinent, when you help someone who has a urinary tract infection, when you assist a person with a urinary catheter, and when you collect and test urine specimens.

Providing Special Care for a Person Who Has Urinary Incontinence

Because she has Alzheimer's disease, Shirley McDay is often confused about where she has been and what she has done. She often forgets whether she has used the toilet and even forgets where the bathroom is. As a result, she often doesn't get to the bathroom in time to void. She has episodes of incontinence. To help Mrs. McDay, do all the things you normally do for any person in your care. In addition,—

❖ Offer her fluids frequently throughout the day. Increasing fluid intake dilutes the urine so that it is less irritating to the bladder, which results in a decrease in the problems of incontinence, urinary dribbling, and urinary tract infection.

❖ Help her if she has trouble rising or walking to get to the bathroom.

❖ Offer her frequent opportunities to go to the bathroom, particularly if she is confused. Give her sufficient time and provide privacy.

❖ Learn about her voiding pattern and offer her assistance just prior to the time she usually voids.

❖ Be sensitive to the embarrassment she may feel about being incontinent. Be aware that she may be concerned about the need to wear adult briefs to protect her clothing. It is important to call the protective underwear "briefs," not "diapers." Adult briefs should be used only when absolutely necessary and not as a convenience for the health care team.

❖ Offer her emotional support and encouragement.

❖ Help her with a bladder training program.

A doctor or nurse may sometimes recommend that a person participate in a bladder training program to help her regain urinary control. The training schedule is written on the person's care plan. Support the person in her bladder training program by taking her to the toilet on a regular schedule or at least every 2 hours, giving her sufficient time to urinate, and following the training schedule 24 hours a day. Supporting a bladder training program means following the schedule during the night as well, although the intervals between using the toilet may be longer during the night.

Helping a Person Prevent a Urinary Tract Infection

The stroke that left Mr. Rivera paralyzed on his right side also left him incontinent of urine. As part of his training program to help him regain control of his bladder, you encourage him to be patient and to take the time he needs to completely empty his bladder. But Mr. Rivera becomes irritated and impatient about this part of the training program. You think he may be embarrassed about all the attention he is getting about urinating. So he always insists that you take away the urinal immediately. As a result of his failure to completely empty his bladder, Mr. Rivera develops a urinary tract infection.

To help a person prevent the development of a urinary tract infection, do all the things you normally do for any person in your care. In addition,—

❖ Offer him fluids frequently.
❖ Provide time for him to completely empty his bladder when eliminating urine.
❖ Encourage a woman to wipe from front to back.
❖ If the person is incontinent, change adult briefs often.

Helping a Person Who Has a Urinary Catheter

Sometimes when a person has a urinary problem, he or she needs a **urinary catheter** to help eliminate urine from his or her body (Figure 13-6). A person also may need a urinary catheter if she has nerve damage following a stroke or spinal cord injury, if she is incontinent (and is prone to developing sores on the skin), or during or after certain kinds of surgery. (You may hear health care professionals refer to the catheter by other names, such as a Foley catheter or an indwelling catheter.)

urinary catheter
(YUR-uh-nair-ee/KATH-uh-ter)   A small tube (ordered by a doctor) that is inserted (usually by a nurse or doctor) through the urethra into the bladder. A small balloon at the end of the tube on the bladder end is blown up, or inflated, to hold the tube in place. On the other end, the tube connects to a bag that collects the urine.

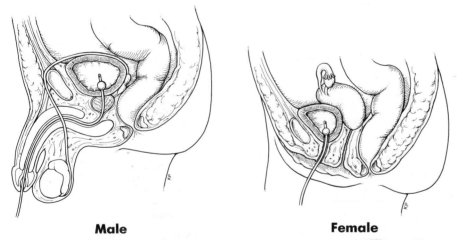

Male   **Female**

Figure 13-6
An indwelling urinary catheter is inserted through the urethra and into the bladder. It is held in place by a small balloon inflated in the bladder.

To show special concern and provide special care for someone who has a urinary catheter,—

❖ Offer fluids frequently to help dilute urine, which decreases the chance of developing a urinary tract infection.
❖ Provide perineal care on a regular schedule and whenever the person is soiled with secretions or feces. Use universal precautions and infection control procedures when providing perineal care for a person who has a catheter, which includes wearing gloves. Make sure the perineal area is kept clean, dry, and free from skin irritation. Clean the perineum from the front to the back.
❖ Keep in mind that a catheter can be uncomfortable, and without proper care a person can develop an infection.

When providing perineal care for a person who has a urinary catheter, follow the specific procedure that is explained step by step in Skill 43 in the skills book.

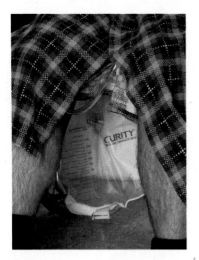

Figure 13-7

When positioning a urinary drainage bag, make sure the bag is always placed lower than the person's bladder so that urine can flow into it. Also, make sure the tubing is not kinked or hanging below the bag.

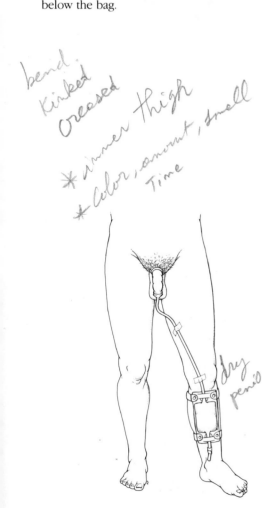

Figure 13-8

An external urinary catheter is less likely to interfere with body function or to cause a urinary tract infection than an indwelling catheter.

Taking care of a urinary catheter. In addition to providing care for the person who has a urinary catheter, you must take care of the catheter in the following ways:

❖ Maintain the urinary drainage flow by keeping the drainage bag below the person's bladder (urine flows downward by the force of gravity) and making sure the catheter tubing is not kinked, bent, or creased. If the tubing kinks, urine backs up into the bladder. An infection or serious damage to the bladder could occur if the tubing kinks for a long time. Also make sure that extra tubing does not loop down below the bag (Figure 13-7).

❖ For security, make sure the catheter tubing is taped or secured by a fastener to the top part of the person's thigh. Securing the tubing prevents it from rubbing and pulling at the entrance to the urethra.

❖ Keep the tubing or drainage bag from touching the floor, because the floor is dirty.

❖ When transferring a person to a chair, move the drainage bag before moving the person. If you do not move the bag first, the catheter could be pulled, causing injury and pain to the person.

❖ Notify your supervising nurse if you learn that the catheter has come out.

❖ Empty the drainage bag and note the color and volume of the urine.

When emptying a urinary drainage bag, follow the specific procedure that is explained step by step in Skill 44 in the skills book.

Applying an external urinary catheter to a male. An external urinary catheter is used for many of the same reasons as an indwelling catheter. Used only for males, it consists of a condom-like device, tubing, and a drainage bag (Figure 13-8). The condom fits over the man's penis and is attached to tubing, which is attached to the drainage bag. The bag may be the same type as the indwelling catheter drainage bag, or it may be designed to be strapped to his calf or thigh. This smaller leg bag is useful to wear under pants. Because it is smaller, it must be emptied every 2 hours.

When applying an external urinary catheter, make sure the condom is completely unrolled so that it does not interfere with the person's circulation. Also, make sure the tubing does not get twisted at the tip of his penis. When attaching the condom catheter to the drainage bag, make sure the bag is lower than his bladder, but not touching the floor, for proper urine flow. When attaching the tubing to his calf or the top of his inner thigh, allow some extra tubing so that the catheter isn't pulled taut. Check the person frequently to make sure the condom isn't too tight and that circulation is good. If you notice any swelling or color change in his penis, remove the condom and report your observations to your supervising nurse.

Remove the catheter once each day for bathing and then apply a new catheter. After bathing or perineal care, make sure the person's penis is dry so that the tape will stick.

When applying an external urinary catheter, follow the specific procedure that is explained step by step in Skill 45 in the skills book.

Emptying a urinary drainage bag.   To measure output from a urinary drainage bag, release the clamp on the drainage bag and let the urine flow from the tube into the graduate (Figure 13-9). Never let the tip of the tube touch the graduate or your hands. When all the urine has emptied out of the bag, secure the clamp.

Record the amount collected in the graduate on the intake and output sheet. Also note any important observations, such as cloudy or foul-smelling urine, a change in the amount of urine, a change in the color of the urine, and any complaints of pain by the person. To learn more about measuring and recording urinary output, read the worksheet in the skills book.

* don't let your hands or tube or the graduate touch the graduate

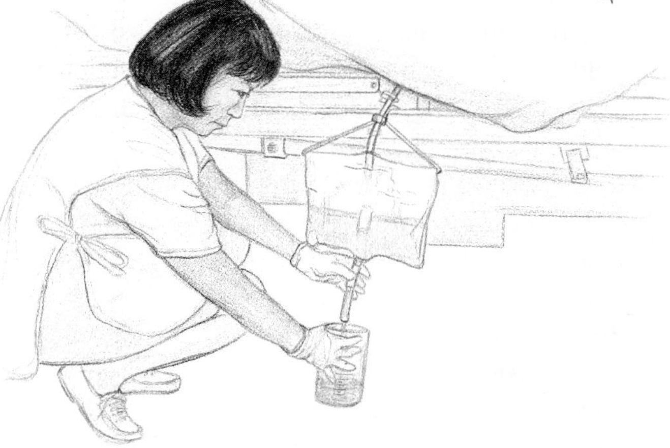

Figure 13-9
When emptying a urinary drainage bag, use good body mechanics and proper infection control techniques.

Collecting and Testing Urine Specimens

In addition to measuring and recording urinary output, you may collect urine when a doctor orders other laboratory tests. These tests, to be performed on a person's urine, help the doctor make decisions about his medical treatment. When you collect urine, you use one of three methods and, for people who have diabetes, you may actually perform one of the tests on the urine.

Collecting urine specimens.   Three methods of collecting urine specimens are routine urine collection, clean catch or midstream collection, and 24-hour collection. Each method is ordered by the doctor for a particular purpose, so use only the method ordered. Follow your supervising nurse's instructions for specimen collection. Also, observe the principles of infection control and wear disposable gloves.

❖   **Routine urine specimen collection.** A routine urine specimen is collected for lab tests or to test for sugar and acetone in the urine of a person with diabetes. This specimen can be collected while the person is using the bathroom toilet, portable commode (Figure 13-10), bedpan, or urinal by having him void

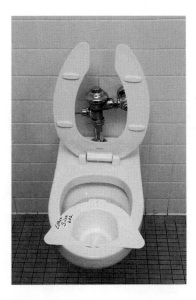

Figure 13-10
A urinary collection device, often called a "hat," is placed in a toilet or commode to collect and measure urine output.

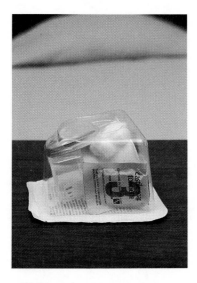

Figure 13-11
To collect a clean catch or midstream specimen of urine, gather the following supplies: a labeled sterile specimen container, cotton balls or gauze pads, and an antiseptic solution, such as povidone-iodine. Your employer may have all these supplies packaged in a container.

directly into a specimen container or into a collection device. The specimen can also be collected by emptying urine from a portable commode, bedpan, or urinal into a collection container.

❖ **Clean catch or midstream urine specimen collection.** A clean catch or midstream urine specimen is collected to determine if the person has an infection. The urine is analyzed for white blood cells and bacteria. Because the test is for bacteria, it is important that you do not touch and contaminate the inside of the container, because contamination would affect the results of the lab test.

This type of collection is called a "clean catch" because the opening of the urethra is cleaned before the person starts to void (Figure 13-11). The cleaning removes any bacteria that may be around the opening so that it is not confused in the lab with the bacteria that may be in the urine. This type of catch is also called a "midstream" collection because the person starts to void, then stops, then voids into the container. The initial flow of urine washes away additional bacteria around the urethral opening, giving the lab a more accurate specimen for the test. A clean catch urine specimen is often used to test for urinary tract infection. A clean catch specimen can be collected while the person is using the bathroom toilet, portable commode, bedpan, or urinal.

❖ **24-hour urine specimen collection.** A 24-hour urine specimen is collected over 24 consecutive hours (Figure 13-12). The specimen is used to check for particular things in the urine. For example, a person with kidney problems may have to provide urine over a 24-hour period so that the doctor can ask the lab to check for protein in the urine. Too much protein present in the urine shows that the kidneys aren't working properly.

When you begin the collection, label and store the container according to your employer's policy.

A 24-hour urine specimen can be collected like a routine urine specimen while the person is using the bathroom toilet, portable commode, bedpan, or urinal.

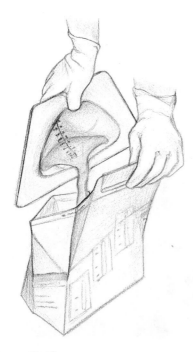

Figure 13-12
When a person is on a 24-hour urine collection, be sure to collect the urine each time the person voids.

Collecting urine specimens for people in isolation. For people in isolation, take special precautions when collecting urine specimens. After putting on appropriate protective clothing, go into the person's room and place the labeled specimen container on a clean paper towel. Remove the lid of the container and place it on the paper towel. Collect the urine specimen and transfer the urine from the collection container into the specimen container, taking care not to touch the outside of the specimen container or spill any urine on the outside of the specimen container. Use a clean paper towel to replace the lid on the specimen container. When you have finished the procedure, remove your protective clothing and dispose of it properly. Take the specimen container outside the isolation room and double-bag it according to the techniques indicated for the person's type of isolation. Put the specimen container in a designated area at the nurses' station, in the refrigerator, or on a special tray, and wash your hands.

When collecting urine specimens, follow the specific procedure that is explained step by step in Skill 46 in the skills book.

Testing urine specimens for sugar and acetone.   Although there is not yet a cure for diabetes, it can be controlled through diet, exercise, and medication therapy. To maintain the proper balance among these controls, it is important to know how much glucose, or sugar, is in the blood of the person with diabetes or how much sugar and acetone are in his urine. Testing blood for glucose is the most common method for keeping track of the condition of someone with diabetes, but urine is still tested for sugar and acetone. It is very important that you report your sugar and acetone findings to your supervising nurse, because the person's diet and insulin may have to be changed, depending on urine sugar and acetone results.

The doctor orders a test for sugar and acetone and specifies in the person's care plan what time of day to do the test, as well as how often to do the test. Three different ways of testing urine for sugar and acetone are with Clinitest, TES-TAPE, and Keto-Diastix (Figure 13-13).

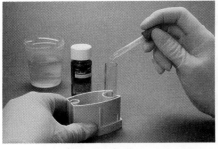

Clinitest

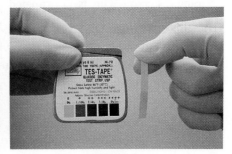

TES-TAPE

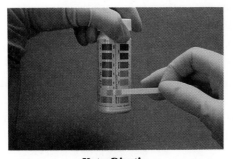

Keto-Diastix

Figure 13-13
These products are used for testing the urine of people who have diabetes to determine the amounts of sugar and acetone in their urine.

When testing urine for sugar and acetone, follow the specific procedure that is explained step by step in Skill 47 in the skills book.

Special Bowel Elimination Needs

Because Mr. Rivera's stroke resulted in loss of feeling, he does not feel the urge to have a bowel movement, and, as a result, is often incontinent of stool, or feces. You have learned his bowel elimination pattern and are alert to when he normally has a bowel movement. Every other day, just after lunch, you ask him if you may help him to the bathroom or bring him the bedpan. He usually complains and says he doesn't have to go, but after you convince him to at least try, he admits that you were right.

Some people need assistance with special bowel elimination needs. As a nurse assistant, you play a key role in identifying potential bowel elimination problems by observing and reporting changes in elimination patterns. For example, you would alert your supervising nurse if someone in your care usually has a bowel movement every day after lunch and then doesn't have one for 3 days.

Because of problems with the digestive system, people sometimes suffer from constipation, fecal impaction, diarrhea, or bowel incontinence, which are the most common bowel elimination problems. Also, because of these conditions and other health problems, some people need to have stool specimens collected and tested. When you respond to people who have special bowel elimination needs, it is important for you to remember that the people in your care cannot meet their own needs. They rely on you to help them and to offer support and encouragement.

Helping a Person Who Is Constipated

The difficult elimination of a hard, dry stool is called constipation. It occurs when stool moves too slowly through the intestine and too much water is absorbed by the intestine. The following factors contribute to constipation:

❖ Not drinking enough fluid
❖ Ignoring the urge to eliminate
❖ Not exercising enough
❖ Changing the diet
❖ Aging
❖ Having certain diseases
❖ Taking some types of medication

A person who is constipated probably feels uncomfortable and may be irritable. He may complain that his abdomen feels hard. When he tries to move his bowels, he may feel pain, which is due to straining to get the hard stool to move through the rectum and out the anus.

When a person in your care is constipated, offer him fluids frequently and encourage him to eat high-fiber foods. Also encourage him to get more exercise and help him take more walks. In addition, help him maintain normal elimination patterns and report any changes to your supervising nurse. It may be necessary for the person to receive medication or an **enema** to help relieve constipation.

Bowel habits

enema
(EN-uh-muh) A solution introduced into the rectum and lower colon to relieve fecal impaction or constipation.

As a nurse assistant, you may or may not be permitted to give someone an enema. When giving someone an enema, follow the specific
procedures that are explained step by step in Skills 48 and 49 in the
skills book.

Helping a Person Who Has Fecal Impaction

A more serious form of constipation is fecal impaction, a hard stool
that remains in the rectum. It occurs when feces become too hard
and too large to pass through the anus (Figure 13-14).

A person with fecal impaction may have pain, discomfort, and abdominal swelling. He also could have a mucus and water discharge
that looks like diarrhea, which occurs because liquid stool is oozing
around the hard stool.

The nurse sometimes provides treatment for fecal impaction by
manually removing stool. The manual removal of stool is called dis-
impaction. Sometimes fecal impaction is treated with an enema,
which the doctor orders and the nurse or nurse assistant gives to the
person with a fecal impaction.

Helping a Person Who Has Diarrhea

When Josie had diarrhea, you reported this condition to your supervising nurse, because diarrhea usually indicates that something is
wrong. Diarrhea may be caused by a bacterial or viral infection, food
allergies, or poor nutritional habits. A person with diarrhea usually
has frequent, watery stools, sometimes accompanied by cramping.
She probably feels weak, tired, frustrated, embarrassed by the smell,
and sore because of the irritation of the anus. Continued diarrhea
can cause a serious fluid loss called dehydration. For example, a
person with HIV infection or AIDS may become dehydrated due to
frequent bouts of diarrhea. The diarrhea may be the result of opportunistic bowel infections or problems associated with tube feedings
and is one of the most difficult complications of HIV/AIDS. Read
again the information about dehydration in Chapter 12.

Sometimes a doctor prescribes no medical treatment for diarrhea
but just lets it run its course. Other times a doctor may prescribe a
clear liquid diet and a medication. Because Josie is so frail and cannot risk becoming dehydrated, the doctor prescribes medication for
her diarrhea.

As a nurse assistant, you can help the person who has diarrhea if
you understand the discomfort associated with it. Respond immediately to her call signal, place a portable commode by her bedside,
offer clear liquids, provide good skin care, and suggest more rest
time. Keep her and her environment very clean. Make her room
more pleasant by using a room deodorizer to mask unpleasant odors
and by increasing air circulation with a fan or open window.

When providing care for a person with HIV/AIDS, encourage the
person not to eat foods, such as spicy and greasy dishes, that may
irritate the bowel. Encourage her to drink fluids, such as juice, bouil-
lon, or commercial products that contain vital substances that are lost
as a result of having diarrhea (Gatorade, for example).

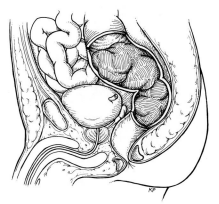

Figure 13-14
Fecal impaction is very painful. To
reduce the possibility of fecal
impaction, help the person in your care
maintain normal elimination patterns
and, when instructed, treat constipation.

Report any occurrence of diarrhea to your supervising nurse. The very young and the elderly are especially susceptible to becoming dehydrated quickly from diarrhea. Also, because diarrhea can be contagious, pay special attention to the principles of infection control when helping a person who has diarrhea. Make sure the person understands and practices good personal hygiene, especially handwashing, as she cares for her own needs.

Helping a Person Who Has Bowel Incontinence

Loss of control of the bowels, like loss of control of the bladder, is called incontinence. The following factors can lead to bowel incontinence:

❖ Damage to the brain that keeps the individual from feeling the urge to have a bowel movement
❖ Weakness of the anal sphincter muscle
❖ Medications
❖ Confusion about where to go to the bathroom
❖ Limited mobility that makes it hard to get to the bathroom
❖ Not having a call signal answered immediately
❖ Diarrhea
❖ Fecal impaction (liquid feces leak out from around the hard, impacted mass of feces)
❖ Presence of HIV infection and AIDS

Note that many of these factors are similar to those that lead to urinary incontinence.

To help support a person who has bowel incontinence,—

❖ Respond quickly to his elimination needs.
❖ Offer him fluids frequently throughout the day. Increasing fluid intake decreases the problem of incontinence and may prevent stool from hardening and becoming impacted.
❖ Encourage a high-fiber diet.
❖ If he has trouble rising or walking, help him get to the bathroom.
❖ Offer him frequent opportunities to go to the bathroom, particularly if he is confused. Give him sufficient time and provide privacy.
❖ Learn his pattern of bowel elimination to determine how often you should offer assistance. For example, one person's regular pattern may be daily. Another person's regular pattern may be every 2 to 3 days.
❖ Treat each person based on his individual needs.
❖ Be sensitive to the embarrassment a person may feel about being incontinent.
❖ If the person wears adult briefs, change them as soon as they become soiled to minimize skin breakdown.
❖ Perform perineal care as often as the person needs it, especially for people who have diarrhea as a result of HIV infection and AIDS.

❖ Offer emotional support and encouragement.

❖ Help with a bowel training program. A doctor may sometimes recommend that a person participate in a bowel training program to help regain control of his bowel movements. As with a bladder training program, the schedule for the program is written on the care plan. In addition to the steps above, you can help support the person in his bowel training program by taking him to the toilet on the regular schedule set up by the program.

Collecting Stool Specimens

A doctor orders a stool specimen to be collected when laboratory tests have to be run. The doctor uses the results of these tests to make decisions about a person's medical needs. Your responsibility is to collect the stool specimen. A stool specimen can be collected when the person uses the bathroom toilet, portable commode, or bedpan.

Check with your supervising nurse to see if she has specific instructions regarding the collection or handling of the stool specimen. Observe the principles of infection control and wear disposable gloves. Before collecting the stool specimen, have the person void first to avoid getting urine into the stool specimen.

When collecting stool specimens, follow the specific procedure that is explained step by step in Skill 50 in the skills book.

To learn about providing care for children's elimination needs in hospitals and home health care, please read the next section. Otherwise, turn to the end of this chapter to read "Information Review" and "Questions to Ask Yourself."

Providing Care for Children's Elimination Needs

When you work in a hospital or in home health care, you often provide care for children. You help infants and toddlers with special elimination needs, such as diapering, and use a different procedure to collect urine specimens.

Diapering

When you go the Clark's apartment today, one of the first things you notice is that Dominic's overalls are wet and that he needs to have his diaper changed. Ms. Clark is so frustrated because she cannot chase after her active child to try to get him to hold still while she changes his diaper. Her neighbor usually comes over to help her, but this morning her neighbor has a doctor's appointment.

Before changing his diaper, you gather together all the things you will need: clean disposable diaper, wipes, plastic trash bag, laundry bag, lotion, and clean overalls. You also get a couple of toys for him to hold and play with while you change him. As you are changing him, you talk to him about what you are doing and sing him a little song, which makes him laugh.

When providing care for a child, always stay with him. Never leave

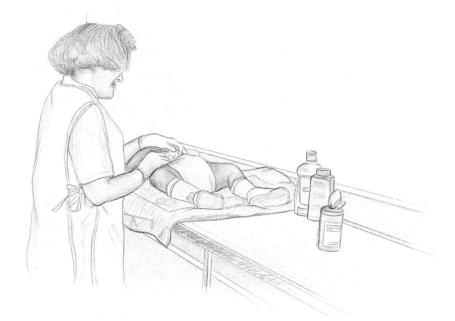

Figure 13-15
When diapering a child, always keep one hand on him. A child can twist and turn very quickly, even if he hasn't yet learned how to roll over.

him unattended. For example, when diapering a child, make sure all the supplies you need are within reach so that you do not have to turn your back or walk away from him (Figure 13-15).

If you are using disposable diapers, lay the diaper with absorbent side up and the closure tabs at the back.

If you are using pins to fasten cloth diapers, place the pins in a place where the child cannot reach them. Place the thick part of the diaper toward the back for a girl and toward the front for a boy. When you fasten the diaper, place your fingers between the diaper and the baby to help guide the pin through the cloth. Also, make sure you have allowed enough room by checking to see if two of your fingers can fit between the child's abdomen and the diaper.

Use diapering time as an opportunity to talk and play with the child, making it a fun time. After completing the procedure, report any rashes from the diaper area or any liquid stools to your supervising nurse.

When diapering a child, follow the specific procedure that is explained step by step in Skill 51 in the skills book.

Collecting a Urine Specimen from an Infant

Obtaining a urine specimen from an infant, or a child who is not toilet trained, requires applying a special self-adhesive collection bag, called a pediatric urine collection bag, to the infant's perineal area or over the infant's penis. First provide perineal care, cleaning from front to back in girls and from the urethra outward in boys.

To apply the collection bag, position the infant on his or her back and spread the knees apart, exposing the genitals. If the child is very active, you may have to ask a co-worker or the child's parent to help hold the child. For a boy, position the penis through the opening at the top of the bag and press the adhesive securely around the base of the penis and the scrotum, taking care not to cover the anus. For a girl, position the bag over the urethra and press the adhesive area over the labia to create a seal, taking care not to cover the anus.

Reapply the diaper over the collection bag. If the infant is young enough so that he cannot pull off the bag, cut a slit in the disposable diaper before reapplying the diaper and pull the bag through the slit so that you can see when the infant has voided. Check every 15 minutes to see if the infant has urinated (Figure 13-16).

To remove the bag, loosen the adhesive and gently remove the bag. Seal the top by folding the adhesive area over and placing it in the sterile specimen container. Do not leave the infant unattended to do this. Instead, set the specimen bag down on the crib, and put the collection bag in the specimen container later. Some pediatric urine collection bags have a port, or opening at the bottom of the bag to empty the urine into the container.

Record that you have collected the specimen and report any important observations, such as cloudy or foul-smelling urine or blood in the urine.

When collecting urine from an infant, follow the specific procedure that is explained step by step in Skill 52 in the skills book.

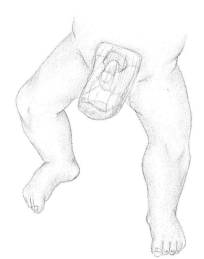

Figure 13-16
To collect urine from a small child, place a collection bag over the urethral opening for a short period of time. Observe the child frequently until you obtain the specimen.

Information Review

Circle the correct answers and fill in the blanks.

1. ____Drinking fluid_____ aids elimination by diluting the urine and keeping the stool soft.

2. Learn about the person's elimination pattern by asking him or a family member, or by checking his ____CARE_____

   _____PLAN_____ to find out when and how often he urinates or has a bowel movement and if there is anything special about his elimination habits.

3. Incontinence is—
   a. The inability to control the release of urine.
   b. The inability to control the release of feces.
   c. The inability to control the release of urine, feces, and perspiration.
   d. The inability to control the release of urine or feces.

4. A portable commode is—
   a. A bedpan.
   b. A special toilet seat.
   c. A chair with a toilet seat and a container to collect waste.
   d. A collection container to put into a standard bathroom toilet.

5. When a person is sitting on a bedpan, it is important to help him into a position that best resembles sitting on a

   _____toilet_____ and to check on him every

   _____5_____ minutes.

6. Burning on urination, frequent but scanty urination, cloudy or dark-colored urine, or milky mucus threads in the urine are signs of urinary _infection_ _____.

7. When a person in your care has a urinary catheter, prevent infection by providing _perineal_ care on a regular schedule and whenever the person is soiled with secretions or feces.

8. An external catheter should be removed—
    a. Once daily.
    b. Only when the adhesive loosens and the catheter is ready to fall off.
    c. Twice daily.
    d. Every other day.

9. When testing a person's urine for sugar and acetone, check his _CARE_ _PLAN_ to find out when and how often to do the test.

10. Symptoms of fecal impaction include—
    a. Abdominal pain and a diarrhea-like discharge from the anus.
    b. Burning on urination and an increased frequency to void.
    c. Passage of hard dry stool and blood in the urine.
    d. Excessive thirst and nausea.

Children's Elimination Needs

1. When diapering a child, which one thing would you *not* do?
    a. Give him a toy to play with
    b. Leave him for just a second to get supplies
    c. Talk and sing to him
    d. Keep one hand on him at all times

2. To obtain a urine specimen from a child who is not toilet trained,—
    a. Apply an external catheter.
    b. Use a bedpan.
    c. Apply a self-adhesive collection bag.
    d. Use a hat.

Questions to Ask Yourself

1. When assisting a person onto the toilet or portable commode, how would you use good body mechanics?

2. How can you make someone feel safe and secure when you leave him alone to eliminate in private?

3. How can you make a person feel respected when you help him with elimination?

4. What can you do to help a person become more independent about his elimination needs?

5. What can you do to show your professionalism when you assist with elimination?

6. During one of Shirley McDay's incontinent times, you follow the care plan and put adult briefs on her. She begins to cry and says she doesn't want to be treated like a baby. What should you do?

7. You have helped Josie onto the portable commode. While you are waiting outside the curtain for her to signal that she is finished, her roommate asks you to help her get back into bed. What should you do?

8. Mr. Smith is expecting company. He is sitting in a wheelchair with his urinary collection bag hanging on the side. What can you do to enhance his self-esteem and protect his dignity and privacy?

9. What is different about collecting a urine specimen from Mrs. Wang, who is in isolation, and collecting a urine specimen from someone who isn't in isolation?

10. You are changing Dominic's diaper when Ms. Clark calls for you from the living room. What should you do?

14

Providing Restorative Care

Goals

After reading this chapter, you will have the information to—

Promote independence, self-care, and good health habits.

Help a person be active.

Provide care for a person with hearing problems.

Provide care for a person with vision problems.

After practicing the corresponding skills in the skills book, you will be able to—

Help a person with passive range-of-motion exercises.

Help a person walk.

A   young man came to a master craftman's shop, lugging behind him an old, water-marked chest of drawers. He leaned it up against the wall because it had a broken foot and could not stand well on its own. The chest was crafted from a beautiful piece of oak, but years ago it had been ruined in a flood. It also bore the marks of a fall, as it had a deep gouge in its left side. The five drawers either stuck or fell open. Three of them were each missing a drawer pull. "Please, sir," he asked the master craftsman, "Could you possibly fix up this old chest? It was mine when I was a child, and now I would like to give it to my new-born son." The master craftsman grumbled and shook his head at the damaged piece of furniture and told the young man to come back in 2 weeks.

Later, when the young man returned to the shop, he could hear the sounds of the master craftsman gently sanding and rubbing in the back room. While he waited for the craftsman to come to the front of the shop, the young man looked around anxiously for his old chest of drawers. He hoped the craftsman had been able to repair the foot and fill in the gouge. He wondered if he had been able to replace the drawer pulls. Soon he was filled with anxiety. He did not see his chest anywhere. Perhaps the master craftsman had not had time to work on it. Perhaps it was too worn and old to be fixed.

Just then the master craftsman came into the front room and said, "Well, young man, what do you think of it?"

"Of what?" asked the young man.

"Of your chest of drawers, of course," said the craftsman, pointing to a beautiful, shining, smooth chest of drawers that stood proudly on its own feet in the center of the shop.

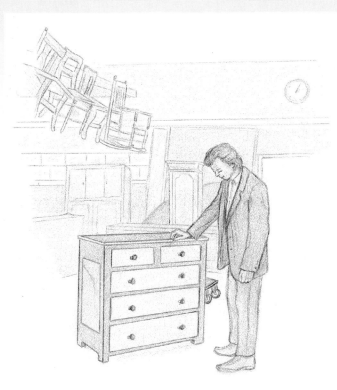

The young man could not believe his eyes. "This is it?" he stammered. "I can't believe it." He could see ever so slightly where the gouge had been. The drawer pulls were not an exact match, and one of the drawers still stuck a little when he opened it. But the rough edges had been smoothed, and the old dirt had been rubbed out with oil to make the inner color of the wood shine with a rich luster. "I was afraid that you couldn't fix it," he finally said.

"I didn't fix it," said the old man, with the same dignity that the chest now wore. "I restored it."

The Art of Restoring

The master craftsman saw his task not as fixing, but as restoring. As a nurse assistant, your work is similar. You do not merely patch up people and keep changing their bandages. Instead, you help people find their inner strength, stand on their own again, and find dignity in their lives, even though they are not like new. This kind of caregiving is called restorative care. When you provide restorative care, your goal is to help a person become as fully functional as possible and to help her be able to enjoy her life.

When to Provide Restorative Care

Restorative care is part of basic nursing care that you apply every day as you perform your other duties. It is the extra effort that you give to help a person reach her highest level of wellness. When you follow the doctor's or supervising nurse's orders for the amount and type of restorative care for each person, you can prevent disabilities and promote self-esteem, independence, and dignity in each person.

When a person functions as well as possible in all areas of life, she has reached her best overall health. By encouraging her to do as much for herself as possible, you help increase her self-esteem and sense of purpose.

How to Respond to the Person's Needs

When providing restorative care, also called rehabilitation nursing, you use rehabilitation techniques and procedures. In addition to monitoring the person's vital signs and using good body mechanics, you promote her independence in daily living and emphasize communicating with her. You also enable a person to enjoy life more fully. Enable is an important word in restorative care. Enabling a person gives her the power to do something (Figure 14-1). How do you give a person such power? If you apply the following principles of rehabilitation, you enable a person to stand on her own, just like the chest of drawers, in less than perfect condition, but shining and full of dignity.

As a nurse assistant, you enable a person when you—

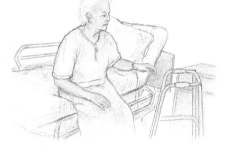

Figure 14-1
Mrs. Garcia can get out of bed more independently if her walker is placed where she can reach it. This enables her to go to the bathroom or visit with others when she wants to, instead of having to call for assistance.

atrophy
(AH-tro-fee)   A condition in which a part of the body, such as the leg muscles, wastes away or shrinks due to disuse or inadequate nutrition.

❖ Emphasize her abilities rather than her disabilities. Recognize what she can do for herself and encourage her to do it.
❖ Begin her rehabilitation program early, according to the doctor's and supervising nurse's orders. Decreasing the amount of time she spends in bed prevents complications such as pressure sores; urinary tract infections; muscle weakness, tightening, and shortening; **atrophy**/disuse syndrome; and respiratory infections.
❖ Keep her active by helping with exercise whenever possible, because activity strengthens and inactivity weakens.
❖ Treat the whole person, not just the affected part of her body. Consider her emotional, social, spiritual, vocational, and physical being. Assist with developing her care plan and make sure that it meets her specific needs.

Promoting a Healthy Lifestyle

Views on being healthy have changed during this century. People once believed that being healthy was a matter of luck. After the discovery of antibiotics and vaccines, people believed that taking these medicines was the way to control disease and illness.

Today, evidence shows that many diseases are caused by unhealthy habits, like smoking cigarettes or eating fatty foods. Many things that affect health can be controlled. As a caregiver, you can help a person reach his best overall health by encouraging him to adopt good health and lifestyle practices. You encourage him by promoting independence, self-care, and good health habits; teaching important skills to help him gain independence; and measuring his progress in the areas of independence and self-care.

Promoting Independence, Self-Care, and Good Health Habits

Because the process of restorative care requires the help of all the health care team members, many people are involved in helping the person in your care become more independent and healthier. The physical therapist and occupational therapist may be key players. A speech therapist, dietitian, or other health care worker also may play active roles. All health care team members depend on you to report how the person progresses with activities. As a nurse assistant, you have many opportunities to encourage the person to take control of his life and health.

Independence.   When you help a person do things for himself to gain independence, your goal is to teach, retrain, motivate, and encourage him to do as much as he is physically and mentally able to do by himself.

How can you promote independence in a person? In the following scenario, notice what the nurse assistant does to promote independence in Mr. Lightfoot.

Mr. Lightfoot has breathing difficulties and gets tired even when dressing. Although he moves very slowly, he likes to choose his clothes and dress himself as much as possible. Today, he selects a warm turtleneck sweater.

The nurse assistant has six other people to help with dressing. He thinks he does not have time to stand by waiting for Mr. Lightfoot to put on the turtleneck. However, knowing how much it means to him to dress himself, the nurse assistant holds up the sweater for him. Then he asks him to draw it down over his head while he begins to make the bed. As he does his bedmaking tasks, he talks to Mr. Lightfoot about his son. He also notices that Mr. Lightfoot becomes tired while pulling down the body of the shirt (Figure 14-2).

The nurse assistant praises Mr. Lightfoot for completing the difficult task of putting on his sweater this far and asks him if he would like help to finish the task. He says that he would, and the nurse assistant finishes pulling down the shirt and straightens the sleeves. He lets him rest a minute as he finishes the bed, and then helps him with the rest of his clothes.

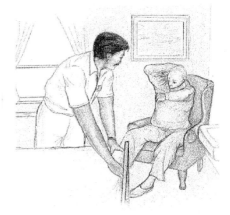

Figure 14-2
The nurse assistant encourages Mr. Lightfoot to do all that he can for himself. He also notices when Mr. Lightfoot gets tired and needs assistance.

What did the nurse assistant do to promote independence for Mr. Lightfoot?

* ❖ While giving care, he paid attention to the whole person—mind, body, and spirit. He understood how much it meant to Mr. Lightfoot to do things for himself. Because Mr. Lightfoot felt physically able to take care of himself, it was important to encourage him to do it.
* ❖ The nurse assistant explained to Mr. Lightfoot what he would do *for* him and *with* him.
* ❖ He encouraged and praised him for even his smallest successes.
* ❖ He focused on Mr. Lightfoot's abilities, not his disabilities.
* ❖ He was patient.

Self-care through personal care.   A person who is encouraged to help provide his personal care feels positive about becoming independent and improving his appearance. A person may need to use self-help devices to maintain his independence. The most commonly used personal care items are—

* ❖ A built-up handle toothbrush, which makes it easier for a person to grasp when brushing his teeth (Figure 14-3).
* ❖ A long-handled device with a hook on the end, which helps a person take off his shoes (Figure 14-4).
* ❖ A zipper pull, which attaches to a person's zipper, making it easier to grasp when she zips and unzips her clothes by herself (Figure 14-5).
* ❖ A long-handled shoe horn, which enables a person to put on his shoes (Figure 14-6).
* ❖ A washcloth with self-fastening fabric, which enables a person to hold onto the mitt while washing or bathing himself (Figure 14-7).
* ❖ A sock aid, which helps a person with weak hands and a limited range of motion to put on socks (Figure 14-8).
* ❖ A grabbing device (long-handled scissors-like device) that helps a person pick up things (Figure 14-9).

By encouraging people to use these self-help devices, you help them increase their independence. People who think they are becoming self-sufficient feel better about themselves, have improved energy levels, and are happier, because they believe their lives are more productive.

You may feel frustrated when it takes more time for a person to do something using a self-help device than it does when you provide the care. It is important to be patient because, as a person becomes more self-sufficient, the time he needs to do a task decreases. Both you and the person should feel very proud of your hard work and accomplishments.

Good health habits.   A person is never too young or too old to adopt good health habits. Everyone, including you and the people in your

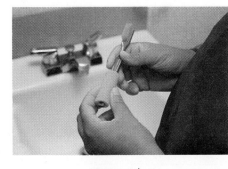

Figure 14-3

Figure 14-3
An inexpensive way to build up the handle of a toothbrush is to put a foam curler around the handle. This makes the handle larger and provides a non-slip surface.

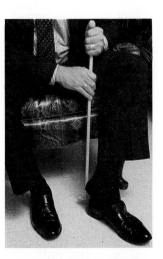

Figure 14-4

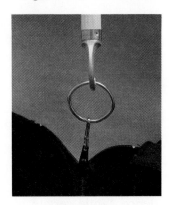

Figure 14-5

Figure 14-4
A person who has difficulty bending over can use this device to help remove shoes.

Figure 14-5
A person who can't grasp small items can attach a zipper pull to a zipper. She can then fasten the zipper by pulling on the zipper pull.

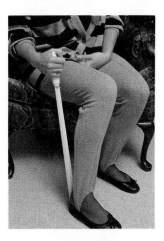

Figure 14-6

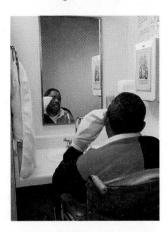

Figure 14-7

Figure 14-6
A person who is confined to a wheelchair or who has difficulty bending over can use a long-handled shoe horn to help put on shoes.

Figure 14-7
A mitt makes it easier for a person who doesn't have good control of his hands to wash by himself.

Figure 14-8
Using a sock aid helps people who have trouble bending over or have hand problems to put on socks.

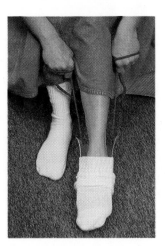

Figure 14-8

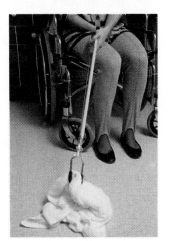

Figure 14-9

Figure 14-9
A person in a wheelchair or someone who can't bend over can use a grabbing device to pick up things from the floor or reach light items on shelves.

Box 14-1   How to Maintain Good Health Habits

❖ Eat a well-balanced diet.	❖ Visit with family and friends.
❖ Exercise regularly.	❖ Do rewarding activities.
❖ Do not smoke.	❖ Talk about your feelings.
❖ Get yearly check-ups from a doctor.	❖ Follow safety rules.
❖ Receive routine dental care.	❖ Wear a seat belt.
❖ Examine your breasts or testicles regularly.	❖ Use a car seat for young children.
❖ Make time for daily relaxation.	

care, can benefit from making healthy lifestyle choices. What good health habits can you suggest to the people in your care? You can suggest that they gain control of their own well-being by following the ideas in Box 14-1.

Teaching Independence Skills

Some people need to learn new ways to do old things so that they can do as much for themselves as possible. For example, Mrs. Garcia needed to learn how to walk with a walker to maintain her independence. While certain members of the health care team may begin to teach or retrain a person, the nurse assistant is often asked to continue or reinforce the teaching.

In Chapter 5, Communicating with People, you read about effective teaching techniques. The same principles apply to helping a person learn how to maintain his independence.

❖ Explain the task you want a person in your care to complete. Use short, concise statements.
❖ Give clear instructions.
❖ Ask the person to repeat your instructions. (This feedback lets you know if she understands.)
❖ Repeat the instructions, if necessary.
❖ Give an example, if necessary.
❖ Demonstrate the procedure.
❖ Explain why the activity is important.
❖ Ask the person if she has any questions.
❖ Have patience. Progress may be slow, but if you become impatient, there may be no progress.

prompting
Using a simple statement to help someone remember.

In addition, use a method called **prompting** to reinforce something that has been taught. It is a way of reminding a person of what to do without actually telling her. For example: Mrs. Garcia is about to stand up by herself and use her walker. Her walker is to the left of where she is going to stand, not right in front of her. By asking Mrs. Garcia if her walker is where she wants it, you remind her that it is not in the right place. If a person hesitates to do something you know she can do, it is better to prompt her than to do it for her.

Or, when a person who is doing a task gives you a questioning look, do not assume she has forgotten what to do. She may be worried about doing the task wrong in front of you. Help by asking, "What do you think you should do next?" The person may tell you and then go on with the task. If necessary, tell her what step should come next, but encourage her to do the task independently.

Measuring Progress

Rehabilitation can be a long, slow process. A key part of your job is observing even the smallest changes and improvements. Telling the person in your care about her progress encourages her to continue (Figure 14-10). Use your senses when observing a person for positive changes. What you observe depends on the goal of the restorative nursing care plan. You may have to watch to see how far a person walks, how well she eats, or how far she can bend a joint. Listen to the person's descriptions of how much effort it took to do the task, or touch the person's skin to see if it is warm, cool, moist, or dry. Her skin can provide a clue about how much effort she exerted. For example, if she exerted a great deal of effort, her skin may be warm and moist.

Keeping track of small successes is important. If you say, "Mr. Lightfoot, you were able to do all but the sleeves on your turtleneck today, and last week you could only get it over your head before getting tired," he will probably want to try to pull on the entire turtleneck by next week. Your expressed observations encourage him to try harder.

Always remember to record your observations about the progress of the person in your care. This information helps the other health care team members.

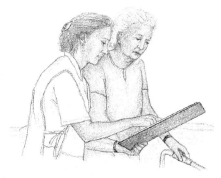

Figure 14-10
When she first entered the nursing home, Mrs. Garcia was a little depressed about the amount of progress she made while learning to walk better with her walker. The chart helps her keep track of her walking distance. Even though some days are not as good as others, Mrs. Garcia knows she is making steady progress.

Promoting Activity

Activity helps people attain or regain independence. Have you ever heard the expression, "Use it or lose it"? This condition really can happen. Many physical problems occur when people do not get enough exercise (Box 14-2). Their muscles become weak, flabby, and tired. Their joints and muscles may atrophy, causing their joints to become permanently contracted or bent. People may become **immobile** if muscles and joints aren't used.

Lack of exercise also can cause problems in almost all the other body systems. For example, a person may become constipated when the movement of the intestines slows down or may develop pneumonia from secretions that pool in the lungs. When circulation slows

immobile
(im-MOW-bul)   Unable to move.

Box 14-2   **Physical Problems Resulting from Inactivity**

❖ Decubitus ulcers	❖ Blood clots
❖ Constipation	❖ Pneumonia
❖ Contractures	❖ Osteoporosis
❖ Atrophy	❖ Decreased sense of well-being and independence

down, a person may develop dangerous blood clots. Without exercise, bones lose minerals and become brittle, making it easy for them to break. Even the immobile person who cannot move on his own needs to be active.

People feel better physically and emotionally when they exercise. Without exercise, people may feel depressed, angry, helpless, and lonely. To help a person reach his highest capabilities, you must encourage and guide him to exercise. As a person exercises, he starts feeling better.

ambulation
(am-byoo-LAY-shun)   The medical term for walking.

As a nurse assistant, you help a person stay active and mobile with range-of-motion exercises and **ambulation**. The medical abbreviation for range of motion is ROM. Range of motion is the amount of movement possible in a joint such as the elbow, knee, or hip. It is also how far a person can move a joint comfortably. For example, one person may be able to bend his elbow and touch his shoulder with his hand and another person may only be able to bend his elbow an inch or two.

For the person in your care to get the most benefit, he needs to do each kind of exercise regularly. For example, you may help a person do range-of-motion exercises three times a day and help him walk four times a day. This regular exercise helps keep the person's muscles, joints, and other body systems working.

Helping a Person with Range of Motion

The range of motion a person has can change within a day and from day to day. For example, a woman who has arthritis may not have much range of motion in the early morning because her muscles are stiff. But in the late morning, after her bath, she may have more range of motion or mobility in her joints.

Range-of-motion exercises can be active, which means the person moves his joints. They also can be passive, which means another person moves the person's joints for him. You may be asked to help teach family members how to do passive range-of-motion exercises.

contracture
(kun-TRACK-tyur)   A condition in which unused muscles cause a person's joints to become permanently bent.

Passive range-of-motion exercises are important for people who cannot move much on their own. If you do not move the person's joints, his muscles shorten, which may cause the joints to become permanently bent. This condition is called a **contracture**. Bend your wrist so that your palm moves toward the inside of your arm. This bending is the position of a common contracture. Imagine what it would be like to try to eat, dress, and go to the bathroom with your hands and arms bent in this position.

When helping someone with passive range-of-motion exercises, follow the specific procedure that is explained step by step in Skill 53 in the skills book. When you do passive range-of-motion exercises, begin at the top of the person's body and work your way down. Exercise seven sets of joints each time you do the exercises. Do all seven sets of joints on one side of the person's body, and then move to the other side and start at the top again. Figure 14-11 shows the number of exercises for each set of joints.

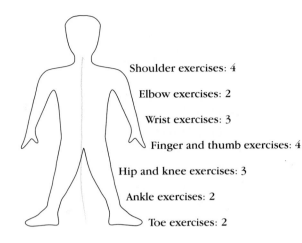

Shoulder exercises: 4

Elbow exercises: 2

Wrist exercises: 3

Finger and thumb exercises: 4

Hip and knee exercises: 3

Ankle exercises: 2

Toe exercises: 2

Figure 14-11
Do a specific number of passive range-of-motion exercises for each of the seven sets of joints.

Helping a Person Walk

Walking is good exercise. Because of a disability, someone may need to use a device that helps her walk, such as a walker, cane, or crutches. Using such a device helps give the person a way to exercise independently. The physical therapist or nurse teaches the person how to use the device, and you reinforce what she learns. A person in your care may need your assistance because she is learning how to use a device or because she may be unsteady when walking with a device (Figure 14-12). When a person is dizzy, sweaty, in pain, or short of breath, encourage her to sit down and rest. When helping someone walk, follow the specific procedure that is explained step by step in Skill 54 in the skills book. If a person begins to fall, help that person by following the specific procedure that also is explained in Skill 54.

When a person has an IV or catheter, make sure this equipment is cared for properly so that treatment is not disrupted and the person is not harmed as you help her walk. Make sure an IV bag or bottle is always higher than the IV entry site. Also make sure a urinary catheter bag and tubing are always lower than the person's bladder. Find out how the physical therapist taught the person to use the device to help her walk. Make sure the person's shoes or slippers fit well and have nonskid soles. Encourage her never to walk barefoot. Help her put on her footwear, if necessary.

Helping a person walk with a walker.   A person uses a walker when she needs support on both sides. When a person uses a walker, make sure the rubber tips are in good condition. The height of the walker should be at about the same height as the person's hip bones (Figure 14-13).

The person in your care may use one of the following three kinds of walkers:

❖   **Pick-up walker**. A person who is unsteady on her feet, but does not need to lean heavily, uses this type of walker. She can pick up the walker when she doesn't need to lean on it.

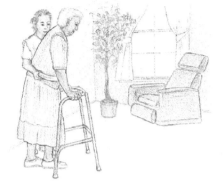

Figure 14-12
A chair placed in the hallway gives Mrs. Garcia a place to sit down and rest if she becomes tired.

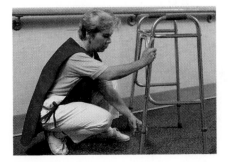

Figure 14-13
Many walkers have adjustable legs so that a walker can be fitted to a person's height.

❖ **Four-wheeled walker**. A person who needs constant support when walking uses this type of walker.

❖ **Semi-wheeled walker**. A person who lacks strength and endurance uses this type of walker, which has two front wheels and two back feet. The person can stop and lean on the walker. When she thinks she is ready, she can pick up the back feet of the walker and roll it forward on the wheels.

Helping a person walk with a cane. A person uses a walking cane when he needs support on one side but is able to walk without much difficulty. When a person uses a cane, make sure the rubber tips are in good condition. Put the cane near the person's stronger hand. Ask him to put his hand on the cane handle. Be certain that when the cane is at his side, the top of it is even with his hip bone and the bottom is 6 inches from his foot. Walk on the person's weaker side and help him, if necessary.

Three kinds of walking canes are pictured in Figure 14-14.

Figure 14-14
Three types of walking canes are single tip, tripod (with three legs), and quad (with four legs).

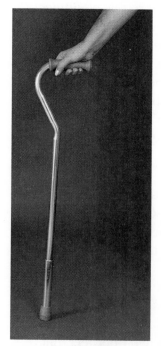
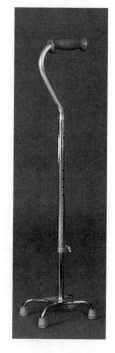

Single-tip   **Tripod**   **Quad**

// **Helping a person walk with crutches.**   A person uses crutches when he cannot use one leg or when both legs are weak and need support. The nurse or physical therapist adjusts the crutches to the proper height for the person (Figure 14-15). The person should not lean on a crutch with his armpit because he may injure himself. He can walk with crutches in several different ways, depending on how much weight he can bear on each foot and how strong his upper body is. The physical therapist teaches the person how to use the crutches, and you reinforce what he has learned.

Helping a person walk without a device.   Put a safety belt on the person. (Review the information you read about safety belts in Chapter 9, Positioning and Transferring People, and review Skill 18 in the skills book.) Never use a safety belt if the person has—

Safty Belt

❖   Had a colostomy or ileostomy recently.
❖   Severe heart problems.
❖   Had abdominal, chest, or back surgery recently.
❖   Severe respiratory problems.
❖   A fear of safety belts.

   If the person is weaker on one side than the other, stand on the weaker side, unless you are instructed otherwise, so that you can support the person's ambulation. Gradually increase the distance the person walks to help build his confidence.

Helping a Person with an Artificial Limb

Any device that replaces a natural body part is called a prosthesis. An artificial limb is a prosthetic device that replaces a missing leg or arm and helps a person with balance and movement. The following tips help you and the person in your care to take care of an artificial limb:

prosthesis

❖   Handle the artificial limb with care.
❖   Check the artificial limb to be sure no parts are worn, loose, bent, or broken. Check to see if the hinges are stiff or the straps or laces are worn. If you observe any of these defects, report them to your supervising nurse.
❖   Be sure the person wears a stump sock, a special sock designed to prevent irritation and swelling, when wearing an artificial arm or leg.
❖   Check the stump sock for worn areas, which may be a clue that the artificial limb does not fit correctly. Report worn spots in stump socks to your supervising nurse.
❖   Check the person's stump for signs of irritation, swelling, sores, or breaks or tears in the skin. Report any such problems to your supervising nurse.
❖   Store the artificial limb in a safe place where it won't get damaged.

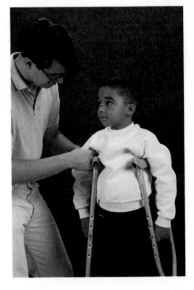

Figure 14-15
Crutches fit properly when you can measure two finger widths of space between the person's armpit and the top of the crutch and when he can comfortably grasp the hand grip with his elbow extended.

You are responsible for helping to take care of a person's artificial limb, for observing how well he uses it, and for documenting his improvement. You also report on the person's progress and recommend additional equipment when he needs it.

Providing Care for a Person Who Has Hearing Problems

Do you know a person who cannot hear well? Is it easy for him to communicate? Does he struggle to hear and understand what you are saying? Does he miss some words? Does he sometimes miscommunicate because he cannot understand what you have said to him? Does he get frustrated trying to hear?

A person may become depressed as he finds he is losing his hearing. His speech may change because he cannot hear himself talking. He may become self-conscious or embarrassed and may not want to be around other people. Or he may try to dominate the conversation to avoid the embarrassment of giving the wrong answer to a question. Have you seen these behaviors in the people you know who have a hearing loss?

Suppose you are a home health aide and have been assigned to provide care twice a week to Mr. Smith. The chart states that Mr. Smith has a severe hearing loss. As you carry out the plan of care, it is important to focus on communication. You play a special part in making sure that he is able to communicate his needs and feelings to you. How can you communicate with Mr. Smith so that he understands you and you understand him? When providing care for Mr. Smith or any person who has a hearing loss, use the following ideas:

❖ Gently touch the person on the hand or arm to gain his attention before speaking.

❖ Reduce background noise as much as possible. If you are trying to carry on a conversation, the television or radio can be very distracting.

❖ Face the person when you are speaking so that he can see your mouth move and see your facial expressions.

❖ Do not cover your mouth while speaking. Often hearing-impaired people learn to read moving lips and rely on watching your mouth move.

❖ Speak slowly, clearly, and a little louder than normal. Do not say words unnaturally, exaggerate syllables, or shout. Speaking in a slow, clear manner makes it easier for a person who is reading your lips to understand what you are saying.

❖ Use gestures and body movements to help explain what you are saying. Or write messages on paper if the person does not understand you.

❖ If the person does not seem to understand what you said, change your words, not the volume of your voice. Shouting sometimes creates more distress for the person, and he still may not understand what you are saying. High-pitched tones also may be difficult for the hearing-impaired person to hear.

❖ In an emergency, be sure to identify and help people who have hearing loss, because they may not hear alarms or directions telling them what to do.

❖ If the person has a hearing aid, help him use it properly, store it away from metal, store extra batteries, and take care of it according to the manufacturer's directions.

You may have to help a person with a hearing aid. A hearing aid is a device that helps people with impaired hearing to hear better. Some hearing aids are small enough to fit entirely in the ear. Others may be part of a person's eyeglasses. The following tips help you and the person in your care to take care of the device:

❖ Keep the hearing aid dry, making sure that the person does not wear it when bathing, showering, or washing.

❖ If you notice wax in a person's ears when helping her insert the hearing aid, report this condition to your supervising nurse.

❖ If the person is going to be in a large group where there may be many irritating sounds, suggest that she turn down the hearing aid.

❖ Make sure the hearing aid is turned off when the person is not using it to keep the batteries from running down.

❖ Keep the hearing aid in a safe place when the person is not using it, and take special care not to drop it (Figure 14-16).

❖ To prevent possible crackling sounds, check tubing for cracks or poor connections and correct if necessary.

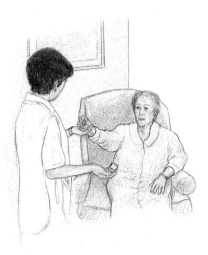

Figure 14-16
When Mrs. Wang removes her hearing aid, she always asks you to place it in its case and put it in her drawer.

When helping to take care of a person's hearing aid, observe how well she uses it, document her improvement, and report her progress to your supervising nurse.

Providing Care for a Person Who Has Vision Problems

Think how the world might seem to a person with a vision problem. Have you ever been in a room or dark tunnel where you could not see? How did you feel? Were you afraid? Did you lose your sense of balance? Were you nervous about taking the next step for fear you would fall? When you provide care for a person with vision problems, it is important to put yourself in her place and be sensitive to her feelings and fears.

Sarah Andrews, a person in your care, has cataracts, a clouding of the lenses of the eyes that causes a gradual decline of sight. Cataracts may be caused by aging, injury, or other diseases. A cataract may develop in one eye or in both eyes. Mrs. Andrews has blurred vision. She says she feels as if she has a film over her eyes.

You also provide care to Jake Wilson. Mr. Wilson's diabetes has caused changes in his eyes that have resulted in blurred vision.

Imagine what it must be like for Mrs. Andrews and Mr. Wilson. They cannot move around at will because they cannot see clearly what is in front of them. They are unable to read a newspaper or watch television comfortably. Most vision problems are chronic conditions that do not go away. When planning care for a person with vision problems, the important points to consider are safety and communication so that the person's life is as pleasant as you can help make it.

When carrying out the plan of care for a person with vision problems, do the following things:

❖ Stand where the person can see you.
❖ Call him by name and say who you are. "Good morning, Mr. Wilson, this is your nurse assistant (or home health aide)."
❖ Describe what you are going to do. "It's time for dinner and I'm going to help you get to the dining room."
❖ When serving food, describe the items on the plate by location, using a clock as a reference point. "Your meal is chicken, green beans, and potatoes. The chicken is at 12 o'clock on your plate, the potatoes are at 4 o'clock, and the beans are at 8 o'clock." (Review Figure 12-11 in Chapter 12, Healthful Eating.)
❖ If you are serving the person's meal on a tray, remove hot drinks from the tray and serve them separately. "Here is your hot tea. I'm putting it at the top of your tray at 1 o'clock."
❖ When helping a person move around, encourage him to hold your arm just above your elbow for support. Describe where you are going, and mention things that are in your path. "We are going up three steps now." (Figure 14-17)
❖ Keep the room well lighted. Open the curtains to let in daylight and turn on lamps in the early evening.
❖ Keep furniture and belongings in the same place all the time to help the person keep a mental picture of where things are and to avoid injuries.
❖ If the nursing home or hospital has raised numbers or symbols on doors, show him how to find them.
❖ Describe people, surroundings, or events in a way that would help the person create a picture. "Mr. Wilson, your daughter Susan is here and she is wearing a beautiful red dress. Today is a sunny day and the patio is open, if you would like to sit outside."
❖ If the person wears eyeglasses, be sure to keep them clean. Smudges on his glasses can cause more blurring.

Helping a Person with Eyeglasses

Eyeglasses help people with limited vision see better. Some people need to wear them only for reading. Others need to wear them all the time. Some people have eyeglasses with hearing aids built in and wear them for seeing and hearing. Eyeglasses may not correct a person's vision completely, but they should improve it enough to allow him to function better. The following tips help you and the person in your care take care of eyeglasses:

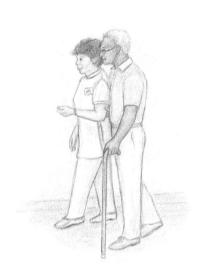

Figure 14-17
Mr. Wilson, who is visually impaired, feels more independent when he holds the nurse assistant's arm than when the nurse assistant holds his arm.

❖ Clean the eyeglasses by holding them under warm water. Use a gentle soap, if necessary, and then rinse with warm water. Dry them with a clean, soft cloth or towel.

❖ Check the person's eyeglasses to be sure they fit. If the glasses slip down on his nose, he may not be able to see well. If they pinch, his nose or ears may become reddened or sore. If a person's glasses do not fit properly, report this observation to your supervising nurse.

❖ Store eyeglasses in a case so that they do not break or become scratched. If you have to put them down when they are not in a case, be sure to place the eyeglasses with the lenses facing up. Placing the glasses with the lenses face down on a surface may scratch them. Store eyeglasses where the person can reach them.

❖ Encourage the person to wear his eyeglasses when he appears to need them.

When helping to take care of a person's eyeglasses, observe how well he uses them, document his improvement, report on the person's progress, and recommend additional eyeglasses or cases when he needs them.

Helping a Person with an Artificial Eye

An artificial eye is a prosthetic device that fits into a person's eye socket after his eyeball has been removed. When providing care for someone who has an artificial eye, be sure to handle the eye with care.

To remove the eye for cleaning, depress the person's lower lid until the edge of the artificial eye slides out. To help prevent dropping it, catch the artificial eye in a clean washcloth or small towel. To clean the eye, use soap and water or the prescribed solution. Always rinse the eye before returning it to the person's eye socket. Never use chemicals or alcohol to clean an artificial eye. After replacing the eye in the person's socket, check the eye to make sure it is fitting properly. If the person has any complaints, report them to your supervising nurse.

When helping to take care of a person's artificial eye, observe how well the person uses it, document his improvement, report on the person's progress, and recommend additional equipment when it is needed.

Information Review

Circle the correct answers and fill in the blanks.

1. To help people become as fully functional as possible and to help them be able to enjoy life, you provide _____Restorative_____ care.

2. To encourage a person's independence, you would—
   a. Feed the person yourself so that his food does not get cold.
   b. Set the food in front of him and leave the room.
   c. Give him 5 minutes to feed himself and then feed him the rest of the meal to save time.
   d. Encourage him to use a self-help eating utensil so that he can feed himself.

3. A built-up handle toothbrush, a long-handled shoe horn, a zipper pull, and a stocking aid are examples of _____Self-help_____ devices.

4. Inactivity can cause—
   a. Atrophied muscles.
   b. Blindness.
   c. Fractures.
   d. Arthritis.

5. Mrs. Clymer has arthritis and needs to do range-of-motion exercises. When you go to her room to help her, she says that she can't do them today because she hurts too much. The best way to respond is to say,—
   a. "You need to do them because the doctor ordered them. Let's just do them and get them over with."
   b. "If we do them quickly, we'll finish up faster."
   c. "Okay, we'll do them tomorrow."
   d. "It's so important for you to do these exercises to keep your joints flexible. Let's try to do them very slowly, and you can let me know when you need to rest or stop."

6. The physical therapist teaches a person how to use crutches, and the nurse assistant _____reinforce_____ what has been taught.

7. A _____prosthesis_____ is any device that replaces a natural part of the body.

8. To take good care of a hearing aid,—
   a. Store it in a glass of water so that it doesn't dry out.
   b. Make sure it's turned off when the person isn't using it.
   c. Store it in its case on top of a radiator.
   d. Keep it turned on all the time so that it is always ready to use.

9. When serving food to a person who has vision problems, describe items on the tray by location, using a _____clock_____ as a reference point.

10. If you must put eyeglasses down on a surface, place them with the lenses facing _____up_____.

Questions to Ask Yourself

1. Mr. Rivera had a stroke, which resulted in right-side paralysis. What suggestions do you have for Mr. Rivera to help him increase his activity?

2. Mr. Roberts has severe arthritis in his hands. He struggles, but he usually manages to feed himself at lunch and breakfast using his adaptive spork. His wife feeds him dinner every night. What do you think you should do about this situation?

3. Ms. Jones complains about not being able to do things or get around like she did before the car crash that left her with a below-the-knee amputation. She has a prosthesis, but she does not like to wear it. She wants you to take her to the bathroom in her wheelchair. What do you think would be the best thing for you to do?

4. How can you help maintain independence for a person who needs to use a walker?

5. How can you help maintain good body mechanics for someone who uses a cane to walk?

6. Mrs. Garcia is upset because she couldn't reach the end of the hallway today. "Yesterday I walked twice as far with this stupid thing!" she says, and angrily pushes away her walker. What can you do to help her feel better?

7. Name some of the body parts that are exercised when you help someone with passive range-of-motion exercises. Why are these exercises important for providing restorative care?

8. Why must you be especially careful to maintain the skin integrity of someone who uses crutches?

9. Mr. Sanders is 79 years old and wears a hearing aid. His memory is not as good as it used to be, and he often misplaces the hearing aid. What can you do to help make sure the device is always ready for use?

10. Ever since he developed contractures, Mr. Hudson has lost weight. "I'm just not as hungry as I used to be," he tells you at lunch. One day you overhear Mr. Hudson telling his roommate that he doesn't want to be a burden to anyone. What can you do to make sure Mr. Hudson receives adequate nutrition and maintains his independence?

15

Admitting, Transferring, and Discharging

Goals

After reading this chapter, you will have the information to—

Help people when they are admitted to a nursing home, hospital, or home health care agency.

Help people when they are transferred within a nursing home or hospital.

Help people when they are discharged from a nursing home, hospital, or home health care agency.

One day in the lunch room, you talk with another nurse assistant about a resident that you helped discharge that morning. You talk about how difficult it was to say good-bye to someone that you had helped for several months.

"I always have mixed feelings about admitting and discharging residents," says your co-worker, Kathy Barnes. "When a resident first arrives, I feel a little nervous. I really want the person to be as comfortable and relaxed as possible. I know how important my role is in making the person feel that way.

"I remember when I first started working, a woman I'll call Mrs. E. was admitted. One of the other nurse assistants was out sick, so the rest of us split up her work load. I was rushing around trying to get everything done. I even rushed through Mrs. E.'s admission. Just before I was getting ready to leave at the end of my shift, I checked on her one more time and saw that she was crying. When I asked her how I could help her, she snapped back at me, 'Well, I certainly wouldn't want to bother you. You obviously have too many other things to do without having to worry about me.' I felt terrible. She was right. I hadn't even taken the time to make her feel welcome, because I had so much to do. Now, I always think about Mrs. E. whenever I help with someone's admission. I learned from her how important it is to slow down, work in an unhurried manner, and treat each person as if she's the most important person at that moment.

"When the time comes to discharge residents whom I've gotten to know fairly well, I often have mixed feelings. I'm glad that they are well enough to go home, but at the same time, I'm sad to see them go. I know I'll miss them."

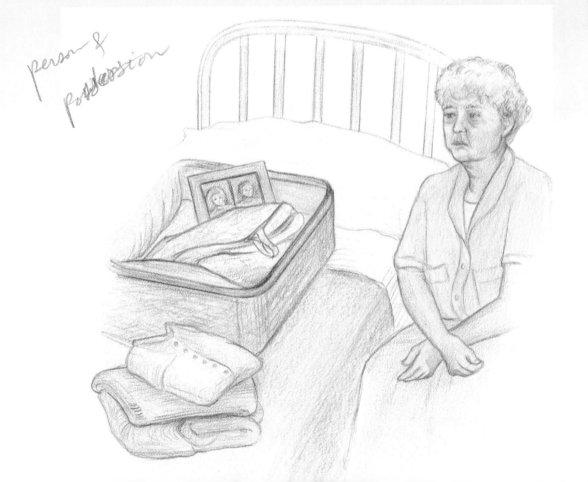

Admitting, Transferring, and Discharging a Person

Have you ever had to spend time away from home in a strange place? What do you remember as being important? Were you made to feel comfortable, or did you feel unwelcome or ill at ease? Did you plan to stay for a short or long time? Were things ready for you when you arrived, or did you have to wait for arrangements to be made? Thinking about your own answers to these questions may help you understand what people feel when they are admitted to health care. In addition to emotional uncertainties, people may experience physical pain or discomfort at the time they are admitted.

As a nurse assistant, how you perform your role in admitting a person to health care may influence her attitude about the care she receives. One of your tasks is to make the admission process as smooth as possible. Another is to help a person transfer from one part of a hospital or nursing home to another part of the facility as easily as possible, ensuring that the person and her possessions are moved safely and completely. The care that you provide in helping to discharge a person when she leaves a health care situation may leave a lasting impression about the care she received.

Each employer and each health care facility has its own procedures for admitting, transferring, and discharging people. Some procedures, such as taking vital signs, are basic to all situations. And in most situations, the role of the nurse assistant is basically the same: to look after and help ensure the safety of the person and her possessions as she is admitted, transferred, and discharged.

Looking After the Person

Make the person feel welcome as she is admitted into care by introducing yourself to her. To help her feel less anxious about her health care experience, explain what is happening and what is going to happen.

When a person is first admitted to health care, take and record her vital signs. (Review the information in Chapter 8, Measuring Life Signs.) These measurements at admission are important for other health care workers to use as a baseline reference point when vital signs are taken at other times. Perform your tasks in a warm, unhurried manner to help her relax and feel better about being in a health care situation (Figure 15-1).

One way to help ensure the safety of the person in your care is to interview her. In addition to asking her the questions on the admission form, encourage her to tell you anything that would make her stay more comfortable. Ask about special preferences, habits, or problems. One way to organize the interview is to ask questions, working your way from head to toe. The admission form often prompts you to work this way. For example, you might ask the person: "Do you wear glasses? Is there anything special I should know about them? Do you have a hearing aid? Is there anything special I should know about it or about your hearing in general? Do you wear dentures? Do you have trouble sleeping at night?" Continue asking

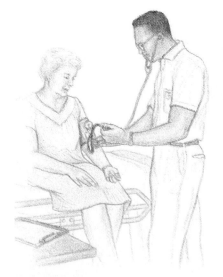

Figure 15-1
Take vital signs in an efficient and competent manner to reassure a person who is being admitted.

similar questions about diet, mobility, and elimination. Record her answers and report important information to your supervising nurse.

It also is important to remember the person's needs and feelings when you transfer her from one room of a nursing home or hospital to another and when you discharge a person to a nursing home or hospital, or to her own home. Even in the home health care setting, it is important to think about how the person may feel about having you in her own home, doing the things that she once did for herself.

Looking After the Person's Possessions

An important part of looking after a person's possessions in a nursing home or hospital is filling out the admission checklist, which also may include an envelope for valuables and a personal belongings list. Following your employer's guidelines, fill out the admission checklist, noting valuables and personal belongings. When describing valuables such as jewelry, use words that do not assign value to the object. For example, describe a ring as a yellow metal ring with one clear stone, being careful not to use words like gold, silver, or diamond. When describing a watch, write down the brand name found on the watch face. Encourage the person to send as many valuables home as possible. If necessary, you can arrange for valuable items to be locked in the facility's safe. After completing the checklist, give it to your supervising nurse.

When you help a person transfer within a nursing home or hospital, you must take special care of her possessions to make sure that they arrive safely with her in her new room. (Sometimes a person is moved from one area of the nursing home or hospital to another. Other times a person is moved only from room to room.)

Admitting, Transferring, and Discharging a Nursing Home Resident

When helping with someone's admission to a nursing home, it is important to focus on the needs of a person who enters this health care situation knowing she may stay for a few months or perhaps for the rest of her life. Because of the long stay, it is important to find out about her individual habits and preferences. And because she may never go home again, it is important to be sensitive to her feelings.

As one of the first people to have contact with a new resident, you can help her feel comfortable and trusting in her new environment. Because her first impression of the nursing home may influence how she feels about being there, your approach and consideration can help make her experience pleasant and give her confidence in the care she is about to receive. To ensure a good first impression, take some of the following steps:

❖   Each time you greet a new resident, smile, call her by name, and be attentive to her feelings. Find out her needs. Does she need to use the bathroom, be repositioned, or have a drink of water?

❖ If family members are with her, use this opportunity to talk with her and her family about mealtime, activities, using free time, and making positive use of visiting time.

❖ Always include the resident in conversations that concern her.

At times, a resident may have to be transferred from one section of the nursing home to another. For example, a resident who receives rehabilitation therapy may no longer need therapy. At that time, she may be transferred to a different unit in the nursing home.

Some nursing home residents also are discharged. Some are discharged to a hospital to receive medical treatment that is not available at the nursing home, and others are discharged to their homes for further recovery.

Admitting a Resident to the Nursing Home

Today, you prepare for the arrival of 72-year-old Alma Garcia, who is recovering from surgery and who will be transported from the hospital to the Morningside Nursing Home by ambulance. To get ready for Mrs. Garcia's arrival, follow the admission sheet and instructions from your supervising nurse. Gather and bring to her room the equipment and materials you need for admission: blood pressure cuff and stethoscope, thermometer, and any other items listed by your supervising nurse. Put a pitcher of water and a cup on the nightstand. Put a gown, washcloth, and towel in the nightstand, and be prepared to put a washbasin, bedpan, emesis basin, soap, and soap dish in the nightstand if she doesn't bring these items from the hospital. Also bring a laundry marker, personal belongings sheet, pen, and paper to her room. Prepare Mrs. Garcia's bed. (In some nursing homes, the nurse assistant fan-folds the top linens down to the bottom of the bed so that the bed is ready for the new resident when she arrives.) (Figure 15-2)

Your supervising nurse has already told you a little about Mrs. Garcia and her physical condition, so you know that she broke her hip and will be receiving physical therapy. You think about other

Figure 15-2
When you fold the top bed linens down in preparation for a new resident, you are making an "open bed."

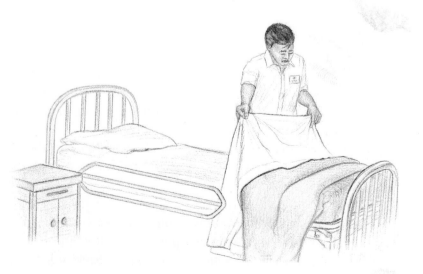

things to explore when she arrives, such as how she feels about being in a nursing home. Entering a nursing home can be a very emotional experience, and people may react in many different ways. They may be sad, frightened, anxious, relieved, or withdrawn. It is important for you to recognize and support new residents' feelings and to report any extreme behaviors that you observe to your supervising nurse.

When a new resident is admitted to the nursing home, you and other members of the nursing home staff follow a planned series of events. If you are admitting the new resident, knock on the door, smile at her, and greet her with a friendly "hello." Check her name band and introduce yourself to her and anyone who is with her. Remove the hospital name band and replace it with one that your unit secretary has prepared. Explain that you are the nurse assistant who will be providing care for her. Ask her what she would like to be called, and be sure not to use her first name unless she gives you permission. Introduce her to her roommate. (Sometimes an admissions clerk or social worker manages the admissions and introduces the new resident to the nurse assistant.) Ask her if she needs to use the bathroom before continuing with the admissions process.

Help the new resident fill out a personal belongings list, and help her label her clothes with the laundry marker. Be sure to mark the clothes in an area where the ink won't show through to the outside (the label is often a good place). Encourage her to send any valuables home. If she decides not to send them home, list them and lock them in the safe. Help her put her things away.

Explain nursing home policies, schedules, and visiting hours to the new resident and her family. Also, ask about her food, bathing, and activity preferences. Show her how the call signal works and ask her to demonstrate her understanding of its use. Demonstrate how to raise and lower the bed and overbed table.

After explaining the surroundings to the new resident and her family, measure her vital signs, height, and weight, and record them. Then offer to take her and her family on a tour of the facility. If she wishes to go, introduce her to other members of the staff and to other residents.

After the tour, help the new resident get comfortable in her room and put the call signal within her reach. Ask her if she needs anything. If not, wash your hands, tell her when you will return, and report your completion of the admission checklist, as well as any observations about the new resident's physical condition and emotional status, to your supervising nurse.

Transferring a Resident Within the Nursing Home

Two weeks ago, Mrs. Eastman broke two vertebrae in her back and was admitted to Morningside Nursing Home to receive physical therapy. From the first day that she arrived, she refused to cooperate with the physical therapist and, eventually, refused to leave her room to go to physical therapy. Today, when she tells the doctor that she won't go to physical therapy, he reports this situation to the nursing home administrators. Because the unit where she now resides is specified for residents who receive physical therapy and nursing care, they arrange for Mrs. Eastman to be transferred to a unit where she will receive only basic nursing care.

When you help transfer a resident to a different unit in the nursing home, go to her room, greet her, and wash your hands. Explain to her that you are going to help her get ready for her transfer. As you help her pack her belongings, check the closets, drawers, and nightstand for personal items. Pack all of her equipment, such as the washbasin and bedpan, to take to the new room. As you help gather her things, talk with her about the transfer. Ask her if she wants to share her feelings about what is going to happen and answer any questions she may have (Figure 15-3). Give her time to say good-bye to her roommate.

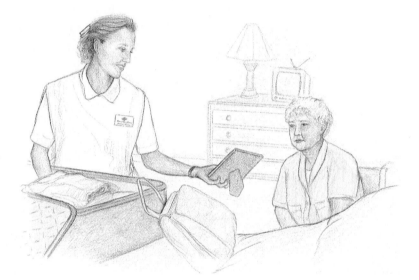

Figure 15-3
Any move may have an emotional impact on a resident. Whether the resident moves down the hall or to another floor, it is important to tell her why she is being transferred, encourage her to talk about her feelings, and reassure her if necessary.

Ask your supervising nurse for the records and charts that must go with the resident, and ask the unit secretary to inform the staff on the new unit that you are bringing the resident from your unit. It may be necessary to adjust the time of her arrival in the new unit so that the nurse assigned to her is available to receive her.

Help the resident into a wheelchair. (Some facilities prefer that you move the resident in her bed from one room to another.) Ask a co-worker to help you, if necessary. Move the resident and her possessions to her new room, and introduce her to her new nurse and nurse assistant. Report important information, as necessary.

To help the resident make a comfortable transition from one nursing home unit to another, and as a courtesy to her new nurse assistant, you may stay and assist her new nurse assistant with some of the tasks to help get her settled in her new room. Then spend a few minutes talking with her about how you enjoyed helping her. Wish her well in her new room and say good-bye to her.

Return to your own unit. Remove any equipment that the resident did not take from her old room. Since she wasn't moved in her bed, strip it of dirty linens. Follow your employer's policy for preparing the room for use by another resident.

After finishing these tasks, wash your hands. Report to your supervising nurse that the resident's transfer has been completed. Provide important information, such as the time of the transfer, her mode of transportation, how she responded, and any important observations.

Discharging a Resident from the Nursing Home

A resident may be discharged from the nursing home to a hospital or to her own home. In either situation, you must help her make the transition as smoothly and safely as possible.

Discharging a resident to a hospital.   Mr. Wilson has been doing very well at Morningside Nursing Home. Suddenly his temperature goes up, he complains of pain in his chest, and he develops a cough. His doctor writes orders to send him by ambulance to the hospital, and your supervising nurse notifies his family of the decision to hospitalize him. As his nurse assistant, you help him get ready to be transferred.

Pack only the clothing and belongings that he needs for the hospital stay (robe, slippers, and personal care items such as a comb, brush, toothbrush, toothpaste, eyeglasses, and dentures). Help him dress appropriately. In this case, pajamas, a robe, and slippers are appropriate, because the ambulance crew will make sure that he is covered and warm.

Check with your supervising nurse to make sure that the proper forms are filled out and are ready to go with the resident. (It is helpful to send a detailed description of his physical needs and personal habits, as well as medications and usual vital signs, to the hospital.) Stay with him and comfort him until he is in the ambulance, because he may be very frightened.

Check the resident's name band and introduce him to the ambulance crew. If they need assistance, help the ambulance attendants transfer the resident to the stretcher. Make sure that his belongings and forms are in the ambulance with him. Follow your employer's policy for listing and storing his personal belongings that he didn't take to the hospital, and make sure that his room is clean.

Report to your supervising nurse that the resident's discharge has been completed. Provide important information, such as the time of the discharge, his mode of transportation, how he responded, and any important observations.

Discharging a resident to her home.   For several weeks, Mrs. Garcia has been receiving physical therapy at the nursing home to help strengthen her hip. You have helped her with bathing, dressing, and walking, as well as with special exercises that she learned from the physical therapist. Over time, Mrs. Garcia has become strong and independent enough to walk with a walker. Today, her doctor explains to her that she is well enough to go home but says that she will need

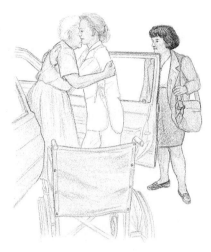

Figure 15-4

When discharging a resident, provide for her safety by transporting her out of the building in a wheelchair and carefully helping her into the waiting vehicle.

help at home for a while. He refers her to a home health care agency.

On the day that a resident is ready to go home, help her gather all her belongings and pack her suitcase. Check items against the personal belongings sheet to make sure that she has everything she brought with her. After your supervising nurse gives verbal and written instructions to the resident and her family members, help the resident into a wheelchair and transport her to the nursing home exit where her family's car is waiting (Figure 15-4). Tell her how much you have enjoyed helping her. Wish her well in her recovery and say good-bye.

Return the wheelchair to your unit, clean it, and return it to the proper place. Then strip the discharged resident's bed, pick up discarded items, and report important observations to your supervising nurse.

To learn about admitting, transferring, and discharging a hospital patient and admitting and discharging a home health care client, please read the next two sections. If you do not plan to work in a hospital or home health care, turn to the end of the chapter and read "Information Review" and "Questions to Ask Yourself."

Admitting, Transferring, and Discharging a Hospital Patient

Although some hospitals may have similar admission procedures, it is important to know your role, as well as your employer's policies and procedures, and follow them. The following example illustrates your role in one particular hospital setting.

Admitting a Patient to the Hospital

Preparing for the admission of a new patient in a hospital is similar to preparing for a new resident in a nursing home. Today you are admitting Dora Creed, age 55, who is entering the hospital for surgery to repair her knee that she injured in a car collision several months before. To get ready for Mrs. Creed's arrival, gather the equipment and materials that you need for admission and bring them to her room: a urine specimen container, blood pressure cuff and stethoscope, thermometer, and scale. Also gather personal care items such as a washbasin, bedpan, emesis basin, lotion, soap, and tissues (these items may be contained in an admissions pack) and put them in the nightstand. In addition, put a gown, washcloth, and towel in the nightstand. Place a water pitcher and glass on top of the nightstand. Fanfold the top linens down to the bottom of the bed so that the bed is ready for Mrs. Creed when she arrives. To prepare yourself, bring an admission checklist (which also may include an envelope for valuables and a personal belongings list) and pencil and paper.

When a new hospital patient arrives, greet her, introduce yourself, introduce her to her roommate, and make an effort to be warm and friendly and not to rush her as she gets settled. Your goal is to make her feel as comfortable and relaxed as possible.

After washing your hands and pulling the privacy curtain, ask the new patient to change into the hospital gown, helping her if she needs assistance. When she is in her gown, bathrobe, and slippers and is comfortable, fill out the admission checklist, noting valuables and personal belongings according to the policy of the hospital. Encourage her to send home any valuable items, such as jewelry, wallet, and credit cards.

Familiarize the new patient with her surroundings by explaining which nightstand, closet, and chair are hers. Explain to her how to use the call signal and have her demonstrate her understanding of its use. Put it within easy reach (Figure 15-5). Show her how to adjust the bed and overbed table and how to operate the TV, if the room has one. Explain hospital policies regarding visiting hours, meals, and where she may go within the hospital. Also, explain to her whether her care plan permits her to get out of bed to use the bathroom (if not, place the bedpan within her reach), whether she has any other activity restrictions, and if she may eat or drink anything. If she is not permitted anything by mouth, explain the NPO sign and place it above her bed.

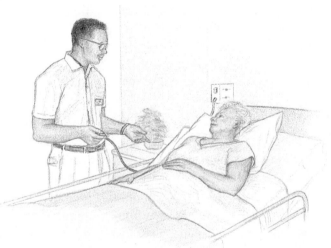

Figure 15-5
Explain to a new patient how the call signal works and the location of anything else she might need.

Your supervising nurse may ask you to do some other steps in the admission process, such as measuring and recording the new patient's vital signs, height, and weight and asking her to provide a urine specimen. Make sure to complete the rest of the checklist carefully.

NOTE: Usually the checklist has questions about allergies, medications (which your supervising nurse probably records), and food preferences. Make sure that you complete and record each item accurately.

If the new patient can have water, fill her water pitcher. Ask her if she needs anything. When you have completed all your tasks, wash your hands. Then report to your supervising nurse the things you have completed on the admission checklist and tell her about the status of the new patient's physical and emotional condition when you left her room. Share any important information or observations with your supervising nurse.

Transferring a Patient Within the Hospital

In a hospital, patients may not always be admitted directly into your department from outside the facility. Sometimes a patient may arrive at your department from another department within the hospital. For example, someone may be transferred from the emergency room to the surgery department for recovery. Likewise, a patient receiving care in the surgery department may be transferred to the rehabilitation unit.

When a patient is transferred into your department.   A person such as Alma Garcia, who fell and broke her hip at home, was taken by ambulance to the hospital and admitted to the emergency room. There the doctor examined her and determined that she had broken her hip and needed to have surgery. Because the operating room was not immediately available, the emergency room doctor transferred her to the surgical department.

As a nurse assistant in the surgical department, you prepare the bed and room just as you would if the person were being admitted from outside the hospital. In most hospitals, you don't fill out the valuables list for a transferred patient, because it is included in the paperwork that comes with her from the other department. But you may have to sign the list when the person arrives. Your signature indicates that you've checked the items that came with the person when she arrived in your department against the information written on the form.

When a patient is transferred out of your department.   A week after Mrs. Creed's surgery, the doctor explains to her that she is going to be transferred to the hospital's rehabilitation unit, where she will spend several hours a day learning to walk again. Your assignment is to transfer Mrs. Creed to the rehabilitation unit. The transfer procedure is similar to that of transferring in the nursing home.

In preparation for a patient's transfer, your supervising nurse gathers records and charts that must go with the patient and calls ahead to report the patient's status and care needs to the nurse in the new unit. Just before you are ready to take the patient to her new room, ask the unit secretary to call and inform the staff that you are ready to bring her. Transport the patient and her belongings in a wheelchair or in her bed, according to the hospital's policy.

Discharging a Patient from the Hospital

In many hospitals, discharge planning starts as soon as the person is admitted. Special nurses, called discharge planners, often have the responsibility to plan a patient's discharge. They assess the need for referral services, make follow-up appointments, and discuss the doctor's plan for medications, treatments, diet, and activities with the patient and interested family members. Discharge planners also act as resource people whom patients can call after they leave the hospital.

Discharging a patient to a nursing home.   A patient who is discharged from a hospital to a nursing home to continue recovery and rehabilitation may be transported by ambulance. The patient's doctor and social worker will contact the nursing home and arrange for her care.

The procedure for discharge is similar to the procedure for discharging a resident from a nursing home to a hospital. The main difference is that all the person's belongings must go with her or must be taken home by a family member or friend.

Discharging a patient to her home.   When a hospital patient is discharged to her own home, her doctor writes discharge orders, and the nurse (or discharge planner) talks with the patient about her discharge plan. She discusses medications and activities the patient can and cannot do and explains treatments, diet, and doctors' appointments. She then asks you to help the patient get ready to leave.

To prepare her for discharge, bring a wheelchair to transport her. (For safety reasons, all patients must leave the hospital in a wheelchair, even if they can walk.) Ask the patient's family member or friend, who is driving her home, to bring the car to the appropriate exit. Then, after all matters are completed with the business office and the discharge slip is in the patient's hand, check to make sure that she has the information that the nurse gave her regarding medications, activities, and appointments. Wheel her to the exit and help her into the car.

To learn about admitting, transferring, and discharging people in home health care, please read the next section. If you do not plan to work in the home health care setting, turn to the end of the chapter and read "Information Review" and "Questions to Ask Yourself."

Admitting and Discharging a Home Health Care Client

Have you ever had someone come into your home to do repairs? What did it feel like to have a stranger in your home? Were you afraid that he might break something? Were you concerned that he would leave a mess from his work? Did you feel that your home was no longer private? Thinking about your own responses to these questions may help you understand what people experience when they are admitted to home health care and have new people help them in their homes.

Because a home health aide often takes care of both the client and her home, it is important to remember how valuable a person's possessions are to her. In a client's home, it is important to treat all her belongings with special care. Everything in her home may be a special treasure to her. When a person is discharged from a nursing home or hospital to her home, you may have to help her put away her belongings. It is important to put them where the client wants them, even if you think another place would be better.

A person who receives health care at home is admitted into the care of a home health care agency and, when she no longer needs to receive care at home, she is discharged from the care of the home health care agency.

Admitting a Home Health Care Client

Before Mrs. Garcia is discharged to her home, the discharge planner at the nursing home calls a local home health care agency to arrange for services. After Mrs. Garcia arrives home, the nurse from the agency assesses Mrs. Garcia and her needs and, based on her doctor's orders and conditions in her home, develops a plan of care. The nurse then discusses the plan with other members of the health care team, and together they coordinate their activities, including the scheduling of a home health aide. Mrs. Garcia needs a home health aide for personal care, a homemaker for housekeeping, a physical therapist to continue her exercises, and a social worker to plan for her health care needs.

On the first day that you arrive in a new client's home to begin providing care, you must try to help her feel comfortable and relaxed about your being in her home. Talk with her, ask her about her interests, discuss her preferences and habits that are in her plan, and help her understand what you will be doing in her home.

Discharging a Home Health Care Client

After several weeks, Mrs. Garcia no longer needs home health care. The social worker puts Mrs. Garcia in touch with community resources that can offer ongoing assistance with needs such as transportation.

Although you will not be directly involved with Mrs. Garcia's discharge from home health care, be sure to talk with her on your last visit to tell her how much you enjoyed providing care for her. Wish her well and say good-bye to her.

Information Review

Circle the correct answers and fill in the blanks.

1. When a person first enters a health care setting, you help with a procedure called _Admission_.

2. When a person moves from one unit in a nursing home or hospital to another unit, you help with a procedure called _transfering_.

3. When a person leaves a health care situation, you help with a procedure called _discharge_.

4. When a person moves into and out of health care situations, the nurse assistant looks after the person and the person's—
   a. Family.
   b. Pets.
   c. Doctor.
   d. Possessions.

5. One of the basic tasks performed in all admitting procedures is measuring ___vital signs_____.

6. In a nursing home and hospital, it is important to keep records of a person's personal—
   a. Belongings.
   b. Thoughts.
   c. Desires.
   d. Remarks.

7. You can help a resident or patient feel more comfortable in her new health care setting by introducing her to her
   _____roommate_____.

8. When you admit a new resident to a nursing home, one of your tasks is to use a laundry marker to label—
   a. Her new bed.
   b. Her clothing.
   c. The back of her hand.
   d. Her bed linens.

9. The nurse who sometimes helps with discharging a person from a nursing home or hospital is called a
   ____discharge_____ planner____.

10. When a patient is discharged from a hospital, she may go to a
    _____Nursing_____ home_____ or to her
    own ___home_____.

Questions to Ask Yourself

1. Mrs. Marker insists on wearing her opal and diamond ring in the nursing home. One day, after Mrs. Marker has become very ill and is slipping in and out of consciousness, the ring slips off her finger onto the bed. What would you do?

2. Mr. Yoder, a patient with diabetes, has been admitted to the hospital so that doctors can try to regulate his blood sugar levels. As you help him unpack his suitcase, you notice that he brought along a stash of cookies and cupcakes. What would you do?

3. After Mrs. Garcia has been transferred to the nursing home, you clean her hospital room. As you are changing the bed linens, you find a picture of a small boy just under the bed. What would you do?

16

Providing Care for People with Specific Illnesses

Goals

After reading this chapter, you will have the information to—

Describe the nature of acute and chronic conditions.

Describe common chronic conditions of several body systems.

Describe some of the characteristics or symptoms of several chronic illnesses.

Focus care to meet the specific needs of people with chronic illnesses.

Describe some of the chronic illnesses that begin in childhood.

Focus care to meet the specific needs of people who have cancer.

The first time you went to Gene and Sue Conrad's house to provide care for 63-year-old Mr. Conrad, he had recently been diagnosed with heart disease and needed help with personal care. When you arrived, you could see that Mrs. Conrad's eyes were red and puffy and that her eye makeup was smudged.

After hanging up your coat on the hall coat rack, you asked Mrs. Conrad what you could do to help her. "Nobody can help me!" she said in a loud, high-pitched voice. Then she sat down in a chair and burst into tears. You put your hands on her shoulders to try to comfort her. When she calmed down, she said, "I'm sorry. It's just that Gene's disease has made everything so difficult. We can't go out together because I'm not strong enough to handle his wheelchair and oxygen tank, and I'm afraid to leave him alone. I feel like a prisoner. I never get out of this house. All I do is take care of Gene. I don't mind taking care of him, because I love him. But I'm so tired. I don't see how we can continue to live like this."

As with many other families living with chronic disease, the Conrads had a hard time accepting a new lifestyle. However, over time, with help from several caregivers, the Conrads have adapted to living with Mr. Conrad's disease. He has learned how to do many things for himself, and Mrs. Conrad arranges for help so that she occasionally can go out by herself, go to the store, or enjoy a movie with her husband. They have learned how to adjust to their new lifestyle so that they can once again enjoy their life together.

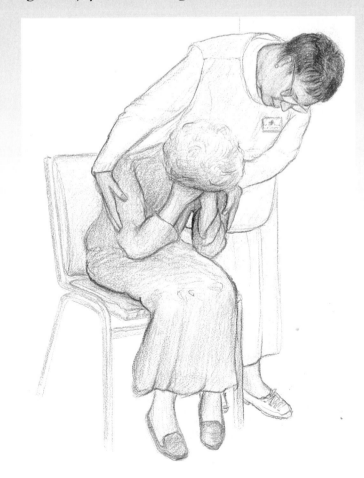

Providing Care for People with Acute and Chronic Illnesses

Think about the last time you were sick. Did the illness occur suddenly? Perhaps one day you felt fine, and the next day you were ill with a cold or an infection. Or perhaps someone you know had surgery to remove an infected appendix (appendicitis). In both of these cases, the illness is considered an acute condition. That is, the illness happened fairly suddenly and lasted a short time. When your cold ran its course, you felt well again. And when the person received treatment for appendicitis, he felt well again.

Some other illnesses occur gradually and last a long time. These illnesses are chronic conditions. In many cases, a person who has a chronic condition lives the rest of his life with an illness or condition that never really goes away. Do you know someone who has a chronic condition, such as heart disease, diabetes, or arthritis? Sometimes a person can have a chronic condition that continues for years without many serious symptoms, and then suddenly it flares up. When it flares up, the chronic condition is in an acute phase. The person feels ill and may need to consult a doctor. After treatment, the acute phase goes away, and the person continues to live with the chronic condition.

Think about some of the emotional events a person goes through when he has an acute condition. The illness disrupts his normal life. He cannot continue with daily activities. He may have to cancel plans or make an appointment to see the doctor. Has your life ever been disrupted by illness? Did you go to the doctor for an examination and go home hoping the illness would go away soon? Did your family and friends support you and try to make you feel comfortable? If you had an acute illness, you probably were able to go back to your normal way of living after a few days or weeks.

What do you think it would be like to live with a chronic condition? A chronic condition lasts a long time, and may never go away. It often affects the activities of daily living. For example, a person who has arthritis may not be able to walk without a walker or cane, or a person who has heart disease may have to change his diet. A chronic condition also may impact a person's emotional health. He may be depressed or unhappy about not being able to do the things he once did, or he may be short tempered because he is in pain. As a health care provider, you must focus your care so that you can help a person with a chronic condition to live the fullest life possible.

Family members and friends also are affected by a chronic condition. If a person's diet changes, his family may have to eat differently, too. If the person cannot move without help, he may need assistance with a variety of tasks. Family members and friends also may be sad, angry, or depressed about the change in the person's health.

As you read this chapter, you will learn mainly about providing care for people with chronic conditions. Remember, it can be very difficult to cope day to day with a condition that may prevent a person from ever feeling really well.

Chronic Conditions of the Skeletal System

In Chapter 9, Positioning and Transferring People, you read about the bones, muscles, and joints that provide a framework for your body and give you the flexibility to move. Two chronic conditions that affect the skeletal system are arthritis and **osteoporosis**. When providing care, remember that a person with a bone disease has a chronic illness. She may feel depressed with her inability to move without pain and her need to be more dependent on others. Your role is crucial. You can give her emotional support and encouragement.

osteoporosis
(os-tee-oh-per-OH-sis)   A condition of the skeletal system in which the bones become weak and fragile.

Providing Care for a Person Who Has Arthritis

Mrs. Chatterjee hardly looks up at you from her wheelchair. She rarely speaks and she eats little. You see on her chart that she is a 55-year-old woman who has had arthritis for the last 20 years. She has stiffness in her hips, knees, and fingers, and these joints are tender and swollen. When she moves, she feels a great amount of pain. She often is depressed because of her inability to move without pain and because of how deformed her joints have become.

Characteristics and symptoms of arthritis.   Arthritis is a condition of the skeletal system that causes joints to become inflamed, swollen, stiff, and painful. A few or many joints may be affected. The smooth, slipping tissues that cover the ends of bones become rough or wear away, causing painful friction between bones when they move. The remaining tissues around the joints swell, which causes stiffness. This stiffness makes normal movement difficult. Even an activity such as unscrewing the lid of a jar or walking upstairs can be difficult and cause pain (Figure 16-1).

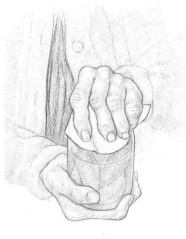

Figure 16-1
Adaptive devices, which make tasks easier, may be as simple as this rubber jar lid opener.

The plan of care.   Mrs. Chatterjee's plan of care should focus on relieving her pain and helping her move. Imagine what it might be like not being able to move without pain or being in constant pain. When you provide care for a person with arthritis, such as Mrs. Chatterjee, focus on the following things:

❖ Let the person know that you understand how painful movement is for her and that you are there to help her. Let her know you are concerned for her well-being. Ask her about the things that make movement easier for her.

❖ If the person takes medication, plan her daily morning care after she takes her morning dose. When she has less pain, she may be more in control and able to participate in her own care.

❖ Because warm water is soothing to the joints and helps reduce stiffness and pain, give her tub baths as often as possible. Make sure the water temperature is not too hot.

❖ To reduce stiffness and pain, encourage the person to wear warm clothing that covers the affected joints.

❖ Do gentle range-of-motion exercises to prevent contractures. Never move a joint that is painful, red, or swollen.
❖ Handle the person's joints carefully and support the areas above and below the joint when you move her. This care decreases the pain that accompanies movement of the joints.
❖ Encourage the person to exercise her affected joints on her own. This activity promotes independence and keeps her joints more flexible.

A person who has an arthritic jaw joint may not be able to open her mouth or chew food comfortably. If she has arthritis in her hands, she may not be able to hold a toothbrush or comb. Personal care, especially mouth care, needs to be assessed for a person who has arthritis. Depending on which joints are affected, encourage a person with arthritis to maintain her independence through the use of joint-protection techniques, such as—

❖ Attaching cloth loops to drawer handles to make them easier to open.
❖ Pushing doors open with the side of her arm instead of her hand and outstretched arm.
❖ Using the palms of both hands to lift and hold items such as cups, plates, and pots and pans.
❖ Using a cart to transport heavy items from place to place, instead of carrying them in her arms.

Providing Care for a Person Who Has Osteoporosis

When you first meet Charlotte Bryan, a delicate-looking woman of 68, she tells you how, for the past several years, she had been feeling pain in her back. "But I told myself, 'I don't have time to feel pain. I have too much to do,' so I ignored the pain," she said. "Then my favorite dresses seemed too long, and they didn't seem to hang right across my shoulders. 'Am I growing shorter?' I wondered. One sunny October morning, I began opening my bedroom window. Suddenly, I felt a great pain in my back and I fell to the floor. Slowly I inched across the floor to the telephone and called for help.

"After doing a series of tests and x-rays, my doctor told me I had osteoporosis. He said that, when I opened the window, the bones in my spinal column were not strong enough to support my muscles, and some of them broke. From now on, I have to be very careful not to fall because all the bones in my body have become weak and brittle."

Characteristics and symptoms of osteoporosis. Osteoporosis occurs mainly in women as they get older, often striking women who are in their 60s and 70s. The disease is caused by a gradual loss of minerals, especially calcium, in the bones. Calcium helps make bones hard and strong. When calcium is lacking, bones become soft and weak, and they break more easily. The spinal column of a person with osteoporosis shrinks, and the person becomes shorter. She may have a rounded upper back and stooped posture (Figure 16-2). As the disease progresses, she may have severe pain in the parts of the body that support her weight. She often tires easily and fears falling while walking.

The plan of care.   Imagine how a person with osteoporosis might feel. Imagine how you would feel about losing the ability to move without pain, having to depend on others, and always fearing that you are going to break a bone. When providing care for a person who has osteoporosis, such as Mrs. Bryan, focus mainly on safety. In addition, do the following things:

❖   Help the person exercise as much as she is able to do comfortably. Gentle exercise may help slow down bone loss.

❖   If the doctor orders a safety belt for the person, use it when helping her walk or move. The safety belt helps to support her and prevent falls. Use the belt very carefully. Remember, her bones are very fragile.

❖   Clear the paths and hallways near the person's room. Make sure that chairs are the proper height for her and that grab bars are fastened in appropriate places. This precaution helps reduce the risk of injury.

❖   Help her choose clothes that do not emphasize posture changes.

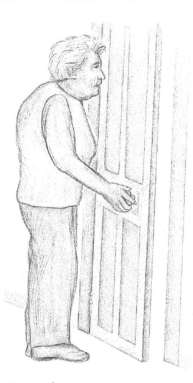

Figure 16-2
A person who has osteoporosis often has a hump at the base of her neck. This happens when the bones of the upper spine weaken and collapse.

Chronic Conditions of the Cardiovascular System

In Chapter 8, Measuring Life Signs, you read about the cardiovascular system and its pumping system—the heart and blood vessels—that transports nutrients and oxygen to all the tissues of the body and then carries away the wastes from these same tissues. You may know someone who has heart disease, because disease of the cardiovascular system is the leading cause of death in the United States.

Two chronic illnessess that result from poor functioning of the cardiovascular system are **angina pectoris** and **congestive heart failure**. Someone who has either of these illnesses may be afraid to do certain things, such as walking or working, for fear of making his condition worse. Your role is crucial because you can provide encouragement and help in alleviating fears. When providing care for someone who has a cardiovascular condition, you should always be on the lookout for the signs of a heart attack, which are described in Box 16-1 on p. 356.

angina pectoris
(an-JY-nuh/PEK-to-ris)   The medical term for heart pain.

congestive heart failure
(kun-JES-tiv)   A condition of the cardiovascular system in which weakened heart muscles prevent the heart from working effectively.

Providing Care for a Person Who Has Angina Pectoris

Today, when you go to 67-year-old Max Richardson's room, you knock on the door several times, but there is no answer. You knock again, call his name, and go in. Inside, you find Mr. Richardson slumped in a chair, clutching his chest. You approach him, softly call out his name, touch him gently on the arm, tell him who you are, and ask him what is wrong and if he is in pain.

Mr. Richardson whispers, "I need my medicine. I have pains in my

Box 16-1   Signs of a Heart Attack

When providing care for people who have heart disease, it also is especially important to recognize these signs of a heart attack:

❖ Persistent chest pain that is not relieved by resting, changing position, or medicating with nitroglycerin or that may travel to the jaw or down the arms
❖ Difficulty in breathing or shortness of breath
❖ Flushed, pale, or slightly bluish skin
❖ Profuse sweating
❖ Change in pulse rate (faster, slower, or an irregular beat)

If you think a person in your care may be having a heart attack, stay with him and signal for help. The nurse will assess the situation and use appropriate emergency procedures. If you provide care in a home to a client who is having a heart attack, call for emergency medical assistance. Help the person remain as calm and quiet as possible until help arrives. Notify your supervising nurse as soon as possible.

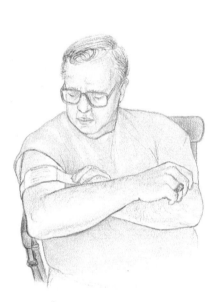

Figure 16-3
A person with angina may receive a continuous supply of nitroglycerin through a patch on the skin. The patch is replaced on a regular schedule.

chest." You signal your supervising nurse and tell her about Mr. Richardson. She brings the medicine, and Mr. Richardson places a tablet under his tongue. After a few minutes, you are relieved to see that he is sitting up and feeling better.

Characteristics and symptoms of angina pectoris.   Mr. Richardson suffers from angina pectoris, an illness that causes chest pain because the heart is not getting enough oxygen. An angina attack can be caused by activity, exercise, or stress. The medication that Mr. Richardson takes to relieve the chest pain is nitroglycerin. He takes it in a pill form under the tongue, although some people take it in the form of patches, which they apply to their skin (Figure 16-3). People suffering from angina who receive home health care usually have a supply of nitroglycerin with them and should know when to take it. In a hospital or nursing home, the medication policy of the facility may allow a person to keep his own supply of nitroglycerin.

The plan of care.   When you provide care for an individual who has angina, encourage him to be as independent as possible without pain by doing the following things:

❖ Provide care in a relaxed and unhurried manner.
❖ Encourage the person to relax and breathe slowly if chest pain occurs. The increase of oxygen produced in the heart muscle reduces the pain.
❖ Tell him to stop an activity if he feels any chest discomfort. This decrease in activity reduces the need for oxygen.
❖ If he smokes, encourage him in his efforts to stop smoking.

Providing Care for a Person Who Has Congestive Heart Failure

Sarah Rogers requires a great deal of care in the nursing home. When she walks from her bed to the chair in her room, when she tries to bathe herself, or even when she eats a meal, she becomes short of breath. Mrs. Rogers is a 60-year-old woman who, for the last 10 years, has lived with congestive heart failure.

Characteristics and symptoms of congestive heart failure.   Congestive heart failure is a chronic heart disease. Because the heart no longer pumps strongly, the person with congestive heart failure may have high blood pressure and a buildup of fluid throughout her body. Some of the symptoms of congestive heart failure are difficulty in breathing, a weight gain due to fluid buildup, and swelling of the feet, legs, hands, and face. The person may feel anxious and restless as a result of her difficulties in breathing, and her symptoms may be worse at some times and milder at others.

The plan of care.   When providing care for a person who has congestive heart failure, focus on helping her with her breathing and monitoring her fluid intake. In addition, do the following things:

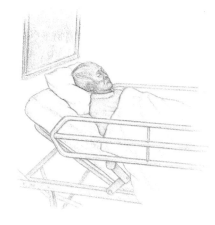

Figure 16-4
A person with congestive heart failure will often find it easier to breathe while sitting up in a Fowler's position. A person with this disease also may sleep this way or with pillows to prop her up.

❖   Provide frequent rest periods when helping the person with daily care activities. People with congestive heart failure often become tired after only a little exertion.

❖   Help her maintain a comfortable position, preferably a sitting position supported by pillows, that allows her to breathe more comfortably (Figure 16-4). Keep her legs elevated to reduce swelling of the legs and feet.

❖   Provide special mouth care. A person with congestive heart failure may breathe through her mouth or receive oxygen, which makes her mouth dry.

❖   Provide frequent opportunities for her to use the toilet. Medication for an individual with congestive heart failure can increase both urinary output and frequency of urination. As always, answer call signals immediately.

❖   Measure and record intake, output, and weight every day. These measures are used to determine how well the person is eliminating excess fluid. A person with congestive heart failure may also have a fluid-restricted diet.

Because congestive heart failure is a chronic disease that Mrs. Rogers must live with for the rest of her life, she may be depressed sometimes. She needs encouragement and support. Involve her in her plan of care. Help her see that by pacing her activity during the day, she accomplishes more.

Chronic Conditions of the Endocrine System

You read about the endocrine system in Chapter 4, Understanding People. When glands in the endocrine system fail to function properly, certain conditions and diseases may result. One very common disease of the endocrine system is diabetes, or diabetes mellitus. When providing care for a person who has diabetes, remember that she has a chronic disease. She may feel frustrated with the way her body fails to function properly, and she may have a hard time adapting to a new diet and demanding schedule. Your role is crucial. You are the one who can help the person turn this intrusion on her life into an acceptable way of living.

Providing Care for a Person Who Has Diabetes

As a home health aide, you regularly visit Dorothy Roth, a 73-year-old woman who developed **Type II diabetes** when she was 65 years old. Mrs. Roth says she has "sugar in the blood." She used to control her diabetes with a special diet, but recently she started taking an oral medication as well. Two of your responsibilities are to monitor her diet and remind her to take her medication.

Characteristics and symptoms of diabetes.   Diabetes mellitus occurs when the body is not producing enough insulin to help it break down, store, and use the sugar and starches in food for energy. As people grow older, they have a greater chance of becoming diabetic. There is no cure for diabetes, but it can be managed through diet, exercise, and medication. The medication may be pills that help the body produce and use insulin, or it may be insulin injections. People may develop **Type I diabetes**, or they may develop the type of diabetes Mrs. Roth has.

Several years ago, Mrs. Roth began feeling tired constantly, even though she was getting enough sleep. She always felt thirsty and needed to urinate more often than usual. She told her doctor about these symptoms and, after a few tests, he told her she had diabetes. Other symptoms of diabetes may include the following:

❖ Itching all over the body
❖ Numbness in the hands and toes
❖ Slow healing of a sore or infection
❖ Blurred vision

Diet is the most important part of managing diabetes. Mrs. Roth, like all people with diabetes, is on a special diet that is low in sugar and fat. She must eat only foods specifically prepared for her. She should not have candy, cookies, or other sweets. Her diet and medication help control the amount of sugar that is in her blood at any one time. This balance is important to her well-being. Too little sugar in the blood (called hypoglycemia) can cause—

❖ Dizziness.
❖ Shakiness.
❖ Sudden change in behavior (combative, argumentative, aggressive, or angry).
❖ Cool, clammy skin.
❖ Seizures.

If you notice someone who has diabetes having any of these symptoms, tell your supervising nurse immediately.

Too much sugar in the bloodstream (called hyperglycemia) can cause—

Type II diabetes
(dye-uh-BEE-tez)   A form of diabetes in which the output of insulin from the pancreas is inadequate for the body's needs. Also called maturity onset or insulin-independent diabetes, Type II diabetes often develops later in life.

Type I diabetes
A form of diabetes in which the pancreas produces very little or no insulin. Also called juvenile onset or insulin-dependent diabetes.

❖   Tiredness.

❖   Grogginess.

❖   Hot, dry skin.

❖   Breath that has a fruity smell.

❖   Coma.

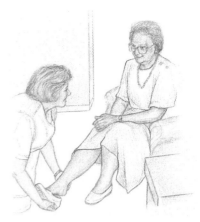

Figure 16-5
A person with diabetes often has poor circulation and may not realize that her shoes don't fit properly until a sore develops. To detect early signs of trouble, regularly inspect the tops and bottoms of her feet for red or sore areas.

If you notice any of these symptoms in someone who has diabetes, tell your supervising nurse immediately.

A person with diabetes can have many complications, such as vision problems and poor healing of any cut or wound, especially on the hands or feet.

The plan of care.   When you carry out a plan of care for a person with diabetes, such as Mrs. Roth, focus your care on the following things:

❖   Provide good skin care to prevent pressure sores. Keeping the skin clean and dry is important.

❖   Provide good foot care. Examine her feet each day for small cuts or breaks in her skin. In people who have diabetes, cuts do not heal well because of decreased circulation, and even the smallest cut can become badly infected. The sensation of touch also may be impaired, and a person with diabetes may not feel an injury (Figure 16-5).

❖   Inform your supervising nurse when the person's toenails need to be cut. Because of the risk of injuring the person, only a doctor, licensed nurse, or podiatrist may cut her toenails.

❖   Tell your supervising nurse if the person is not eating her food or is eating food brought in by friends or relatives. She should follow her diet strictly to avoid complications of the disease.

❖   If urine testing is ordered, make sure you test for sugar and acetone accurately and on time. Regular testing helps monitor sugar levels daily. Some people test their blood for glucose levels at regular intervals during the day.

❖   Report any change in the usual amount of exercise, activity, or stress in the person's life. Diet and dosage of insulin may have to be adjusted to help maintain balance.

❖   Encourage the person to exercise, because it improves circulation and helps the person keep a positive attitude.

❖   In home health care, be prepared to assist a person who has symptoms of hypoglycemia or hyperglycemia. If the person is conscious and can take food or fluids, give her sugar—dry sugar, sugar dissolved in water, candy, fruit juice, or a nondiet soft drink. If the person has hypoglycemia, the sugar will help quickly. If the person has hyperglycemia, the excess sugar will do no further harm. If the person does not respond within 5 minutes, or if her condition worsens, call EMS personnel immediately. If the person is unconscious, do not give her anything by mouth. Call EMS immediately and monitor her vital signs while waiting for their arrival.

Chronic Conditions of the Respiratory System

In Chapter 8 you read about the respiratory system and how the lungs supply your body with oxygen and rid your body of carbon dioxide. Two disorders of the respiratory system are chronic obstructive pulmonary disease, or **COPD**, and **tuberculosis**, or **TB**. When providing care for a person with a respiratory illness, remember that she has a chronic condition. She may be afraid because she can't breathe well. Your role is crucial, because you can help her stay calm and learn to live with her illness.

Providing Care for a Person Who Has COPD

You are ready to help a new patient, Mrs. Reilly, a 75-year-old woman who is being admitted to the hospital because she is suffering from dyspnea, has difficulty breathing, and is perspiring. Both her feet are swollen, and she is afraid. You try to imagine what it would be like to have difficulty breathing and to be afraid that you are not going to be able to catch your next breath or that you may die. You know how important it is to try to calm Mrs. Reilly, because extreme fear increases shortness of breath and difficulty in breathing.

When you observe Mrs. Reilly, you notice cyanosis: Her skin has a bluish-gray color, her fingernails look bluish, and her lips look dark. These signs mean that not enough oxygen is circulating in her body.

Characteristics and symptoms of COPD.   Mrs. Reilly has been diagnosed with an acute flare-up of COPD. Many lung diseases are grouped together in this category, including chronic bronchitis, emphysema, and asthma.

Symptoms of COPD include the following:

❖   Coughing up a great deal of mucus
❖   A tendency to tire easily
❖   Little appetite
❖   Bent posture with shoulders elevated and lips pursed to make breathing easier
❖   A fast pulse
❖   Round, barrel-shaped chest
❖   Confusion (caused by lack of oxygen circulating in the body)

The plan of care.   Mrs. Reilly tells you that she has been a smoker for years. In fact, she still smokes. Even though she has great difficulty breathing, she tells you she would really like to have a cigarette. She tells you she has had chronic respiratory infections over the past 20 years and is now trying to live with COPD (Figure 16-6).

When providing care for a person who has COPD, focus on helping her breathe more easily and do the following:

❖   Encourage the person to take four or five deep breaths often during the day. Deep breathing helps fill the lungs with air and maintains flexibility in the chest wall.
❖   Encourage her to relax and breathe slowly but as deeply as possible. Relaxation and slow, deep breathing increase the flow of

COPD
An abbreviation for **c**hronic **o**bstructive **p**ulmonary **d**isease, a condition of the respiratory system, which includes emphysema, asthma, and chronic bronchitis — diseases that are long term and interfere with the body's ability to breath efficiently.

tuberculosis
(to-ber-cue-LOW-sis)   A contagious bacterial infection of the lungs.

TB
An abbreviation for **tub**erculosis.

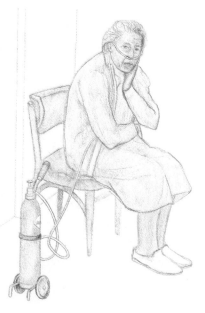

Figure 16-6
A person with advanced COPD spends much of her energy breathing. She may not be able to say long sentences or express an entire thought without stopping to take a breath.

oxygen to the lungs. Often the person learns special breathing exercises that improve her ability to relax and breathe slowly.

❖ Provide special mouth care. A person with COPD may breathe through her mouth or receive oxygen, making her mouth dry.

❖ If a person is receiving oxygen therapy, check regularly to see that tubes are in place and not kinked. Follow your employer's rules about oxygen. If a person is using a nasal **cannula**, provide skin care to the skin around her nose.

cannula
(KAN-you-luh)   A tube placed under the nostrils to deliver oxygen.

❖ Provide a bedside commode when the person needs it. Sometimes using the commode is easier than getting to the bathroom. A commode is also more comfortable than a bedpan.

❖ Offer small, frequent meals if necessary. This meal plan ensures adequate nutrition and reduces fatigue.

❖ Encourage a person with COPD not to smoke. Remind her that no smoking is permitted if a person is receiving oxygen.

❖ Encourage her to cough to help clear air passages of excess mucus.

To help maintain her independence, let Mrs. Reilly set her own pace for activities. When she has some control over her life, she feels better about herself and is better able to cope with her illness.

Providing Care for a Person Who Has TB

You learn from Jim Minton's wife that he is 39 years old and works long hours, and that they live in a crowded apartment with nine other family members. Often there isn't enough food to go around. Several months ago, Mr. Minton began to cough. At first, she says, it was just in the morning, but lately he coughs throughout the day and often coughs up blood-tinged mucus. Mrs. Minton says that her husband complains of feeling tired all the time and she learned that, instead of eating during his lunch break, he sleeps. It's obvious to her that he's losing weight, and she worries because he wakes up at night soaked through with sweat. His whole family is concerned about him, she says, and they finally convinced him to come to the clinic to see a doctor.

After running some tests and taking x-rays, Mr. Minton's doctor tells him he has TB.

Characteristics and symptoms of TB.   TB is a bacterial infection of the lungs. Before the discovery of appropriate antibacterial drugs, TB almost always was fatal. In the 1950s, it was considered one of the nation's most pressing public health problems. An aggressive battle to conquer the illness through a network of clinics, outreach workers, and screening programs was very successful in steadily lowering the spread of the disease. Partly because of its success, money to continue the effort became less available.

Today the United States is seeing a large number of new cases of TB. Many of these new cases appear among the homeless and people whose immune systems have been weakened, such as people with AIDS. Lack of treatment for people with TB has increased the seriousness, as well as the spread, of the disease. People who could have been treated with a course of medication are requiring repeated hospital stays, and people who would not have been infected are becoming infected.

The standard treatment for TB is a course of medicines taken for 6 to 9 months. When hospitalization is required, it is for the initial evaluation, the treatment of side effects from the medicine, or the treatment of the disease itself or another illness and usually not for an extended time as in the past. Of rising concern to public health officials, however, is the occurrence of new strains of the organism that causes TB. These new strains are not responding to the usual drugs and treatment of the disease, resulting in lengthy or repeated hospitalizations to gain control of the disease.

Mr. Minton's doctor tells him that he must take medicine for a long time, 6 to 9 months, and that his family also must be checked, because some of them might have to be on medicine too. The good news is that, after a period of time to rest and regain some strength and to allow the medicine to work, Mr. Minton can return to work. It is essential, however, that he continue to take the medicine regularly and not skip doses, because the organism could become resistant to the medicine. If the organism changed, the medicine would no longer be able to fight the disease.

TB is highly contagious and is spread by droplets sprayed into the air by coughing, talking, or sneezing. Droplets can contain active bacteria even after being in the air for 9 hours. In a few days after starting the medication, a person's sputum generally won't spread infection. But until then, the person and caregivers must take precautions to prevent the spread of the disease.

The plan of care.   Because TB is highly contagious, you should focus on infection control when providing care for a person newly diagnosed with the disease and do the following things:

❖   Wear a mask when assisting with personal care. Wearing a gown isn't necessary unless your clothing might possibly be contaminated.

❖   Ask the person to cover his mouth with a tissue when coughing so that bacteria are not sprayed into the air. Have him discard the tissue into a plastic bag. Arrange for the contents to be burned.

❖   Early in his treatment, have the person wear a mask when he is in close contact with other people. This mask prevents droplets from being spread into the air, where they can be breathed in by someone else (Figure 16-7).

❖   Install and use a window fan to circulate the air in closed rooms.

❖   Practice good handwashing techniques.

❖   Make sure the person's plan of care includes good nutrition and adequate rest.

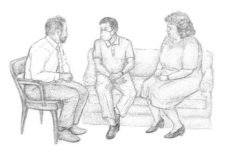

Figure 16-7
Early in his treatment, a person with tuberculosis wears a protective mask when he is with his family and friends to reduce their risk of catching TB.

❖   Make sure his diet is well balanced and adequate in calories to promote good healing and rebuilding of lost body mass.

❖   Plan rest periods for the person during the day to minimize fatigue.

People may have fears and misconceptions about TB. These feelings and ideas may interfere with their following the doctor's instructions about treatment and follow-up. By encouraging the person and the family to talk about their fears, the caregiver may be able to identify and correct misconceptions and lessen fears.

Chronic Conditions of the Urinary System

In Chapter 13, Elimination, you read about the urinary system, the body's filtering system that eliminates waste in the form of urine. When that system fails to function properly, several conditions can result. **Kidney failure** is an example of a chronic condition of the urinary system. When providing care for a person who has kidney failure, remember that he has a chronic illness. He may feel depressed about his need for regular treatment. In your role, you can give him emotional support and encouragement to adapt to his illness.

kidney failure
A condition of the urinary system that occurs when the kidneys no longer function and are unable to get rid of the body's waste.

Providing Care for a Person Who Has Kidney Failure

Sam Green has had diabetes since he was 9 years old, and now, at the age of 50, his doctor has ordered him to go on peritoneal dialysis to filter wastes from his blood. His kidneys no longer function. When Mr. Green has dialysis, a solution is introduced into his abdomen, where it absorbs the waste, and then it is drained out. Mr. Green has been told that, like most people on dialysis, he will no longer urinate through the urethra, and he feels like he has lost a normal body function.

Before going on dialysis, Mr. Green had retired from his job because of his progressing illness. He had begun to experience increased fatigue, nausea, increased blood pressure, and decreased urine output. His diabetes also was becoming increasingly difficult to control.

Now that he is on dialysis, he doesn't have as many food and fluid restrictions as he did before he started the treatments, and he feels better. He and his doctor also have been talking about the possibility of a kidney transplant. But he worries. He often worries about his uncertain future and about the cost of the treatment and medications. Sometimes he resents the restrictions his illness places on his independence, and sometimes he feels guilty about his wife's having to do more of the work around the house. He always talks to you about these feelings when you come to his house to provide care.

Characteristics and symptoms of kidney failure.   Kidney failure, also called renal failure, results from the kidney's inability to get rid of

ESRD
An abbreviation for **e**nd-**s**tage **r**enal **d**isease, a condition of the urinary system.

waste products. In its late stage, it is often referred to as end-stage renal disease, or **ESRD**. Renal failure can be the result of an acute disease or of an injury that causes the kidneys to stop functioning temporarily. Renal failure also can be a complication of certain chronic diseases such as diabetes.

When waste products accumulate in the body, they produce some of the following symptoms:

❖ Fatigue, weakness, and confusion
❖ Muscle twitching or cramping
❖ Nausea, vomiting, and an unpleasant taste in the mouth, which often lead to poor nutrition
❖ Itching skin, often severe
❖ High blood pressure
❖ Extreme thinness with little muscle mass, if the renal failure goes on for a long time

People with renal failure often need dialysis, a process that filters waste products from the blood using a special filtering solution. Two types of dialysis are peritoneal dialysis and hemodialysis. Peritoneal dialysis involves injecting a solution through the abdominal wall and then withdrawing it after a period of time. The peritoneum, the membrane lining the abdominal cavity, acts as a filter for waste products. Usually the person has a permanent catheter in place through which the dialyzing fluid is administered and withdrawn. Hemodialysis uses a machine to clean the blood of waste products. It relies on a permanent "shunt" or port where the machine can be connected. The shunt may be located on the person's forearm or ankle (Figure 16-8). Some forms of dialysis can be done in home care. Dialysis can be used to maintain the health of the person with renal failure in preparation for a kidney transplant.

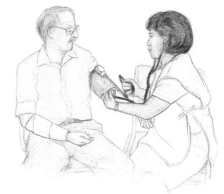

Figure 16-8
If a person has a hemodialysis shunt on his arm, take his blood pressure on the other arm to avoid damaging the shunt.

The plan of care.   When providing care for a person with kidney failure, such as Mr. Green, focus on the following things:

❖ Encourage the person to rest.
❖ Carefully monitor and report his food and fluid intake. Encourage his food intake in accordance with his diet plan.
❖ Plan activities of daily living to conserve the person's energy and to provide for periods of rest, because a person with kidney failure may frequently have periods of wakefulness at night.
❖ Take increased care to prevent infections. If the person is on dialysis, pay special attention to keeping the access site (either for peritoneal dialysis or hemodialysis) clean and dry. Keep his skin in good condition without breaks or sores that could become infected.

Help Mr. Green retain his independence by encouraging him to perform as many of his activities of daily living as possible. Encourage him and his family members to talk about their concerns.

Chronic Conditions of the Nervous System

A variety of conditions affects the nervous system. You read in Chapter 4 that the nervous system is like a communication center. Messages are sent to the brain from all parts of the body and, after organizing the information, the brain tells the body what to do.

One kind of problem with the nervous system results from an interruption of activity in the nerves or spinal cord, usually caused by an injury. Parts of the brain also can be damaged. The condition occurs when it becomes impossible for messages to get back and forth from the brain to other parts of the body.

Mental retardation and mental illness also are considered conditions of the nervous system because they involve the brain. Multiple sclerosis, stroke, paraplegia, quadriplegia, Parkinson's disease, and mental depression also are chronic conditions of the nervous system. When providing care for a person who has a disorder of the nervous system, remember that he has a chronic illness that may be difficult for him and his family to deal with. In your role, you can support and encourage the person, as well as his family.

Alzheimer's disease is one of several diseases classified as cognitive impairment. These diseases impair a person's thinking and reasoning abilities. You will read more about cognitive impairment in Chapter 18, Providing Care for People Who Have Alzheimer's Disease.

Providing Care for a Person Who Has Multiple Sclerosis

You just finished visiting with Charlene Hunter, a 35-year-old mother who has had multiple sclerosis for the past 5 years. Mrs. Hunter has some difficulty walking, and she often loses her balance. She also has muscle tremors and muscle weakness, so sometimes she drops a plate or glass. Over the past few months, she has had problems with bladder control and she says she feels embarrassed when she loses control. Today she told you that the bladder problem is getting worse.

You think about how frustrating it must be for Mrs. Hunter to cope with this disease. She says she sometimes feels depressed. She knows the disease will get worse, and she says she feels helpless and out of control. She is afraid of becoming more disabled and unable to take care of her 2-year-old son (Figure 16-9).

Characteristics and symptoms of MS.
Multiple sclerosis, or **MS**, is a chronic disease that gradually destroys the coating on nerve endings in the brain and spinal cord. This condition creates a situation like a short circuit or crossed wire. Nerves cannot communicate with each other or with the brain. The disease usually begins when a person is between 20 and 40 years old. What makes MS different from other diseases with similar symptoms is that the symptoms usually appear and disappear over a period of years. During the time that symptoms disappear, the person is said to be in remission There is no cure for MS.

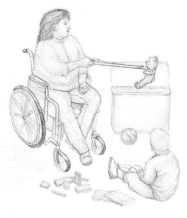

Figure 16-9
Assistive devices, such as the wheelchair and grabber, make it possible for a woman with disabilities to remain at home and help provide care for her son.

MS
An abbreviation for **m**ultiple **s**clerosis.

Symptoms of MS include the following:

❖ Feelings of numbness, tingling, and burning
❖ Overwhelming fatigue at all times
❖ Vision problems (double vision, blurred vision, or both)
❖ Insomnia
❖ Speech problems (slurring, using the wrong name for an object, slowness in replying to others)
❖ Bowel and bladder problems (constipation, incontinence)
❖ Fits of anger or crying (she may shut down her emotions to control her mood swings and may be intensely anxious or fearful)
❖ Paralysis
❖ Forgetfulness and slowness in understanding what is said to her
❖ **Edema** and cold feet due to lack of circulation (parts of the body affected by edema must be massaged to retain joint flexibility)

edema
(uh-DEE-muh)   Swelling of body tissue due to an accumulation of fluid.

The plan of care.   Your role is a challenging one as you carry out the plan of care for a person with MS, such as Mrs. Hunter. Focus on maintaining mobility and bowel and bladder control. Also help the person focus on what she can do, not on what she can't do. Use the following caregiving techniques:

❖ Do passive range-of-motion exercises on the person's affected limbs, and encourage her to do active range-of-motion exercises when possible. Range-of-motion exercises prevent contractures and maintain joint mobility. Encourage her to actively help with exercises.
❖ Encourage the person to eat meals high in fiber. High-fiber foods help maintain healthy elimination. The use of laxatives also may be necessary.
❖ Encourage her to drink lots of fluids. High fluid intake increases urination and helps prevent bladder and kidney infections. High fluid intake is also important for bowel regularity. Often people with incontinence problems think reducing fluid intake solves the problem, but it doesn't.
❖ Encourage warm tub baths when possible, but make sure the water is not too hot. Warm water reduces muscle spasms (cramping), but hot water causes weakness and fainting.

Encourage Mrs. Hunter to do as much as possible for herself so that she can be more independent. Remind her to pace herself and rest as needed so that she doesn't overdo it. Listen to Mrs. Hunter, and encourage her to express her feelings to you. Also encourage her to participate in activities and maintain friendships outside her home so that she doesn't isolate herself.

Providing Care for a Person Who Had a Stroke

You provide care regularly for Bernie Avery, a 65-year-old resident at Morningside Nursing Home. He had a stroke 5 years ago and, as a result, is paralyzed on his right side. You often think about how it must feel to be unable to move your arm and leg on one side of your body, or how frustrated he must feel when he wants to say something, but the words won't come to him. Thinking about his feelings helps you understand why Mr. Avery is often depressed.

Characteristics resulting from a stroke.   Stroke is another term for a **cerebrovascular accident**, or **CVA**. A stroke can cause paralysis, usually on one side. This condition is called hemiplegia. A stroke can result in weakness on one side instead of paralysis. This condition is called hemiparesis. Other possible characteristics resulting from a stroke are the following:

❖ A decreased sense of pain, touch, and temperature on the paralyzed side
❖ Bowel and bladder incontinence
❖ Difficulty speaking, reading, or writing (he may want to say something, but the words won't come to him, or he may not be able to understand what other people say—a condition called aphasia)

The plan of care.   When carrying out the plan of care for a person who has had a stroke, such as Mr. Avery, focus on the characteristics of his condition. This focus will help him regain function of his arm or leg. Also promote safety issues related to his loss of sensation, encourage his independence, and do the following things:

❖ Do passive range-of-motion exercises on the person's affected limbs. Range-of-motion exercises prevent contractures and maintain joint mobility. Encourage him to use the unaffected side of his body to exercise his paralyzed side as much as he is able (Figure 16-10).
❖ Supervise the person while he eats. If you have to feed him, always put food in the side of his mouth that is not affected by paralysis. Make sure no food is left in his mouth after a meal is finished. Not being able to feel food in the mouth increases the risk of choking. Make sure he sits up while he eats so that he can swallow food more easily.
❖ Since the person may drool on the paralyzed side and his skin may become irritated, keep his face clean and dry. If possible, apply a protective skin cream.
❖ Supervise the person while he shaves. He may miss spots that he cannot feel, or he may cut himself and not feel it.
❖ Offer to help complete any personal care activities that may be difficult because of his weakness or paralysis.
❖ Help him walk, following the physical therapist's directions. Walk at his weaker side unless the physical therapist directs otherwise. He may need a walker or cane to steady himself.
❖ Raise the person's paralyzed arm on a pillow when he is in bed. Support the arm with a sling when he is out of bed. Paralyzed

cerebrovascular accident (suh-ree-bro-VAS-kyu-ler) An interruption of blood flow to a part of the brain, which results in the death of a few or many brain cells.

CVA An abbreviation for **c**erebro**v**ascular **a**ccident.

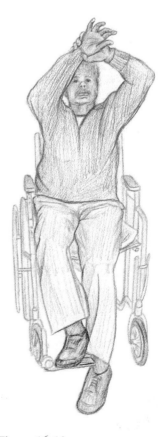

Figure 16-10
This man, with paralysis on his right side, maintains his independence by taking responsibility for his range-of-motion exercises.

limbs have poor circulation, and raising the arm helps keep blood from pooling. Supporting the arm also prevents swelling and may help him feel that he has better balance.

❖ Put articles that the person needs, such as eyeglasses, hearing aid, telephone, and glass of water, within reach on his unaffected side.

❖ Put the call signal within reach on his unaffected side.

Encourage Mr. Avery to do as much as possible for himself so that he can be more independent. If the dominant side of his body is affected, he may have to relearn how to do activities using his other hand. Encourage Mr. Avery to use adaptive devices for eating, mouth care, and other activities to maintain his independence. Give him encouragement and support. He needs to feel good about himself.

Providing Care for a Person Who Has Paraplegia or Quadriplegia

When you visit Karen Bowman, she often asks you to turn the pages of her scrapbook, which is filled with pictures and mementos of her glorious days of swimming competition. She started competing in swimming events when she was 6 years old. Now, at age 22, she sits at home in a wheelchair—a quadriplegic, with no feeling in her arms, legs, or lower trunk.

Some days, Miss Bowman becomes very angry and tells you about how stupid she was to go drinking and swimming with her sorority sisters. "If I hadn't been drinking, I would have noticed that the water was too shallow for diving. Now, look at me. Useless. Absolutely useless."

Characteristics of paraplegia and quadriplegia. Paralysis is a loss of the ability to move parts of the body that results from a brain or spinal cord injury. Paralysis can affect one side of the body (hemiplegia), two legs and the lower trunk (paraplegia), or both arms, both legs, and the lower trunk (quadriplegia), depending on where damage has occurred on the spinal cord or in the brain and how severe it is. The area affected with paralysis depends on where the spinal cord has been injured. An injury in the lower back or at waist level can result in paraplegia. An injury in the neck or upper back can result in quadriplegia.

Often this kind of injury happens suddenly, as in an automobile collision. Many broken necks also result from diving into shallow water. If a person breaks her neck, her spinal cord can be severely damaged, although her brain works and thinking is not impaired. However, the brain cannot send messages to the body, and it cannot receive messages from the body.

In paraplegia or quadriplegia, the affected parts of a person's body lose the following body functions partly or completely:

❖ Sensation (pain, temperature, pressure, touch, vibration)
❖ Fine motor movement (small movements, such as writing, sewing, and using a fork and knife)

* Gross motor movement (large movements, such as lifting arms or legs)
* Ability to maintain body temperature
* Balance
* Bladder and bowel control
* Breathing, without some form of assistance

The plan of care.   When providing care for someone with paraplegia or quadriplegia, focus your caregiving on promoting independence and safety related to the person's difficulty in movement and loss of sensation. Also do the following things:

* Keep the skin clean and dry and use lotions on rough or irritated areas. Provide good skin care to prevent pressure sores. Turn or reposition the person every 2 hours. Assure proper body alignment. Be sure to elevate the hand of the affected arm above the elbow. Use rolled towels or a pillow to ensure that the affected leg does not rotate outward. Use footboards or special boots when necessary.
* Be aware that the person's ability to feel is impaired. He is unable to recognize pain and temperature and loses awareness of how his affected body parts are positioned.
* Encourage a person with paralysis to use self-help devices for eating, walking, or mouth care. He may have a spoon or fork with a special grip, or a brace or splint on a paralyzed limb. Using crutches or a walker also may help (Figure 16-11).
* Help with a bladder or bowel training program. (See Chapter 13 for more information on bladder and bowel training programs.)
* Encourage a person with paralysis to do as much as possible for himself so that he can be as independent as possible.
* Provide emotional support.

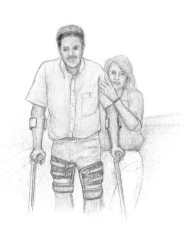

Figure 16-11
After strengthening his arms and shoulders, a person with paraplegia may be able to walk with crutches.

Providing Care for a Person Who Has Parkinson's Disease

Patrick O'Malley is a 70-year-old man who has had Parkinson's disease for the past 20 years. He has muscle weakness and his arms shake (muscle tremors). He has a tremor that causes his hands to move in a "pill-rolling" motion. His posture is slumped, he bends forward, and he shuffles when he walks. Because his balance is poor, he falls frequently.

When you first provided care for Mr. O'Malley, he was able to do many things for himself, although with great difficulty. Now, his hands shake uncontrollably, and he can barely grasp and hold onto anything. He also drools and has difficulty chewing his food.

Characteristics and symptoms of Parkinson's disease.   Parkinson's disease is one of the most common nervous system disorders that affects older people. In Parkinson's disease, the parts of the brain that control movement are gradually destroyed. A person with Parkinson's disease has stiff muscles, moves very slowly, and has muscle tremors, which cause shaking or repetitive motions of the muscles, especially those of the hands (Figure 16-12). As the disease progresses, the person's **gait** is affected, and greater physical effort is required to do even the smallest task. As a result, the person easily becomes tired and frustrated. The disease usually appears when a person is in his 50s or 60s. The cause is unknown.

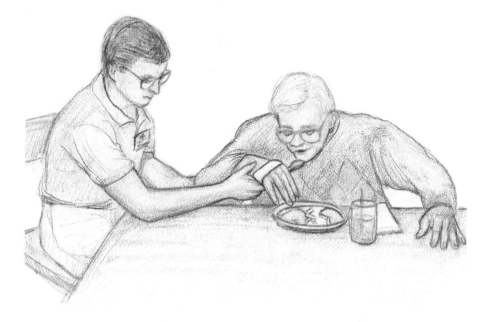

Figure 16-12
Even though a person with Parkinson's disease may have constantly shaking hands, he can feed himself with an assistive device and a little help from the nurse assistant.

Symptoms of Parkinson's disease include the following:

- ❖ Lack of facial expression
- ❖ Difficulty chewing and swallowing
- ❖ Drooling
- ❖ Low-pitched, soft, slow, and monotonous speech
- ❖ Constipation
- ❖ Confusion
- ❖ Mood changes
- ❖ Depression and loss of interest

The plan of care. When providing care for a person who has Parkinson's disease, such as Mr. O'Malley, think about his symptoms and focus your caregiving on safety, good nutrition, and mobility by doing the following things:

- ❖ Encourage the person to rest often. Resting prevents him from getting too tired or frustrated.
- ❖ Avoid rushing him. Muscle tremors increase when the person becomes anxious.
- ❖ Give him warm tub baths to help relax his muscles and reduce muscle spasms.
- ❖ Encourage the person to use any self-help devices he may have

for activities of daily living. For example, he may have a comb,
razor, or toothbrush with an extended handle or grip.

❖   When he is walking, remind him to think about standing tall,
swinging his arms, raising his feet, and putting his feet down on
the ground heel first and then rolling up to the toe. A person
with Parkinson's disease has to make a conscious effort to do
what comes naturally to people who can control their movement.

❖   Use a high toilet equipped for use by disabled people, because a
person with Parkinson's disease may have difficulty changing
from a standing to a sitting position.

❖   As the person eats, remind him to think through the process of
swallowing. For example, you might say, "Try keeping your lips
and teeth closed." Or, "How about changing the side that you
chew on so that one side does not get too tired?" Or, "Try lifting
your tongue up and then back, and then swallow."

❖   Offer small, frequent meals and snacks. People with Parkinson's
disease usually lose weight because they become tired before
they finish a meal. They also may be embarrassed by the mess
they make or by how slowly they eat, and they may lose interest
in eating.

❖   Provide emotional support and be especially patient with his
self-help efforts.

Providing Care for a Person Who Has Mental Illness

Rick Baskin's sister Beth told you that things began to happen after
Rick moved back home after college. "He became more and more
withdrawn," she explained. "And when friends approached, he often
would yell, 'Leave me alone.' Sometimes he would get angry for no
reason at all or accuse people of trying to do things to hurt him. One
night, when I came home, I found Rick hiding in the closet. He
seemed very frightened. 'Enemy are all around us,' Rick whispered.
'Do you hear them talking and loading their guns? Hide before they
see you and kill you.' He tried to pull me into the closet with him. I
felt then that my fears were true: Rick was showing signs of mental
illness."

Characteristics and symptoms of mental illness.   Just as our bodies can
become sick, so can our minds. Like a physical illness, mental illness
can last a short while, or it can be a chronic condition that affects a
person for many years, or for his entire life. As with a physical illness, a person with a mental illness may recover if he follows his
prescribed treatment program and is in a supportive and caring environment.

Scientists are still working to find out what causes mental illness.
They think that some kinds of mental illness are caused by the body's
lack of a chemical it needs to function properly. They think other
kinds of mental illness may be caused by extremely stressful experi-

ences. No one knows for sure why some people become mentally ill (Figure 16-13).

A person with mental illness has trouble thinking clearly and realistically, and he may act differently from what is normally expected in a given situation. The symptoms vary, depending on the severity of the mental illness. A person with mental illness may have the following common symptoms:

❖ Confusion about time, places, or people
❖ Difficulty in making decisions
❖ Inability to follow through with routine tasks, including grooming and other self-care activities
❖ Nonsense speech (speaking in sentences that do not fit together or make sense)
❖ Withdrawal (spending much more time alone than usual)
❖ Suspiciousness (being wary of people and things)
❖ Seeing, hearing, smelling, and feeling things that aren't real and talking to people who aren't there

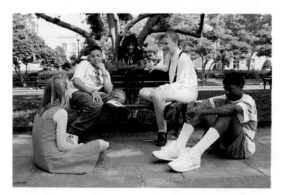

Figure 16-13
It is impossible to tell by looking at this group of young people that one of them may be wrestling with depression, a form of mental illness.

The plan of care.   Providing care for someone with a mental illness is difficult. One person may have mild symptoms and be very receptive to care. Another person may have very severe symptoms and not be responsive to care. A person with mental illness may receive care in an acute care setting or in a specialized hospital. If you choose to work in such a hospital, you will receive special training.

Providing care for a person with mild-to-moderate mental illness.   When providing care for a person with mild-to-moderate mental illness, such as Rick Baskin, focus on treating the person with respect and dignity and on maintaining a routine by doing the following things:

❖ When the person is talking, let him know that you care and are listening to what he is saying. Make eye contact when possible.
❖ Let the person know that you understand what he has said or what he is feeling. For example, you might say, "You look as though you might be feeling sad." Use appropriate facial expressions and have an attentive body posture.
❖ If you cannot take the time to pay attention to what a person is saying, do not pretend to listen to him, but explain that it is not

a good time to talk. This message lets the person know that you *do* care but you cannot give him your full attention at the moment.

❖ Talk to the person in your care about familiar objects, people, or events that are important to him to help him keep track of reality (the season, time, place, and people around him). When the person picks out clothing to wear for the day, talk about how the clothing fits with the weather outside and the person's planned activities.

❖ Praise the person for even the smallest accomplishment. For example, say, "You picked just the right sweater for a cold winter day."

❖ Be consistent. Follow ground rules created by the health care team for how to treat the person. If the person experiences visual or auditory hallucinations, changes in behavior or speech, or increased confusion, report these changes to your supervising nurse.

❖ Help the person keep in touch with what is real. Encourage him to look out the window and watch people coming and going to remind him where he is. Ask him to check clocks and calendars and read newspapers and magazines.

❖ Keep familiar objects close by and avoid changing the person's room or bed position in the room.

❖ Introduce change slowly. When introducing new people or activities, give the person plenty of time to get used to them before introducing other new things. These gradual introductions limit uneasy feelings he may have about change.

❖ Help the person keep a structured routine of meals, medications, personal care, and activities.

❖ If the person becomes loud, angry, or abusive, try to keep your voice calm and your body relaxed. Also, if the person is especially sensitive about other people getting too close, give him space so that he does not feel threatened.

❖ If a person appears likely to hit someone or become violent, get help to handle the situation. Observe safety precautions by clearing the area, keeping distance and objects between you and the person, and removing sharp instruments. (For additional information about providing care to a person who might harm himself or others, read the next section.)

❖ Try to help the person focus on positive things about himself. For example, you might say, "Remember how much your granddaughter enjoyed the pretty picture you painted?" Encourage him to socialize with others and to participate in recreational activities. Staying physically and mentally active is important for him.

Providing care for a person who might cause harm.   To ensure the safety of some people with mental illness who may be at risk of harming themselves or others when left alone, you may be required

suicidal
(sue-uh-SIDE-uhl) A tendency to intentionally and voluntarily harm oneself with the intent to take one's own life.

homicidal
(hom-uh-SIDE-uhl) A tendency to harm other people with the intent to kill.

to provide continuous observation. This is commonly called one-to-one observation. A person who needs one-to-one observation may be confused, **suicidal**, or **homicidal**. Think of how you would feel if you were alone with a person you didn't know who was watching you constantly.

Being sensitive to the person's feelings is important. Talk to him calmly. Treat him with respect. Explain that you are staying with him to ensure his safety. If he feels like talking, encourage him to talk. Allow him quiet time if he prefers. Be a good listener and observer.

Always be aware of the person's actions. If you observe any potentially harmful behavior, act to prevent it. If you think you cannot succeed alone, call for assistance immediately.

Be ready to give your supervising nurse your report when she arrives to check the person (every 1 to 2 hours). Contact your supervising nurse more frequently if you think it is necessary.

Remember, you are doing a lot more than just sitting. Your continuous observation and reporting are crucial to the care and safety of the person.

Review your employer's policy with your supervising nurse before providing care for the person. Learn the following guidelines for a person on one-to-one observation:

❖ Always stay with the person—never leave him alone for any reason. If a person is suicidal, you must be close enough to him to reach out and touch him. You must escort him to the bathroom and stay with him.

❖ Inspect the person's belongings for potentially harmful objects. Remove and label them, and store them in a secure place out of his room.

❖ Remove all potentially harmful objects and substances from the area, including objects the person might throw. Examples of potentially harmful objects are scissors, razors, matches, belts, glass objects, and all liquids.

❖ Make sure visitors have checked in with the nurse before visiting. Make sure all packages and items are inspected for potential risks. Your supervising nurse will tell you who may be alone with the person. This may be a family member who has a full understanding of the person's condition.

❖ Use only plastic forks and spoons at mealtime. Never give any type of knife to suicidal or homicidal people.

❖ Allow smoking only in designated smoking areas and only with staff supervision. Never allow the person to have matches or a cigarette lighter.

❖ Make sure the person wears a hospital gown and slippers.

❖ Make sure a suicidal or homicidal person stays in his room. If he must leave his room for a procedure, you or another person must accompany him.

❖ Give your complete attention for one-to-one observation. Avoid activities, such as reading or watching television, that would distract your attention.

Providing Care for a Person Who Has Mental Depression

Letitia Carpenter never talks to you when you go to her room to provide care. When you try to involve her in conversation, she just turns her head away. Most of what you know about Mrs. Carpenter's condition, you learned from her husband LeMar. He told you that every January Mrs. Carpenter, who is now 43 years old, became depressed but always "snapped out of it" with the first signs of spring. But this year nothing seemed to help—not sunshine, not warmth, not flowers. When Mr. Carpenter found a bottle of sleeping pills and some razor blades in his wife's bedside table, he took her to the hospital and had her admitted.

Characteristics and symptoms of mental depression. Depression is a common mental disorder. It can be defined as a persistent feeling of sadness. Sometimes the depression can be triggered by an event, a trauma, or a loss, but often it is not related to a single event. Signs of depression may be similar to those of a physical illness, and often the person is treated for the physical illness while the depression goes untreated. If a person becomes extremely depressed, she may try to take her own life. Depression is a common problem in the elderly that often is mistaken for confusion or Alzheimer's disease.

Signs of depression include the following:

❖ Sadness
❖ Crying spells
❖ Decreased memory
❖ Inability to concentrate
❖ Low energy
❖ Fatigue
❖ Sleeping problems (too much or too little)
❖ Eating problems (too much or too little)
❖ Isolation and unwillingness to participate in social activities
❖ Irritability
❖ Feelings of helplessness
❖ Feelings of hopelessness
❖ Expression of wanting to kill self
❖ Headaches, muscle aches, backaches, abdominal pain, or nausea
❖ Preoccupation with bodily functions and illness

The plan of care. For a person with depression, a mental health worker usually directs the efforts of the staff. When providing care for a depressed person, such as Mrs. Carpenter, focus on maintaining her safety and increasing her self-esteem. To accomplish this,—

❖ Give the person appropriate positive feedback and reinforce her accomplishments.
❖ Help her express her own strengths and functional abilities.
❖ Work with the person to set simple, attainable goals. Be sure to praise her when she meets the goals.

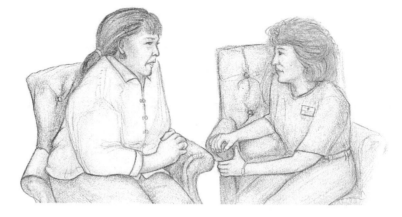

Figure 16-14
Sometimes, if you sit and listen, a depressed person may feel better.

❖ Listen when she expresses sadness (Figure 16-14).

❖ Provide time for the person to cry.

❖ Because her energy level is low, schedule rest periods throughout the day.

❖ Monitor her food intake to make sure that nutrition is adequate.

❖ Provide fluids frequently, because the person may not drink enough fluids on her own.

❖ Report all complaints of pain so that her symptoms do not get overlooked.

❖ Encourage the person to use a prescribed hearing aid or eyeglasses so that she is more in touch with the world around her.

❖ Encourage her to participate in activities, especially those that involve contact with another person and those that are physical, within her limitations. Avoid overly stressful or tiring activities.

❖ Encourage independence to try to build her feeling of self-worth.

Take all comments about suicidal thoughts seriously and report them to your supervising nurse. Report to your supervising nurse when the person—

❖ Shows a dramatic change in mood or behavior, such as increased withdrawal or elevation of mood. Sometimes a person who is deeply depressed and struggles with thoughts of suicide does not have enough energy to carry out a suicide plan. However, once she has finally made the decision to commit suicide, she may feel temporary relief and increased energy so that she can actually follow through with her plan.

❖ Hoards medication or purchases a gun or other weapon.

❖ Gives away her belongings.

❖ Increases her use of alcohol.

❖ Becomes preoccupied with inner thoughts.

❖ Becomes secretive.

Report any sign. Do not conclude that a suicide threat or attempt is just a way to get attention. Especially vulnerable are the very old, a person who has just been diagnosed with a terminal illness, such as cancer or AIDS, or a person who has suffered a severe loss or multiple losses.

Chronic Conditions That Begin in Childhood

Providing care for sick children can be very exhausting and often overwhelming for parents and family members, because sick children require so much attention. They need a parent or other adult around almost all the time to provide care for physical needs and to provide company and activity. This constant need for care can be very taxing on the adults, who also must continue with their other responsibilities of maintaining the household, perhaps taking care of other children, and working at their professions.

In addition, sick children create additional strain on families because of the financial burden that often accompanies acute or chronic illnesses. Parents also may find it difficult to cope emotionally with children's illnesses and often feel guilty or helpless. If the illness results in death, this situation creates yet another emotional hardship on the family.

When providing care for children with muscular dystrophy, cystic fibrosis, cerebral palsy, and mental retardation, remember that you help provide care for the sick child. In addition, you also provide emotional support for the family by keeping them involved in the day-to-day caregiving for the child, by offering them reassurance about the care they are providing, and by listening to their concerns.

Providing Care for a Person Who Has Muscular Dystrophy

One client you provide care for is Jimmy Becker, a 9-year-old boy with muscular dystrophy. Jimmy developed muscular dystrophy when he was 4 years old. He had a waddle when he walked, was very clumsy, and frequently fell. In a few years, he will get weaker and probably will need a wheelchair.

Characteristics and symptoms of muscular dystrophy.   Muscular dystrophy is an illness that results when the nerves in the muscles do not function. This condition causes the muscles of the body to become smaller and weaker. The most common form of muscular dystrophy develops in young boys ages 3 to 7. There is no cure for this disease at this time.

The plan of care.   Your focus as a caregiver is to help maintain muscle strength and give emotional support to a child like Jimmy and his family. To accomplish this—

❖ Do passive range-of-motion exercises to prevent contractures and to strengthen muscles.
❖ Encourage the child to be as active as possible. Activity helps delay the decrease of muscle function and also makes him feel more independent.
❖ Monitor the child's diet to prevent obesity, which is an additional burden on the muscles.
❖ Encourage the family to contact an organization that will provide them with resources to help them and with the emotional support of other parents and professionals.

Providing Care for a Person Who Has Cystic Fibrosis

Another child that you provide care for is Jennifer Leaming, a 7-year-old girl with cystic fibrosis. She cannot breathe well enough to run in the park or ride a bike. Her parents always worry that Jennifer might catch a cold that could turn into **pneumonia**. They watch her diet carefully. She can't eat hot dogs, french fries, and ice cream, like most children can, because they contain too much fat for her body. On a hot day, she can sweat so much that she loses too much salt and fluid and becomes ill.

pneumonia
(nuh-MOAN-yuh)   An infection in the lungs.

Imagine how Jennifer must feel because she cannot be like the other children who run and play and do not worry about feeling sick. Imagine how Jennifer's parents must worry about their daughter's day-to-day health and whether they can afford the care that she needs. Imagine how they must feel, knowing that children with cystic fibrosis have a shortened life expectancy.

Characteristics and symptoms of cystic fibrosis.   Cystic fibrosis is a disorder that involves the mucus and sweat glands and results in lung problems. Thick mucus secretions block the air passages in the lungs and make it difficult to breathe. Cystic fibrosis is considered the most serious lung problem in children in the United States.

Mucus secretions also affect the pancreas by blocking necessary enzymes that flow from the pancreas to the small intestines. Fats cannot be broken up and used by the body. Even though the child with cystic fibrosis may have a good appetite, she has a hard time maintaining a proper weight. Medication can be given to replace the pancreatic enzyme.

A person with cystic fibrosis also experiences an increase in the amount of sodium and chloride (salt) excreted by her sweat glands. As a result, the sweat glands, tears, and saliva become very salty. Many years ago, before the development of sophisticated medical tests to diagnose cystic fibrosis, mothers of affected children reported to doctors that their children's skin tasted salty when they kissed them.

The plan of care.   When providing care to a child with cystic fibrosis, such as Jennifer Leaming, focus on assisting with her breathing and nutrition and with providing the family with emotional support. Carry out a plan of care that may include the following:

❖   Encourage the child to take four or five deep breaths often during the day. Deep breathing helps fill the lungs with air and helps the chest wall stay flexible. Help her with her breathing exercises.

❖   Encourage her to relax and breathe slowly but as deeply as possible to increase the flow of oxygen to the lungs.

❖   If the child is receiving oxygen therapy, check regularly to see that the tubes are in place and are not kinked. If she uses a nasal cannula, provide skin care around her nose.

❖ Encourage the child to cough to loosen mucus secretions. The respiratory therapist uses special exercises that involve tapping on the child's chest and back (Figure 16-15).

❖ Encourage her to eat all the foods recommended. A child with cystic fibrosis is usually on a high-calorie, fat-restricted diet.

To help maintain the child's independence, let her set her own pace for activities. Listen to her and encourage her to express her feelings. Also listen to the parents and other family members who may need extra support in providing care for a child with cystic fibrosis.

Providing Care for a Person Who Has Cerebral Palsy

Mark Bentley is a 2-year-old boy with cerebral palsy. At first you found it hard to provide care for Mark, who has "jerky" movements in many of his muscles. When he tries to move one way, his muscles involuntarily move another way. It is difficult for Mark to crawl or to eat. When he brings his hand to his mouth, it jerks away. When he tries to speak and form words, the muscles tighten and the words cannot be formed correctly, and people do not understand him.

Characteristics and symptoms of cerebral palsy.   Cerebral palsy is a disorder that affects the centers of the brain that control movement. A child may be born with the condition or may acquire it because of problems during the birth process. A person who has cerebral palsy may have a wide range of conditions, ranging from mild to severe. Cerebral palsy is one of the most common crippling conditions seen in children.

Cerebral palsy delays a child's physical development. He usually doesn't sit, crawl, or stand at the age expected. Think about the parents as they anticipate their child's achieving each milestone as other children do. How often have you heard or even asked the question, "How old was your child when he first sat up?"

Sometimes, when people see a child with cerebral palsy, they think he is mentally retarded, because he has difficulty coordinating body movement and communicating. Often children with cerebral palsy have normal intelligence, but they may have vision and hearing problems.

The plan of care.   When you carry out the plan of care for a child with cerebral palsy, focus on what the child can do and encourage these activities. Your activities may include the following:

❖ Provide good skin care to prevent pressure sores. It is important to keep the child's skin clean and dry.

❖ Turn or reposition the child every 2 hours. Use rolled towels, hand splints, and foot splints, as prescribed, to ensure proper alignment.

❖ Do gentle, slow range-of-motion exercises to prevent contractures and to strengthen muscles.

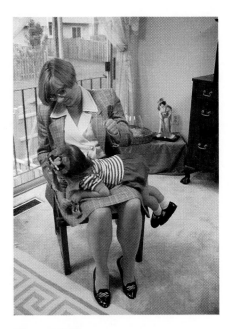

Figure 16-15
A therapist can teach the parent of a child with cystic fibrosis how to rap on the child's chest and back with cupped hands to loosen the mucus and enable the child to cough better.

❖ Encourage the child to use any self-help devices he may have for talking, walking, or eating such as a spoon or fork with a special grip.

To help a child with cerebral palsy, such as Mark Bentley, become as independent as possible, encourage him to do as much as possible for himself. As he gets older, listen to him and encourage him to tell you how he is feeling. You can provide emotional support by listening to him and accepting his feelings. Also, listen to the parents' concerns, as they may have feelings, including thoughts of guilt, about their child's illness that they need to talk about.

Providing Care for a Person Who Has Mental Retardation

One day when you go to the Button's house to help provide care for their 12-year-old daughter Alice, Mrs. Button talks with you about Alice's mental retardation. She says that for one reason or another, she and Mr. Button had waited for a long time to have a second child. During the pregnancy, she watched her diet carefully and got plenty of exercise.

But when Mrs. Button and her husband saw newborn Alice, they knew at once that something was wrong. Alice's head looked very large for her small size, and her facial features were unusual. She did not look like a normal, healthy baby. "Alice won't develop at the same rate as healthy children do," the doctor told them. "In many ways she'll be like a very young child all her life. She can learn to do some things for herself, but teaching her will require much patience. She may have problems with her vision and with her heart. She may require full-time care."

Characteristics and symptoms of mental retardation. A person who is mentally retarded may behave like a baby or a young child, even though she is a teenager or an adult. Sometimes people feel uncomfortable being around someone who is mentally retarded, because she looks unusual and her behavior seems strange. Some people may treat the person unkindly and laugh at her or tease her. Some people are afraid of a mentally retarded person. Imagine how the person must feel when people laugh at her. It is important for you to understand that the person cannot help being the way she is. Like all other people, a mentally retarded person needs to be shown respect and to live in a nurturing environment where she can learn, grow, develop to her fullest ability, and make choices about her life.

A person can be born with mental retardation. For various reasons, the baby's brain does not develop normally during the pregnancy. One reason could be a defect in the egg or sperm cell. The way the baby's brain develops can also be affected by the mother's health habits or an illness during pregnancy. The developing baby's brain can be damaged by the mother's poor diet or by her use of even extremely small amounts of alcohol, tobacco, and drugs. For this reason, a pregnant woman never should take a drug of any kind without her doctor's permission, even a prescription drug or an over-the-counter drug, such as aspirin.

Brain damage at birth, during infancy, or in early childhood also can impair a person's ability to think and learn. If a baby's brain does not receive enough oxygen during birth, she may become mentally retarded. If a child nearly drowns and her brain is damaged from lack of oxygen, she may become mentally retarded.

Mental retardation is a condition that can range from mild to very severe. In a supportive environment that supplies a good education, a person who is mildly retarded usually learns to take care of herself. A moderately retarded person takes longer to learn things and needs help taking care of herself. A person who is severely retarded probably will be totally dependent on others for care. In addition to mental retardation, the person may also have speech, vision, heart, and hearing problems.

Compared with other people her age, a person who is mentally retarded is more limited in what she can learn, how fast she can learn, and how independent she can be. Severely retarded people need the same kind of nurturing, loving care that is given to a baby or very young child.

Imagine how you would feel if you had a difficult task or idea to learn and your teacher would not give you the time you needed to learn it. Then think about the kind of environment that helps you learn best. A mentally retarded person's need for a good environment for learning is the same as any other person's. Learning to do tasks as simple as washing hands, putting on shoes, or pouring a glass of milk can be very difficult for a mentally retarded person. But with gentle, patient encouragement, a mildly or moderately mentally retarded person can take pride in learning to take care of many of her own needs. With each new task she masters, the mentally retarded person's self-confidence grows, and she has the courage to try to do more and more for herself.

The plan of care.   The plan of care for a person with mental retardation is based on how mild or severe the retardation is and whether the person also has other health problems. It focuses on treating the person as normally as possible within her limitations and incorporates the following ideas:

❖   Act as an assistant or associate, not as a parent. Help the person learn to do as much as possible for herself.

❖   Encourage the person to make choices if she is able. For example, offer her two leisure-time activities to choose from, or give her a choice of bedtimes.

❖   When helping to groom and dress a person with mental retardation, treat her the same as you would treat any other person. Provide privacy while giving care, encourage her to do all that she can for herself, and help her select clothes and a hairstyle that other people her age would wear.

❖ To help develop social skills, encourage the person to participate in social and recreational activities.

❖ Give praise for even the smallest accomplishment. What may
seem like a small change or gain to the average person may
seem like a large accomplishment to a mentally retarded person.
The sense of accomplishment gives her the courage to try to do
new things.

❖ Talk or sing to a severely retarded person. Put brightly colored
objects where she can see them. Play soft music. Even though
she may not be able to respond to you, it is important to treat
her as a person worthy of respect.

A frequent cause of mental retardation is Down's syndrome, sometimes referred to as mongolism because the person's eyes are slanted
and the bridge of his nose is flattened. In addition, he may tend to
hold his mouth open because of a large, protruding tongue. His
hands are short and broad, with short fingers. In many cases, a child
with Down's syndrome can have a heart defect. Life expectancy, due
to heart disease and susceptibility to leukemia and accelerated aging
process, is 40 or 50 years. Mental ability ranges from severely
retarded to functioning independently. Although the majority of children with Down's syndrome are born to older mothers, the syndrome occasionally occurs in infants of younger mothers. An infant
who has Down's syndrome generally is very quiet and calm and
rarely cries. Providing care for a person with Down's syndrome is
similar to providing care for others with mental retardation.

Cancer

Providing Care for a Person Who Has Cancer

As Elizabeth Little is recovering in the hospital from surgery, she
begins to talk to you about her illness. "One day, while bathing, I
found a lump in my breast and immediately went to my doctor. After
a series of tests, the doctor determined that the lump was a malignant tumor. I felt shocked and angry. I'm just 34 and I eat properly
and exercise every day. I love my job and I'm good at it. My fiancé
and I planned to get married next month. I just felt good about my
life. I don't deserve this."

Characteristics and symptoms of cancer.   Odds are you know someone
who has or has had cancer, because cancer is the second leading
cause of death in the United States. Cancer is the abnormal growth of
new cells that can spread and crowd out or destroy other body tissues. The abnormal growth can be in the form of a malignant tumor,
a solid mass or a growth of abnormal cells that can grow anywhere
in the body. A tumor can be noncancerous (benign) or cancerous
(malignant). Benign tumors usually grow slowly and do not spread to
other areas of the body. Malignant tumors can spread, or metastasize,
to other parts of the body.

Malignant tumors can grow fast and invade and destroy other body tissue. In the early stages, a malignant tumor does not cause pain or other symptoms, and the person may not suspect she has cancer. Sometimes cancer is detected during a routine physical examination. If a cancer is detected before it has begun to spread, there is a good chance that growth of the cancer can be controlled or stopped.

Once cancer is detected, it can be treated. Typically, cancer is treated in one of three ways, depending on the kind of cancer, the location, and whether the cancer has spread. Often the first treatment is to remove the tumor surgically. The other two treatments are **chemotherapy** and **radiation**. A doctor determines the best treatment for each person and sometimes prescribes all three.

A doctor gives a person chemotherapy in the hope that the drugs can stop or slow the rate of growth of the cancer cells. The drugs used to treat cancer are so powerful that they affect all the systems in a person's body. As a result, the person may feel far worse than he felt before he was given the drugs. Common side effects include nausea, diarrhea, loss of hair, and extremely dry skin. A person having chemotherapy may have some or all of these side effects.

The goal of radiation treatment is to destroy the cancer cells through the use of x-rays. A person usually does not feel pain during the treatment, but she can experience unpleasant side effects from it.

With her doctor's guidance, Ms. Little had decided to have surgery and a combination of radiation and chemotherapy to treat her breast cancer. But she felt frightened and worried. How would her fiancé react to the news? Would he still feel the same way about her after the surgery? Would she be able to wear the beautiful new bathing suit she had bought to wear on her honeymoon? What if the chemotherapy caused her hair to fall out? Would her job be held for her while she was recovering from surgery? Would she feel well enough during chemotherapy and radiation treatment to keep working? What if the treatment did not work and she died?

The plan of care.   When providing care for a person who is being treated for cancer, such as Ms. Little, carry out the prescribed plan of care and incorporate the following suggestions:

❖   The most important thing for you to do is to be there for the person, listen to her, support her, and show her you care by being positive and hopeful. Many people believe that having a positive, hopeful attitude helps in the healing process.

❖   During your caregiving, remember that infection control becomes of utmost importance. Chemotherapy and radiation affect a person's immune system, the system responsible for fighting off infection. Exposure to germs may cause infection. Therefore, follow strict handwashing and universal precaution rules.

❖   Provide good mouth care to reduce the spread of germs. Perform mouth care every 2 hours, because some drugs can cause a person to have a very dry mouth or serious oral infections. A doctor may recommend the use of an antibacterial mouth rinse.

chemotherapy
(key-mo-THER-uh-pee)   Treatment with one or more drugs that stop cancer cells from multiplying.

radiation
(ray-dee-AY-shun)   Treatment in which x-rays are focused on the part of the body where cancer cells are growing.

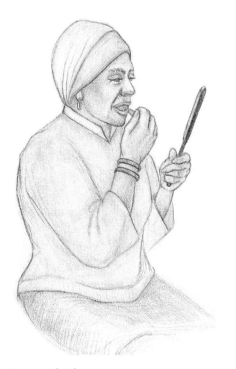

Figure 16-16
A common side effect of chemotherapy is hair loss, which may lead to self-image problems. To help maintain her self-esteem, encourage a person receiving chemotherapy to try new styles and to maintain her appearance.

❖ Observe the mouth and other parts of the body for redness or irritation.

❖ Maintain adequate nutrition and proper rest.

❖ Generally, a person receiving treatment loses her appetite. For a day or so after the person has chemotherapy, she often has nausea and diarrhea. Chemotherapy also can affect the person's sense of smell and taste so that nothing seems appetizing. Yet, she still needs nutritious foods to aid in the healing process and to give her strength. Some ways to provide good nutrition to a person who has lost her appetite are: Provide fluids frequently, especially nutritious fluids such as milk shakes and broth; provide good, nutritious foods anytime a person feels hungry and make sure the food looks appetizing; make mealtime as pleasant and relaxing as possible; provide small, more frequent meals and offer snacks frequently; offer foods the person enjoys.

❖ *Never* provide care for a person who is receiving cancer treatment if you have a cold or flu, because you may pass your illness on to the person.

❖ You can help a person who begins to lose her hair feel better about herself by reassuring her that her hair will grow back after treatment is completed. Suggest that she wear a scarf, wig, or even a favorite hat, if she wishes (Figure 16-16).

❖ If the person receiving chemotherapy or radiation treatment feels tired, explain to her that she feels tired because of the treatment. (Sometimes when you know why you feel a particular way, you cope with your feelings better and allow yourself to rest.) She may be on a treatment schedule that lasts weeks or months. It takes a great deal of physical and emotional energy for her to fight the disease.

❖ Encourage the person to rest more, take naps, or go to bed earlier than usual. You may want to ask if you can help her into a comfortable position to maintain proper body alignment and comfort.

❖ If the person's skin changes and she gets a rash from a drug she has received, or she reddens or burns from radiation treatment, provide good care by inspecting her skin often and keeping it clean. Also, give her frequent backrubs, especially if she is in bed a great deal, which causes fatigue. A backrub increases circulation to the skin. *Never* massage the area that receives the radiation treatment. Often this area has semi-permanent marks on it that the radiologist put there to focus the x-rays. To prevent skin breakdown and to avoid undue pressure, reposition the person frequently.

When providing care for a person who has cancer, report any changes to your supervising nurse without delay. Chemotherapy and radiation can cause a variety of side effects, which may alter the plan of care. The plan of care differs for each person, based on the person's special needs.

The most important things to remember when providing care for a person with cancer, such as Ms. Little, is that she needs a positive attitude and kindness. She is going through an extremely stressful time, as are her family members, friends, and also the health care team members who have grown to love and provide care for her. A great many support services are available for people with cancer. Your supervising nurse or the social worker can find out what is available in your community.

Sometimes a person completes the treatment only to find out that the cancer has reappeared or spread to different areas of the body. Depending on the nature of the recurrence, this situation may be particularly difficult for the person and family to accept. Often they believe that the person might die and they take steps to deal with the possibility.

As you will read in Chapter 22, Providing Care for People Who Are Dying, a person goes through many stages when she faces a terminal illness, often moving in and out of these stages. Your support, compassion, and skillful care are essential to providing comfort to the person and her family.

Information Review

Circle the correct answers and fill in the blanks.

1. Someone with arthritis should be encouraged to—
    a. Avoid the pain by not moving.
    b. Take cold showers to reduce swelling of joints.
    c. Exercise strenuously to keep joints flexible.
    d. Do active or passive range-of-motion exercises regularly.

    Active & Passive range motion

2. All of the following are signals of an impending heart attack except—
    a. Pain in the lower legs.
    b. Persistent chest pain that is not relieved by changing position, resting, or medicating with nitroglycerin.
    c. Shortness of breath.
    d. Sweating.

3. A person with congestive heart failure generally is most comfortable when he is—
    a. Lying flat.
    b. Sitting up.
    c. Lying on his left side.
    d. Lying on his right side.

4. Someone with diabetes—
    a. Needs to eat extra sugar and protein to maintain his strength.
    b. May have reduced sensation in his feet.
    c. Needs to eliminate exercise completely.
    d. Needs to have the nurse assistant cut his toenails daily so that they don't become too long.

5. Someone with COPD should be encouraged to—
   a. Eat one large meal per day instead of several smaller meals.
   b. Lie flat after eating.
   c. Breathe deeply often during the day.
   d. Smoke to relieve tension.
6. Tuberculosis—
   a. Is always fatal.
   b. Is spread by touching the person.
   c. Always requires hospitalizaton.
   d. Is spread by breathing in droplets that have been sprayed into the air by an infected person's coughing.
7. When providing care for someone who has had a stroke, you must—
   a. Place the call signal within reach of the person's unaffected side.
   b. Position the person so that he is lying flat when he eats, since he may have paralysis and drool.
   c. Place food in the person's mouth on the affected side.
   d. Keep the paralyzed arm or leg lower than the rest of his body to keep blood flowing into it.
8. When providing care for someone with paraplegia or quadriplegia, focus your caregiving on promoting _____independence_____ through the use of assistive devices.
9. When a person is depressed, he may have thoughts about suicide. You must report any of the signals of suicide such as dramatic _____change_____ in mood or behavior, giving away _____belongings_____, preoccupation with _____inner_____ thoughts, or hoarding _____medicine_____.
10. Mary's cystic fibrosis causes _____mucus_____ to accumulate in her lungs.
11. People with cerebral palsy may have difficulty walking and talking, but they often have _____good normal_____ intelligence.
12. A person who is being treated for cancer may have a decreased ability to fight off _____infection_____.

Questions to Ask Yourself

1. You provide home health care for Agnes Tilgard, who has osteoporosis and lives on the fourth floor of an apartment building that doesn't have an elevator. Ms. Tilgard hardly ever leaves her apartment because she is afraid of slipping on the stairs. What can you do to help her maintain her independence?

2. Today, while providing home health care for Mrs. Roth, who has diabetes, her hands start shaking. You ask her if she is okay. "I'm fine!" she snaps, "so leave me alone!" What do you think might be happening? What should you do?

3. Martha Boswitch has MS. When you bring her breakfast tray one morning and ask her how she slept, she replies that her feet and hands were cold all night. What should you do?

4. Mrs. Reilly, who has COPD, is very short of breath. She has difficulty with any amount of exertion and needs to rest frequently. Today Mrs. Reilly's daughter is bringing her 6-month-old son to visit at 10:30 A.M. Mrs. Reilly wants to look especially nice, but she also doesn't want to be too tired to enjoy the visit. How would you help her plan her morning care so that she can accomplish both goals?

5. Do you know anyone who is quadriplegic? How does the person spend his day? If you don't know anyone with quadriplegia, imagine how you would spend your day if you had no feeling in your arms and legs and had to remain in a wheelchair?

6. Ruth Linquist is a new resident at Morningside Nursing Home. Because of her depression, she often doesn't sleep at night. When her husband stops by for afternoon visits, she usually is too tired to spend time with him. What might you do to make this situation better?

7. If you were told today that you had an illness that would require you to change your lifestyle completely, how would you react? Think of some possible changes and how you would respond.

8. You provide care for 7-year-old Jennifer Leaming who has cystic fibrosis. Today Jennifer begs you for an ice cream sundae with chocolate syrup, whipped cream, and nuts. What should you do?

9. Nine-year-old Scott Epter has Down's syndrome and has been admitted to the hospital for heart surgery. You are wiping Scott's face after lunch when his mother brings a new picture book for her son. She hands the book to Scott, who promptly rips a page from the book and puts it in his mouth. "Scott! I just bought that book!" shrieks Mrs. Epter. Scott begins to cry. What would you do in this situation?

17

Providing Care for People Who Have AIDS

Goals

After reading this chapter, you will have the information to—

Explain which ideas about AIDS are untrue and which are true.

Explain what AIDS is.

Define HIV and explain how it is transmitted.

Explain how the HIV infection and AIDS are related.

Identify behaviors that can transmit HIV, the virus that causes AIDS.

List behaviors that cannot transmit HIV.

Describe some medical problems of people who have AIDS.

Describe the people who are living with AIDS.

Explain how to provide care for a person who has AIDS.

Explain how to provide care for a child who has AIDS.

Today you go to the home of Mrs. Mary Hill to provide care for her and her 3-month-old daughter Melissa. Mrs. Hill's mother answers your knock at the door of the old, two-story row house and explains that her daughter is having a bad day. You can smell the odors of vomit and diarrhea. In the living room, Mrs. Hill rests on a make-shift bed made up on the sofa. Her ankles appear swollen, as well as the glands in her neck. You observe how dry and sore her mouth is as she speaks.

"I'm so glad you're here," she says. "I don't have the strength to even get out of bed. I feel so helpless. I can't even hold my baby." In the next room, you can hear Melissa fussing in her crib. Mrs. Hill's mother heads toward the baby's crib to take care of her while you get ready to help Mrs. Hill.

Before beginning Mrs. Hill's personal care, you ask her what she would like to drink. When she says she doesn't want anything to drink, you suggest that she try sucking on some ice. You explain that fluids will help her dry mouth feel better and will also help reduce her bouts of diarrhea. She agrees to try the ice.

As you provide personal care for Mrs. Hill, you handle her skin with extreme gentleness because you know how fragile it has become. After you complete her bed bath, help her dress in a clean sweat suit, and put fresh linens on the sofa, Mrs. Hill thanks you. "I feel so much better now that I'm fresh and clean. But, I'm so tired."

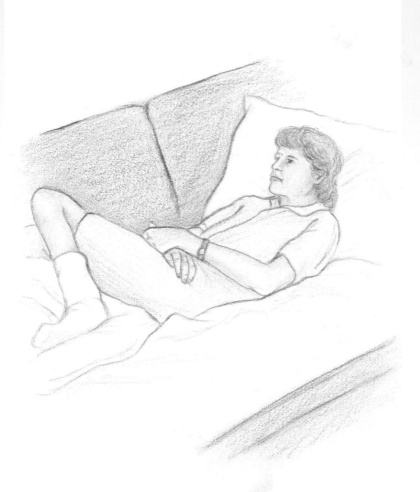

opportunistic infection
(op-or-too-NIS-tik)   An infection caused by germs that normally would not make a person sick. Any person whose immune system is weakened may develop opportunistic infections.

antibodies
(AN-ti-bah-dees)   Special proteins or chemicals the body produces when an infection is present.

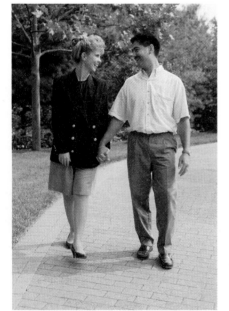

Figure 17-1
You *cannot* get AIDS from holding hands.

Facts About AIDS

Mary Hill has AIDS. Her daughter Melissa tests positive for HIV, the virus that causes AIDS. Mrs. Hill's husband Glen died a few months ago from an **opportunistic infection** associated with AIDS. Glen became infected with HIV when he shared needles with friends to inject drugs. He infected Mrs. Hill with the virus through vaginal sex.

Like many babies born to mothers who are infected with HIV, Melissa had tests that showed HIV **antibodies** in her blood when she was born. At birth, some babies already are infected with HIV. Others only show positive test results for the virus because of the influence of antibodies they receive from their mothers before birth. By the time they are 15 months old, babies lose the effects of maternal antibodies. At this time, if they are not infected with HIV, they will test negative for the virus. About one third of the babies born to HIV-positive mothers are actually infected with the virus. So far, Melissa has no symptoms of HIV infection, and Mrs. Hill expresses hope that she is not infected.

AIDS was identified in 1981. It kills men, women, and children everywhere in the world. The four letters in the word "AIDS" are an abbreviation for **a**cquired **i**mmune **d**eficiency **s**yndrome. If you read the newspaper, watch television, or listen to the radio, you have heard about AIDS. Almost every week the media carry another story about it or about someone who has it. What have you heard about AIDS? Are you aware of the following facts?

❖   In 1981, 152 cases of AIDS were diagnosed in the United States.
❖   Ten years later, nearly 200,000 cases of AIDS had been diagnosed.
❖   The number of people who have AIDS is increasing.
❖   People who have AIDS live in almost every county in the United States, and many of them are very sick.
❖   People with AIDS need the care, kindness, and compassion of health care workers who aren't afraid to help them.

Doctors and scientists are still learning about AIDS, so you don't have to feel embarrassed if you don't know some things about it. Some ideas people have about AIDS are untrue. One false idea is that you can get AIDS from insects. Another is that you can get it from your pets. These statements are not true, but many people are frightened by them. People are less afraid of AIDS when they know the facts (Figure 17-1). The following statements about AIDS are true:

❖   You *cannot* get AIDS from a drinking fountain.
❖   You *cannot* get AIDS from the sweat of an infected person.
❖   You *cannot* get AIDS from hugging someone who has AIDS.

The more you know about AIDS, the virus that causes it, and how the virus spreads, the more in control you are of your own life and health. As you read this chapter, you'll learn the basics about the virus and AIDS so that you can keep yourself safe and provide safe, compassionate care for people who have the disease. You can share this information with your sexual partner, children, family, or friends.

What Is AIDS and What Causes It?

AIDS is a **syndrome** that is caused by a virus. The virus is called HIV, which is the abbreviation for **h**uman **i**mmunodeficiency **v**irus. The word *immunodeficiency* is the key to understanding what AIDS is and what it does to people. If you break the word into two parts, it makes more sense.

syndrome
(SIN-drum)   Several signs and symptoms that occur together and characterize a disease.

❖ **Immuno.** The first part of the word refers to the body's immune system, which contains the special substances that defend the body against germs and infections. White blood cells are one part of this immune system. They rush to the site of a cut or wound and help fight off infection.

❖ **Deficiency.** The second part of the word refers to a deficiency, which means a lack of something that you need. For example, if you don't eat enough, you are deficient in calories and you lose weight. Or, if you don't eat certain foods, you may develop a deficiency in iron, which results in a lack of red blood cells.

When you put the two parts of the word back together, what does immunodeficiency mean to you? Most people explain it as a lack in the body's immune system. Immunodeficiency means that the special cells and substances that fight off infection aren't able to do their job. They have been destroyed or weakened by the virus so that, when other infections or diseases attack, the person gets sick easily. Many symptoms that characterize different diseases develop in a person who has AIDS.

In summary, in the process that leads to AIDS, a person is exposed to the human immunodeficiency virus and becomes infected. This person is HIV infected or HIV positive. A person who is infected with HIV may look and feel healthy and lead a productive life for many years. However, during this time the virus is breaking down the person's immune system. When the immune system is weakened, the person begins to experience some or all of the many and varied symptoms of **acquired** immune deficiency.

acquired
(uh-KWY-erd)   A condition that is not inherited and does not just happen to a person for an unexplained reason.

How Do People Get HIV?

What have you heard about how people get AIDS? What things are you more cautious about now that there is more publicity about AIDS? People do not catch HIV the same way they catch cold or flu viruses. People catch colds or flu by breathing in germs from the air. HIV is not a virus that spreads through the air. People must learn how HIV is transmitted so that they know how to protect themselves against the virus that causes AIDS.

How HIV Is Transmitted in the General Population

Think again about the term "acquired immune deficiency syndrome." AIDS is an acquired disease that is caused by a contagious virus. People develop AIDS because of something they do or something that happens to them that exposes them to HIV.

HIV is not easy to get. It is transmitted through blood and a few other body fluids, the most important of which are semen, vaginal fluids, and occasionally breast milk. HIV is spread in three major ways—through sexual intercourse with an infected partner, through exposure to infected blood, and from an infected mother to her baby. For example, HIV spreads—

❖ From an HIV-infected person to her sexual partner when semen or vaginal fluid is exchanged. (The use of latex condoms can help prevent the spread of HIV during oral, anal, or vaginal sex.)

❖ From an HIV-infected person to anyone who shares a needle with her. Whenever two people use the same needle to inject drugs, get a tattoo, or pierce their ears, they risk spreading HIV if one of them is infected. Some infected blood may remain on the needle and can be passed from one person to another. If you use drugs, get the necessary help to stop using them. If you know people who inject drugs, warn them never to share needles with another person.

❖ From an HIV-infected mother to her unborn baby during her pregnancy or during childbirth. The virus is so tiny that it can pass through the membranes of the **placenta** and infect the blood of the developing fetus. Some babies who initially test positive for HIV antibodies may test negative when they get older as they lose the effects of the maternal antibodies. Other babies who test positive may actually be infected with HIV (Figure 17-2). An HIV-infected mother also may pass the virus to her nursing baby through breast milk, although only a few such cases have been reported. The virus can be present in breast milk and can enter the baby's system through the mucous membranes of the baby's mouth. In most instances, a mother who is HIV positive should bottle feed rather than breast feed her infant.

placenta
(pluh-SEN-ta)   A blood-filled structure through which the unborn child receives oxygen and nourishment and through which it gets rid of carbon dioxide and its other wastes.

Figure 17-2
A mother who is HIV positive can pass HIV antibodies and the virus to her baby. This can happen during pregnancy or during delivery of the baby.

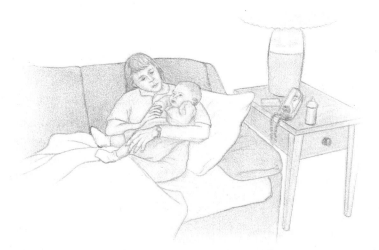

❖ From HIV-infected blood given to a recipient. Organizations that collect blood donations have been testing blood for the virus since 1985. If they find antibodies to HIV, they destroy the blood.

How HIV Is Transmitted in the Health Care Setting

Worldwide studies of people who provide care for those who have AIDS show that the caregivers do not get infected when they provide routine care. Some health care workers often have contact with blood, as do people in their care who undergo certain procedures. For this reason, it is vital for health care workers to follow the universal precautions discussed in Chapter 7, Controlling the Spread of Germs. In a health care setting, HIV may be spread—

❖ From an HIV-infected person to her health care worker, or from an HIV-infected health care worker to a person receiving health care, *only* if infected blood or body fluids come in contact with the blood or mucous membranes of the uninfected person. When an HIV-infected health care worker does not use universal precautions, he or she can infect the person receiving health care.

❖ From an HIV-infected person's blood or body fluids to another person receiving health care, *only* if the virus is transmitted from a health care worker's hands or equipment. When a health care worker uses universal precautions, he or she eliminates the risk of passing the virus from one person to another.

❖ From HIV-infected equipment used for piercing the skin or mucous membranes and from people who use the equipment. Whenever you have a procedure done that requires piercing the skin or mucous membranes, be sure that the person doing the procedure uses sterile equipment and wears gloves.

How HIV Is Not Transmitted

Most interactions between people do not have to change because of HIV. HIV is *not* transmitted by any of the following behaviors:

❖ Hugging, kissing, or holding hands
❖ Rubbing the shoulders, massaging the body, or touching an infected person in a casual way (not in a sexual way)
❖ Sharing food or beverages, pencils, books, tools, eating utensils, or clothes
❖ Being in the same room, sitting on the same chair, or touching the same things

Some other viruses can be spread by doing these things, but HIV cannot be spread in these ways.

Testing for HIV

One day Mrs. Hill tells you about the day she found out that she was HIV infected. "I found out when I had a blood test done during a prenatal examination," she says. "Until then, I didn't know that I was infected. After this discovery, Glen also was tested and found he was HIV positive. The doctor said his HIV infection had already developed into AIDS. Glen had been trying to keep his symptoms a secret, because he didn't want to worry me. I was already worried about his drug use. I never injected drugs and I never had sex with anyone but

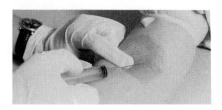

Figure 17-3

Getting a blood test for HIV is a simple procedure. It may be very hard for someone to decide to have this test done because she is scared about what the results will be.

anonymous

(uh-NON-uh-mus)   Not named or identified.

him. I was very angry when I found out that he had gotten this horrible disease from sharing needles with one of his drug buddies and then passed it on to me, and possibly Melissa. I hated his drug use, but I never thought that it would end up killing all of us."

A person can be infected with HIV without knowing it. A simple blood test can detect antibodies in the blood (Figure 17-3). If the test detects HIV antibodies, it is said to be positive, which is why someone who is infected with HIV is referred to as HIV positive.

Many people who think they may have been infected may be afraid to have an HIV test because of what they might find out. Or they may be afraid that their employers or family members and friends might find out about the behaviors that put them at risk. They also may be afraid that they might lose their jobs if their test results are positive. People who have HIV often suffer discrimination, but local, state, and federal laws can provide some legal protection. The Americans with Disabilities Act protects many people who have disabilities, including those who have HIV.

A person who may have been exposed to HIV must have the courage to be tested, because the sooner she knows she is infected with HIV, the sooner she can begin treatment that may prolong the time before she develops AIDS.

Facts about AIDS testing.   A person should keep the following things in mind when considering being tested for HIV:

❖   She should go to a place where pre-test and post-test counseling is available.

❖   She can be tested **anonymously**. A person's test results are confidential. They are identified by a number, not by her name.

❖   A positive HIV test does not mean that a person has AIDS or might develop AIDS any time soon. It simply means she has been infected with HIV. A person infected with HIV should see a doctor immediately, because early treatment can slow the development of the disease and contribute to better-quality and longer life.

❖   A person recently infected with HIV still may have a negative result when tested. It takes from 6 weeks to 3 months after exposure (being open to the risk) for the antibodies to the virus to be detected in a person's blood. If a person whose test results are negative thinks she may have been exposed to HIV, she should have the test repeated after 3 months. In the meantime, the person should prevent the spread of the virus by using latex condoms for every sexual encounter and, if injecting drugs, by not sharing needles.

❖   Getting a negative test result does not protect a person from becoming infected in the future. It means only that the person probably was not infected at the time of the test.

❖   In health care settings, when a worker experiences an occupationally related exposure such as a needle stick, policies may

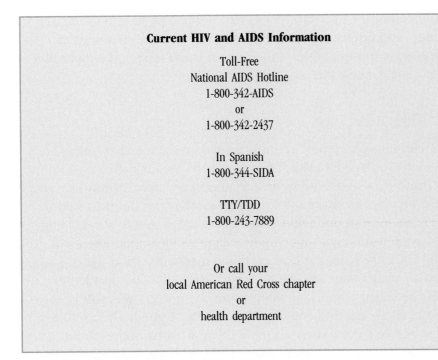

Current HIV and AIDS Information

Toll-Free
National AIDS Hotline
1-800-342-AIDS
or
1-800-342-2437

In Spanish
1-800-344-SIDA

TTY/TDD
1-800-243-7889

Or call your
local American Red Cross chapter
or
health department

576-1414 Parenthood
887-1332 B. Count health
Dep.

include immediate blood testing and then periodic blood tests in the following months. If a health care worker learns that she is infected with HIV, she can begin receiving early treatment that may delay the development of AIDS by months or even years.

When test results are positive.   If a person's blood tests positive for antibodies to HIV, a second test is done to confirm the results of the first test. If the second test is positive, the person is asked to come into the testing facility or clinic. There she receives the test results and is given the opportunity to talk with a counselor (Figure 17-4). The counselor is trained to give necessary support and guidance to help her deal with the information, receive appropriate medical care, and change sexual and drug use behaviors that could infect other people. The counselor reinforces the fact that the person is infected with the virus but doesn't yet have AIDS, if that is the case.

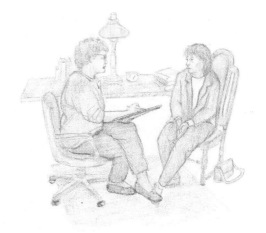

Figure 17-4
When Mrs. Hill found out she was HIV positive, she had many questions for the counselor. She was very concerned about her baby's health and her own.

The counselor also advises the HIV-positive person to tell sexual partners and others who may have been infected so that they can be tested as soon as possible. If the person is embarrassed about telling others, she can ask the counselor for help.

How Does AIDS Affect the Health of an Infected Person?

Most HIV-infected people do not know they are infected because they don't look or feel sick, often for years. This is the case of Rodney Britten, a 41-year-old homosexual client with AIDS whom you visit every day. Mr. Britten told you about the care he had taken in practicing safe sex after he learned about AIDS in the '80s. He knew that having anal sex without using a latex condom put him at risk, so in the late '80s, when he learned that a man with whom he had had a sexual relationship in 1980 had died from AIDS, he decided to have a test. "I was shocked when I found out that I was HIV positive. I had been so careful for all those years. But I guess I became infected before I even knew about AIDS. At least by being careful, I've avoided infecting my current partner. We've been together almost 6 years."

When a person is exposed to HIV, the virus enters his body, multiplies in the blood and other organs, and damages his immune system. It may take a long time for the virus to destroy enough of the immune system to cause sickness. The person can be infected with HIV for 10 or more years without showing any signs or symptoms of AIDS, but he still is able to infect other people during that time.

Symptoms of AIDS

Health professionals think that most people who are infected with HIV will eventually develop AIDS. Their symptoms may vary, but most experience several of the symptoms that are associated with AIDS. Not only do symptoms vary from one person who has AIDS to another, but one person's symptoms and conditions can change from day to day. As a person's HIV infection worsens and the immune system weakens, any or all of the following symptoms can occur:

❖ Hard-to-treat yeast or other fungal infections (caused by tiny organisms that cannot be seen without a microscope and that feed off of other living organisms) in the mouth, throat, or vagina
❖ Repeated episodes of diarrhea
❖ Dry cough or shortness of breath
❖ Swelling in the glands that does not go away
❖ Continual feelings of tiredness
❖ Fevers that occur again and again
❖ Night sweats
❖ Unexplained weight loss of 10 pounds or more
❖ Memory loss or confusion
❖ Pain and difficulty when moving
❖ Red or purplish spots on the skin

Some of these symptoms also occur in other illnesses, so they are not always signs of AIDS. But if a person has any of these symptoms for more than 2 weeks, he should consult a doctor.

Infections and Diseases Associated with AIDS

An adolescent or adult is diagnosed as having AIDS when he is infected with HIV and has one or more of the opportunistic conditions or infections—sometimes called indicator diseases—listed in the Centers for Disease Control (CDC) case definition. The most common opportunistic conditions that are seen in people when HIV infection has weakened their immune systems include ***Pneumocystis carinii* pneumonia (PCP)**, **systemic herpes**, **HIV wasting syndrome**, and **candidiasis** of the esophagus or the respiratory tree. A person with a healthy immune system would not become severely ill with these conditions, as happens in a person who has AIDS. Their bodies would be able to fight off any infections in time. Figure 17-5 shows what happens to people who have healthy immune systems and to those whose immune systems have been weakened by HIV.

Pneumocystis carinii **pneumonia (PCP)**
(NEW-mo-sis-tis/kuh-REE-nee-eye/new-MOAN-yuh)   A parasitic lung infection that makes breathing very difficult. PCP is the leading cause of death for people who have AIDS.

systemic herpes
(sis-TEM-ik/HER-pees)   A type of infection caused by the herpes virus in which sores develop over the entire body, especially the hands, feet, and mouth.

HIV wasting syndrome
An opportunistic condition characterized by the loss of 10 percent or more of total body weight over a short period of time.

candidiasis
(kan-de-DYE-uh-sis)   The growth of painful white patches in the mouth, throat, or vagina caused by a fungus called candida.

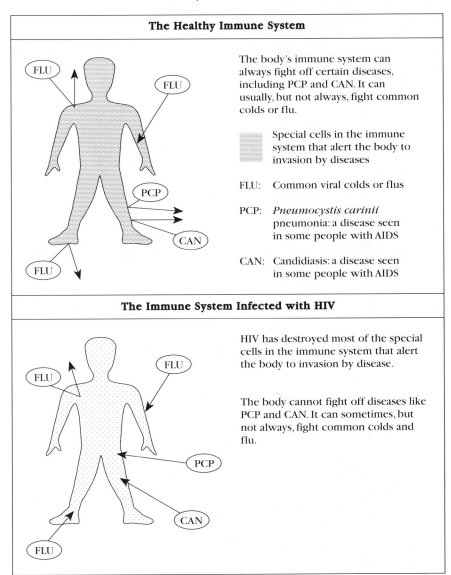

Figure 17-5
How the Immune System Fights Off Infection

From Quackenbush M, Sargent P: *Teaching AIDS: a resource guide on acquired immune deficiency syndrome*, Santa Cruz, Network Publications, 1986.

Kaposi's sarcoma
(KAP-oh-sees/sar-KO-muh)   A rare kind of skin cancer that may attack the skin, mucous membranes, and lymph nodes.

In addition to developing opportunistic infections, people with AIDS may develop unusual cancers. A cancer found in many homosexual people who have AIDS is **Kaposi's sarcoma**. People who have AIDS also may develop a form of tuberculosis (TB) that cannot be controlled by the usual medications. (Review the information on TB in Chapter 16, Providing Care for People with Specific Illnesses.)

Scientists are looking for better ways to treat AIDS. Today, no drug actually cures HIV infection, although several drugs can slow down the development of opportunistic infections or the reproduction of the virus and help an HIV-infected person live longer and more comfortably.

Who Are the People Living with AIDS?

Mr. Britten likes it when you come to provide care. When he feels well enough, he likes to talk with you about all kinds of things: the weather, sports, music, and his disease. He tells you how lonely it is now that he has AIDS. "My partner Owen has stuck by me, but all of my family and many of my friends have just cut me out of their lives. I guess some are afraid that they'll get AIDS. My family used to pretend my homosexuality wasn't real, but when I got AIDS, they had to face it, and they couldn't deal with it. They always seem to be too busy to visit me. You and Owen are the only people who think I'm worth anything."

Who gets AIDS? Many people answer, "Gay men and IV drug users," but that is only partly correct. Anyone who has been infected by HIV, such as Mrs. Hill and Melissa, can develop AIDS. Although the majority of people infected with HIV are homosexual men and IV drug users, other people living with AIDS include—

❖ Married men and women infected by their spouses who may have contracted HIV infection from IV drug use, sex with an HIV-infected man or woman, or the transfusion of infected blood.

❖ Single men and women infected by sexual partners who may have contracted HIV infection from IV drug use, sex with an HIV-infected man or woman, or the transfusion of infected blood.

❖ Babies born with the virus in their blood because their mothers were infected.

❖ Children, teenagers, and adults who were given infected blood or blood products during transfusions before 1985, the year that routine testing of blood supplies began. Today the risk of getting HIV from a blood transfusion is very small.

❖ Small numbers of health care workers who were inadvertently infected while providing care for HIV-infected people, through occupational exposure (needle stick, human error).

❖ Small numbers of people who were infected by HIV-infected doctors, dentists, and other health care workers who did not follow universal precautions.

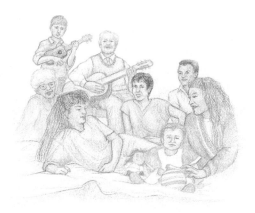

Figure 17-6
Any of these people may one day live with AIDS. Men, women, and children of any race, age, and income bracket may be exposed to HIV, may become infected, and may develop AIDS.

Were you aware that people in all age groups and walks of life are infected with HIV and developing AIDS (Figure 17-6)? By 1991, just 10 years after AIDS was first diagnosed, an estimated one million people in the United States had been diagnosed as being infected with HIV. Many of those diagnosed did not know they were infected and still had no symptoms of AIDS. By the end of 1991, more than 133,000 people had died from infections and cancers associated with AIDS (Figure 17-7). Unless a cure is found, it is expected that all the people infected with HIV will develop AIDS. They need nursing care while they are sick, whether in hospitals, nursing homes, or their own homes. Health care workers are finding that providing care for a person with AIDS is more and more common, whether they work in a small town, a large city, or a rural area.

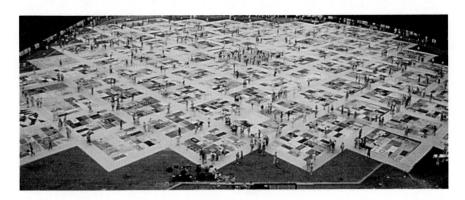

Figure 17-7
This huge memorial quilt represents many of the people who had died from AIDS by mid-1988. Each panel has one or more names on it. By late 1992, the quilt had 21,000 panels, representing about 11 percent of the people who had died from AIDS.

Think about all the things you have read about human beings and human behavior in this book. People who are living with AIDS are people just like anyone else, but they are seriously ill. They have hopes and dreams, but they also fear that they may not live long enough to see them come true. They have pain and sadness, but the caring of a friend or the touch of a caregiver can help them feel better physically and emotionally.

People who are living with HIV infection and AIDS have the same basic human needs that you read about in Chapter 4, Understanding

People. You read that being sick or disabled does not change those needs. You have the opportunity to help meet those needs if you choose to work as a caregiver for any of the thousands of people who have AIDS.

In addition, the person's family, friends, and other caregivers may need emotional support. They may seek you out to talk about the feelings they have about providing care for their loved one who will never get well.

How do you feel now that you have more information about AIDS? Do you feel confident that you can safely provide compassionate care for a person with AIDS? Do you think you can avoid judging someone for the behaviors that may have led to infection of the virus? If you are going to provide care for someone with AIDS, you must first understand how you feel about the disease and the people who have it.

Providing Care for a Person Living with AIDS

People who are living with AIDS need you to provide the same type of thoughtful caregiving that you provide to every sick person. They need you to help with things they cannot do for themselves. They need you to be the best nurse assistant you can be for them. Because they have a disease that has no cure and that often isolates them from other people, they may need more emotional support than some other people in your care and may need extra warmth and kindness from you (Figure 17-8).

The one big difference in providing care for someone with AIDS is that you must remember that AIDS is a syndrome, a collection of different symptoms that may change from day to day. You must change the types of care you provide as the person's condition changes.

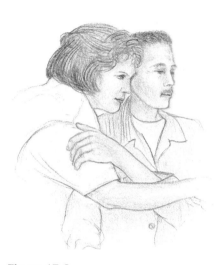

Figure 17-8
Only a few people come to visit Mr. Britten and he often feels isolated. When he feels down, Mr. Britten really appreciates getting a hug from his home health aide.

Practicing the Principles of Care

When providing care for a person living with AIDS, all of the principles of care are important, but four need special consideration.

Dignity.   The person in your care may have been treated unfairly or unkindly because of her disease. Dignity, self-respect, and feelings of self-esteem may have been damaged. You can help restore her dignity by showing respect, compassion, and concern for her feelings and needs while you provide personal care.

Communication.   People living with AIDS may be cut off from friends and family by the disease or by the attitudes of people around them. They may need to talk with someone about their fears and feelings of loneliness. One of the most important things you can do as you provide care is to be a good listener. Think back to the communication bridges you learned about in Chapter 5, Communicating with People. What are some things you may want to remember to do to communicate more effectively when you provide care for someone with AIDS?

Independence.   Often a person with AIDS loses control over many things in her life. Because of the disease, she may have lost her job, her home, her friends and family, and many of her physical abilities. You must provide care in a way that encourages her to stay as independent as possible. You can help her keep as much control as possible over her daily life, but also save as much strength as possible. She needs her strength to fight off the next opportunistic infection.

Infection Control.   Some people who work with those who have AIDS are afraid of getting infected. Universal precautions were designed to protect health care workers and the people they provide care for from contact with possibly infectious body fluids. You must practice good universal precautions when you provide care for someone who has AIDS, just as you should practice them when you provide care for anyone. You don't have to do anything differently for a person with AIDS than you do when you provide care for anyone else. You can safely touch, help, and hug the person, as well as laugh and talk with her.

Because of her weakened immune system, practicing good infection control is very important to the well-being of the person with AIDS. You must be especially careful not to spread germs that could cause the person to develop an infection.

Dealing with the Symptoms of AIDS

Several symptoms commonly occur when a person has AIDS. Descriptions of these symptoms appear in Table 17-1 on p. 402, along with the physical and emotional care you may have to provide.

In addition, as the level of the person's health changes and she spends more time in bed, keep the following suggestions in mind:

- ❖ Change the person's position in bed often.
- ❖ Monitor her skin condition and prevent bedsores.
- ❖ Maintain body movement as much as possible. Do gentle passive range-of-motion exercises as needed.
- ❖ Provide general comfort measures, such as giving a backrub or placing a bell to ring within easy reach.

Risks of Physical Contact for a Person Who Has AIDS

A person who has AIDS is particularly susceptible to infection caused by contact with people who have illnesses (especially chicken pox), foods that have not been handled safely, and pets.

Risks of contagious illnesses.   If someone living in the home with the person in your care has a contagious illness such as a cold, flu, stomach flu, or diarrhea, you and the person who has AIDS should avoid close contact with that person. Your supervising nurse should remind

Text continues on p. 405.

Table 17-1   Symptoms that May Occur with AIDS

Symptoms and Description	Physical Care	Emotional Care
Mouth Infection Sores or white patches in the mouth may cause pain and make it difficult for the person to eat or drink.	Provide frequent mouth care by using a soft toothbrush, a disposable mouth sponge, or a special solution ordered by the doctor or supervising nurse. Leave sores and white patches alone. Trying to scrub them off may cause bleeding. Report to your supervising nurse if the person has difficulty swallowing. She may suggest changing the person's diet to include foods that are easier to chew and swallow and that contain fewer spices. Offer water if the person's mouth is irritated by juice or soda.	Be compassionate. Remember how you felt at a time when you had a cold sore in your mouth, or a toothache, and were unable to eat.
Diarrhea The person may not be able to control frequent, watery stools.	Provide good skin care. Keep the skin clean and dry. Offer liquids often and encourage the person to drink extra liquids to replace the lost fluids. Report to your supervising nurse the frequency of the diarrhea, as well as the color and consistency.	Because being unable to control the bowels is embarrassing to the person receiving care, reassure her that you understand and are not upset by her loose or uncontrollable bowels. Act calm and tell the person it is not a problem for you to help her to the bathroom or help with cleaning after an incident. If you are calm, it helps the person remain calm and feel less embarrassed. Encourage the person to talk to you about how she feels.
Nausea and Vomiting An infection or a medication used to treat the person may cause nausea or vomiting.	Make the person as comfortable as possible. Ask what things would help her feel more comfortable. Reduce odors in the room, if possible. If the person wishes you to, gently wipe her face with a cool, slightly damp cloth. Provide mouth care as often as the person wants it. Wait until the person feels ready before offering food or liquid. Give clear liquids, such as ginger ale or gelatin, in small amounts to a person who is ready to eat again. Report to your supervising nurse whenever the person feels nauseated or has vomited, because she may be able to arrange for a medication that can help. Also be especially careful to report whether the person takes fluids and how much.	Reassure the person that you are nearby to help if she needs anything. Reassure the person that you understand and are not embarrassed or upset if she vomits.

Table 17-1   **Symptoms That May Occur with AIDS—cont'd**

Symptoms and Description	Physical Care	Emotional Care
Breathing Problems A person may have difficulty breathing and may be very nervous because of it.	Limit the person's activity if she has difficulty breathing. Check the person's position frequently. Sitting in an upright position makes breathing easier. Be sure nothing, such as tight pajamas or heavy bedclothes, blocks the person's breathing. Follow the doctor's orders if oxygen is required to help the person breathe. Encourage the person to stay out of areas where people are smoking.	Stay with the person during an episode of difficult breathing. Sit or stand calmly and quietly by the person. Your calmness may help her become calm. Be aware that anything upsetting may make the person's breathing more difficult. Anxiety causes difficulty in breathing, and the difficulty in breathing causes the person to become even more anxious.
Swelling (Edema) Swelling may occur in different parts of the body, including the face.	Apply cool compresses to the swollen area as directed by the doctor or your supervising nurse. Raise the head of the bed or help the person lie on several pillows if her head and face are swollen. Check with your supervising nurse about placing pillows under the person's swollen arms, legs, hands, or feet. Raising a swollen part of her body higher than the level of her heart helps reduce swelling. Observe the person's skin frequently. The skin over a swollen area may become stretched or torn. Provide good skin care by gently applying lotion to the swollen area. This may help keep her skin from drying and tearing.	Be compassionate. Think how you would feel if your face were swollen and misshapen. Tell the person you care, and encourage her to talk to you about her feelings.
Chronic Fatigue Feeling constantly tired is a common symptom of AIDS.	Ask the person how you can help. Involve her in planning her care. Ask what tasks she would like to help with and what tasks you should plan to do. Offer as much assistance as possible with personal care activities so that the person can save her energy. Offer frequent rest periods during activities such as walking or bathing. Plan your care so that the person can be rested and alert at times when there are things she wants to enjoy during the day, such as visitors or a special activity.	Reassure the person that you understand that her tiredness is caused by the disease and that you want to help as much as possible. Be compassionate. Imagine how you would feel if you were so exhausted you were barely able to brush your own teeth.

Continued.

Table 17-1   Symptoms That May Occur with AIDS—cont'd

Symptoms and Description	Physical Care	Emotional Care
Fever Many opportunistic infections may cause a low-grade fever in the afternoon and evening or may cause night sweats.	Encourage the person to drink liquids to replace fluids lost during sweating. As directed by the doctor or your supervising nurse, give a lukewarm sponge bath to help reduce the fever, but keep the person from becoming chilled. Keep her covered with a light blanket during the bath. Change linens and clothing frequently when sweating occurs. Use ice packs when directed by your supervising nurse. Place these in a face cloth or towel (never directly on the skin) and then in the person's armpits or near the genital region, or in both areas. Take the person's temperature often if she receives medications that are supposed to bring the temperature down.	Encourage the person to talk about feelings of anxiety or fear.
Muscle Loss Many people with AIDS lose as much as 20 percent and more of their body weight, which includes both body fat and muscle. This loss makes them even more susceptible to infections and skin problems.	Add high-calorie and high-protein extras, such as butter or margarine and peanut butter, to foods. Spread peanut butter on apple slices or bananas and add honey to tea. Have the person maintain an intake of 2000 to 2700 calories per day. Good nutrition is very important in helping to strengthen the immune system and to counteract weight and muscle loss. To help tone and strengthen the person's muscles, help her with range-of-motion exercises that you learned in Chapter 14, Providing Restorative Care. Because the person may have little fat or muscle between her skin and bones, reposition her every 2 hours to prevent decubitus ulcers, and give good skin care to prevent skin breakdown.	Help the person look her best by helping her with grooming and dressing. Encourage family members or friends to purchase new clothes in smaller sizes, if possible, so that the weight loss is less noticeable.
Mental Difficulties Because HIV often infects the person's nervous system, she may become confused.	Make sure the environment is safe and restful. Decrease clutter and noise. Speak in short sentences and use simple statements. Use memory cues, such as clocks and calendars, to help the person keep track of the time and date.	Stay calm, as your calmness has a tranquil effect on the person.

all people living in the home to make sure their immunizations are up to date.

If the person who has AIDS has not had chicken pox in the past, he should avoid any contact with a person who has the disease, because it can be deadly for a person with AIDS. The person in your care should avoid contact with—

❖ A person with active chicken pox.
❖ A person recently exposed to chicken pox. He should not be in the same room with that exposed person from the 10th to the 21st day after exposure.
❖ A person who has not had chicken pox and who may have been exposed recently.
❖ A person who has shingles, because that disease may cause chicken pox in the person who has AIDS.

If you learn that the person in your care is exposed to chicken pox, report this information to your supervising nurse, who will recommend that the person see her doctor immediately.

Risks of infections through touch.   When providing care for a person who has AIDS, you can help protect her from infections by—

❖ Washing your hands frequently.
❖ Not touching the person or her personal items if you have skin infections, such as boils, cold sores, impetigo, and shingles.

Risks of infections through food.   As you learned in Chapter 11, Providing Care for the Person's Place, and Chapter 12, Healthful Eating, handling food properly is vital for preventing infection and contamination. This proper handling is especially important for a person who has AIDS, as some bacterial infections, carried by spoiled food, are fatal to a person who has a weakened immune system.

When preparing food for a person who has AIDS, be sure to heat leftovers and other foods until they are steaming hot. Separate uncooked foods from cooked and ready-to-eat foods, and don't leave foods out of the refrigerator for more than 2 hours. Advise the person to avoid prepared foods from a delicatessen and soft cheeses such as feta, brie, Camembert, and blue-veined cheeses like Roquefort. Also advise her to avoid Mexican-style cheeses sold as "queso fresco" and "queso blanco." Have the person avoid raw, unpasteurized milk and products made from it, but let her know that cottage cheese, yogurt, and other pasteurized products are safe to eat. Be sure to follow "use by" instructions on food labels.

Foods such as organic vegetables and raw meats are very susceptible to bacteria. Either avoid these foods or handle them with great care. For example, thoroughly wash all fresh fruits and vegetables, and cook all poultry, beef, pork, and eggs until they are well done. Use two separate cutting boards: one for fruits and vegetables and one for meat and fish. Observe the basic rules of sanitation and hy-

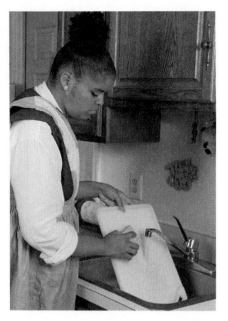

Figure 17-9
Wash a cutting board after preparing meat, chicken, or fish to reduce germs that can grow on the cutting surface.

giene presented in the home health care section of Chapter 12 (Figure 17-9).

Remember, a person with AIDS does not require separate dishes or eating utensils, and dishes used by a person with AIDS don't require special methods of cleaning.

The person with AIDS can prepare food for others, provided that she does not have diarrhea caused by a germ that can be spread by food. Anyone preparing food should wash her hands before beginning the preparation and avoid licking her fingers or spoons used during preparation.

Risks of infections through pets.   When providing care for a person who has AIDS, help protect her from infections through pets by having her avoid all contact with litter boxes or animal stool, bird cage droppings, and water in fish tanks.

Risks of infections through personal items.   It is especially important that a person with AIDS not share razors, toothbrushes, or other disposable items that sometimes draw blood. She also should not share other personal items such as tweezers, cuticle scissors, and pierced earrings that sometimes draw blood.

Providing Emotional Care to a Person Who Has AIDS

It is important to provide emotional care to a person who has AIDS, but it also may be difficult. The following tips may help you:

❖   **Be a good listener.** Try to stop what you are doing, no matter how important it is, and listen to what the person says. Talking may be the person's greatest need at that moment.

❖   **Be trustworthy.** Do not gossip about the person with your family or friends. Living with AIDS is difficult. Respect the privacy of the person in your care.

❖   **Be dependable.** Do what you say you are going to do, when you say you will do it. The person with AIDS has much uncertainty in her life. It helps if she can count on you to be dependable.

❖   **Be positive.** Always try to point out any improvement in the person's health, outlook, energy level, or capability. At the same time, if she is concerned about something, stay in touch with her feelings. Don't try to downplay or gloss over something that is very important and serious to her.

❖   **Don't be fooled by anger.** Remember that the person you are providing care for may be angry at AIDS, not at you. Don't take the anger personally, and don't let it affect the kind of care you give.

❖   **Keep your own emotions out of the way.** You may develop strong emotions as you provide care for a person who has AIDS. You may watch the person waste away and die. You may feel sorrow, frustration, or anger about someone going through such pain, but you must save your feelings for another time and place. Find someone you can talk to, such as your supervising nurse, a social worker, or a counselor in a community organization that helps people who live or work with people who have AIDS. Arrange to take a break from caregiving when you feel overwhelmed.

Think about all you have learned about providing care for a person who has AIDS. What things could you do to help Mrs. Hill live more comfortably? How can you provide for her physical needs? How can you provide care for her emotional needs, especially for her need to be a caring mother for Melissa? What things can you do to protect yourself from infection while providing care for them?

Who Are the Children with HIV Infection?

Providing care for children with HIV infection and AIDS may be challenging for some health care workers. To be most effective as a nurse assistant, you need more information about how HIV infection and AIDS affect children.

Children under the age of 13 who actually have AIDS account for less than 2 percent of the total AIDS cases. In addition, the Public Health Service estimates that, for every child who has AIDS, 2 to 10 children are infected with the virus but show no symptoms. As of December 1991, more than half of the children who had been diagnosed as having AIDS have died.

In comparison, as of December 1991, 789 adolescents ages 13 to 19 had AIDS. The number of adolescents who are HIV infected but have not yet shown symptoms of AIDS are not included in this number. Given the length of time between infection and the appearance of symptoms, experts suspect that many of the people diagnosed with AIDS in their 20s actually became infected while they were teenagers.

Sharing needles and syringes and having sex with an HIV-infected person are common ways that young people become infected. They are especially at risk because they often experiment with sex, alcohol, and drugs. As a result of these activities, many teenagers contract other sexually transmitted diseases—2.5 million cases a year. The potential exists for teenagers to become infected with HIV as well. If infected and sexually active, they may pass the infection to their children.

In the United States, babies with HIV infection who develop AIDS often die before they are 3 years old. On the average, they live only 14 months after being diagnosed with AIDS. Two factors that can determine how long they live are: (1) their age when they develop AIDS, and (2) the types of opportunistic infections they develop. Babies who develop *Pneumocystis carinii* pneumonia generally do not live as long as those with pneumonia caused by other organisms.

Babies and children with HIV infection and AIDS most commonly display the following signs and symptoms:

❖ Various bacterial infections
❖ Malnutrition and "failure to thrive"
❖ Pneumonia caused by organisms other than *Pneumocystis carinii*
❖ Anemia
❖ Shorter time to progress to AIDS
❖ Die in a shorter period of time
❖ Fail to develop Kaposi's sarcoma
❖ Heart, liver, kidney, or skin problems
❖ Nervous system damage, including developmental disabilities

Babies are not born with fully functioning immune systems. Remember that the immune system serves two functions:
1. To make antibodies against disease agents
2. To surround and attack these disease agents

When babies and children have AIDS, both functions of the immune system tend to fail. Adults, however, lose mainly the second function when they develop AIDS. They tend to develop viral, parasitic, and fungal infections. Babies and children with HIV also display—
❖ Weight loss.
❖ Persistent diarrhea.
❖ Recurrent fever.
❖ Swollen lymph glands.
❖ Severe thrush (oral fungus infection).
❖ *Pneumocystis carinii* pneumonia.

How Children Become Infected with HIV

Of the infants and children under 13 who have developed AIDS, the vast majority were born to mothers who were at risk of becoming infected or who had HIV infection, including AIDS. Many of these women did not know they were infected until their children were diagnosed and did not know that they could pass the virus to their babies. Because almost 80 percent of women who are HIV positive are in their child-bearing years, the number of infants with HIV born to infected parents will grow in the next few years.

An infected mother can pass HIV to her baby in three ways:

1. During pregnancy, the mother's blood nourishes the baby. If this blood has HIV, the virus could cross the placenta and infect the baby.
2. During delivery, the baby must pass through the mother's vagina. The baby comes in contact with her vaginal fluid, as well as some blood. If these fluids are HIV infected, they could infect the baby.
3. During breast feeding, the baby could receive milk infected with HIV. Other blood-borne viruses have been transmitted from mother to baby through breast feeding. Relatively few cases of

HIV transmission through breast feeding have been reported, and experts believe that the relative risk of transmission is small.

By December 1991, 8 percent of the children with AIDS had become infected through receiving infected blood, blood products, or body tissues. Five percent had **hemophilia** or some other **coagulation disorder**. These children became infected before the antibody test for HIV was developed and approved. All donor blood is now tested, and blood that tests positive for HIV is discarded. Blood that is used for producing blood products is treated to remove infectious agents, which include HIV, which may be present in small amounts from a recent infection and may not have shown up on the test. Thus, it is unlikely now that a child or adult would become infected by receiving either blood products or transfusions.

Providing Care for Children with HIV or AIDS

Infants and children who are infected with HIV or who have AIDS need the same things as those who are well. Infants need to be held and loved and have all the things that they need to grow physically and emotionally. Older children need to play and have friends and, when able, go to school. When you treat the infant or child as you would any other, the entire family benefits.

The same infection control principles apply to children as to adults. Remember to practice the principles of care that guide all your caregiving. In addition,—

❖ Pay extra attention to any changes in health or behavior and report these observations to your supervising nurse. For a young child with AIDS, these changes could become serious quickly. Watch for breathing problems, fever, exhaustion, diarrhea, and changes in appetite.

❖ Consult the doctor before a child with HIV infection or AIDS receives immunizations or booster shots.

❖ Wear gloves when changing diapers, since blood may be in the child's stool.

❖ Encourage the child to play with plastic and washable toys, because they are easier to clean. Stuffed and furry toys can contain dirt and can be a possible source of other infections to the child with AIDS. If a child plays with stuffed toys, keep them clean and machine washed often.

❖ Keep the child away from litter boxes and sandboxes to which pets or other animals have access.

❖ Ask your supervising nurse what precautions you should take if pets live in the home.

❖ Protect children with HIV infection from getting infectious diseases, especially chicken pox. Report immediately to your supervising nurse if the child has been exposed to chicken pox or shingles. It could be deadly to the child.

hemophilia
(he-mo-FILL-e-uh)   A hereditary blood disease, occurring almost exclusively in males, in which the blood fails to clot and abnormal bleeding occurs.

coagulation disorder
(ko-ag-you-LAY-shun)   An illness identified by problems in the process of blood clotting.

Providing care to a chronically ill child can be especially hard for family and other caregivers. Provide support by being trustworthy, dependable, and positive and by listening. Remember the anger parents express to you may really be directed at the disease, not at you. Also, try to keep your emotions out of the way while you are providing care. Talk with your supervising nurse about your feelings of caring for an infant or child with AIDS.

Information Review

Circle the correct answers and fill in the blanks.

1. Which statement is true? You can get AIDS if you—
   a. Share eating utensils with an infected person.
   b. Are bitten by an infected dog.
   c. Share needles with an infected drug user.
   d. Come into contact with someone's sweat during a basketball game.
2. AIDS is—
   a. A syndrome that has many signs and symptoms.
   b. A type of virus that infects only homosexual men and IV drug users.
   c. A type of bacteria that you can get in foods.
   d. An illness that you can catch by breathing certain germs in the air.
3. The abbreviation HIV represents three words:
   ___Human___ immunodeficiency ___virus___.
4. HIV infection breaks down a person's
   ___Immune___ system, a process that may take years.
5. The use of latex ___Condom___ during vaginal, anal, and oral sex can help prevent the spread of HIV.
6. A person who is exposed to HIV through contact with an HIV-infected person's blood, semen, vaginal fluids, or breast milk may become ___infected___ with the virus.
7. To find out if she is infected with HIV, a person has a simple test that checks for antibodies in the ___blood___.
8. The most common diseases that attack people when HIV infection has weakened their immune systems include *Pneumocystis carinii* pneumonia, systemic herpes, and candidiasis. These are called ___opportunistic___ infections.
9. People living with AIDS may include persons of ___all___ age groups and walks of life.

10. Because a person's ___*Condition*___ may change from
     one day to the next, you must be prepared to change the care
     that you provide each day to a person with AIDS.

11. In addition to providing physical care to a person with AIDS,
     you must provide ___*emotional*___ care.

12. Babies and children with HIV infection and AIDS may suffer
     from failure to ___*thrive*___.

Questions to Ask Yourself

1. A friend tells you that he tried shooting up
    drugs a few years ago, but he no longer
    uses drugs. He says he is afraid to get
    tested for AIDS for fear he might find out
    he is going to die. He also is afraid that his
    employer might find out about the test and
    fire him. How would you feel? How would
    you help him decide what to do?

2. Mrs. Hill is expecting visitors. She has lost a
    lot of weight and her clothes no longer fit.
    What can you do to help her look her best?

3. Mrs. Hill yells at you for fixing her hair
    wrong. You think she is being unfair and
    you are tempted to yell back at her. What
    things would you do to help calm yourself
    and Mrs. Hill?

4. A person with AIDS cuts himself while
    trying to shave. What precautions would
    you take before trying to help him?

18

Providing Care for People Who Have Alzheimer's Disease

Goals

After reading this chapter, you will have the information to—

Discuss cognitive impairment and dementia, including Alzheimer's disease.

Identify the causes of cognitive impairment that can be treated to reverse the symptoms.

Identify the needs and behaviors of a person who has Alzheimer's disease.

Discuss how to meet the needs and respond to the behavior of a person who has Alzheimer's disease.

Demonstrate an appropriate response to a person whose behavior is dysfunctional.

Identify ways that caregivers can make a difference when providing care for a person with Alzheimer's disease.

Discuss how to communicate with a person who has Alzheimer's disease.

Discuss the challenges caregivers face when providing care for a person who has Alzheimer's disease.

Identify the needs of a caregiver who provides care for a person who has Alzheimer's disease.

One day, Shirley McDay's husband asks if you have time to talk. You sit in the nursing home dayroom and listen as he tells you about the person Mrs. McDay once was. "By the time Shirley was 50 years old," he says, "she owned and operated an up-and-coming flower shop with a greenhouse filled with beautiful flowers and plants. She supervised two gardeners, an accountant, a receptionist, and a driver. Sometimes during busy seasons, she also helped make deliveries. She loved being her own boss.

"Three years later, she moved to a larger shop, where she eventually supervised 15 employees. She was more successful than she had ever dreamed. But, little by little, she also became more and more forgetful. Often, she misplaced her keys and forgot to keep appointments. She must have wondered what was happening.

"By the time she was 55, Shirley was acting more and more confused. She accused me and her employees of taking her eyeglasses, jewelry, and other items she couldn't find. She couldn't manage her business, and we became concerned about her driving.

"Shirley always used the same route to drive to the flower shop. But one day she got lost and must have become very frightened. When a police officer saw her weaving in and out of traffic, he pulled her over and asked to see her driver's license. In his report, he wrote that my wife didn't seem to understand what he meant. When he asked Shirley her name, she started questioning him: 'What are you saying? What are those lights on your car? Why did I hear sirens?'

"She agreed to be admitted to the hospital for tests and evaluation. While waiting for the results, we were standing in the room by her bed—my two daughters, my son, and myself. Shirley was sleeping, when suddenly she opened her eyes and

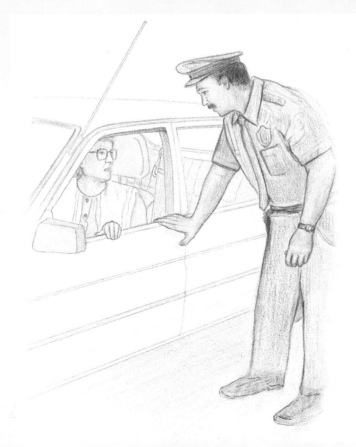

looked around at each of us, searching our faces. When she looked at me, I said, 'Hello, Shirley.' She sat up in bed and kept saying, 'Who are you? Who are you?' I said I was her husband, John. She said, 'No, you're trying to trick me. I don't know you. Where is John? He'll be here. I know he will.' I couldn't believe what I was hearing."

Mr. McDay stops talking and begins to cry.

Why Do People Become Confused?

A person becomes confused when her ability to know, think, understand, remember, believe, solve problems, learn, and create decreases. These mental activities are cognitive functions. Confusion is a symptom of memory loss, a condition that occurs when a person experiences cognitive impairment.

Some people assume that confusion from memory loss is a condition of old age. But most adults over the age of 65 do not behave in a confused way. Healthy older people are able to think and remember about as well as they did when they were younger. Most middle-aged and older adults retain their abilities to learn, remember, and solve problems. A normal adult may forget something, then realize that she forgot, and later remember whatever it was that she forgot.

Cognitive impairment, exhibited by memory loss, is not a normal part of the aging process, but the result of changes in a person's body. For example, a person may become confused when taking a particular medication. A person who has not eaten for a long time may become confused and forgetful. Someone who suffers from vitamin deficiency also may suffer memory loss. All these kinds of cognitive impairment can be reversed. The doctor can change the person's medication, health care workers can give nutrients to the person who has not eaten, and the doctor can provide vitamin therapy to someone with a vitamin deficiency. When these physical needs are taken care of, the person's memory generally returns, and she no longer acts confused.

In addition, cognitive impairment can be caused by certain illnesses, such as lung infections, stroke, heart attack, depression, hypothermia, hypoglycemia, brain tumors, and alcoholism. When these conditions are treated properly, many of the symptoms of memory loss decrease.

Some kinds of cognitive impairment are chronic and cannot be reversed. These chronic medical conditions are commonly called **dementias**. With these conditions, the mind gradually ceases to function as it once did. An affected person exhibits changes in personality, becomes confused, has difficulty carrying on a sensible conversation, becomes increasingly unaware of her surroundings, and ultimately becomes incapacitated. Approximately 50 percent of all residents in nursing homes suffer from some type of dementia. Of all the people diagnosed with dementia, the majority suffer from a condition called Alzheimer's disease.

Alzheimer's Disease

When Mr. McDay regains his composure, he asks if he may tell you more about what happened to his wife. You take time to listen.

"My family and Shirley's co-workers were the first to notice that things weren't exactly 'right' with her," Mr. McDay says. "Her forgetfulness and irritability were not typical of her usual behavior. But none of us realized how serious it was until she was unable to un-

dementia
(de-MEN-she-uh) An incurable disorder of the brain in which there is a progressive loss of memory and other cognitive (thinking) functions.

derstand and communicate with the police officer. In the hospital, the doctor examined her family history, performed a physical examination, tested her memory and reasoning power, and looked for symptoms of some underlying condition, such as vitamin deficiency. He ordered laboratory tests and x-rays, including a **CAT scan** (Figure 18-1). The CAT scan showed signs of brain shrinkage, which explained why she was less and less able to reason and understand. It explained why her personality had changed so much that, not only did she not know her family members, but we didn't recognize the person she had become. The doctor said Shirley had Alzheimer's disease."

Responding to People Who Have Alzheimer's Disease

A person who has Alzheimer's disease has the same basic needs as other people. Because of situations created by her condition, her capacity for meeting these needs often becomes limited, and her behavior becomes **dysfunctional** and may seem inappropriate to you. As a nurse assistant, you must understand these needs and behaviors, and you must know how to respond appropriately to them so that you can ensure the well-being and comfort of a person with Alzheimer's disease.

When you see someone behaving dysfunctionally, think of the behavior as a form of communication: The person is trying to tell you in the only way she can that something is wrong. Your job is to observe and think about the behavior to find out what she is trying to communicate so that you can provide appropriate care.

A person who is confused because of memory loss may behave in ways that seem strange to you. But the dysfunctional behavior of a person who has Alzheimer's disease has some common patterns. She may put up a **social façade**, pace or wander, rummage and hoard, have extreme **catastrophic reactions**, or become more and more restless and confused as evening approaches. She may say things that don't make sense, see or hear things that aren't real, or believe things that aren't true. She may be depressed, angry, or suspicious of people.

Some people who are confused because of memory loss may occasionally exhibit some of the same dysfunctional behaviors as people with Alzheimer's disease. If you know how to respond to these behaviors, you can provide better care. In spite of her dysfunctional behaviors, a person with Alzheimer's disease, as well as any person who is confused, still must be treated with dignity and respect.

Social Façade

Mr. McDay continues to pour out his story about his wife's illness. "You know, at first she was just a little forgetful," he says. "But, now that I look back on it all, I realize that her forgetfulness and confusion gradually were getting worse. When we went out socially, Shirley would only pretend to know the familiar people who talked with

CAT scan
Computerized **a**xial **t**omography, a form of x-ray that produces a three-dimensional picture of sections of the brain or other parts of the body.

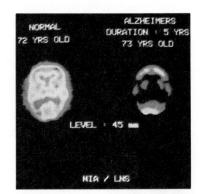

Figure 18-1
Alzheimer's disease is characterized by the death of nerve cells, which causes slight-to-severe memory loss, depression, confusion, and difficulty thinking.

dysfunctional
(dis-FUNK-shun-uhl)   Functioning in a way that is not normal.

social façade
(fuh-SOD)   In a social setting, pretending to know or recognize an unfamiliar person or thing.

catastrophic reaction
(kat-uh-STROF-ik)   Violent and sudden behavior that disrupts order.

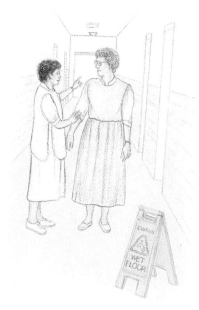

Figure 18-2
If someone who has Alzheimer's disease wanders toward an unsafe area, try to redirect her by suggesting she take part in an activity in the dayroom.

anxious
(ANGK-shus)   The state of being extremely nervous or agitated.

disoriented
(dis-OR-ee-en-ted)   A condition in which a person is unsure of who she is, where she is, and what day or time it is.

her. Soon it became obvious to me that she didn't remember any of them. I guess she put up a front to 'save face' and to hide the fact that she couldn't remember."

Think of a time when you may have pretended to remember someone who remembered you. Why do you think you pretended? Some people pretend to remember so that they can keep their dignity and self-respect. In the earlier stage of her illness, Mrs. McDay was aware of her disability and tried to hide it. She put up a social façade. Because she didn't look ill, she often was able to hide her illness.

It is important to know how to respond to a social façade. At a social event you may meet an old friend who only pretends to remember you. How should you respond? An inappropriate response would be: "You don't really remember me, do you?" A more appropriate response would be: "You may not remember me. I'm Chris Brown. We haven't seen each other since our last high school reunion."

If you know a person has Alzheimer's disease, you can promote good communication by making eye contact. Speak slowly, ask general questions, and use simple sentences. Give her information that she needs to respond appropriately. For example: "Mrs. McDay, your husband is coming down the hall. He looks well today." Keep the conversation brief.

Pacing and Wandering

Sometimes a person who has Alzheimer's disease displays a behavior called pacing and wandering. She walks aimlessly in an area and then walks away. She may pace and wander as a result of several causes. She may be overstimulated by too much talking or noise around her. She may feel uncomfortable, **anxious**, or **disoriented**. She may be looking for someone or something (Figure 18-2). Or she may not like what is happening where she is. Her behavior is a form of communication, but it could be unsafe.

When responding to pacing and wandering behavior, use some of the following suggestions:

❖ Reassure the person. Listen for a clue to what her behavior communicates. Gently ask, "May I walk with you?" and guide her back to where she should be.

❖ A distraction may help. Offer her a snack, take her for a walk, or do something she likes to do to help stop the pacing before her anxiety gets worse.

❖ Take her to use the bathroom. She may have a full bladder and not realize it.

❖ Try to help her remove her shoes. Removing her shoes may prompt an old memory that taking off shoes means a person should sit or lie down. (For safety reasons, replace her shoes if this action doesn't stop her pacing behavior.)

❖ Observe her for signs of anxiety (restlessness, fidgeting). Give her a ball or another smooth object to manipulate in her hands.

❖ Talk to her and listen to what she has to say.

❖ At her room entrance, place a familiar object (perhaps dried flowers or a photo from her past) to help her locate her room.

❖ Take steps to prevent the person from leaving. Some health care facilities have special safety doors to indicate when the door is being opened by a person who is wearing an ankle or wrist bracelet that triggers an alarm as she approaches the door.

❖ If you provide home health care for a person who has Alzheimer's disease, have her wear a metal bracelet imprinted with her name, address, phone number, and the words "memory impaired." Or place a card in her pocket with this information on it.

Rummaging and Hoarding

Mrs. McDay has begun going into other people's drawers and closets, taking items, and hiding them. When a person who has Alzheimer's disease behaves in these ways, these activities are called rummaging and hoarding. She may rummage and hoard because she might be feeling generally lost and confused, or she might not be able to find an item that she wants.

When you respond to Mrs. McDay's rummaging and hoarding behavior, use some of the following suggestions:

❖ Do not scold her, because she may become fearful of you as her caregiver.

❖ Try distracting her. Offer her another activity or a snack. Reorient her to where her personal belongings are.

❖ Take her to the bathroom. (She may have been searching for it when she wandered into someone else's room.)

❖ Learn her hiding places so that you can find lost items.

❖ Use your sense of fun and humor to help Mrs. McDay enjoy her environment, but be careful not to laugh at her behavior.

❖ Label all of her personal items and provide specific places for them. Put valuables away.

❖ Keep a spare set of keys in a safe place.

❖ Provide a rummaging drawer (Figure 18-3).

Catastrophic Reactions

When you greet Mrs. McDay this morning, she ignores you and seems restless. You explain to her that you want to give her a tub bath. After you gather supplies and prepare the bath, you approach Mrs. McDay. You mention again that you are going to help her with her bath. She begins to yell and lash out, and then tries to hit you.

Mrs. McDay is having a catastrophic reaction. Whenever a situation overwhelms her ability to think or react, she tends to overreact because she has lost the ability to control her impulses. At times she

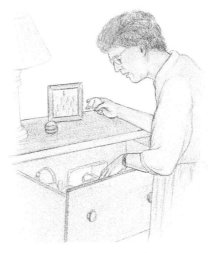

Figure 18-3

A nurse assistant placed inexpensive items in this drawer to satisfy Mrs. McDay's desire to rummage. The nurse assistant learned several of Mrs. McDay's hiding places so that items could be returned to the drawer when necessary.

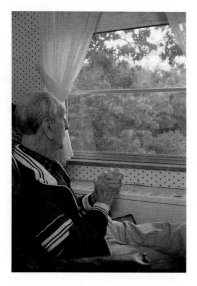

Figure 18-4
Agitation is one aspect of sundowning. Taking an afternoon nap may give a person more energy later in the day and prevent sundowning.

coping
(KOPE-ing) The ability to deal with problems and difficulties.

may strike out at people around her. When such situations occur, what should you do?

When responding to a person in your care who is having a catastrophic reaction, first identify yourself as you approach her. Look for nonverbal cues to her behavior. What nonverbal cues indicated that Mrs. McDay might be uncooperative? Do not take the attack personally. Avoid arguing with her. Keep routines as structured, predictable, and orderly as possible.

Although Mrs. McDay's behavior cannot be controlled when she is having a catastrophic reaction, the situation can. Stay calm. Prevent Mrs. McDay from injuring herself or anyone else but do not restrain her. Acknowledge her anger by saying something like, "You seem very upset. What is upsetting you? Things can get pretty scary when you're alone. What is frightening you? You seem to be uncomfortable. What is making you uncomfortable? Where do you have pain? Let's see what we can do to make you feel better." After each question, wait for a verbal or nonverbal response. What are some ways you can help Mrs. McDay if she is afraid, uncomfortable, or in pain?

Reassure Mrs. McDay that you aren't going to hurt her and won't allow her to hurt anyone. Let her know the limits by saying something like, "It's not okay to hit someone. It hurts." Distract her with her favorite activity. If she remains unable to respond to your request, try giving her a bath later.

Sundowning

As late afternoon or evening approaches, you may notice that a person who has Alzheimer's disease gets more and more restless or confused. He may become more demanding, upset, suspicious, or disoriented. He may be experiencing a behavior called sundowning, which is common to people with Alzheimer's disease. What do you think would cause a person's spirits to go down when the sun goes down?

During the day, as the hours pass, a person with Alzheimer's disease may become tired or less able to handle stress or may have difficulty **coping** with things (Figure 18-4). Approaching darkness may cause him to feel confused or afraid. Instead of communicating his needs, he may exhibit some of the following signals:

❖ Restlessness, anxiety
❖ Worried expressions
❖ Reluctance to enter his own room
❖ Reluctance to enter brightly lighted areas
❖ Crying
❖ Wringing his hands
❖ Pushing others away
❖ Gritting his teeth
❖ Taking off his clothing

These signals may represent real physical needs, such as needing to use the bathroom or being hungry, uncomfortable, or in pain. Or they may represent the need for loved ones who once shared their evenings, other human contact, or control over something. What are some ways you can determine what his needs are?

It is important to know how to respond to a person who is experiencing sundowning. After determining that someone doesn't have physical needs to be met, look for other clues that could tell you what his emotional needs might be. He may have a worried look on his face. He may be frightened of the dark or of unfamiliar sounds, or he might be afraid of being left alone. Accept his feelings.

Provide enough light for him to see his surroundings, but avoid glaring, bright lights. Offer to stay and visit with him. Talk softly to him and rub his arm or back. Comfort him with something to cuddle and play soothing music.

If Mrs. McDay experiences sundowning, try giving her some flowers to arrange to remind her of her former flower work in the flower shop. These measures should improve her feeling of security. If her reaction to approaching darkness includes pacing, provide a secure, visible place for her to pace or take her for a walk.

Find out when Mrs. McDay normally rested and try to follow that pattern. Before she had Alzheimer's disease, Mrs. McDay worked hard all morning in her shop and usually put her feet up after lunch. If you follow that pattern, keep Mrs. McDay active in the morning and let her rest after lunch. Plan fewer activities in the evening. Don't argue and don't ask her to make decisions during her anxious times. A person experiencing sundowning needs to feel calm and secure.

A person displaying any or all of these behaviors is responding to something in her environment. You must remember that she is not behaving this way on purpose to make her caregivers' jobs difficult. Patience and understanding are vital for providing care for people who have Alzheimer's disease.

Making a Difference

"At first, we tried to take care of Shirley at home," Mr. McDay tells you. "The social worker and other health care workers at the hospital helped us make a plan of care for her. They said we needed to have a consistent approach to treatment and that we needed to attend to her carefully to guard against potential disasters, such as turning on the gas stove and forgetting to light it, that may occur when a person is forgetful. So, we organized memory aids, lists, and routines for her. We made sure that she was warm and had regularly scheduled meals. When we needed a break, we arranged to take her to an adult day-care center that accepts people who have Alzheimer's disease. There she received lunch and occupational and activity therapy.

"But one day she wandered away from our house (Figure 18-5). We were frantic. We eventually called the police. For more than 3 days, a search team looked for her. Fortunately, the weather was warm and, when they found her, she was curled up under a bench in a school yard—tired and hungry, but safe. She had given us all

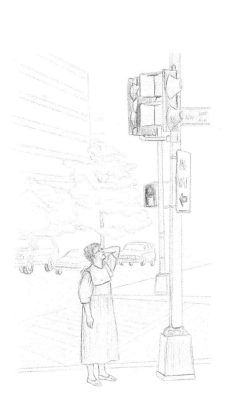

Figure 18-5
Shortly before she was admitted to Morningside Nursing Home, Mrs. McDay left her house and wandered beyond her neighborhood. Nothing looked familiar to her and she couldn't find her way back or ask anyone for directions.

such a scare. I think those were the 3 worst days of my life. That's when we decided to bring her here to Morningside Nursing Home."

Alzheimer's disease progresses through predictable stages and gets worse over time. People who have the early stages of the disease may be able to receive health care at home. However, demands on the caregiver's time increase as the person becomes less and less independent.

Providing care for a person with Alzheimer's disease is a stressful and challenging task. Understanding Alzheimer's disease and the behaviors that accompany it helps you provide care for the person compassionately and safely.

A person with Alzheimer's disease still needs joy and pleasure in her life. Simple pleasures such as a warm comfortable bed, a gentle massage, soft music, sweet smells, and bright colors can add to the quality of a person's life. Even when people are confused and out of touch with reality, compassionate care helps them feel secure. Always remember to celebrate the person's life by looking beyond the disease and seeing the person inside.

When you provide care for a person who has Alzheimer's disease, it is important to remember that—

❖ She does not act the way she does deliberately. It is the condition that causes her behavior.

❖ The person is an adult and must be treated with respect and dignity. Even though her behavior seems childlike, never laugh at inappropriate language or speech. Never talk about her as if she is not there.

When you provide care, keep the following overall guidelines in mind:

❖ Be creative and flexible. Something that works well for one person who has Alzheimer's disease may not work for another. If one thing doesn't work, try something else. Also, after a while, a particular technique may no longer work with the same person.

❖ Avoid situations that call for the person to make difficult choices or have to explain "why."

❖ Keep the environment calm and organized.

❖ Talk about pleasant past events.

❖ Be patient.

Caregiving Tips

Here are some additional tips to remember when you provide care for a person who has Alzheimer's disease.

Tips for communicating.   When speaking to the person,—

❖ Stand directly in front of her and maintain eye contact. Touching her arm or shoulder gently may help keep her attention focused.

❖ Speak softly, slowly, and clearly, using simple words and sentences. If she doesn't understand, repeat the same words.

❖ Use direct statements when you want her to do something. For example: "It's time to eat breakfast now."

❖ Allow extra time for her to understand and answer. Don't expect a quick response to a question or statement. If you don't get an answer, ask the question again using the exact same words, or come back in 5 or 10 minutes to ask again.

❖ Use humor when possible and appropriate.

❖ Because a person who has Alzheimer's disease is more comfortable in her own reality than in the present, don't argue with her or confront her. If she believes that it's 1956 and she's 19 years old, don't tell her she's wrong. Respond to the emotions she expresses.

❖ To help orient her when she is confused, remind her about where she is, what time of the year it is, and what day it is (Figure 18-6).

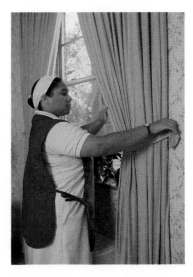

Figure 18-6
In the morning, to help orient someone who is confused, say, "Good morning, Mrs. Jones. Today is Tuesday, and it's a warm, beautiful spring day."

Tips for responding to behavioral problems.   When the person exhibits behavior that seems inappropriate to you,—

❖ Don't accuse her of lying or stealing. Her understanding of the world is different from yours.

❖ Use distraction. A temporary change of subject or scene often solves the problem. Often, distracting the person may cause her to forget what caused the problem.

Tips for maintaining an orderly and safe environment.   To keep the person's surroundings and activities orderly and safe,—

❖ Follow a simple, set routine. Introducing change can be confusing for her.

❖ Avoid situations that could make her angry or frustrated.

❖ Show her how to do things. For example, move your arm in an appropriate motion to demonstrate toothbrushing.

❖ Do activities in small steps. Remember that she is able to pay attention for just a short time.

❖ Remove safety hazards. (Read Box 18-1 on p. 422.)

Tips for promoting dignity and independence.   To show respect for the person and to promote her dignity and independence,—

❖ To help her dress independently, set out her clothes in the order in which she will put them on (Figure 18-7).

❖ Praise her actions as often as possible.

❖ In a nursing home, try to get her involved in scheduled activities that occupy her time, calm her, and give her a feeling of purpose and accomplishment.

❖ Make sure she gets enough exercise.

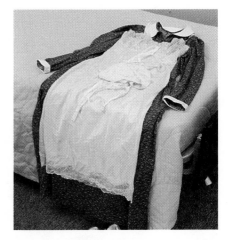

Figure 18-7
Encourage a person who has Alzheimer's disease to choose between two clothing options, and lay the garments out in the order in which she should put them on. Place outer garments on the bottom and underwear on top.

Box 18-1   Reducing Safety Hazards at Home for a Person Who Has Alzheimer's Disease

Reduce clutter.

Keep furniture and other items in the same position.

Lower the thermostat on the water heater.

Place gates or barriers at stairways.

Put away dangerous items (household poisons, guns, knives).

Hide a spare key outside the house.

Use a very large key ring to identify keys easily.

Supervise smoking.

Place locks near the floor on kitchen and outside doors.

Put locks on the windows.

To maintain a sense of independence and freedom for the person, create a space where she can wander.

Caregiving Techniques for Helping with Daily Activities

Use the following techniques when helping a person who has Alzheimer's disease with bathing, oral hygiene, dressing and grooming, mealtime, and elimination.

Bathing.   A person who has Alzheimer's disease may refuse to bathe because it seems too complicated. Or the person may believe that her privacy is being invaded. Respect her need for privacy and dignity.

❖   Find out the person's bathing schedule and stick to it.
❖   Have everything ready before starting. Be calm and unhurried. Avoid discussing whether the person needs a bath. Use expressions such as, "It feels good to be clean."
❖   If the person resists, try distraction, or wait and try again later. Never use force.
❖   Avoid using a shower. Water coming from above may frighten her.
❖   Use only a few inches of water in the tub. If the person objects or seems unhappy, adjust the water level according to her comfort. Keep the bathroom very warm because people who have Alzheimer's disease get chilled very easily. Make sure safety mats, side rails, and grab bars are available.
❖   Use pleasant distractions such as soft music, low singing or talking, massage, and colored bath towels to help the person relax in the tub.
❖   Remove locks from the bathroom door. Remove electrical appliances such as hair dryers and curlers, electric razors, and radios from the bathroom.

Oral hygiene.   Often a person with Alzheimer's disease doesn't brush her teeth or allow anyone to help her brush them. If she fights the procedure, stop and try again later. Use motions and gestures to encourage her to do it alone (Figure 18-8). In some cases, mirror the movements: Pick up a toothbrush to prompt her to do the same, or move a brush in your mouth so that she will do the same. Sometimes seating the person in a recliner and standing to the side while giving mouth care may make her feel less threatened.

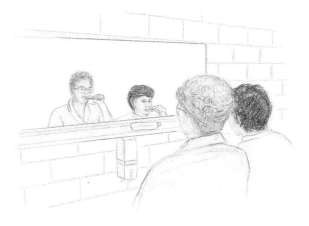

Figure 18-8
Sometimes showing a person who has Alzheimer's disease how to do a very common task is enough to trigger her memory of how to complete the task.

Dressing and grooming.   A person with Alzheimer's disease may not know what clothing is appropriate to wear, which garments to put on first, or how to fasten clothing. She may become frustrated with trying to dress or groom herself.

❖   Avoid forcing decisions. Remove clutter and unused garments from the closet.
❖   Lay out clothing items one at a time in the order in which they are to be put on.
❖   Encourage independence by providing clothing that fastens in the front with large buttons, zippers, or self-fastening fabric fasteners.
❖   Have her wear slip-on shoes with nonskid soles.
❖   Go slowly. Come back to an activity if it becomes too frustrating.

Mealtime.   A person who has Alzheimer's disease may not remember whether she has eaten, how much she has eaten, or what she has eaten. She may not remember how to use eating utensils and may have to be fed or reminded to chew or swallow.

❖   Offer finger foods, because they may be easier for the person to handle and less messy.
❖   If the person chokes easily, grind or chop the food.
❖   Try to serve foods that the person likes.
❖   Use plates without designs on them to avoid confusion. Also, if possible, use plates with colors that contrast with the food. For example, when serving white rice, put it on a dark-colored plate rather than on a white plate.

❖ Fill a drinking glass half full.

❖ Use self-help devices to help the person feed herself. (See Chapter 12, Healthful Eating.)

❖ Serve food warm. Make sure it is not too hot or too cold.

❖ Put only one food in front of the person at a time.

❖ Use simple instructions such as, "Pick up your fork. Put the food on it." Repeat as necessary.

❖ Remind the person to chew and swallow.

❖ Avoid placing things like ketchup, salt, or pepper on the table until the person asks for them, because she may use them inappropriately, or they may distract her.

❖ Keep things that might look like food (dog biscuits, flower bulbs, marbles, beads, etc.) out of sight.

Elimination. A person with Alzheimer's disease may not recognize the signals that tell her she needs to use the bathroom. She may not remember where the bathroom is or what to do once she gets there. It may help to do some of the following things:

❖ Post a picture of a toilet on the door of the bathroom to help the person recognize it (Figure 18-9). Use reflective tape around the door to help her see at night.

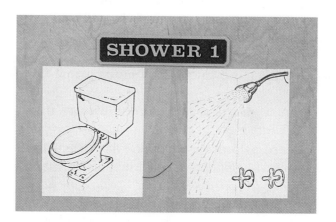

Figure 18-9
Placing pictures on a door shows a person who has Alzheimer's disease what is behind the door. Visual prompts help a person who may be unable to read signs.

❖ Set a regular schedule for going to the bathroom, and include using the bathroom as a regular activity after she has eaten. Maintain a regular routine for using the toilet for as long as possible to minimize the need to use catheters and adult briefs.

❖ Watch for signs, such as restlessness, that may indicate that the person needs to go to the bathroom.

❖ When helping a person get to the bathroom, turn on the light before she enters the room.

❖ A person with Alzheimer's disease may not want to enter the bathroom. She may think her reflection in the mirror is another person. Try removing or covering the mirror.

❖ Help the person remove or adjust clothing as necessary.

❖ Respect the person's need for privacy.

❖ Encourage the person to eat a high-fiber diet. (See Chapter 12.)

Understanding the Needs of Caregivers

Alzheimer's disease is a chronic condition that lasts for the rest of an affected person's life. Because a person with Alzheimer's disease loses her ability to take care of herself, she may need help with eating, bathing, grooming, dressing, and using the toilet. She also may be incontinent of bowel and bladder. She needs reassurance that her caregivers won't abandon her.

Alzheimer's disease can be overwhelming to the person who has the condition and to her family. The loss of the person's ability to think and reason causes dysfunctional behavior that is difficult for caretakers to understand and manage. Often she is confused, depressed, scared, and insecure. Over time, she becomes more and more dependent on her caregivers.

People who have Alzheimer's disease receive care in hospitals (when a person has an acute illness, such as pneumonia), in nursing homes, or at home.

Caregivers of people who have Alzheimer's disease may be family, friends, health care providers like yourself, or any combination of these people. To meet the challenge and handle the stress of providing care to a person with Alzheimer's disease, the caregiver must stay healthy. If you are the caregiver, you must have adequate rest, sleep, nutrition, and exercise, and you must balance work with play. You should ask yourself: What do I like to do for fun? How can I arrange to do these things on a regular basis? What consequences could result from my behavior if my life were all work and no play?

Suppose you are the family member who is the primary caregiver for Mrs. McDay and you have just spent 1 hour bathing and grooming her. She then becomes incontinent of stool and soils herself. You have not had a break from providing care for Mrs. McDay for almost 2 weeks, and you have been too tired to keep up your exercise program or to spend time with friends. Your meals have been inconsistent. You just want to sleep and not have to deal with Mrs. McDay. Because you have not taken care of yourself, you might react to Mrs. McDay in an inappropriate way. In what ways might you react?

Caregivers often fall victim to weariness and anger, as well as feelings of isolation and despair. These emotions can prevent the caregiver from coping with the situation.

Isolation frequently separates the caregiver, often a family member, from others. The caregiver may be overcome with despair, a feeling of hopelessness that robs him or her of energy. Caregivers need support from others. They need to know they are not alone.

Support groups are available to encourage caregivers to share their feelings and experiences and to learn how others cope with similar situations. Support groups also can provide information about available resources. These resources might include respite care to give family caregivers relief from providing care or bereavement counseling to help family members and friends learn to cope with the loss of the person who once was and learn to celebrate the person who remains. To be able to cope and celebrate, caregivers must take care of their own needs.

Information Review

Circle the correct answers and fill in the blanks.

1. Loss of the ability to think and reason is called
    Cognitive impairment.

2. Of the people diagnosed with dementia, the majority suffer
    from _ALZHEIMER_ _DESEASE_.

3. Behavior is a form of _COMMUNICATION_. The person is
    trying to tell you something.

4. Early in the disease process, a person with Alzheimer's disease
    may pretend to remember someone or something when in fact
    she does not. This behavior is called putting up a
    Social façade.

5. Mrs. McDay keeps wandering into other people's rooms and
    taking their personal items. You often find the missing items in
    Mrs. McDay's dresser drawer. What is the best response to this
    behavior? You should—
    a. Scold Mrs. McDay so that she will understand that she can-
        not take other people's things.
    b. Have Mrs. McDay return the items and force her to apolo-
        gize for stealing.
    c. Return the missing items to their owners yourself, and try
        to determine when Mrs. McDay is most likely to wander
        into someone else's room and the reason why she behaves
        this way.
    d. Keep Mrs. McDay confined to her room so that she doesn't
        have the opportunity to take things.

6. Mrs. McDay becomes very upset and starts to scream at you and
    other staff members when you ask her to sit down for break-
    fast. Her extreme reaction is an example of—
    a. Pacing.
    b. Catastrophic reaction.
    c. Sundowning.
    d. Social façade.

7. Which is the best response to Mrs. McDay's behavior? You
    should—
    a. Restrain her so that she doesn't hurt herself or someone
        else.
    b. Walk away.
    c. Tell her that you can tell she is upset and offer to walk
        with her for a while.
    d. Insist that she sit down because she should know better
        than to behave like that.

8. Mr. Lawrence has Alzheimer's disease. Each evening, between 5:00 and 9:00 P.M., he paces the halls and rips at his clothes. He empties his dresser drawers, screams if anyone tries to confine him, and begs visitors to take him home. An approach to managing his behavior that would *not* be beneficial is to—

   a. Keep Mr. Lawrence active in the mornings and encourage him to rest after lunch to minimize fatigue.

   b. Help him into a reclining chair after dinner and put him in a quiet, dimly lit room.

   c. Give him something to hold or keep his hands occupied so that he won't pull at his clothes.

   d. Take him for a walk after dinner.

9. Which of the following would be most useful in helping Mrs. McDay find her own room?

   a. Placing a recent picture of her on the door

   b. Writing her name on a sign on the door

   c. Placing a picture of her family on the door

   d. Placing a picture of her as a young woman on the door

10. Mrs. McDay confronts Mrs. Morgan in the hall and accuses her of wearing her clothes. What is the best thing for you to say?

    a. "You both have such good taste in clothes. I think it's time for lunch now. Come with me."

    b. "Don't be ridiculous. You know that she wouldn't even be able to fit into your clothes."

    c. "Mrs. Morgan, tell Mrs. McDay that you are not wearing her clothes."

    d. "You're absolutely right. I'll make her take them off immediately."

Questions to Ask Yourself

1. How would it feel to be providing care for someone who paces and wanders and has to be watched constantly?

2. How would you feel if you were unable to control your bowels and bladder?

3. What things could you do to give dignity and respect to a person with Alzheimer's disease? How could you give her joy and pleasure?

19

Finding Alternatives to Restraints

Goals

After reading this chapter, you will have the information to—

Describe restraints, what they are, and why they seldom are used.

List the different types of restraints.

State how restraints affect the people in your care both physically and emotionally.

Describe a person's right to be free from restraints and how you must protect this right.

Recognize the dangers of using restraints.

Use alternative methods whenever possible to manage the behavior of the people in your care.

Meet a person's needs rather than use restraints.

Use restraints correctly, when they are ordered by a doctor.

It's been snowing so hard that it looks like a blizzard as you ride the bus to work on Friday morning. You step down into a deep snow drift at the bus stop next to Morningside Nursing Home and grumble to yourself about having to walk all the way around to the main entrance when the emergency fire exit door is just a few feet away. Suddenly you turn your head in the direction of a voice that calls your name and see one of your co-workers standing in the open fire exit door. She motions you to come in that way. As you go through the door, she whispers to you that she taped the automatic lock on the door so that other health care workers can sneak in during the bad weather. You ask her if it's okay and then thank her for the shortcut out of the snowstorm.

During morning report, your supervising nurse assigns you to provide care for eight residents, one of whom is Bernice Klausner, a 65-year-old woman who has Alzheimer's disease. She was admitted to Morningside yesterday. Your supervising nurse tells you that you have to watch Mrs. Klausner closely because she frequently wanders up and down the corridors looking into every room she passes. Your supervising nurse expresses concern that Mrs. Klausner's behavior upsets two other residents. She says she also worries that Mrs. Klausner might get lost or hurt and has been trying to reach the doctor to get an order for restraints to keep Mrs. Klausner from wandering.

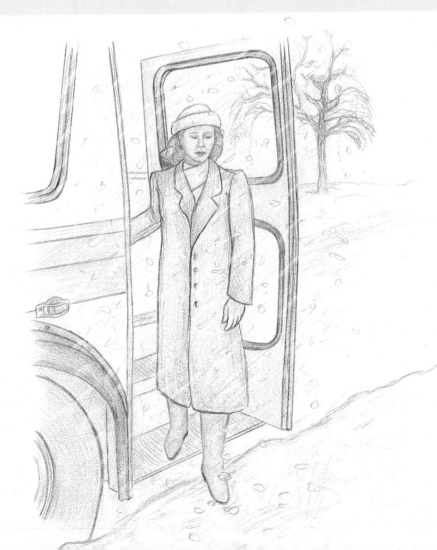

What Are Restraints?

A restraint is any device that inhibits a person's free physical movement or that controls her mood, mental status, or behavior. Until recently, most nursing homes commonly used restraints in the care of people—especially the elderly—to keep them from wandering away from the nursing home, to protect others from their sometimes abusive behavior, and to keep them from falling or injuring themselves. Now, health care workers know that they can use more human alternatives to accomplish the same goals as using restraints, while providing greater comfort and dignity to the person receiving care. Today, health care workers should use restraints only as a last resort and only when ordered by a doctor.

Restraints are classified as either physical or chemical. A physical restraint is any method or device that restricts a person's free movement or does not allow her normal access to her own body. Physical restraints include leg restraints, arm restraints, wrist restraints, hand mitts, soft ties or vests, lap and wheelchair belts, safety bars, and geriatric chairs (Figure 19-1, *A* and *B*). Chemical restraints are drugs that are used to control a person's mood, mental status, or behavior.

Fiction and Facts About Restraints

Health care providers once believed certain myths about physical and chemical restraints. Table 19-1 contrasts how health care workers thought about restraints at one time and what they now know to be true.

Some health care workers once thought that elderly people in their care didn't mind being restrained because they didn't complain and often became passive when restraints were applied. Health care workers didn't know of other ways to make sure people in their care were safe, so they tied them to their beds or in chairs to make sure they didn't fall over or wander around.

The fact is: People *do* care if they are restrained. You can meet their needs in many other ways without using restraints.

What We Now Know About Using Restraints

Today the use of physical and chemical restraints is considered a form of abuse, and a person has the right to be free from restraints. Refer to Chapter 3, Protecting People's Rights, and re-read the section about abuse.

Medical researchers studied the use of restraints and found that being restrained can injure people both physically and emotionally. Physical restraints can cause bodily injury and can rob a person of her dignity and independence. Chemical restraints are just as harmful, because they tie down the person's mind instead of her body.

As you read in Chapter 2, Working in Health Care, the federal government passed the Omnibus Budget Reconciliation Act (OBRA) in 1987. This law states that people receiving care in nursing homes and in their own homes have "the right to be free from any physical or

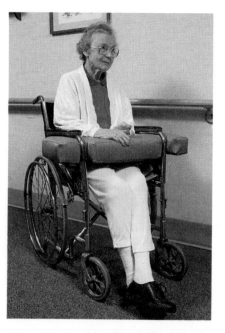

Figure 19-1A

In addition to preventing a person from sliding down in the wheelchair, this cushion provides a comfortable resting place for her forearms. When the person wants to move about freely, she simply removes the cushion.

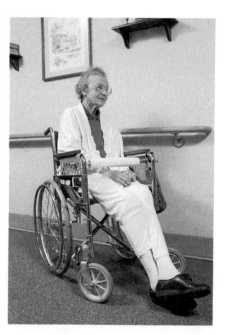

Figure 19-1B

This roll bar prevents a person from slipping out of the wheelchair, but does not rob her of her freedom. She can release the bar and move freely whenever she chooses.

Table 19-1   **Fiction and Fact in Restraints**

Fiction	Fact
Without knowing the facts, health care workers thought that using restraints was a good way to—	*In reality—*
Protect people from harming themselves or others.	More people are harmed than helped when they are restrained.
Make sure that people in their care were safe if no one was available to watch them.	It takes more health care workers to provide care for people who are restrained than to provide care for people who aren't restrained.
Keep people in certain positions, such as sitting up straight in a wheelchair.	Health care workers can use many kinder, safer ways to help people maintain good body mechanics without using restraints.
Protect their employers from law suits if a person injured herself or others.	Many law suits have resulted from injuries and deaths caused by restraints. No law suits have occurred because restraints weren't used.

chemical restraints imposed for purposes of discipline or convenience, and not required to treat the person's medical symptoms."

What this law means is that, with the exception of temporary use for life-threatening emergencies or medical treatments, health care workers can use restraints *only* under certain, specific conditions. Box 19-1 describes these conditions.

Box 19-1   **OBRA: When Restraints Can Be Used**

Restraints can be used only—
❖   With a doctor's order stating when, for how long, and for what purpose.
❖   To ensure the physical safety of the person or others.
❖   After less restrictive measures have been used unsuccessfully. (Less restrictive measures may include pillows, pads, and removable lap trays, which enable a person to retain some dignity and provide restorative nursing care.)
❖   When the person receiving care (or a representative of the person) and family members, if the person desires, understand both the risks and the benefits of restraints. If the person agrees to being restrained, she should receive an explanation of how the device works, why it is needed, and for how long it will be used.

The Problems and Hazards of Using Restraints

People who are restrained often develop physical and emotional problems. In addition, their safety is often jeopardized. Restrained people may panic and fracture or dislocate bones by struggling to get free. Some have died tragically of **asphyxiation** from restraints that squeezed their necks as they tried to escape from beds or chairs.

asphyxiation
(as-fik-see-AY-shun)   Suffocation caused by the lack of oxygen.

Physical Problems Caused by Using Restraints

A restraint can cause injury by keeping the restrained person in an unnatural position that violates good body mechanics. Restricting a person's ability to move can cause many other physical problems. Table 19-2 contains some examples.

Emotional Problems Caused by Using Restraints

In addition to physical problems, restrained people experience many emotional problems. Many people who are restrained experience—

- ❖ A loss of dignity.
- ❖ A loss of self-image.
- ❖ A loss of the ability to socialize with others.
- ❖ Increased dependence on health care workers and others.
- ❖ Increased agitation, confusion, and combativeness.
- ❖ Withdrawal and depression.

Safety Problems Caused by Using Restraints

The use of restraints also causes safety problems. If a person is restrained, an emergency situation can become deadly. Imagine what would happen if a restrained person suddenly needed CPR. Crucial

Table 19-2   **Physical Problems Caused by Restraints**

Physical Problem	Cause
Tissue damage	Restraints applied too tightly, causing pressure and constricting blood circulation, which strains the circulatory system and decreases blood supply to certain parts of the body.
Nerve damage	Restraints applied too tightly or the person fought the restraints after they were applied.
Chronic constipation	Lack of exercise or lack of independent mobility.
Incontinence from loss of bowel or bladder function	Lack of freedom to use the bathroom when needed
Loss of muscle tone and balance	Lack of exercise or lack of independent mobility
Pressure sores and contractures	Restraints applied too tightly
Pneumonia	Activity restricted or lack of independent mobility
Decreased appetite	Mental depression
Injury and death	Person struggled to get free

lifesaving minutes would be lost by having to untie the person before starting CPR.

Imagine the horror of a fire breaking out in a nursing home where people are restrained. Would there be enough time to untie everyone and get them and yourself to a safe place? Think about other people who might have needed your help while your time was spent frantically trying to release the people who were restrained. Restraining people makes them helpless and puts the whole burden of their safety on you and the other health care team members.

Avoiding the Use of Restraints

Mrs. Klausner's doctor believes that her wandering stimulates her circulation and helps keep her muscles active. He also thinks that Mrs. Klausner's wandering is a positive outlet for her energy. He is concerned that restraining her would rob her of this outlet and might redirect her energy toward combativeness and agitation. The doctor asks the health care team to find a kinder, safer way to deal with Mrs. Klausner's wandering.

Because Mrs. Klausner is in your care, your supervising nurse asks you to observe her for clues that might help the team determine some of the causes of her behavior. She says that, because you spend the most time with her, you may be able to observe patterns and behaviors in different situations and to know what is and is not working. She welcomes any observations and suggestions for solutions you can offer.

Accepting the challenge, you decide to spend as much time as possible during the next few days with Mrs. Klausner to watch for clues in her behavior. You notice that after breakfast she becomes very busy, leaves her room, and starts walking down the hall. She looks into every room she passes (Figure 19-2). If any of the other people notice Mrs. Klausner or call out to her, she smiles and waves, but quietly goes on to the next room. When she comes to a closed door, she opens it and looks inside for a few minutes, carefully studying the contents of the room or closet, and then closes the door and moves on. She seems irritated if you try to distract or stop her, but, after she finishes her walk, she is content to return to her room and allows you to help her with her personal care.

Mrs. Klausner's daughter Lisa arrives at the nursing home around noon to help her mother eat lunch. You introduce yourself to Lisa and tell her that you and her mother are just getting to know one another. After talking with her for a few minutes, you ask her what she can tell you about her mother's life before she developed Alzheimer's disease.

"Mother was the principal of the local elementary school for many years," Lisa says. "She was a good principal and was liked by all the teachers and students. She thought it was very important for the students to know her and be comfortable with her. So, every morning and afternoon she would make her rounds, stopping for a moment at

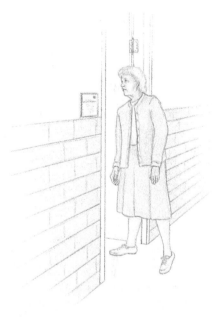

Figure 19-2
As you observe Mrs. Klausner, you realize that her wandering has a pattern. People who have Alzheimer's disease may wander aimlessly or may walk in certain patterns.

each classroom door. She never wanted to be a distraction, but she did want the students to know that she was making sure everything was all right. If any of them noticed her, she would smile and wave.

"When she retired 2 years ago, she received a beautiful brass plaque that said, 'To Our Principal and Friend.' Mother was so proud of that plaque that she hung it over our fireplace. Every now and then, a student would stop by our house just to say 'hello.' It makes me sad that I can't keep Mother at home anymore. I work, and she wasn't safe at home by herself after my father died. But I still bump into her old students when I'm grocery shopping, and they always ask how she's doing."

Suddenly Mrs. Klausner's behavior makes sense to you. You explain your observations to Lisa and thank her for giving you this helpful information. Lisa says she is pleased with your concern and impressed with your detective work. "I'm so relieved that Mother's here," she tells you as she gets ready to leave. "I know she is safe and receives good care."

Looking for Clues About Behavior

You must have reliable information to find ways to avoid using restraints while still providing good care in a safe way. A person in your care may communicate this information to you verbally or through her behavior and facial expressions. The information also might come from family members and friends. As you gather information, look for clues and ask questions. Read Table 19-3.

Table 19-3 **Looking for Behavior Clues**

General Question	Specific Question
What problem does the person in my care have?	Is Mrs. Klausner's wandering a problem for her?
Is there a need behind this problem?	Why does Mrs. Klausner need to wander? What is she looking for? Does she need to see that everyone is safe?
When does this behavior happen? Is there a pattern or routine?	Does Mrs. Klausner's wandering happen at certain times every day?
What circumstances make this problem worse?	Does Mrs. Klausner seem especially restless after taking a certain medication? (If so, perhaps the supervising nurse needs to discuss this reaction with the doctor.)
If a behavior pattern is the problem, is there a connection with a behavior from the person's past life?	Is this behavior similar to the rounds Mrs. Klausner made every day as a school principal?
What is the problem for the health care team involved in providing care for this person?	Is the problem that Mrs. Klausner might fall, get lost, or upset other residents?
Can the health care team members accept her behavior and ensure her safety? Can they put her needs before theirs?	Can the health care team accommodate Mrs. Klausner's need to "make rounds"?
Are there ways to let Mrs. Klausner wander without endangering herself or others?	What alternative to restraints can the health care team use to make sure that Mrs. Klausner is safe?

Helping People Who Are Agitated, Confused, or Wandering

Just as you suspected, after lunch, Mrs. Klausner starts preparing for her afternoon rounds. You feel less concerned about her behavior now that you have information about her past behavior as a school principal. You look down the corridor every few minutes to check on Mrs. Klausner as you provide care for the other residents assigned to you.

One of your co-workers asks you to help reposition a person who has a broken hip. This task takes more time than you thought it would, and it has been 15 minutes since you checked on Mrs. Klausner. You look down the corridor, but she is not in sight. You quickly check the other corridors, but she's not there either. Worried, you tell your supervising nurse that you can't find Mrs. Klausner. You also tell her about the tape on the fire exit door. Your supervising nurse designates who on the team will help search for her. (In some nursing homes, where residents are free to wander, health care professionals have put a process in place for locating residents. The process may include a designated search team and a method for sharing responsibilities for providing care for the other residents.)

Fortunately, you find Mr. Klausner in an unlocked closet (Figure 19-3). When she sees you, she smiles and waves. You take Mrs. Klausner gently by the arm, tell her how glad you are to see her, and lead her out of the storage room. Relieved, you watch her as she continues on her afternoon rounds.

Your supervising nurse calls everyone on the nursing home staff together and tells them what happened. She also tells them about the danger of the unlocked door to the outside, especially since it was snowing. "An important safety rule was broken today and we almost had a very serious problem," she says. Everyone agrees that it would have been much better to take a longer walk through the snow to the main entrance. They also offer ideas on how to help Mrs. Klausner avoid getting lost again.

Often the best way to avoid using restraints is to help people exercise as much as they can or do other meaningful activities, such as singing, moving to music, painting, or doing hobbies they have always enjoyed. These activities provide gentle physical and mental stimulation, help people feel useful, and improve their self-esteem. Each person in your care is an individual who has personal needs and desires. The care you provide must be special for each individual and flexible enough to meet each person's changing needs.

When mental or physical illness keeps people from acting safely and sensibly and causes them to become agitated, confused, or prone to wandering, many common sense measures can be used instead of restraints.

Focus on the environment.   Create a restful, stress-free environment for the people in your care to reduce some of the reasons for using restraints. Part of creating such an environment is establishing good

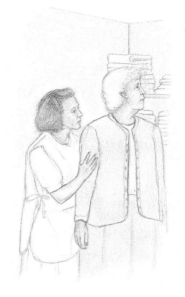

Figure 19-3
People who have Alzheimer's disease may wander into any place that is not secured. This closet doesn't contain anything harmful, but other closets may. Make sure that dangerous materials are kept in locked areas.

communication. As you read in Chapter 5, Communicating with People, people who cannot speak often communicate through their behavior and facial expressions.

Focus on kindness. People who have severe cognitive impairment respond better to caregivers who treat them gently, sensitively, and with respect. As a nurse assistant, you can provide better care for these people if they know that you care about them, are trying to understand them, and are willing to help them.

Focus on quiet. When providing care for an agitated or confused person, talk softly and eliminate as much extra noise as possible. Playing the person's favorite kind of music at a low volume on the radio may help.

Focus on calmness. To help an agitated or wandering person relax and to help satisfy her need for motion, encourage her to sit in a comfortable rocking chair. Give her something soft, such as a stuffed animal, to hug, because this also may help calm her.

Focus on familiarity. Encourage family members to bring in items that are familiar to the person in your care. A person's desire to wander may decrease if she feels at home in her room (Figure 19-4).

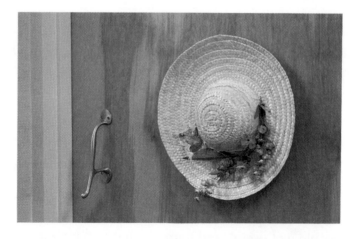

Figure 19-4
Pictures from a person's past or some of her favorite things may help her identify her room. A name plate may not help if the person can no longer read or doesn't recognize her own name.

Table 19-4 contains ideas to discourage people from wandering into inappropriate areas or from leaving the building. You remember that one of these ideas was suggested during the meeting after Mrs. Klausner was found, and you decide to try it.

You get a piece of adhesive-backed black felt from the arts and crafts cart, cut a large circle from the felt, and place it on the floor in front of the storage room door. You walk with Mrs. Klausner toward the door. She stops at the black circle. After studying it for a moment, she turns and walks away. It works!

When she has time, your supervising nurse asks you to tell her about what you have learned about Mrs. Klausner's behavior. You explain to her—

Table 19-4   **Ways to Discourage People from Wandering**

Take This Action	Why?
Place a dark mat, felt circle, or grid made of masking tape on the floor in front of doorways.	People who have impaired thinking often stop and won't use the doors, because they think there are holes or puddles in front of them.
Cover doors with wallpaper or curtains.	Covering the doors makes them less noticeable.
Place mirrors on doors.	Cognitively impaired people often stop when they see the reflection of a person in a mirror, because they don't recognize themselves.
Place a stop sign on a door.	Cognitively impaired people have better long-term memories and respond well to brightly colored safety signs that they remember from the past.
Use self-adhesive fabric to attach an 18-inch strip of fire-proof fabric to a door frame, or hang cafe curtains that swing open.	A cognitively impaired person often stops when he sees the fabric and won't cross through the door.
Encourage a person in your care to help you with simple tasks such as folding napkins, sorting papers, decorating a bulletin board, and pushing a beverage cart.	Keeping busy helps a person feel useful and active.
Suggest that your employer install alarms on all doors leading to the outside or to dangerous areas.	Alarms would alert health care workers if someone is trying to leave.
Suggest that your employer consider using some of the following devices and techniques:.	These devices and techniques enable health care workers to monitor a cognitively impaired person's movement.
❖ A battery-operated alarm, such as an alarm that is attached to a person's leg, that monitors her movements.	This alarm could indicate if she tries to get out of bed.
❖ Movement sensors that are placed in a person's shoes to track her location.	These sensors could indicate her location if she wanders off.
❖ A special call signal that slips through the sleeve of a person's shirt or gown and sets off an alarm if the person gets out of bed and pulls the signal from the wall.	This signal would indicate that the person needs to be redirected.

❖ About Mrs. Klausner's past life and suggest that Mrs. Klausner be permitted to make rounds every day to "make sure that everyone is all right."
❖ That Mrs. Klausner walks well but often needs prompting to find her way to her room or to the dining room.
❖ About the black felt circle and offer to make more circles for any other doors that might pose problems.

You ask permission to call Lisa Klausner to suggest that she bring in the plaque given to Mrs. Klausner by her students and any other items that might make her feel more at home when she is in her room. You also suggest that the residents who are upset by Mrs. Klausner's behavior might feel better if they understand that she looks into their rooms because, in her former job, she used to check in all the rooms.

Your supervising nurse is impressed with your ideas and your plan. The next day she takes Mrs. Klausner with her on her daily rounds, and together they check each room to make sure each resident is all right. In a short period of time, Mrs. Klausner is well known and liked by everyone at Morningside Nursing Home. And the other health care team members often ask your advice about ways to avoid using restraints on the people in their care.

Helping People Who Need Individualized Support

Many elderly and weak people cannot keep themselves in proper body alignment. Some people constantly slump forward, lean to one side, or slide down in their chairs if they are not supported. Instead of using restraints, use the following techniques and devices to help the people in your care maintain proper body alignment:

❖ Use wedge cushions, positioning pillows, beanbag cushion seats placed in wheelchairs, and deep, inclined seats to support people who tend to slump forward, lean to one side, or slide out of chairs.

❖ Try a variety of chairs, such as recliners, lounge chairs, rocking chairs or gliders, and deep-seated chairs with high backs (Figure 19-5).

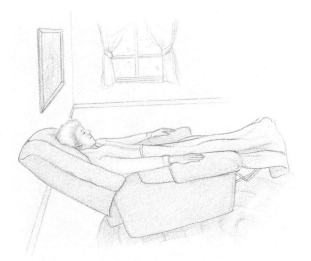

Figure 19-5
Mrs. Klausner can't easily get out of the big chair by herself, but she has freedom to change position and move about in the chair. This is a good alternative to restraining her.

Review your employer's policy on restraints. Policies differ from one facility to another as changes are made to follow the OBRA laws regarding the use of restraints. Because this is a new law, health care facilities may be in various stages of implementing it. Your employer may value your ideas and suggestions. By sharing your knowledge and skills, you play an important role in helping both your employer and your co-workers to monitor the behavior and movement of people in their care in kinder, safer ways with a minimum use of restraints. Show them what you know and how well it works for the people in your care, as well as for other health care team members. And by your example you can show them that you recognize the importance of following the law to maintain safety and provide proper care.

When Restraints Become Necessary

With the passage of OBRA's law restricting restraints, limitations on the use of restraints triggered many questions from health care workers: What are acceptable uses for restraints during medical treatment? What about a woman who receives intravenous fluids and becomes agitated and restless? What is an acceptable use for restraints during a life-threatening emergency? What about a young man who is combative because of a head injury from a car crash?

In their efforts to comply with the law, nursing homes can become predominantly restraint-free, but there are times and conditions when restraints may still have to be used, and OBRA acknowledges these situations. When restraints are ordered by a physician and are used within the law, you must know how to take care of a restrained person.

The Use of Restraints in Hospitals

Health care workers should know the hospital's policy regarding restraints and how they are used. Generally, hospitals follow restraint guidelines that are similar to those used in nursing homes, such as:

❖ Restraints cannot be used without a doctor's order.
❖ As needed or "prn" orders for restraints are not acceptable.
❖ The doctor's order must include time limits for how long the restraint is to be applied.
❖ The restraint and the reason why it was ordered must be explained to the patient.
❖ Restrained patients must be checked at regular intervals, and the maximum time between observations must be noted.
❖ Health care workers must be trained to use restraints correctly and safely before using them on patients.

However, because hospitals are governed by a different set of laws than nursing homes, their policies on restraints are slightly different. In a psychiatric hospital, a violent person's legs and wrists may be restrained. This person may not be released upon request because she may injure herself and others while she is violent. The doctor who ordered the restraints specifies when the patient can be released.

Hospitals have begun to examine their use of physical and chemical restraints, acknowledging that there are alternative ways to provide safety and support for patients. Generally, restraints are used in hospitals only because they are needed on a short-term basis for problems that will improve with medical care.

Providing Care for a Person Who Is Physically or Chemically Restrained

If a doctor orders a physical restraint for a person in your care, you must observe the person carefully and report any problems immediately to your supervising nurse. Physical restraints most commonly used are:

❖ Wrist restraints, which limit the movement of the arms.

❖ Waist restraints, which are designed to keep a person from falling out of bed or out of a chair.

❖ Poncho or vest restraints, which are designed to keep people from standing up or moving around.

If a person in your care is physically restrained, it is your job to help safeguard her well-being. Follow these important rules when providing care for a person who is physically restrained.

❖ Remind the person and her family why the doctor has ordered restraints to be used.

❖ Understand exactly how to use the restraint, making sure to use the right size for the person's height and weight. Secure the restraint properly.

❖ If a person is restrained, check on her every 15 minutes. She may need to be reassured that she hasn't been abandoned. Many people injure themselves by trying to get out of restraints without assistance.

❖ Release the restraints every 2 hours and help the person go to the bathroom, stretch, and do range-of-motion exercises. Inspect her skin for reddened areas and report any concerns to your supervising nurse. Release the restraints more often if the person seems to be anxious, needs to go the bathroom, or is in distress.

If a doctor orders a chemical restraint for a person in your care, you must observe the person carefully and report any physical reactions or changes in behavior immediately to your supervising nurse. Such reactions might be an increase in agitation, drowsiness, or decreased appetite.

Information Review

Circle the correct answers and fill in the blanks.

1. The two categories of restraints are
   _____*physical*_____ and _____*chemical*_____.

2. Chemical restraints tie down a person's
   _____*mind*_____ instead of her body.

3. The Omnibus Budget Reconciliation Act of 1987 is also called
   _____*OBRA*_____. This law states that people in nursing homes have the right to be free from
   _____*restraints*_____.

4. OBRA allows restraints to be used for temporary use—
   a. For mealtimes and sleeping.
   b. For life-threatening emergencies and medical treatments.
   c. For times when you must search for a missing person.
   d. If there aren't enough health care workers available.

5. Two physical injuries that can result from restraints are

    hurt muscle or nerve and _suffocation_ .

6. Besides physical injuries, restraints also can cause

    _____ _emotional_ _____ problems for a restrained person.

7. One way to help protect the safety of a person who wanders
    is—

    (a.) Place a large, dark circle on the floor in front of a doorway
         that leads to danger.

    b. Put a blindfold over her eyes so that she can't see where
        she's going.

    c. Put her on a long leash so that you can hang on to her.

    d. Tie her to a chair.

8. A restrained person must be checked every

    _____ _15_ _____ _minutes_ .

9. Restraints must be released at least—

    a. Every shift.

    b. Every hour.

    c. Every 2 hours, and more often if necessary.

    d. Whenever a relative visits.

10. Three restraint devices are _____,

    _____, and _____.

Questions to Ask Yourself

1. How would you feel if someone tied you
    down against your will?

2. What are some of the physical problems
    that can result from restraining a person?

3. Every time you come near Ms. Cayhill she
    spits at you and tries to hit you. How can
    you help her with personal care without
    restraining her arms?

4. Why have restraints been used so much in
    nursing homes in the past? What is
    different now?

5. Would your job as a nurse assistant be
    easier if you had restrained Mrs. Klausner?
    How might she have reacted?

6. What important things did you learn about
    being a detective for Mrs. Klausner?

7. What are some things you can do to
    prevent a person who has impaired
    thinking from leaving a room?

8. Think of two situations in which a person
    might be restrained in a hospital.

20

Providing Care for People Having Surgery

Goals

After reading this chapter, you will have the information to—

Explain why people have surgery.

Describe the differences among required surgery, emergency surgery, and elective surgery.

Explain what happens during surgery.

Prepare an adult and a child for surgery.

Provide care for a person after surgery.

Support the family and friends of a person undergoing surgery.

After practicing the corresponding skills in the skills book, you will be able to—

Apply elastic stockings to a surgical patient's legs.

Transfer a person from a bed to a stretcher.

Make a postoperative bed.

Steve Henderson is a 55-year-old man who arrived on the surgical floor today in preparation for surgery tomorrow. He has had a great deal of stomach pain, and after several tests, his doctor has decided that Mr. Henderson should have his gall-bladder removed. He has been admitted as an inpatient and will have the surgery in the hospital operating room. Mr. Henderson's chart indicates that he will be in surgery for about 1½ hours and that he will be under general anesthesia.

After he is admitted, Mrs. Henderson stays with her husband for an hour to keep him company. She seems to be nervous and tries to do everything for him. He keeps reassuring her that he is okay and that everything will turn out all right. He pats her hand and tries to make her smile. You notice that he talks almost non-stop with her and the hospital staff, making jokes and laughing. Later, on her way out of the surgical department, Mrs. Henderson says to you, "Well, I'm glad he's taking this better than I am. I worry about him, and I just don't know what I would do without him."

After his wife leaves, you notice that Mr. Henderson's mood changes radically. He stops laughing and joking and doesn't say much at all. He sits on the edge of his bed rubbing his hands together and staring out the window. You have to call his name several times before he realizes that you are talking to him.

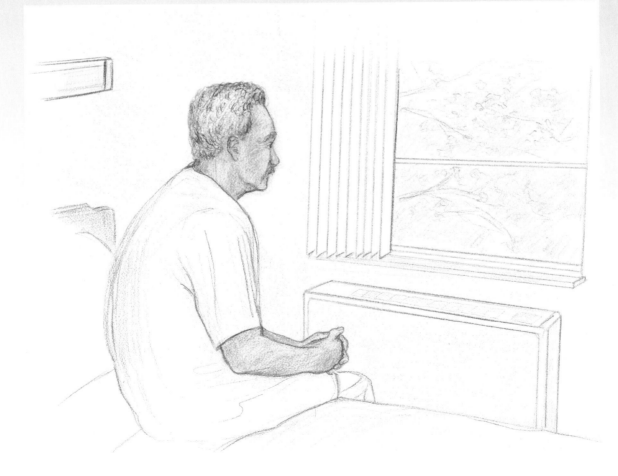

surgeon
(SER-jin)   A medical doctor who uses medical instruments to perform procedures to restore a person's health.

incision
(in-SIZH-un)   A cut made during surgery.

preoperative
Before surgery.

postoperative
After surgery.

Have you ever had surgery? Have you ever known someone who had surgery? Surgery, also called an operation, is a procedure in which a **surgeon** uses medical instruments to improve or restore a person's health. Unlike medical care, which focuses on the use of medicine to improve or restore health, surgery is an invasive procedure. The surgeon cuts into a person's body with a sharp instrument, making an **incision**. Because the inside of a person's body is exposed during surgery, the risk of infection increases.

As a nurse assistant, you may work in the surgical department of a hospital. There, you help your supervising nurse prepare people for surgery by providing **preoperative** care. After the patient has surgery and returns to a room in the surgical department, you help provide **postoperative** care.

Why People Have Surgery

A person may have surgery to repair, remove, or replace a part of his body or to change the way a part of his body looks. A person with a broken leg may need surgery to repair the bone. A person such as Mr. Henderson, who has gallstones, may need surgery to remove his gallbladder. A person with severe arthritis of the hip joint may need surgery to replace the joint. A person who wants to change his appearance may elect to have surgery to alter the shape of his nose.

Urgency of Surgery

Factors such as the person's needs and the condition of his health determine whether the surgery is emergency, required, or elective.

Emergency surgery.   To save a person's life, doctors may perform emergency surgery. They perform the surgery as soon as possible after the person is admitted to the hospital. For example a person who has been in a car crash may need emergency surgery to stop internal bleeding.

Required surgery.   To maintain a person's proper bodily function, a doctor performs required surgery, which can be scheduled in advance for a condition that is not immediately life threatening. A doctor schedules required surgery for a person who needs to have a lens removed to improve his sight, for a person who needs to have a tumor removed from his intestines, or for a person such as Mr. Henderson who needs to have his gallbladder removed.

Elective surgery.   A person may choose to have elective surgery for a condition that is not life threatening and does not harm bodily function. Elective surgery always is scheduled in advance. A person may choose to have this type of surgery to change the shape of his nose or chin.

What Happens During Surgery

Doctors perform surgical procedures in the outpatient surgical clinic and in the inpatient operating room, also called the OR (Figure 20-1). They select the location for surgery based on the kind of surgery to be performed and on the condition of the patient's health.

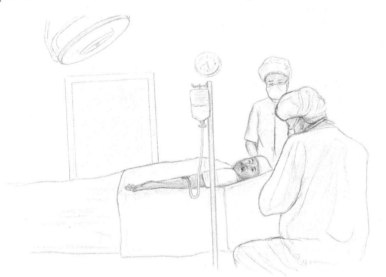

Figure 20-1
Lights, machines, and other operating room equipment can be frightening to a patient lying on the operating table. Before the patient goes into the operating room, health care providers can ease some of his anxiety by telling him what to expect.

When doctors perform minor surgery for less complicated procedures in the outpatient surgical clinic, they usually discharge the patient to his home the same day. When they perform major surgery for more complicated procedures, they admit the patient to the hospital, because it takes longer to perform the surgery and the person needs more time to recover.

Before surgery, the patient receives an **anesthetic** so that he does not feel any pain during the surgery. Two basic types of anesthetics are:

anesthetic
(an-es-THET-ik)   A special medication that causes a loss of feeling in part or all of the body.

1. Local or regional anesthetic, which causes a loss of sensation in a specific part of the person's body. An example of a regional anesthetic is a spinal anesthetic. The person receiving a local or regional anesthetic is awake and aware of the surgery being performed, but cannot feel pain in the anesthetized area.
2. General anesthetic, which causes a loss of feeling or sensation in the person's entire body. The person receiving a general anesthetic is unconscious, or asleep.

During surgery, people on the health care team constantly observe the patient. They monitor his vital signs to make sure his body keeps working correctly while the doctor performs the surgical procedure.

After major surgery, health care workers closely monitor the patient's pulse, respirations, blood pressure and the site of the incision in the **recovery room**, watching for immediate complications. The doctor writes orders for the patient to be transferred back to the surgical department when his condition is stable, which means that his vital signs are steady.

recovery room
A room in a hospital used to observe and treat patients who have just had surgery.

Preparing a Patient for Surgery

After Mr. Henderson's wife leaves, you tell him that you have come to talk to him about some of the things you will do to help him prepare for surgery. Mr. Henderson turns away and stares out the hospital window.

You ask him if there is something you can do to help. "Not really," he says. "I'm just worrying about all of this surgery stuff." When you ask him if the doctor and nurse have explained the procedure and follow-up care, he says, "Yeah. It's not that. It's just that I'm gonna be laid up for several weeks and Lola—that's my wife—she's never had to take care of everything at home by herself, and well, what if my company finds out that they can get along fine without me?"

Emotional Preparation

Providing specific knowledge and emotional support is an essential part of surgical care for both adults and children.

Preparing an adult emotionally for surgery. Sometimes a person is afraid because he doesn't know what is going to happen to him. This operation may be his first surgical procedure, or he may have known someone who had a bad experience with surgery. He also may be afraid because the surgery may confirm the presence of a serious disease, such as cancer. If you were going to have surgery tomorrow, what would you want to know? What would you have to have explained so that you felt prepared? How would you feel about having surgery?

Doctors and nurses give the patient information about the events that occur before and after surgery. The doctor explains the surgical procedure and the expected outcome to help lessen the patient's anxiety.

The evening before surgery, the nurse talks with the patient about what happens before, during, and after the procedure (Figure 20-2). The nurse tells the person—

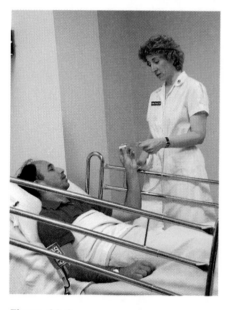

Figure 20-2
During her preoperative talk with a patient the night before surgery, the nurse shows him some equipment that may be used during and after surgery.

incentive spirometer
(in-SEN-tiv/spy-ROM-uh-ter) A small device that encourages a person to take deep breaths to help clear his lungs after surgery.

❖ About the specific treatments he will have before and after surgery.
❖ What to expect in the operating and recovery rooms.
❖ Information about surgical dressings, drains, tubes, and IVs.
❖ How to do coughing exercises.
❖ How to do deep-breathing exercises using an **incentive spirometer** (if he is having a general anesthetic).
❖ What activities are acceptable after surgery.

Sometimes a person is afraid of postoperative pain that he may experience. Another person may be afraid of dying during surgery or of never waking up from the anesthesia. Many people worry about who can provide care for their family members or their homes while they are in the hospital. Others wonder whether they will still have jobs after they recover from surgery and whether they will be able to pay their bills.

How can you help a person feel less anxious about his situation? As a nurse assistant, you can listen to the patient, talk to him, show him you care about his feelings, and let him know that you are interested in him. Communicate his questions and concerns to your supervising nurse and make sure he receives the answers to the questions. He will probably feel better when he knows that someone cares about him.

Preparing a child emotionally for surgery.   To prepare a child for surgery, determine the child's age, ability, and developmental level (review the section on developmental milestones in Chapter 4, Understanding People), as well as his physical condition. Having an understanding of these factors will help you match your activities and communication to the child's level of comprehension. Assess the child's emotional state so that you can support him through the surgical experience. For example, if a child has had previous surgery, that experience may influence his reaction to his current hospitalization. Or if he has experienced a recent life change, such as the birth of a brother or sister, a divorce, or the death of a family member, this event may add to the stress of the surgery.

Encourage parents to participate during teaching sessions or tests whenever possible, because their presence can be comforting to the child. Parental participation also can help the parents feel more involved in the care of their child.

Certain events surrounding surgery are predictably stressful to the child. These common stress points typically are the following:

❖ Admission to the hospital
❖ Blood tests
❖ The afternoon of the day before surgery when preparation for surgery may include special tests or procedures
❖ Preoperative injection of medication
❖ Transport to the operating room
❖ Return from the recovery room

Recognize these stress points and act appropriately to reduce the child's anxiety. Your care and concern will have a beneficial effect on the child's ability to cope with the stress of surgery. In addition, if you provide the child with information about what he will see, hear, smell, and feel, he will be more prepared to cope with surgery. Think about the child's concerns so that you are more sensitive to his needs (Box 20-1 on p. 448).

Whenever possible, the child's physician and the parents begin the preparation before the child enters the hospital. Once in the hospital, the nurse often uses dolls, medical equipment, and pictures to explain to the child what to expect. Encourage the child to talk freely about his fears and feelings and offer information whenever possible to make him feel more comfortable. Encourage his parents to be available for him as much as possible.

You can even help prepare an infant for surgery by playing peek-a-

Box 20-1   Common Concerns of Children Who Experience Surgery

Before, During Transport to, and in the Operating Room	*After Return from the Operating Room*
Feelings	**Feelings**
Fear (of waking up during the operation, pain, being alone, "falling off the stretcher," death)	Dizziness, nausea
Helplessness	Pain
Hunger	Cold
Thirst	Fear
Dizziness or nausea from preop medication	Relief that it is over
	Inability to move
	Helplessness
	Sore throat from intubation
	Hunger or thirst
Smells	**Smells**
Hospital smells	Gases, medications
Antiseptic cleaning solutions	Cleaning solutions
Sights	**Sights**
Strangers in uniforms, masks, gowns	Parents
Unfamiliar surroundings	IV equipment
Stretcher, rails, straps	Monitors
Elevators	BP cuff
Ceilings of strange rooms	Dressings
Strange equipment, bright lights, monitors	Changes in body at site of surgery
	Drainage tubes or bottles
	Blood
	Side rails
Sounds	**Sounds**
Strange voices as the stretcher is rolled along the hallways	Voices of transporters and others in hallways and elevator
Clang of side rails	Parents' voices
Sound of wheels	Beeps, hums, clicks
Automatic door sounds	Clang of side rails
Beeps, hums, clicks	
Strange people talking to each other	
Voices muffled under masks	
Tastes	**Tastes**
Often a dry mouth due to preop medication	Dry mouth
	Perhaps ice chips
Touch	**Touch**
Straps to "hold you still"	Pressure of BP cuff on arm
People "helping you move"	People's hands touching, examining, and helping to move
Cold, hard operating table	IV
	Dressings and tape

boo with surgical masks and caps, and by encouraging him to touch equipment such as IV tubing or stethoscopes. This involvement helps to satisfy his curiosity.

Physical Preparation

A person having surgery requires physical preparation that begins the evening before surgery and is completed on the morning of the operation. You assist your supervising nurse in preparing the person for surgery in a variety of ways.

Assisting the evening before surgery.   The evening before surgery, the doctor may order specific treatments for the person, such as an enema, vaginal douche, or skin prep. (See Box 20-2 to learn more about skin preps.)

Box 20-2   **Skin Prep**

> Skin preparation for surgery involves cleaning the patient's skin and shaving hair from the area of the body where the surgery is to be performed. Most often the skin prep is done in the operating room, although sometimes it is done in the patient's room the evening before surgery.
>
> Follow your hospital's specific procedure for doing skin preps. Doing a skin prep requires special training. If you are asked to do a skin prep, be sure you are first trained.

He also may require that the patient wear elastic stockings (Figure 20-3) to improve the flow of blood from the veins in the legs back to the heart and minimize problems with blood clotting. During surgery blood flow slows, and the chance for blood clot formation increases. Apply elastic stockings only when a person's legs have been elevated for at least 15 minutes, and check his toes every hour for signs of good circulation. When helping someone put on elastic stockings, follow the specific procedure that is explained step by step in Skill 55 in the skills book.

Generally, after midnight the night before surgery, a person is not permitted to eat or drink anything, because there is a chance that he might vomit and aspirate his stomach contents during surgery.

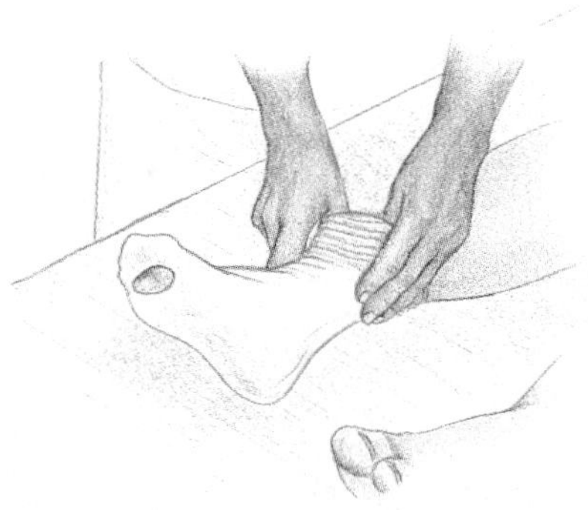

Assisting with the preoperative check.   Before the patient has surgery, your supervising nurse prepares a hospital form called a preoperative checklist. On the form she lists the tasks that must be completed the evening and morning before surgery. Your supervising nurse tells you which tasks she wants you to complete. She may ask you to assist with—

Figure 20-3
Elastic stockings are tight hosiery that are used to help increase blood flow and to minimize circulation problems.

❖   Checking and recording the patient's vital signs.
❖   Making sure the patient wears a correct name band.
❖   Helping the patient remove all his clothing, including underwear, and put on a gown and slippers.
❖   Helping the patient remove makeup, nail polish, dentures, artificial teeth, a wig, hairpins, eyeglasses, a hearing aid, a prosthesis (an artificial leg, arm, or eye, for example), and jewelry. Make sure all valuables are listed and placed in the facility's designated place. It may be best to send expensive jewelry home with

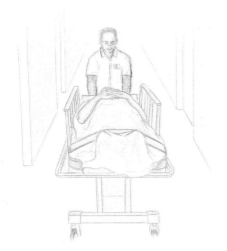

Figure 20-4
When transporting a person on a stretcher, protect the person's head by wheeling the stretcher feet first.

a family member. Usually, you may tape a wedding band in place on the person's finger.

❖ Repositioning the patient every 2 hours before surgery, if he is susceptible to developing decubitus ulcers.

❖ Making sure the patient voids before going to the operating room. (If a person has a urinary drainage bag, make sure to empty it at this time.)

❖ Taking the patient to the operating room. You will transport a patient to and from the operating room on a stretcher (Figure 20-4). To transfer a person from a bed to a stretcher (and vice versa), you must have the help of three other nurse assistants. Be sure to ask for help early in your shift. When co-workers need help transferring the people in their care, you can return the favor. Be sure to lock the brakes on the bed and stretcher, use safety straps and side rails, and use proper body mechanics. When transferring someone from a bed to a stretcher, follow the specific procedure that is explained step by step in Skill 56 in the skills book.

While a Patient Is in Surgery

While Mr. Henderson is in surgery, you make his postoperative bed according to the specific procedure that is explained step by step in Skill 57 in the skills book. You also assist your supervising nurse with a postoperative check to find out what equipment may be needed after he returns from the recovery room. Some of the equipment you may need includes the following:

❖ Emesis basin
❖ Tissue wipes
❖ Vital signs equipment
❖ IV pole
❖ Special equipment, such as a trapeze on the bed
❖ Suction devices and drains
❖ Oxygen equipment

Depending on the type of surgery a patient has, he may not return to the general surgical floor after surgery. He may be placed in a critical or intensive care unit. If he is transferred to such a unit, your supervising nurse will ask you to pack his belongings and transfer them to the new unit.

Providing Care for a Patient After Surgery

You see two people from the recovery room staff wheeling Mr. Henderson on a stretcher down the hall toward his room. When you arrive at his room, your supervising nurse asks you to help her and the recovery room staff transfer him from the stretcher to the bed.

When you first see a person after he has had surgery, you may feel nervous. He may have tubes and machines attached to his body that do not look natural to you. But each item has a purpose and is an important part of a patient's recovery. You must know how to provide care for a patient who is bandaged and has tubes and machines attached to his body. After surgery, you must comfort him, position him properly, measure his input and output, and help him with ambulation, when directed by your supervising nurse. Also after surgery, you may be asked to help the person with coughing exercises and breathing exercises using an incentive spirometer.

Special Postoperative Conditions

Depending on the type of surgery a patient has, you may have to provide care for someone who has surgical dressings, an IV, or a surgical drain; a patient who receives oxygen; or a person who has a cast. It is important to exercise special precautions when positioning and transferring people with these devices, as well as when providing personal care.

Surgical dressing.   Mr. Henderson is now in the postoperative phase of his recovery. Your supervising nurse performs a physical assessment and obtains his vital signs. Mr. Henderson has an abdominal dressing, which you and your supervising nurse observe for signs of bleeding or leakage. Your supervising nurse reminds you—

❖   To report immediately any change in the dressing.
❖   To use caution when helping Mr. Henderson with his bed bath so that you keep the dressing dry.

IV.   Mr. Henderson has an IV in his arm (Figure 20-5). Your supervising nurse adjusts the rate of the drip. She reminds you—

❖   To observe any bleeding or drainage at the **insertion site**.
❖   To make sure the IV is dripping, and, because a pump is being used, to note the rate at which it is set.
❖   To avoid pulling on the tubing and to make sure that the bag is never below the IV insertion site.
❖   To be especially careful to keep the bag high enough to avoid reversing the flow into the bag when helping Mr. Henderson get dressed.

Tell your supervising nurse whenever—

❖   Mr. Henderson complains of pain at the IV site.
❖   You notice redness, swelling, or pus at the IV site. Usually a clear dressing is placed over the needle site so that you can observe these possible conditions.
❖   You see blood in the IV tubing.
❖   The alarm on an IV pump goes off.
❖   Fluid stops flowing from the drip chamber.
    NOTE: First ask the patient to adjust the position of his arm.

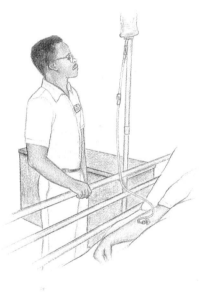

Figure 20-5
If a person in your care has an IV, be sure to monitor the IV site and drip and report any changes to your supervising nurse.

insertion site
The place on a person's body through which a nurse puts an IV needle.

Sometimes this will start the fluid dripping again. If it does not, tell your supervising nurse immediately.

❖ The system is damaged in any way.

When someone in your care has an IV,—

❖ Take his blood pressure in the arm that does not have the IV. Never take blood pressure in the arm with an IV.
❖ Keep the bag above the level of the IV insertion site.
❖ Make sure he is not lying on the tubing, especially when you transfer or reposition him.
❖ When transferring him to a wheelchair, stretcher, or other place, move the IV bag to the other pole first.

Review the section on helping to dress a person who has an IV in Chapter 10, Assisting People with Personal Care.

Surgical drains.   Mr. Henderson also has two surgical drains in his abdomen. Your supervising nurse checks the placement and function of the drains and empties them. She reminds you to—

❖ Be careful to keep the drainage bag lower than the area where the drain is inserted so that the liquid doesn't drain back into Mr. Henderson's body.
❖ Closely observe the drains and immediately report any bleeding or leakage from them.
❖ Be careful not to pull at the drains when helping to remove Mr. Henderson's gown. Occasionally, the drains are pinned to the gown.

She explains to Mr. Henderson that he should take care not to sit, pull, or lie on the drains.

Oxygen.   Mr. Henderson receives oxygen through a nasal cannula. You check to make sure that the oxygen is turned on and note the rate before checking to make sure the cannula is positioned correctly in his nose (Figure 20-6). Your supervising nurse regulates the amount of oxygen entering the cannula. A surgical patient across the hall receives oxygen through a mask instead of a nasal cannula.

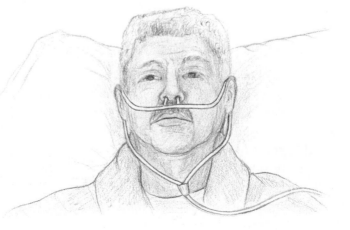

Figure 20-6
When you check someone who is receiving oxygen through a nasal cannula, make sure the prongs are just inside the patient's nostrils.

Cast.   A patient may return from surgery with a cast. The cast may be made of fiberglass, which dries quickly, or of plaster of Paris, which takes up to 48 hours to dry completely. The plaster of Paris cast generates heat and feels warm to the patient while it is drying.

When providing care for a person who has a newly applied cast—

❖   Keep his body in good alignment and support it with pillows or folded blankets. Avoid putting pressure on one area of the cast, which may create a dent, since it is still drying.

❖   Observe the area of the person's body above and especially below the cast for swelling, discoloration (bluish), and temperature (cold). Be aware of the patient's complaint of increased pain and numbness. Observe the person's skin areas for irritation around the edges of the cast. Report any of these conditions to your supervising nurse.

❖   When the cast is dry, cover rough edges with adhesive strips to prevent irritation. Cover areas of a cast around the person's genitals with plastic to prevent soiling the cast with urine and feces.

❖   Always support the cast when positioning or transferring the person.

Providing Comfort to a Surgical Patient

After a patient returns to his room following surgery, check his vital signs, color, awareness, position, and comfort frequently. Let him know that you are there to help and let your supervising nurse know if he is in pain or has swelling, discoloration, drainage, or problems with breathing. Reassure him. If he can turn over or turn onto his side, rub his back to help him relax. Be prepared to relieve his discomforts, such as pain, dry lips and mouth, and nausea and vomiting.

Pain.   A patient often experiences pain from the surgical procedure. The doctor ordered pain medication for Mr. Henderson, and your supervising nurse administers it. When Mr. Henderson tells you he feels pain from the incision site, report his concerns to your supervising nurse.

Dry lips and mouth.   Since returning to his room, Mr. Henderson complains of having a dry mouth. Before giving him anything to drink, check with your supervising nurse to make sure his care plan is no longer marked NPO, or nothing by mouth. Then offer him ice chips or a wet washcloth to relieve his dry mouth or provide mouth care. Putting petroleum jelly on his lips may help make them feel less dry and chapped.

Nausea and vomiting.   Mr. Henderson becomes frustrated with the ice chips and washcloth and asks you for a glass of water. Because anesthesia can make a person nauseated, it is important not to give the person liquids that might cause him to vomit. Tell your supervising nurse that Mr. Henderson wants water to drink.

Keep an emesis basin and tissues within Mr. Henderson's reach. If he vomits, keep his head turned to the side to prevent aspiration and, afterward, wash his face with a washcloth. Report the amount, color, and appearance of any emesis to your supervising nurse.

Positioning a Patient After Surgery

The best postoperative position for a patient depends on the type of surgery and anesthesia he had. Sometimes you may assist your supervising nurse with positioning a person after surgery. Other times, after you feel comfortable using the correct techniques you have learned, you may position him by yourself. Always check with your supervising nurse for instructions about special positioning.

Taking precautions to avoid spinal injuries. If a person has had spinal anesthesia or spinal surgery, she may have to lie flat for a period of time. If the person must spend more than 2 hours in the supine position, arrange for a co-worker to help you turn her, using the log-rolling technique that is explained step by step in Skill 58 in the skills book (Figure 20-7). The patient's spinal column must be maintained in a straight alignment, because flexion of the back may cause injury to the spine. When moving the patient, make sure her whole body, except her legs, moves in one piece and is kept rigid. After positioning the person on her side, bend her legs slightly and place a pillow between them. If the person has to use a bedpan, give her a fracture pan, which has a thinner rim and is lower than a bedpan.

Figure 20-7
A person who has had a spinal anesthetic or spinal surgery needs to lie flat to prevent severe headaches and other complications. If you need to reposition the person, use the log-rolling technique to position her on her side.

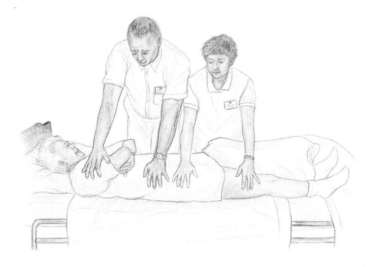

Helping patients who have difficulty breathing. If a patient has minor difficulty breathing, and the care plan does not prohibit it, elevate his head so that he is in a semi-upright position. Reposition him every 2 hours to improve his breathing and circulation and also to help prevent the development of decubitus ulcers. (Using special mattresses to relieve pressure also helps prevent the development of decubiti.) Use pillows to support the patient's body, back, arms, and legs. To lessen discomfort and protect the person from injury, move him slowly and gradually. Explain to him how you plan to make the move so that he can cooperate and help. (Review the procedures in Chapter 9, Positioning and Transferring People.)

If a patient has sudden, severe breathing problems, report this situation to your supervising nurse immediately. Remain calm and reassure the patient until help arrives.

Positioning a patient who has other complications. If a person experiences complications after surgery, such as bleeding or low blood pressure, your supervising nurse may ask you to put him in Trendelenburg position (Figure 20-8), in which the foot of the bed is raised so that the person's head is lower than his feet. This position uses gravity to increase blood flow to the brain.

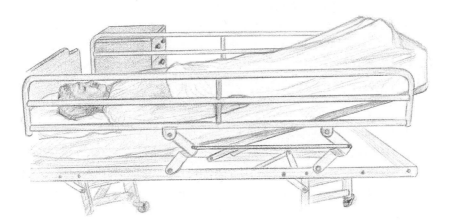

Figure 20-8
A patient is placed in Trendelenburg position to help increase blood flow to his head.

Measuring a Patient's Input and Output

Immediately after a person has surgery, record all intake and output. It is especially important to note when the person first voids after surgery. (Review the procedures for measuring and recording input and output in Chapter 12, Healthful Eating, and Chapter 13, Elimination.)

Helping a Patient with Coughing and Breathing Exercises

Coughing and deep-breathing exercises help prevent breathing difficulties after surgery. During surgery, mucus can accumulate in the lungs and block small air passages. If mucus is not removed, it can lead to a lung infection, or pneumonia. Deep breathing helps move air into the small air passages of the lungs, and coughing helps remove mucus from the lungs.

Helping a person with coughing exercises. Coughing may be painful for a patient who has had abdominal or chest surgery. You can help reduce the amount of abdominal or chest pain and discomfort during coughing exercises by supporting or splinting the abdominal area or incision site with a pillow. To assist a patient who has had abdominal surgery with coughing exercises,—

❖ Support his back by leaning him against the bed, a chair, or your body.

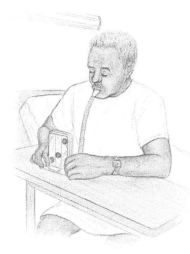

Figure 20-9
The incentive spirometer encourages Mr. Henderson to breathe deeply by giving him a visual cue of his progress. By keeping track of how far the ball rises, he knows if his deep breathing is improving.

❖ Have him place a pillow or folded blanket across the abdominal or chest area.

❖ Have him apply pressure to the pillow or blanket by holding it firmly against his abdomen or chest. The pressure should be applied slowly and gradually, as too much can cause discomfort.

❖ Ask the person to cough while pressure is applied.

Helping a person with breathing exercises. You may be asked to help a patient use an incentive spirometer as part of his deep-breathing exercises (Figure 20-9). The technique for using this device is similar to the technique for using a straw. The patient places his mouth over the mouthpiece of the incentive spirometer and inhales. As he inhales, a small plastic ball rises in the tube. The deeper the person breathes, the higher the ball rises in the tube. When the person exhales, the ball falls back down. The movement of the ball allows the patient to see how well he performs his breathing exercises. After he finishes his breathing exercises, ask him to cough to remove mucus from his lungs. Your supervising nurse will tell you how often each patient should use the incentive spirometer.

Helping a Patient with Ambulation

Mr. Henderson's postoperative activities begin as soon as possible after surgery. His activity level increases from the first stage— sitting on the edge of the bed—to the last stage—ambulating by himself. Early ambulation minimizes the accumulation of secretions in the lungs, which could lead to pneumonia.

Your supervising nurse will tell you when to start helping someone ambulate. She monitors the patient's progress and, based on your observations and hers, lets you know when the person can progress from one stage to the next.

Later in the afternoon on the day of Mr. Henderson's surgery, help him into a sitting position on the side of the bed with his feet dangling over the edge. Sitting and dangling his feet is the first step of the ambulation process.

Then move the bedside table in front of him, lock the brakes, and place a pillow on the table for support. Encourage Mr. Henderson to sit for the amount of time recommended by your supervising nurse.

After Mr. Henderson dangles his legs successfully, your supervising nurse asks you to help Mr. Henderson into a chair, making sure that you use the proper chair and sitting position (Box 20-3).

PRECAUTION: If you help a postoperative patient sit at the edge of the bed and he becomes dizzy or faint, help him back into bed and report the situation to your supervising nurse.

By the next day, Mr. Henderson is ready to progress from sitting in the chair to walking a short distance with assistance. At first, you need the help of a co-worker to help Mr. Henderson ambulate. But, as he progresses, you are able to help him by yourself. Soon he walks without your assistance.

Box 20-3   **Helping a Postoperative Patient to Sit Up**

Proper postoperative sitting position:
❖ Select a chair with a straight back and arm rests.
❖ Make sure the patient's lower back is against the back of the chair.
❖ Make sure his hips and knees are at right angles and that his feet are flat on the floor.
❖ Make sure his forearms rest on the arm rests.

Providing Care as a Member of the Team

As a member of the health care team, you assist in providing care for Mr. Henderson. Your supervising nurse is responsible for planning and evaluating his care, and you are responsible for following her instructions and assisting her. Your supervising nurse is always there to help you, teach you, and answer your questions. Because asking questions is an important part of learning, there are no wrong questions.

Because new procedures and devices are continually introduced into hospital care, periodically every member of the health care team may be learning about something new. Sharing information among health care team members results in better care for the patient.

Supporting Family and Friends of a Surgical Patient

As the health care provider who most often enters and leaves a patient's room, you may be the one who becomes aware of the needs of family members and friends visiting the surgical patient. Before surgery, they may want to know—

❖ What time the person is premedicated, when he leaves the room for surgery, and when he returns from surgery. Visiting friends and family also may want to know visiting hours and other visiting regulations.
❖ Where to wait during the surgery.
❖ Where to find food or coffee while waiting.
❖ Where to find public bathrooms.
❖ What, if anything, they should bring from home for the person.

Family members or friends may find visiting in the hospital to be stressful. The hospital environment may be very new and frightening to some people or may prompt unhappy memories for others. People may not ask questions because they don't want to bother anyone. As a nurse assistant, you can help a person's family members by showing hospitality. You may notice that they need an extra chair or that someone has been in the room all day without eating. When you offer assistance, your hospitality and caring manner can mean a great deal to a worried family member.

Information Review

Circle the correct answers and fill in the blanks.

1. A person who has postoperative pain—
   a. Has pain only in his legs.
   b. Has pain only on the right side of his body.
   (c.) Has pain after a surgical procedure.
   d. Needs to sleep.

2. A person who needs surgery to correct a problem that is not immediately life threatening is scheduled for _____required_____ surgery.

3. Mrs. Jones has always hated her large nose and wants to have surgery to shorten it. This type of surgery is called _____elective_____ surgery.

4. Before surgery, a patient receives an _____anesthetic_____ to prevent him from feeling any pain during the procedure.

5. In the recovery room, the patient—
   a. Is prepared for surgery.
   (b.) Is closely watched for immediate complications.
   c. Is permitted to watch television.
   d. Is given an anesthetic.

6. A device called an _____incentive_____ _____spirometer_____ helps a person to breath deeply, which helps clear his lungs.

7. A surgical patient may receive oxygen through a _____nasal_____ _____cannula_____ or through a _____mask_____.

8. Mr. Smith had surgery several hours ago and says he is "dying of thirst." You check with your supervising nurse and then bring him—
   a. A milkshake.
   b. A large glass of sports drink.
   (c.) Some ice chips in a paper cup.
   d. A cup of black coffee.

9. When placing a surgical patient in a Trendelenburg position—
   a. Place him flat on his back.
   b. Help him sit on the side of the bed.
   c. Make sure his arms are elevated above his body.
   (d.) Raise the foot of the bed so that the person's head is lower than his feet.

10. The friends of a person who is having surgery may not ask questions about the procedure because—
    (a.) They don't want to bother anyone.
    b. They aren't permitted to ask questions.
    c. They think they know everything.
    d. The patient told them everything they need to know.

Questions to Ask Yourself

1. Jennie Smith is a 6-year-old girl who has had surgery to repair a broken arm. She wakes up at night crying with pain. What would you do?

2. Mr. Hopkins is scheduled to have surgery. You have been asked to help get him ready. You ask him to remove his earring. He says he wears the earring for good luck and refuses to remove it. What would you do?

3. While bathing a person, you observe fluid leaking from his surgical drain. What would you do?

4. Mrs. Gordon is waiting for Mr. Gordon to return from surgery. He entered the emergency room early last evening. Mrs. Gordon stayed with him all night. It is now 2:00 P.M. What would you do to help Mrs. Gordon?

5. Brian is 13 years old and thinks it's "sissy" to have his leg shaved for surgery. He scowls when you describe the skin prep procedure to him. What can you do to make him feel better?

21

Providing Care for Mothers and Newborns

Goals

After reading this chapter, you will have the information to—

Describe the physical and emotional changes a mother experiences after giving birth and ways to help her with these changes.

Discuss how to help a mother breast feed a newborn baby.

Discuss how to help parents bottle feed a newborn.

Demonstrate how to hold a newborn safely.

Describe how to provide cord care and circumcision care for a newborn.

Describe how to bathe a newborn.

Explain how to provide care for an HIV-infected mother and her newborn.

After practicing the corresponding skills in the skills book, you will be able to—

Demonstrate how to sterilize baby bottles.

Demonstrate how to bathe a newborn.

Today at Metropolitan Hospital Center your assignment includes three new mothers. You go to their room and introduce yourself. Maggie Ranson is 23 years old and has just delivered her first baby, a girl weighing 7 lb., 3 oz. Mrs. Ranson tells you that she and her husband Jim chose the name Megan for the baby, naming her after her maternal grandmother. When you congratulate her on her new baby and suggest how excited she must be, Mrs. Ranson says, "Thanks. It's wonderful. Jim and I are excited about being parents, but we're also worried about all these new responsibilities, and about how expensive it is to raise a child."

You then introduce yourself to 17-year-old Janice North, one of the other new mothers, who delivered a 6-lb., 7-oz. baby girl last night. Miss North tells you that she is single and has decided to raise her new daughter Jessica with help from her parents. As you provide care, Miss North and Mrs. Ranson talk about their fears and the little things they've noticed about their newborns.

You introduce yourself to the third mother in the room, Cecile Thornbird, who is 42 and has just delivered her third child, a 9-lb., 4-oz. baby boy. Mrs. Thornbird tells you that her other children are 19 and 21 years old. "Gordon and I hadn't intended to have another child at this point in our lives," she says, "but now that Jeremy is here, we're very happy—although I'll admit that I'm a little concerned about how the rest of the family will respond to the new baby, and to me. I also feel anxious about how I'll manage motherhood and my career. I stayed at home with my other two when they were babies, so this experience is going to be very different."

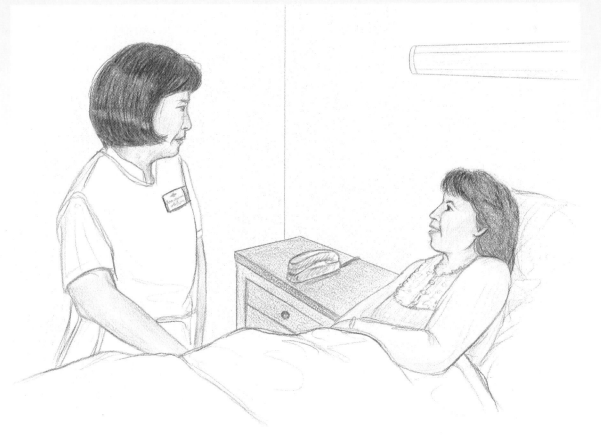

Providing Care to Mothers of Newborn Babies

If you work in the maternity department of a hospital, you provide care for women who have just delivered babies. Or if you work as a home health aide, your clients may include mothers of newborns who need additional care after going home from the hospital. Some of the women may be first-time mothers, and others may already have children. Some may be teenagers, and others may be in their early 40s. Some may be married and others single. Some may be infected with HIV. Each of them experiences physical and emotional changes in her body, and each needs to receive professional, compassionate care while her body heals and returns to its normal state.

Physical Changes

During pregnancy, a woman experiences many physical changes. Visibly, her breasts and stomach become larger. Her body retains extra fluid. Inside, her reproductive organs change. (Review Body Basics, The Reproductive System, in Chapter 4, Understanding People.) Her uterus stretches to accommodate the growing baby.

Within 6 weeks after the baby is born, a woman's uterus returns to its normal size. However, it may take longer for the mother to feel "normal" again. After delivery, she may have an intravenous line until her body fluids stabilize. As with a surgical patient, monitor her vital signs. Observe and record the time and amount of her first voiding after delivery and continue to monitor her output for a period of time following delivery, according to your supervising nurse's instructions.

During the first few days after delivering the baby, the mother loses much of the extra fluid she gained during pregnancy, and she may have to void frequently. She also has a vaginal discharge that begins as bright red blood. After time, the discharge fades to pinkish brown and then becomes clear or white. Although the discharge may resemble a menstrual period, it is not. (If a mother doesn't breast feed her baby, menstruation resumes in 6 to 8 weeks. For women who breast feed their babies, menstruation resumes at varying times.) The mother should wear a sanitary napkin, not tampons, during this time. While she is in the hospital, provide her with special sanitary napkins called perineal pads, which are larger and more absorbent than sanitary pads purchased in retail stores.

After the baby is born, the mother may experience after-pains in her lower abdomen. These pains are caused by uterine contractions that occur as her body tries to return to its normal state. These contractions help her uterus to shrink. Uterine contractions may be more uncomfortable if the mother is breast feeding because additional hormones released during nursing cause the contractions to be stronger.

Episiotomy care.   When you go to Mrs. Thornbird's bedside in response to her call signal, you see that her face looks as if she feels a lot of pain. "I'm so miserable," she says. "The incision is so sore. Is there anything you can do to help me?"

Mrs. Thornbird had an **episiotomy**, and the incision is causing some discomfort (Figure 21-1). You can provide relief by gently bathing the perineal area with warm water and drying it completely.

Encourage her to follow these procedures for perineal care:

❖ Rinse the perineum with warm tap water after voiding or defecating. (Many hospitals provide the mother with a squeeze bottle for this purpose.)

❖ When cleaning the perineum, gently pat, rather than wipe, the area, to avoid irritation. Use a clean wipe or tissue for each pat, and pat from front to back.

❖ Practice infection control when handling the perineal pad: Wash your hands before touching a clean pad and wear gloves when touching a used pad.

If you provide care for a new mother in her home, you must continue providing perineal care for a week or two. If the mother tells you that the episiotomy area has not healed within 2 weeks after delivery, or if you observe that she has swelling, redness, or a fever, report these conditions to your supervising nurse.

A woman who has had an episiotomy may find it difficult to sit because of the **suture line**. Instruct the mother to squeeze her buttocks together as she begins to put weight down in a chair. Then, tell her to slowly relax the buttocks muscles. This movement takes the pressure off the suture line.

Cesarean care.   You must provide special care to Miss North because her baby was delivered by **cesarean section**, also called a C-section. For a variety of reasons, some women are unable to deliver their babies through the vagina. When this situation occurs, the doctor performs a cesarean section. Because this procedure is major surgery, these mothers need the same special care that surgical patients receive. (Review Chapter 20, Providing Care for People Having Surgery.) It also takes a longer time for them to recover from delivery than it does for mothers who have vaginal deliveries.

Just like mothers who have vaginal deliveries, a mother who has a cesarean section has a vaginal discharge to rid her body of the lining that her body created for the **fetus**. She also needs perineal care and a supply of perineal pads.

Breast care.   Any time within a few hours to a couple of days after delivery, the new mother's milk "comes in." This change makes her breasts feel heavier than normal due to milk **engorgement**. Encourage the new mother to wear a good, supportive bra both day and night. If she decides to breast feed, encourage her to nurse her baby very often during the first weeks. If she doesn't breast feed, her doctor may recommend using ice packs on her breasts. He also may order medication to help her breasts return to their normal condition, as well as pain relievers as needed. (Read additional information about breast care later in this chapter in the section on breast feeding.)

episiotomy
(uh-piz-ee-AH-tuh-mee)   An incision in the mother's perineum sometimes made during labor to widen the opening of the mother's vagina for easier delivery of the baby.

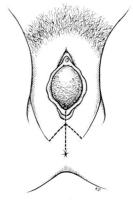

Figure 21-1
An episiotomy is an incision that enlarges the opening of the vagina to ease the delivery of a baby. The episiotomy is stitched together after the baby is delivered.

suture line
(SUE-tyur)   The seam of stitches created when an incision is closed.

cesarean section
(suh-ZARE-ee-en/SEK-shun)   An operation in which the doctor makes a surgical incision in the mother's abdomen through into the uterus, through which a baby is delivered.

fetus
(FEE-tus)   A developing human baby, from 12 weeks after conception until birth.

engorgement
(en-GORJ-ment)   A condition in which the breasts of a new mother become tightly swollen and sore due to her milk supply.

Ambulation.   As with any surgical procedure, help the mother to ambulate progressively from dangling her feet on the side of the bed to walking unassisted. (Review the section on ambulation in Chapter 20.)

Emotional Changes

The day after delivery, when you remove Mrs. Ranson's lunch tray, you notice that she is crying. You ask what you can do to help her. "I feel like I'm on a roller coaster," she says. "One minute I'm full of energy and excitement, and the next minute I'm crying and feeling just awful."

These emotional changes often are caused by the physical and hormonal changes in Mrs. Ranson's body. When she goes home from the hospital, lack of sleep and the stress of providing care for her new baby also may continue to influence her emotional state. To help relieve her anxiety, explain to her that these emotions are normal at this time and, as her body heals, her feelings and moods will even out. Encourage her to rest whenever the baby does, if possible, and to eat well-balanced meals. If the mother seems overwhelmed, advise her to talk to her doctor and notify your supervising nurse. If both parents are available, encourage joint participation in child care.

Breast Feeding or Bottle Feeding?

Each mother decides whether to breast feed or bottle feed her baby. Whatever she decides, you must support her efforts and reinforce what she has learned about feeding her baby.

Breast Feeding

Maggie Ranson decides to breast feed her daughter, Megan. She read about the many advantages of breast feeding and thinks that it is best for her daughter and herself (Box 21-1).

Helping the mother with breast feeding.   Give a breast-feeding mother positive reinforcement and encouragement, especially if she has difficulties in the beginning. Reinforce the advantages, rewards, and satisfaction of being close to the baby (Figure 21-2). When helping a mother breast feed her baby, practice the following guidelines:

Figure 21-2
It is a mother's choice to breast feed or bottle feed her baby, unless a medical reason prevents her from breast feeding.

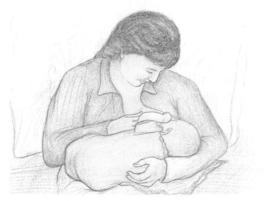

Box 21-1   **Advantages of Breast Feeding**

❖ Breast milk is more easily digested than formula and contains the right balance of
    nutrients for the baby.
❖ Breast feeding helps the baby avoid allergies.
❖ Through breast feeding, the mother's antibodies transfer to the baby, which helps
    keep the baby from getting sick.
❖ Breast-fed babies tend to have fewer colds and milder illnesses.
❖ Breast feeding is convenient. The milk is always available and requires no prepara-
    tion.
❖ Breast feeding is less expensive than bottle feeding.
❖ Breast-fed babies can suckle milk as often as they're hungry without becoming over-
    weight.

❖ Change the baby's diaper, if necessary, before bringing the baby
   to her mother for nursing.

❖ Before giving the baby to the mother to nurse, help her to the
   bathroom and then help her wash her hands with soap and water. Instruct her to wash her nipples with plain water, because
   soap irritates tender skin.

❖ Encourage the mother to sit or lie in a comfortable, relaxed position.

❖ Tell her to hold the baby so that the baby's chest faces her
   breast and the tip of the baby's nose and chin touch the breast.
   Remind her to bring the baby up to the breast rather than bending over the baby. If necessary, position a towel or pillow on
   her lap to support her arms.

❖ To encourage the baby to reach for the breast, tell the mother to
   tickle the baby's cheek with her nipple so that the baby's head
   reflexively turns toward the breast.

❖ When the baby opens her mouth, tell the mother to place her
   entire nipple in the baby's mouth, including most of the **areola**.
   (The **milk pools** are located behind the areola and must have
   pressure on them to release the milk.) (Figure 21-3)

❖ Tell the mother that she will feel a tingling sensation in her
   breasts when the milk "lets down."

❖ Encourage the mother to begin nursing the baby on each
   breast for 5 minutes per feeding on the first day, 10 minutes
   per feeding on the second day, and 15 minutes per feeding on
   the third day and thereafter (or longer, depending on how
   long the baby wants to nurse). Tell her that, at each nursing
   period, she should alternate the breast she starts with, because the baby usually sucks more vigorously on the first
   breast.

❖ Tell the mother that, to remove the breast from the baby's
   mouth, she should put one finger into the corner of the baby's
   mouth, between the gums, to break the suction and gently pull
   out her nipple.

areola
(uh-REE-oh-luh)   The dark area surrounding a woman's nipple.

milk pools
Breast tissue that stores milk.

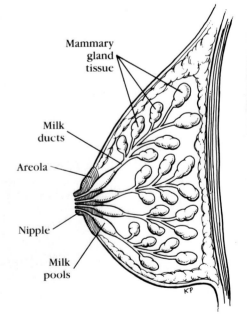

Figure 21-3
The mammary glands produce and
store milk. When the baby nurses, milk
flows (lets down) into the milk pools.
The sucking pressure of the baby's
mouth squeezes the milk through the
ducts and out through the nipple.

Helping the breast-feeding mother take care of her breasts. As a home health aide, you may have to help the mother with any problems she may have as she continues to nurse her baby. For example, if the mother's nipples become sore, help her by suggesting that she—

❖ Ensure that the infant has the whole nipple in her mouth.

❖ Feed the baby more frequently and limit nursing to 5 minutes on the sore nipple. Also, encourage her to begin each feeding on the less sore nipple, since the baby sucks more vigorously on the first nipple.

❖ Keep her nipples dry between feedings.

❖ Just before feeding, briefly apply a cold cloth to the sore nipple to decrease pain sensation and to make the nipple erect and easier for the baby to grasp.

❖ If the mother's breasts become swollen, which may occur even with frequent nursing, instruct her to put warm compresses on her breasts and then **express** some milk by hand just before the baby nurses.

express
To press or squeeze out.

Sometimes a nursing mother may experience a clogged milk duct, which can cause a painful lump or swelling in the breast. If this condition develops, tell your supervising nurse, who will advise the mother to contact her doctor. The doctor will probably tell her to breast feed more often and for a longer time on the affected side. Have her change position for each feeding so that pressure is applied to all parts of her breast equally and the ducts are emptied. Instruct her to relieve pain by applying warm compresses several times a day.

At times, a clogged milk duct can lead to a breast infection called mastitis. Inform your supervising nurse if—

❖ The lump doesn't go away in 3 days.

❖ The lump becomes hot, red, and tender to the touch.

❖ The mother begins to have a fever or headache.

Helping the breast-feeding mother with nutrition. Encourage a nursing mother to eat all the food that comes to her in the hospital and to eat well after she goes home. Remind her that her diet is planned for a nursing mother, who needs about 200 extra calories a day beyond her nutritional needs when she was pregnant to maintain her milk supply. In addition, she needs to drink 6 to 8 glasses of fluid daily. She also should avoid—

❖ Alcoholic beverages.

❖ Large amounts of caffeinated drinks.

❖ Over-the-counter or prescription drugs.

Bottle Feeding

Cecile Thornbird decides that bottle feeding is best for her and baby Jeremy. She tells you that she made her decision because—

❖ It gives her husband the opportunity to feed the baby.

❖ She can return to work sooner and without any worries about feeding Jeremy.

❖ She can take medication without affecting the baby. (Taking medication is important because she suffers from allergies and hay fever and would like to be able to take her prescription medicines.)

❖ She wants to begin dieting as soon as possible. (If she dieted while breast feeding Jeremy, he might not receive adequate nutrition.)

Helping new parents with bottle preparation. Babies who are not breast fed receive **formula**. The type of formula is determined by the doctor. Commercial formula comes in three forms: ready-to-feed; concentrate, which needs to be mixed with water according to the instructions on the container; and powder, which also needs to be mixed with water according to instructions on the container. If you work as a home health aide providing care for a mother or baby who needs special care, you may be responsible for preparing the bottles of formula.

When helping new parents with bottle feeding, reinforce the following safety and infection control precautions:

❖ Because formula provides an excellent place for germs to grow, it is necessary to carefully wash, rinse, and sterilize bottles and nipples before use. Some plastic bottles have disposable liners that do not have to be sterilized, although you still must sterilize the nipples, rings, and caps. Review the information on sterilization in Chapter 11, Providing Care for the Person's Place, and follow the specific procedure that is explained step by step in Skill 60 in the skills book.

❖ To warm the bottle of formula, heat a pan of water on the stove. Remove the pan from the burner. Place the bottle in the pan. Periodically, shake the bottle to distribute the heat, and test the temperature of the formula on the inside of your wrist.

❖ When you heat bottles of formula in a microwave oven, gently shake the bottle to distribute the heat and test the temperature of the formula on the inside of your wrist, because heat distribution in the microwave oven is not even, and the baby may be burned.

❖ Do not take a bottle out of the refrigerator to warm at room temperature. Warming it slowly can cause germs to grow in the formula. If a bottle is unrefrigerated for more than 1 hour, discard it.

❖ To prevent choking, always hold the baby to feed him and never prop a bottle in his mouth. Holding the baby also allows for the parent and child to bond and provides the baby with a secure feeling while he eats (Figure 21-4).

❖ Do not put extra water, honey, sugar, cereal, or other liquids or solids in the baby's formula. (Review the section on nutrition for children in Chapter 12, Healthful Eating.)

formula
(FOR-myou-lah) Milk-based or soybean-based liquid mixture given in bottles to babies.

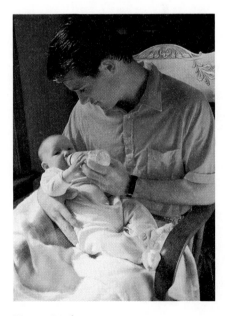

Figure 21-4
After they learn the correct way to hold the baby and the bottle, fathers, other family members, and friends may participate in bottle feeding.

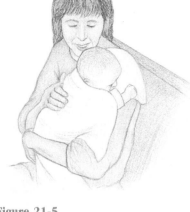

Figure 21-5
A good way to burp a baby is to hold the infant over your shoulder and gently rub or pat her back. If the infant tends to spit up when burping, protect your clothing with a piece of cloth.

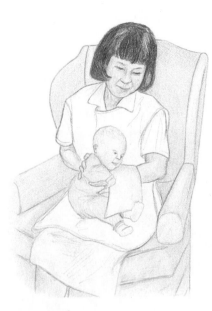

Figure 21-6
Another good way to burp a baby is to hold her on your lap and gently rub or pat her back.

Helping new parents with bottle feeding. When assisting a mother or father with bottle feeding the baby,—

❖ Instruct the parent to keep the baby's head higher than the body.
❖ Tell him or her to make sure that the bottle is positioned so that the nipple is full of milk.
❖ Encourage the parent to hold and cuddle the baby during the feeding.

Burping

All bottle-fed babies and most breast-fed babies swallow some air while sucking. Burping helps the baby get rid of the air. Burp a breast-fed baby when she finishes one breast and before she starts on the other. Burp a bottle-fed baby halfway through a feeding and again afterward. When feeding a baby who gulps air, burp her more frequently. Figures 21-5 and 21-6 show positions for burping a baby.

It is normal for both breast-fed and bottle-fed babies to spit up a little after feeding. The spitting up usually diminishes as the baby gets older. If you work as a home health aide, you have to observe the baby over time to see if she often spits up most of the feeding. If you observe that she does, report this observation to your supervising nurse.

Providing Care to Newborn Babies

Even though Mrs. Ranson and Miss North took classes to learn how to take care of their expected babies, both are uneasy about how to handle them. You help them feel more comfortable with their babies by reminding them of some of the things they learned. You tell them some of the things you have learned and experiences you have had taking care of newborns.

If you know how newborns respond to their environment, it is easier to provide for their needs. Even though newborns are totally dependent, they are aware of the world around them. Their senses of touch, sight, hearing, taste, and smell are active from the moment of birth.

When Miss North's baby Jessica becomes restless, you show her how to wrap the baby snugly in her receiving blanket. You remind her that a newborn's sense of touch is very sensitive and that Jessica likes to be held softly but securely and likes to be warm. You suggest that she hold Jessica closely, wrapped in a blanket, and perhaps rock her so that she calms down.

In the nursery, the nurse assistants sometimes rock Miss North's baby when she is restless. They also sing to her. A newborn's hearing is well developed, and babies especially like high-pitched voices and sounds that are soft and rhythmic, like a lullaby.

Mrs. Ranson tells you how amazing it is that her baby Megan stares at her face when she nurses. She says she remembers learning that a newborn sees most clearly at a distance of 8 to 12 inches, or just about the distance between their faces when the mother cuddles or feeds her. "They said in our class that babies like to look at human faces," says Mrs. Ranson. "And they sure were right about that. They were also right when they said babies prefer sweet tastes and have a sense of smell. Just look at this baby nuzzling to get more milk!"

As a caregiver, you have to know how to respond to babies, because they can't talk and tell you what they want. Babies are born with certain behaviors and reactions that are meant to help them survive outside the womb. If you know these behaviors and reactions, you can respond. Some of these behaviors and reactions are—

❖ The startle (Moro) reflex. A baby who is surprised by sudden changes in light, noise, movement, or position flings out her arms and legs, then quickly pulls them back onto her chest while curling her body as if to cling.
❖ The rooting reflex. If you stroke a baby's cheek or lips, the baby's head turns in the direction of the stroking, and her mouth searches for a nipple.
❖ The sucking reflex. If you touch a baby's mouth or cheek with your finger or a nipple, the baby tries to suck. This response helps the baby latch onto the nipple and feed.

Baby Body Mechanics

When you help Mrs. Ranson with her baby, you remind her that a newborn's head is large in proportion to the rest of her body, and her neck is too weak to support her head. For this reason, you tell her, she should always use both hands to lift the baby and to support her head. Three ways to hold a baby securely are as follows:

❖ The cradle hold (Figure 21-7)
❖ The football hold (Figure 21-8)
❖ The shoulder hold (Figure 21-9)

Cord Care

Before birth, the umbilical cord, which is attached to the placenta in the mother's uterus, provides blood, oxygen, and nutrients to the developing fetus and carries wastes out of the fetus. After the baby's birth, the doctor clamps and cuts the cord. It takes from 7 to 10 days for the remaining section of cord to dry up and fall off the baby. While the cord is still attached to the baby, it is important for the baby's caregiver to—

❖ Keep the umbilical area clean and dry so that bacteria do not cause an infection.
❖ Use an alcohol wipe or cotton ball moistened with alcohol to clean the base of the cord each time you change the baby's diaper.
❖ Keep the diaper below the area of the cord to promote drying.
❖ Look for signs of infection, such as redness, foul smell, or drainage from the cord. Report these observations to your supervising nurse.

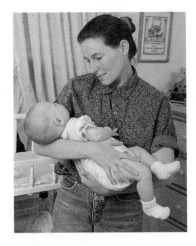

Figure 21-7
When you hold the baby close to you, the baby feels warmth and security.

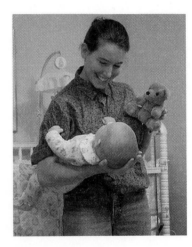

Figure 21-8
Holding an infant in the football hold allows you to properly support the baby with one hand while freeing the other hand to provide care.

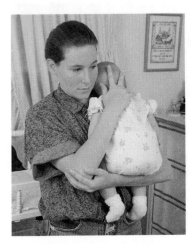

Figure 21-9
Holding an infant upright enables her to look at her surroundings.

❖ Not give the baby a tub bath until the cord has fallen off and the area is dry and healed.

Circumcision Care

Many newborn boys are circumcised while they are in the hospital. Circumcision is the surgical removal of the foreskin on the penis. After circumcision, the baby's penis looks red and swollen. For the first 24 to 48 hours, the site of the circumcision may be covered with a dressing. The nurse will change the dressing as necessary. The baby's penis may bleed slightly when his diaper is changed. It takes from 10 to 14 days for the area to heal. During this time, the baby's caregiver must be careful to prevent infection. After circumcision, when changing the diaper,—

❖ Keep the tip of the penis dry and do not remove the dressing, because this may cause the penis to bleed.

❖ After the baby has had a bowel movement, gently wash the penis with soap, water, and cotton balls. Rinse with clear water to remove all traces of soap, which can irritate the baby's skin.

❖ Use a cotton swab to apply petroleum jelly to the penis to prevent the diaper from sticking and also to provide a barrier against urine and feces.

❖ Put the diaper on loosely.

❖ Look for signs of infection, such as redness, a foul smell, or drainage from the area. Report these observations to your supervising nurse.

If you observe that the baby is not passing urine, report this observation to your supervising nurse.

Bathing

navel
(NAY-vuhl)   The area in the middle of the abdomen where the umbilical cord once was attached.

In the hospital and for the first few weeks after a baby goes home, she should be given a sponge bath, until the cord has fallen off and the **navel** is completely healed. When helping a new mother learn to bathe her baby, tell her that bathing involves more than cleaning the baby. It also provides an excellent opportunity to provide stimulation for the baby, and touching, holding, and talking to the baby are important for her social development (Figure 21-10). Also demonstrate how to give a newborn baby a sponge bath by following the specific procedure that is explained step by step in Skill 61 in the skills book. While demonstrating the bath, highlight the following information:

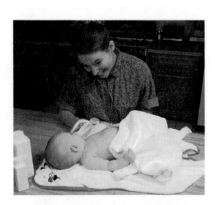

Figure 21-10
For the first weeks after birth, a baby is given sponge baths to help prevent infection of the cord. Bath time is a good time to talk or sing to the baby.

❖ Before bathing a baby, make sure the room is warm.

❖ Be sure to have bathing supplies within reach before starting the bath, because you cannot leave the baby after you begin to bathe her. Also gather supplies for cord and circumcision care, as well as the baby's clean diaper and clothes.

❖ Wash the baby from the cleanest to the dirtiest part, cleaning her face first, then her torso, then her arms, legs, and bottom. Be sure to wash the baby's face and ears with a washcloth and wa-

ter, but no soap, and do not use cotton swabs to clean the
baby's ears.

❖ During the bath, keep the baby covered with a towel to keep
her warm.

❖ To give a sponge bath, put water in a bathtub, pan, or sink. Use
water that is warm to the touch (test on the inside of your
wrist).

Providing Care for HIV-Infected Mothers and Newborns

In Chapter 17, Providing Care for People Who Have AIDS, you read
that the number of babies born to HIV-infected mothers will increase
in the next few years because almost 80 percent of women who are
HIV positive are in their child-bearing years. Many of the women become pregnant, not knowing that they are infected and may pass the
virus to their babies. HIV-infected mothers and their babies require
special care.

When an HIV-Infected Mother Gives Birth

Infected mothers do not always pass HIV to their babies. Studies
show that 30 to 50 percent of babies born to infected mothers become infected with HIV. Scientists have not discovered why some
babies become infected and some do not. They believe the following
factors may influence the chances of a baby's becoming infected:

❖ Whether the mother has other infections

❖ Whether the mother has symptoms of HIV infection during pregnancy

❖ At which stage of pregnancy the mother was when she became
HIV infected

❖ The number of pregnancies the mother has had while infected
with HIV

❖ Whether the mother has had repeated exposure to HIV

Just before a baby is born, she normally receives a variety of her
mother's antibodies to help protect her after birth. If a mother is HIV
infected and has developed HIV antibodies, one of three things could
happen to her baby during pregnancy:

1. The baby could receive HIV and HIV antibodies and become infected.

2. The baby could receive HIV antibodies, but not the virus itself.

3. The baby could receive neither HIV nor HIV antibodies. Only
those babies who are infected with the virus may develop AIDS.

If an infant receives HIV from her mother, she will develop her
own antibodies. However, the HIV-antibody tests cannot tell the difference between the infant's or the mother's antibodies. Because a
mother's antibodies (including HIV antibodies) may stay in the baby's
blood for as long as 15 months, most current HIV-antibody tests on a
baby may be inaccurate until that time has passed. If a baby contin-

ues to test positive for HIV after 15 months of age, doctors know that the baby probably received both HIV and HIV antibodies and is HIV infected. If a baby born to an HIV-infected mother develops symptoms of AIDS, doctors can assume, even without testing, that the baby is infected with HIV.

If the HIV-antibody test is negative on a baby's blood test, it usually means that the baby is not infected with HIV.

When an HIV-Infected Mother and Newborn Need Health Care

As you provide care for an HIV-infected mother and her newborn, remember the six principles of care that guide any care you give. You read about infection control and universal precautions in Chapter 6, Controlling the Spread of Germs, and about people with AIDS in Chapter 17, Providing Care for People who have AIDS. You also read in this chapter about the care you would provide to mothers and newborns. When providing care for an HIV-infected mother and her newborn, you also need to provide additional support by listening and by being trustworthy, dependable, and positive, regardless of how the mother reacts to her disease. The mother may be angry or may appear not to care. How she reacts may depend on many factors. Keep your emotions out of the way. Seek someone, such as your supervising nurse, to talk with about the feelings you have when providing care for an HIV-infected mother and newborn.

Information Review

Circle the correct answers and fill in the blanks.

1. After a mother gives birth to her newborn, she experiences two kinds of changes: ___emotional___ and ___physical___.

2. After giving birth, a woman experiences after-pains in her lower abdomen because her ___womb / uterus___ is contracting.

3. When a woman has a normal delivery through the vagina, her doctor sometimes makes an incision, called an ___episiotomy___ to widen the opening of the vagina.

4. A woman who has just delivered a baby uses ___perineal___ pads to take care of vaginal discharge.

5. If a woman cannot deliver a baby by the normal method through the vagina, the doctor performs a procedure called a ___C-Section___ _____ and delivers the baby through an opening in the abdomen.

6. The emotional changes a woman experiences after giving birth are caused by—
    a. Physical and hormonal changes.
    b. Her own need to become a baby again.
    c. The episiotomy.
    d. Her desire not to be a mother.

7. A breast-fed baby gets antibodies from the mother's milk, which—

   a. Keep the baby's body from getting too big.

   (b) Help keep the baby from getting sick.

   c. Keep the mother's breasts from getting too large.

   d. Help keep the baby from burping.

8. Bottle-fed babies drink ____Formula____, which is poured into sterilized bottles.

9. A newborn baby has to be held in a special way because her ____neck____ is too weak to support her ____head____.

10. All newborn babies must receive ____Cord____ care, and some boy babies must receive ____Circumsion____ care.

Questions to Ask Yourself

1. Mrs. Ranson's mother pulls you aside and tells you that she thinks Maggie's baby is starving on breast milk. She says she thinks Maggie's breasts are too small for breast feeding and wants you to talk her into bottle feeding her baby. What would you do?

2. Miss North says that her incision from the cesarean section is too sore for her to be able to hold her baby and that she doesn't want you to bring the baby to her. What would you do?

3. Mr. Thornbird seems to enjoy helping with baby Jeremy. He changes his diaper and then picks up the bottle to begin feeding him. You notice that he didn't wash his hands after changing the diaper. What would you do?

4. As a home health aide, you go to the home of Janet Ray, who had a cesarean section, to help provide care for her and her newborn baby. You begin to sterilize the bottles for the baby's formula when Mrs. Ray tells you not to bother with all that mess. "That's old-fashioned," she says. "I just put the formula into a bottle, pop it in the microwave, put the rest of the can back in the refrigerator, and feed the baby. In these busy times, one has to keep up with modern technology." What would you do?

5. When you arrive at Tara Kelly's house to provide care after she has given birth to her first baby, Mrs. Kelly is crying. "I'm not going to be able to breast feed my baby," she says. "It hurts too much." What would you do?

6. You provide care for Gina Fiorello who had complications after a cesarean section delivery 2 weeks ago. She is still weak and needs help with her own personal care, as well as with the baby. In spite of her complications, she has managed to breast feed her baby, an accomplishment that makes her very proud. Today when you arrive at her home, you notice that she is drinking a glass of wine and that there is a half-empty bottle on the floor next to her chair. When you ask her about the wine, she says that it's the only painkiller she has, since breast-feeding mothers are not supposed to take over-the-counter or prescription drugs. What would you do?

22

Providing Care for People Who Are Dying

Goals

After reading this chapter, you will have the information to—

Discuss factors that influence a person's reaction to death.

Discuss the five emotional stages of death.

Discuss the needs of the family and friends of someone who is dying.

Describe your role in providing for the needs of a person who is dying.

Define hospice care.

Recognize signs of approaching death.

Recognize signs that death has occurred.

Discuss the needs of the dying person and her family and friends in three health care settings: nursing home, hospital, and home.

Describe the loss experienced when a child dies.

Provide care for a person with AIDS.

Provide postmortem care.

After practicing the corresponding skills in the skills book, you will be able to—

Provide postmortem care.

As you move around Josie's bed, tightening the sheets and making sure that she is warm and comfortable, you listen to her sister Arlene as she holds Josie's hand and talks to her. "The last few months have been good, Josie," says Arlene. "What fun we've had talking about growing up, the boys we both liked when we were in high school, Mom and Pop, and Connie. She may be my daughter, but she acts just like you! We've laughed a lot, Josie, but I'm glad we've also talked about some serious things, like the fight we had 12 years ago, and I'm happy we can even laugh about that now." Without opening her eyes, Josie smiles at Arlene's last comment.

Arlene turns to you and says, "I'm glad you're working here tonight. You're Josie's favorite nurse assistant and mine, too. Remember when I first started visiting here with Josie and how we'd sit in silence watching the television? Your suggestion that I read to her and talk with her instead of watching TV made a world of difference to both of us."

You and Arlene hear a big sigh and, when you turn to look at Josie, you see that her head is drooping to the side. Her eyes are shut. Arlene takes Josie's wrist and searches for her pulse. With a pleading look on her face, she gives Josie's wrist to you. You feel no pulse and observe no breathing. You look at Arlene and shake your head.

After signaling for your supervising nurse and moving to the other side of the bed, you silently put your arm around Arlene's shoulder and squeeze ever so gently. "She died when I turned away for just a moment," Arlene says. A wave of sadness hits you as you look at Josie's lifeless face.

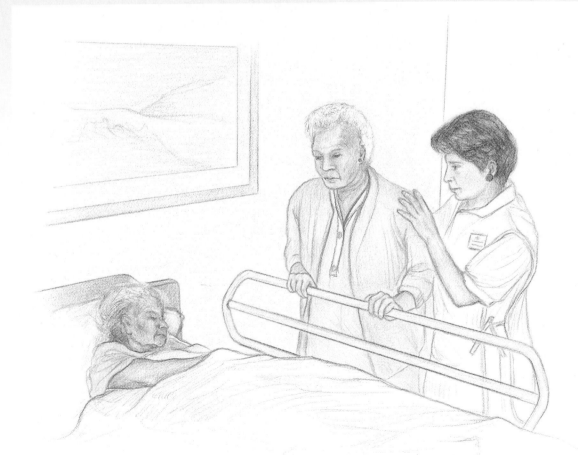

Facing Death

As a nurse assistant, you help people as they deal with illness, injuries, and medical conditions. You work with people to help them gain strength and to encourage them to become as active as they can be so that they can improve their health and, if possible, become well again. But illness is not always followed by improved health or recovery. Sometimes death occurs suddenly and sometimes at the end of a long struggle.

Because you may have to face the death of a person in your care, it is important for you to understand certain things about death and dying. You must recognize feelings you may have, and you must have particular information so that you can help someone through the dying process and provide emotional support to grieving family members and friends.

Factors that Influence a Person's Reaction to Death

How do you think you might feel if someone you know were to die? You might feel sad, angry, powerless, or guilty. When you have these feelings, you might try to ignore them because they make you uncomfortable or because they are too painful to deal with. It is a natural and normal reaction to want to distance yourself from the things that make you sad or uncomfortable or give you pain.

During past centuries, most people died at home with their families around them. Death and dying were a normal part of life. Many popular stories and songs were written about the death of a loved one. But in this century, as doctors learned more and more ways to save lives, many people began thinking of death as unnatural and frightening. Talking about death became **taboo**. It was almost as if people believed they could keep death from happening if they didn't talk about it. How healthy do you think this attitude was?

taboo
(tah-BOO)   Forbidden.

Before the 1960s, health care workers were not trained to talk with people in their care about death. As a result, people with terminal illnesses often felt isolated in a health care setting. In fact, they frequently were put in private rooms so that their dying wouldn't upset other people receiving care. Health care workers didn't tend to stop by to visit with them as they might with people who were getting better. Dying people were sometimes viewed as the failures of the medical profession. As a result, a dying person felt uncomfortable about discussing her feelings about death and dying with caregivers. In the 1960s, health care professionals began to realize that people needed help in dealing with these feelings. And so the "death awareness" movement began.

Death, like birth, is part of life. Dying can take place in the presence of loving family, friends, and health care workers. Or a person may die alone. As a nurse assistant, you may be the only one with the person who is dying. The person may not have a family, her relatives might live too far away, or she may no longer be close to them.

Many people are exposed to death for the first time when an older person, such as a grandparent who has lived a long life, dies. With advances in medicine, Americans now live well into their 70s and 80s. Death in the later years of life is much more expected, accepted, and understood, and it generally causes less stress for family members than the death of a younger person or child. As you read in the section on human development (Chapter 4, Understanding People), dealing with death is something that an older person attends to in that part of the life cycle. However, it is not something young adults, adolescents, or children normally do.

But death can occur at any stage of the life cycle and can be either expected or sudden and unexpected. Although the death of an older person, especially if she has had a long, debilitating illness, is not pleasant, the death of a newborn, child, or young person is generally seen as an unjust tragedy.

Talking about death is frightening to some people because it is so final and because it causes them to think about their own dying (Figure 22-1). The more you understand your feelings about death, the better prepared you are to help others make the transition from life through death. Being comfortable with your own feelings about death might help you to listen, touch, and respond appropriately to the dying person and to the family and friends who also may be struggling with painful feelings.

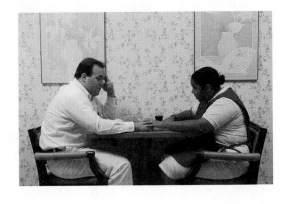

Figure 22-1
Talking with friends or co-workers can help you sort out your feelings about death.

The age of a terminally ill person is one factor that influences how a person reacts to being told of her own approaching death or that of a loved one. Some other factors that may influence her reaction are her culture, sense of fulfillment, religion, and family and friends. To gain insight about how the person feels about death and how you feel about death, ask yourself the questions listed after each of the following factors.

Culture

What stories about dying did the person learn when she was growing up? Was she taught that death is part of life or that it is to be feared? How do people in your family talk about death?

Fulfillment

Did the person live her life fully, with little regret? Were her basic needs met? Was she able to fulfill her hopes and dreams? Was her life purposeful, meaningful, and rewarding? (Figure 22-2) Are you doing what makes you feel good about yourself and your life?

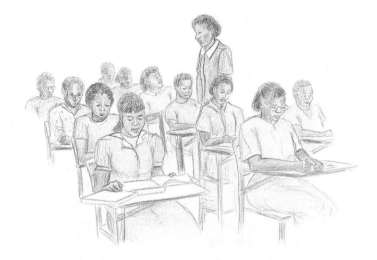

Figure 22-2
Josie felt she had led a very fulfilling life. As a schoolteacher, she watched many of her students become husbands, wives, laborers, doctors, skilled craftsmen, and lawyers. When she entered the nursing home, she had a few things she still wanted to do, but she tried to make peace with herself about those things she knew she would never get done.

Religion

Does the person hold a belief in a spiritual being and an afterlife, which provides additional support and meaning? Or does this belief (or lack of it) cause a feeling of dread for what comes after death? What do you and the people in your family believe about an afterlife?

Family and Friends

Does the person feel loved and connected? Has she been able to finish any "unfinished business" in her life? If not, does this situation make her feel angry about death? (Unfinished business may mean needing to talk about unresolved guilt, regret, or resentment; sharing messages of love and appreciation with significant others; or just simply saying good-bye to someone.) What unfinished business would you want to take care of with the people who are important in your life?

Five Emotional Stages of Dealing with Dying

The factors that you just read about show how our past experiences with living affect our view of death. Dr. Elisabeth Kubler-Ross, an early pioneer in the death awareness movement, identified five stages of emotions that the dying person may experience: denial, anger, bargaining, depression, and acceptance. Each person goes through these stages at his or her own pace and may move back and forth among them, instead of progressing straight through them.

Denial

The dying person cannot accept that something so terrible is happening to her. For example, she cannot accept that she has a terminal illness. A period of denial is a time when the shock of the information makes the dying person put it away so that she can delay dealing with it until she is more emotionally ready. Sometimes a person starts out by acknowledging her illness and the likelihood of death and then slips into denial, which becomes a crutch that supports her until she is ready to deal with this harsh and frightening reality. Some people flip-flop back and forth between denial and reality.

Anger

What kinds of things do you say when you are angry? Often the dying person expresses anger, which is an expression of other underlying emotions: fear, resentment, and frustration. If her anger seems to be directed toward you, it is important that you don't take her emotional expressions personally. She may really be angry at her situation, not at you. She may not be able to express her angry feelings to her family, and so she goes through this critical stage by expressing her anger at you or other caregivers, perhaps over some insignificant thing you said, did, or didn't do. It is most helpful to try and look *beyond* the anger to the emotion that is behind it. Looking at the underlying emotion may give you a better understanding of what she is really expressing and may help you to know how to handle it best.

Another person may become angry with the higher spiritual being that she worships. She may ask, "Why me?" or "What did I do to deserve this? Am I being punished?"

Bargaining

A person may try to bargain for more time by making a deal, usually with her higher spiritual being. For example, she may think or say, "If I just make it to my daughter's wedding, I'll be ready to go. I won't ask for anything else." What is promised, however, is not what is important. What is important is that the person uses this time to take care of unfinished business. Listen to what the dying person says but make no judgments.

Depression

If you have ever felt depressed, what did you think about during that time? Depression in this stage of the dying process can take two forms: (1) grief over past losses, disappointments, and unfulfilled dreams, and (2) preparation for the losses to come. For example, Rodney Britten wants to talk with you about the losses he feels as his death approaches. It is important to listen to and accept this sorrow, because it is a sad time. A time of depression is not the time to try to cheer him up, to try to distract him from his grief, or to try to convince him that he has much to be grateful for in his life. You may be the only person the dying person can talk to about preparing to die, because his family may not be available or may be fearful of talking about the person's losses (Figure 22-3).

Another behavior you begin to see at this stage is withdrawal or detachment. The person's interests begin to decrease. He may no longer show an interest when people talk about home, politics, or

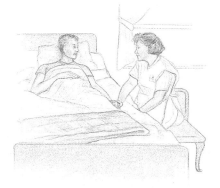

Figure 22-3
A person who wants to talk about his approaching death may not give you many verbal cues. When you think you hear one, ask the person if he wants to talk and then sit and listen.

business. He gradually loses interest or detaches from everything around himself except for his needs for comfort and his concern for the people he loves. This stage may be harder for some men who are dying, because they may believe that they do not have permission to cry or grieve.

Acceptance

Think back to a time in your life when you may have finally accepted something after a difficult struggle. This acceptance may have been a time of calm for you. That does not necessarily mean that you were happy, but perhaps you felt more peaceful. The dying person feels peaceful when she reaches this emotional stage in the dying process. Her acceptance allows her to "let go" of the need to fight the inevitable movement from life into death. It is a time of peaceful resignation.

Not all people go through all five of these stages, and even if they do, they may move back and forth among the stages. It is not your job to help the person move through these stages toward acceptance. Your role as a nurse assistant is to listen, be kind, accept the person's feelings, and try to be understanding. Helping a person who is dying means providing her with emotional support while she deals with this tragedy in her own personal way and at her own emotional speed.

Elisabeth Kubler-Ross said that dying people teach us how to live, how to look at our own lives, and how to see every day as a precious gift. This is what we receive from the people in our care.

When a Person Is Dying

The approaching death of a person affects many lives. Family members and friends begin to experience their own grief. Caregivers, particularly those who spend a great deal of time with the dying person, also experience feelings about the impending death. All these feelings must be recognized and dealt with so that they do not interfere with the quality of care the dying person receives.

Providing for Needs of the Family

When dealing with the approaching loss, family and friends experience emotional stages similar to those of the dying person. They may feel denial, anger, resentment, a need to bargain, depression, and ultimately, acceptance and recovery. This grieving process often begins before the loss occurs and continues for many months afterwards. In the case of the loss of a spouse or a child, the grieving period may take years. The person who is grieving eventually begins to resume normal activities, but the grieving process continues.

You must accept and not judge the family members' feelings of sadness, anger, or relief. You can be supportive by listening and giving physical comfort and by asking about their personal needs for food, water, coffee or tea, or rest. Encourage family members to talk with you about their feelings for the person. Let them know that other members of the health care team, such as social workers, also are available to talk and listen.

Encourage family members to touch the dying person. Your comfort and ease in touching the person as you provide care is an example that the family may follow. Even an unconscious dying person can still hear and feel and may find it very consoling if family members hold her hand and talk about happy times they shared with her. As a nurse assistant, you can help family members feel comfortable about sharing memories by asking questions about the dying person's life. You might encourage them to bring the family album in so that everyone can see the photos and talk about them (Figure 22-4). This activity helps the dying person and the family to review the accomplishments and happy times of her life.

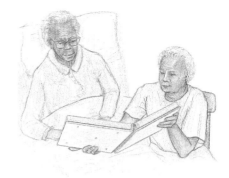

Figure 22-4
As Josie and Arlene looked over their family photo album, they shared memories of the trip their church choir made to the state capital, the Fourth of July picnic when Josie won the pie-baking contest, and the celebration of Arlene's daughter's wedding.

Providing for Needs of the Dying Person

Death is an intimate and personal experience. You play a major role as a caregiver for the dying person. As a nurse assistant, you may be asked to help a person who is nearing death. By applying the principles of care and your knowledge about what the person and her family are experiencing and by expressing your compassion, you can make a difference in how people experience the dying process. Table 22-1 lists the principles of care and some examples of what you can do for the dying person.

Table 22-1   Doing Your Best for a Dying Person

Principle of Care	What You Can Do
Safety	Provide care as usual. Even though the person may not be as mobile as before, you must make sure that she is safe. Keep the room comfortable, lighted, well ventilated, clean, and neat.
Privacy	Provide care quickly and efficiently to allow her maximum private time with her family and with her clergy, if requested.
Dignity	Treat the person as an individual. Continue to offer choices and ask permission to provide care.
Communication	Talk about what the person wants to talk about. Be open and accepting of beliefs and ideas that may be different from your own. Respect the person who may not want to talk at all, recognizing that your nonverbal communication becomes even more important than usual. Make eye contact and stay in touch by making physical contact. When you stand at the bedside, put your hand on her hand, arm, or shoulder. Talk in a normal tone of voice and avoid whispering. Even if the person is unconscious, don't say anything you would not want her to hear. Listening and touching are your two most important tools. Do not isolate the person or leave her alone for long periods of time. She may feel that you have given up on her if she finds herself alone. However, check occasionally to see if she wants to be alone, because a person who is dying may want time alone to think or pray.
Independence	Give the person the opportunity to do as much for herself as she is able and willing to do. A dying person does not lose her pride or her need to be in control.
Infection Control	Practice universal precautions as always. You can prevent unnecessary discomfort by providing proper skin care and by meeting the person's nutritional and elimination needs. Provide excellent personal care, especially mouth care, because the person's mouth may be extremely dry.

Consider and respect the person's religious and cultural preferences. She may or may not wish to have a priest, rabbi, or minister present. She may wish to have a favorite passage from a book read to her, or a favorite piece of music played. Specific rituals may have to be performed before or at the time of death. A person of the Roman Catholic faith who is near death may want to have a priest called in to administer the Catholic ritual for the dying. If the person is an Orthodox Jew, it is important to know that the body must not be handled or touched after death until after the prescribed ritual is performed by a rabbi.

Many religions and cultures have their own customs and rituals relating to death. Be sure to ask the person in your care or her family members, ahead of time, if something special needs to be done and make sure this information is recorded in her care plan. It may be difficult for family members if the religious or cultural practices are not followed. Then the family has to deal not only with the loss of a loved one but also with the guilt or anger associated with not performing a required ritual. For example, a family who believes that a baby's soul won't go to heaven without baptism may suffer if a baby dies before it is baptized.

As a nurse assistant, you have an opportunity to provide needed attention and support to a dying person, as well as to her family and friends. Your caring should focus on their basic human needs and respect their dignity, privacy, and individuality. You may feel rewarded and fulfilled knowing that you have helped others through a difficult time.

Working with the dying, their families, and their friends also can be stressful and can trigger many feelings. To effectively help others, you must understand your own feelings about death. Just as you encourage people to talk about their feelings, you also must talk about your feelings. You may have formed a close relationship with the dying person and her family, and you may experience the loss with sadness or relief. Talk with your supervising nurse or social worker and, after the person dies, attend memorial services, if possible.

Hospice Care

Some terminally ill people receive care through a health care delivery system known as hospice care. Many years ago, the word hospice meant a place of hospitality and caring for travelers. Today, hospice is a word that refers to the philosophy of giving special care to those who are dying. Hospice care is a system of providing the dying with care by health care teams and volunteers.

Central to the hospice way of thinking is the idea that the dying person is an individual who should not be separated from the family or support system, and that dying is a normal and expected part of the life cycle. The family is encouraged and trained to participate in the care. The focus is on keeping the person as comfortable and pain free as possible, because the fear of pain greatly contributes to the stress of the person, his family, and the caregivers. The emphasis is not on curing the illness, but on providing physical, emotional, social, and spiritual comfort to the dying. The hospice philosophy also provides practical assistance, emotional support, and **bereavement care** to the dying person's family.

The hospice philosophy also allows the person to die in her own way, surrounded by the people she loves. The person is able to participate in the rituals that hold special meaning for her.

Most hospice programs provide care for the dying in their homes (Figure 22-5), although some have facilities in which care is provided. Some hospitals have hospice units.

bereavement care
(buh-REEV-ment)   Care provided for people who are grieving after someone dies.

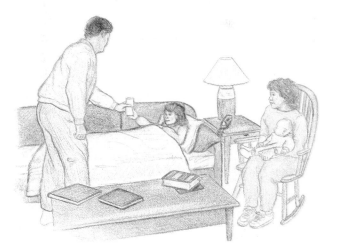

Figure 22-5
Many people prefer to be at home when they are dying. In home health care, family members like Mary Hill's brother and sister often are on hand to help provide care for the person who is dying.

When Death Comes

After a few minutes of crying, Arlene asks if you would help her select a dress for Josie's burial. You tell Arlene that you will and say that you know how much choosing a pretty dress would please Josie, since she was always so particular about her appearance (Figure 22-6). Arlene says, "I know Josie was angry and difficult when she first moved in here. After she was diagnosed with the heart condition, she hated leaving her apartment and didn't want to admit that she couldn't take care of herself anymore. The doctor told her she probably didn't have long to live. She wouldn't believe him and worked very hard at not liking this place or anybody in it. But you were the first one to win her over. You were so patient and understanding of her feelings."

Signs of Approaching Death

As death approaches and the body systems of the dying person wind down, you begin to see many changes. These changes may occur

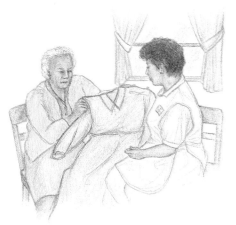

Figure 22-6
As Arlene begins to think about making funeral arrangements, she asks for your help in choosing a dress for Josie.

Box 22-1 Signs of Approaching Death

- ❖ Elevated temperature
- ❖ Rapid, weak, or irregular pulse
- ❖ Decreased blood pressure
- ❖ Skin feels cool and moist and looks pale
- ❖ Hands and feet feel cold and look pale
- ❖ Increased perspiration
- ❖ Incontinence
- ❖ Periods of increased, shallow respiration followed by periods of decreased respiration
- ❖ Mucus in back of the throat may cause a gargling sound with breathing
- ❖ Loss of, or a drifting in and out of, consciousness
- ❖ Loss of movement
- ❖ Loss of the ability to communicate

gradually or rapidly. The signs may not necessarily occur in the order listed in Box 22-1, and not all the signs may occur in everyone.

Signs that Death Has Occurred

A person is considered to be dead only after a doctor has examined her and pronounced her dead. When a person has died,—

- ❖ She has no pulse, respiration, or blood pressure.
- ❖ The pupils of her eyes are fixed (no movement) and dilated (widened).
- ❖ Her skin shows areas of dark discoloration as the blood pools on the side on which she is lying. This condition is called lividity.
- ❖ Her body becomes cold.
- ❖ Her bladder and bowels may empty.
- ❖ Her extremities become rigid within 6 to 8 hours. This condition is called rigor mortis.

Providing Postmortem Care

The word postmortem means after death. Even after death, a person and her family have the right to be treated with dignity and privacy. It is very important to respect the family's need to have time with the person who has died before any postmortem care is started. Some families may not want to see the body at all after death, but some may need time to be with the body. This need should be respected, and family members should not be rushed.

Handle the person's body with care and respect. If someone is helping you to provide this special service, your conversation should be respectful and appropriate. Sometimes when people are uncomfortable with a new situation, they may laugh or joke as a way of dealing with their feelings. If you are uncomfortable, be sure to talk to your supervising nurse and ask for assistance if necessary. Feelings are not right or wrong, but as a good nurse assistant, you don't want your feelings to get in the way of doing your job well. It is helpful to think of what the loss of this person's life means to the family and the community.

When providing care for the body of a person who has died, you must know the policies and procedures followed by your employer. When providing care for a dead person's body, follow the specific procedure that is explained step by step in Skill 62 in the skills book. You also must be sensitive to the feelings of others who share the room with the one who just died. They may feel frightened and sad and may need your attention and reassurance.

Death and Dying in the Nursing Home

After you and Arlene select a dress for Josie to wear for her burial, Arlene looks at the picture of Mr. Wilson and Josie on Josie's nightstand. "And you were the one who brought Jake in to meet her," Arlene says to you, smiling. You say that you think it was love at first sight with Mr. Wilson and Josie and you chuckle. "They were quite a pair, weren't they? They were always together," says Arlene. Suddenly, Arlene says, "Oh no, poor Jake. He doesn't know Josie has died. He'll be heartbroken." She says that she'll go and tell him right away, before he finds out from somebody else.

With tears welling up in her eyes, Arlene takes the framed picture of Josie and Mr. Wilson off the nightstand and says, "I know Josie would like Jake to have this picture." Arm in arm, you and Arlene walk together toward the dayroom, where he spends much of his time. You want a few minutes to watch as Arlene gently breaks the news to Mr. Wilson.

The death of a person in a nursing home can greatly sadden staff and other residents, as well as their families and friends. The residents know each other and usually have had time to develop friendships (Figure 22-7).

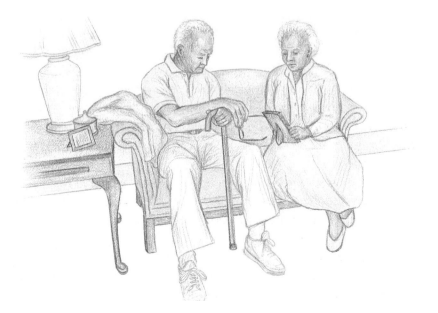

Figure 22-7
Mr. Wilson is very shaken over Josie's death. He knew she had been very ill, but the news is still hard to handle.

As a nurse assistant in a nursing home, you probably are one of the people who knows the dying person very well, and the person may feel closer to you than to other people in the facility. Therefore, you may have both a personal and a professional desire to provide care for the dying resident. It is a special privilege for a nurse assistant to help a resident come to the end of her life with peace, dignity, and a feeling that someone cares. You may experience anger about the person's extended suffering, relief that her suffering has ended, and sadness at the loss of a relationship. If you cannot work through these or other feelings, or if old memories of your own have been triggered, talk about them with your supervising nurse or social worker. Coming to terms with these feelings within yourself is important so that they do not interfere with your ability to support and help dying residents.

Be sure to tell other residents that the person has died so that they do not wonder and worry. Encourage residents to talk about their memories of the person who died and help them to remember the good things. When you give information about the person's death to other residents, you may say whether she died peacefully, where she died, what she was doing at the time of death, and who was with her. Encourage other residents to talk about their own fears about death or their sadness about losing a friend, and encourage them to attend religious or memorial services, if possible. Those residents affected by the death may pass through the emotional stages of grieving and need your ongoing attention.

To learn about death and dying in hospitals and home health care, read the next two sections. If you do not plan to work in hospitals or home health care, please turn to the end of the chapter to read "When a Child Dies" and "When a Person with AIDS Dies."

Death and Dying in the Hospital

Most people in the United States die in hospitals. As a nurse assistant in a hospital, you may deal with the death of people in all stages of the life cycle, ranging from a stillborn infant to an elderly person admitted from home or a nursing home. Some people die outside of hospitals from injuries, heart attacks, suicide, and other causes.

The dying process can occur over a long period of time, with numerous hospital admissions, as in lingering illnesses like cancer. The final admission focuses on providing and maintaining comfort, while previous admissions may have focused on treatments for improvement or a cure.

Death often comes quickly to people in hospitals. You may form only a limited attachment to a patient and wonder if something is wrong with you because you don't feel anything. The degree of feeling or grief often is related to the amount of time you have known the person and the intensity of your involvement. You may find that the family's grief affects you more because of your interaction with and support of them in this situation.

Because the time from admission to death may be short, the patient may not have the opportunity to experience the full range of feelings in response to her own dying. People in hospitals may die in emotional shock, denial, or anger if there has not been enough time for them to go through the emotional stages of dying.

Death and Dying at Home

Some dying people choose to stay at home where they are in familiar surroundings and where they have greater independence and freedom of choice, fewer rules and regulations, and family and friends involved with care. The home health aide may provide care only on a part-time basis.

A hospice program, if accepted by the person and his family, can help avoid stress and allow him to die at home. If the stress or care needed at home becomes too difficult, often the person is admitted to a hospital, nursing home, or an inpatient hospice program. Moving the person out of the home may be a relief for both the person and the family.

The age of the person and the makeup of the household determine the kind and amount of stress that the client and his family may experience. For example, you might be providing home health care to the dying father of a 4-year-old child. What do you think he might be feeling about not being able to see his child grow up, go to school, get a job, get married, and have children? What do you think his wife might be feeling about being a single parent? What kind of feelings might the child have? What do you think you might feel about the death of a young husband and father?

Home health care for a dying person can be both challenging and rewarding. Your relationship with the client and with his family and friends can be special. The family may look to you for guidance on how to provide care for and behave around the dying person. They may be afraid to touch or hug him for fear of hurting him. You can help them feel more comfortable with these actions by showing them through your behavior. Perhaps you could ask them to help you turn or position him. The family's involvement in touching and providing care for him may give them good feelings about how they helped bring comfort to their dying loved one (Figure 22-8). Even young children benefit by feeling that they were helpful and loving

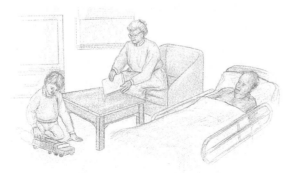

Figure 22-8
To prevent a dying person from feeling isolated, place his bed in a main room of the house. This way, daily activity happens around him, and he can take part in as much of it as he wants.

to the dying person. Maybe a young grandson could comb his grandfather's hair, or a young granddaughter could hold his juice glass and straw if he is too weak to enjoy this refreshment without help. Children need help with their grieving just as adults do. Your support and caring can make it possible for the family and friends to enjoy special times with the dying person through this last stage of life.

When a Child Dies

The loss of a child is difficult for any family to accept. You may feel a great deal of anger yourself and be unable to understand why something like this happened. The family experiences intense, acute grief and requires your understanding, support, caring, and, most of all, your willingness to be there and listen.

A dying child may be too young to communicate as clearly as an adult might. His messages may be sent nonverbally. You may be afraid of not knowing what to do or what to say. Sometimes it's best to say nothing, but instead, stay, listen, and touch the child. Hold, hug, and rock him. Get help with dealing with your own feelings so that you can be there emotionally for the child and for the family.

Although age is a factor in the pain of losing a child, when elderly parents loose an adult son or daughter, their pain also is intense. They may think, "I should have died instead." As a nurse assistant, you can play an important role in providing understanding and emotional support to any parent who loses a child, whether the child is young or old.

When a Person with AIDS Dies

The person with HIV infection or AIDS may go through several episodes of "near death." He may have all the signs of approaching death and then recover. In some cases, the person remains weak, but in others, he may recover enough to provide for his own care. This "roller coaster" ride of events causes emotional turmoil for the person, as well as for his caregivers. Several times the person may move through the five emotional stages of dealing with dying.

Because of his changing health status, a person with AIDS may begin making plans for his death and funeral, plans that would not have occurred until a later time in his life. You already read that talking about death can be uncomfortable, but you must be open to the person and listen to him. It is important for him to be able to make his desired plans and discuss these plans in advance. Your role as a nurse assistant is to provide emotional support as the person and his family make difficult decisions. As the person approaches death, continue to provide care to him and his family, practicing the principles of care, especially focusing on dignity, privacy, independence, and infection control.

The person with AIDS who is dying will experience many of the same signs of approaching death as those listed in Box 22-1 on p. 484. The care that you provide will focus on—

❖ Continuing personal care activities; keeping the person's skin clean and dry.

❖ Continuing communication; speaking calmly, slowly, and reassuringly.

❖ Keeping the person from getting too hot or too cold.

❖ Elevating the head of the person's bed if breathing is difficult for him or if the person experiences an increase in secretions.

❖ Changing the person's position in bed frequently and using pillows for support.

❖ Frequently moistening and cleaning the person's mouth.

❖ Monitoring the person's urinary output, since kidney function decreases and fluid intake may have lessened.

If the person dies in the hospital or nursing home, follow your employer's policy and procedures. If the person dies at home, you may be the one to contact the county or city medical examiner's office to determine what procedures must be followed. Discuss these topics with your supervising nurse.

Discuss your fears and feelings about death with your supervising nurse and seek support for your own grief.

Information Review

Circle the correct answers and fill in the blanks.

1. Factors that influence how a person reacts to being told of her own approaching death or that of a loved one are—
   a. Listening, touching, and responding.
   b. The presence of health care workers and family members.
   c. Death awareness and taboo.
   d. Age, culture, fulfillment, religion, and family and friends.

2. The five emotional stages of dealing with dying are—
   a. Denial, anger, bargaining, depression, and acceptance.
   b. Denial, delivering, bargaining, esteem, and acceptance.
   c. Preparing, experiencing, depression, elation, and acceptance.
   d. Posturing, preparing, anger, knowing, and acceptance.

3. People in the denial stage of dealing with their own impending death may—
   a. Acknowledge that they are going to die, but that they need more time to finish writing a will and settle financial affairs.
   b. Express outrage at the unfairness of having a terminal illness.
   c. Express that they have finished up old business and are ready to die.
   d. State that their doctors are wrong and have made a mistake.

4. Family members of a person who is dying should be—
   a. Encouraged to talk about their feelings and their needs.
   b. Discouraged from participating in the care of the person, because it is too upsetting.
   c. Encouraged to visit with the person who is dying for only a few minutes because it is too tiring for her.
   d. Discouraged from expressing how they feel.

5. Some terminally ill people receive care at home through a health care delivery system called _____.

6. Areas of skin discoloration caused by pooling blood after death are called _____.

7. Providing care for a person's body after death is called _____ care.

8. The body of a person who has died should be handled with care and _____.

9. Parents feel intense, acute _____ and _____ when a child dies.

10. A person with AIDS may experience several episodes of _____ _____ in which he has all the signs of approaching death but then recovers.

Questions to Ask Yourself

1. How do you think Mr. Wilson will react to the news of Josie's death? What are some things you can do to help him with this loss?

2. Mr. Wilson discusses Josie Miller's death with a group of residents the day after her death. You notice that Mrs. Casey looks very upset and doesn't say anything. What should you do?

3. After Josie's death, Arlene calls the nursing home director to ask if she can bring the flowers from Josie's funeral to the nursing home. How do you think the other residents will react? Arlene also asks if it would be a good idea to have a short memorial service in the dayroom for the residents who knew Josie. What do you think about Arlene's idea?

4. Mr. Calloway, a 90-year-old nursing home resident, is dying after a long illness. He is a widower whose three children visit him at various times. Two of the children visit regularly to talk with him and comfort him. The third child, a son named Mike, seldom visits, seems quiet and withdrawn, and stays for only a short time. One day when you are bathing Mr. Calloway, he says he is concerned about Mike. He says that Mike does not seem to care that he is dying, but that he often seems to be hurt, angry, or upset. How would you respond to Mr. Calloway? What, if anything, would you report to your supervising nurse about Mr. Calloway's conversation? Why do you think Mike is behaving the way he is?

23

Managing Your Time

Goals

After reading this chapter, you will have the information to—

Describe how to schedule your time each working day.

Discuss how to adjust your time if unplanned events occur.

Explain how to communicate clearly to help you stay in control of your time.

"I hate days like this," Nora Fuentes says to her friend and neighbor, Sylvia, as she sinks into a seat on the bus. "Why can't I get my act together? Just when I think I have a morning routine all worked out and I'm feeling like a super single mom, something unexpected happens. First the iron stops working before I've finished ironing my uniform. Then Ginny says her sweater doesn't match her pants and she needs me to help her pick out another outfit. Eight years old and she's already worrying about how she looks! Then, to top it all off, Emmy throws up her breakfast—everywhere. All over the kitchen floor. All over her clothes. And then, after I clean her up, she insists on getting dressed and going to school, because the first-graders have a special program today.

"Right now it seems almost impossible that I'll be able to concentrate on the residents in my care today. What if the school nurse calls to say that I need to pick up Emmy, who shouldn't have been sent to school in the first place? And if Ginny's clothes-conscious now, what will she be like when she's a teenager? And where am I going to find the money to pay for a new iron?

"All this when I woke up feeling great about beginning my second month as a nurse assistant. I sure hope I can manage my day at the nursing home better than I've managed my time at home today. It's a miracle that I'm even on the bus!"

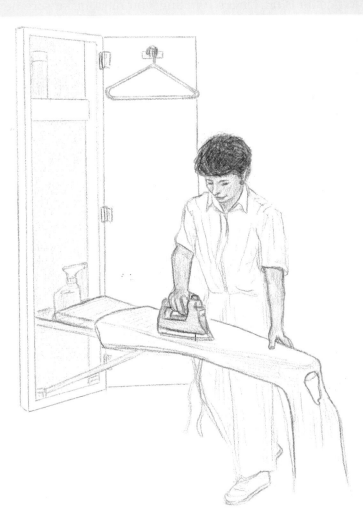

Looking Ahead to the Working World of Caregiving

While you are in training as a nurse assistant, someone else plans your time for you. When you work as a nurse assistant, you plan much of your own time. In training, you provide care for a few people. In your work experience, you may have to juggle your time to provide care for many people at once. As you gain experience, you perform your duties more quickly and with more confidence. Learning to make the most of your time enables you to give people the best care possible.

The world of learning and the world of work are different. They *must* be different. When you learn new ideas and skills in a training program, you learn to perform every step of a task—such as giving a complete bed bath—in a specific, uninterrupted way. By learning the ideal way to perform these skills, you master how to perform each step.

When you work in a health care setting, the situations aren't so specific and ideal. They are more complex. Unplanned events happen when you least expect them. For example, you may be giving a bed bath when the person you are bathing becomes nauseated and begins to vomit. You have to stop what you are doing and sit the person up or turn his head to the side so that he doesn't aspirate. Then, once the person is no longer vomiting, you must make sure he is okay, report the situation to your supervising nurse, and determine new actions.

You may have to consider the safety hazard of vomitus on the floor. The person may have to be bathed again, and the entire bed may have to be changed. You must make decisions based on the new situation. No matter what you do, the bed bath will take longer than normal.

Each day you make many decisions that affect the care you give and the time you have planned for the tasks you must perform.

Other people and situations influence how you use your time. For example, someone else makes decisions about how many people are in your care. Conditions, such as how sick a person is, determine how much time you must spend with the person and what kind of care he needs. A person's mobility is another factor that determines how much time you spend giving him care (Figure 23-1). Your responsibility is to plan how to get all your work done, regardless of the number and needs of people in your care.

Figure 23-1

It takes more of your time to provide care for a person who must stay in bed than to help someone who is somewhat mobile and can do some things for himself.

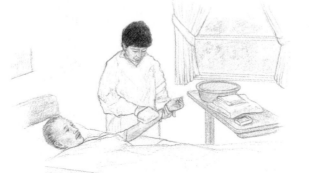

As you move from the role of student to employed nurse assistant, you move into areas of greater responsibility. You must handle this transition thoughtfully and carefully. You can make this transition smoothly if you know how to—

❖   Plan your time.
❖   Balance your scheduling needs and the needs of the people in your care.
❖   Stay in control of your time.

Planning Your Time

Every day on your new job, you have many tasks to accomplish and details to remember. So far, you have been learning specific skills. Now you have to know how to put them all together. You must create a **schedule** to guide you through the day. At first, scheduling your time is difficult. As you gain experience, you find the best way to plan your day.

schedule
(SKED-yule)   A written plan that lists the time and order of several tasks.

Planning your time in hospital and nursing home settings.   At the beginning of each shift, you find out how many people are in your care and who they are. The nursing care plan and a verbal report from either the caregivers who worked on the previous shift or from your supervising nurse give you information about the kind of care that each person needs. You also learn about prescheduled activities or treatments. As you listen to this report, take notes, being careful to write down—

1.   Daily tasks that have to be done at specific times, such as measuring vital signs, providing treatments, serving meals, and turning and positioning.
2.   Daily tasks that must be done but have no set time, such as bathing, dressing, and oral hygiene.
3.   Special things that have to be done or considered that day for the people in your care, such as a nursing home resident's scheduled trip to the beauty shop, a person's appointment with the physical therapist or an appointment for an electrocardiogram, a hospital patient's scheduled surgery, and special treatments or procedures.

After listing the tasks that you must do that day, think about the order in which to do things and jot down a tentative schedule. Often you feel pressured to begin the day's activities, but it will save you time in the end if you take a few minutes to create a plan before you start.

Some tasks might involve important preparation steps. For example, you may have to schedule time to use the tub room before you can give a person a tub bath. When you make your schedule, be sure to include each step of your larger tasks.

Your employer may provide a worksheet on which you add notes to remind yourself of each person's needs. For example, you may want to note that Mr. Wilson had an upset stomach yesterday, or that Mr. Britten is worried because his partner is flying to Australia on business today. You may want to note the tasks that will require the assistance of your co-workers. You need the help of one or more nurse assistants when you transfer a person who—

❖   Weighs a lot.
❖   Is frail, weak, or in pain.
❖   Is much taller or larger than you.
❖   Has bedsores.
❖   Is unable to bear his own weight.

You also may need a co-worker's assistance when you do not have the experience needed to work with a specific person.

After you finish your schedule, put a star next to each task that must be done at a specific time. Then **prioritize** the remaining tasks by marking the most important ones to remind you to do them first, if possible. Now, when you look at your schedule, you know *what* must be done and *when* it must be done. Unscheduled events always occur. But when you know what has to be done, it is easier to read-just your schedule.

As a nurse assistant, you spend a great deal of time with the people in your care. Because of this constant involvement, you often are the person most familiar with their desires and special needs, and you learn how to accommodate their needs into your schedule.

For example, you may have learned that Mrs. McDay becomes agitated if she is rushed through her morning care, or if her usual routine is changed. You know that when Mrs. McDay becomes agitated, it takes much longer to provide comfort and care for her. So it makes sense, as much as possible, to stick to her routine and be relaxed when providing care for her.

What do you do when you need additional time to properly care for Mrs. McDay? Or how do you cope when an assignment is too risky for you to handle alone or too time-consuming for you to do your best job? How might you feel when it seems like you are being asked to do the impossible, or when asking for help seems like "dumping" on your co-workers who already are dealing with their own heavy loads? These questions are difficult. But, in the real world, these situations can happen.

If members of the health care team are dependable and honest in handling their responsibilities, it makes it easier to handle unexpected situations. For example, when one member of the team decides to "play hooky" and calls in sick, or when she doesn't "pull her weight," her workload has to be split up and given to the team members who are there until a substitute becomes available. This places an unfair burden on everyone and causes resentment. But sometimes a health care team member really is sick and needs an unexpected day off. If each team member is honest and considerate at times when special needs arise, the other members of the team willingly work harder to carry the work load.

prioritize
(pry-OR-uh-tize)   To list items or tasks in order of importance.

When an assignment seems too risky to handle alone or too time-consuming for you to do a thorough job, it is important to discuss this problem with your supervising nurse. Perhaps your supervising nurse doesn't realize how much time you must have for the special needs of a person like Mrs. McDay. Or perhaps you don't realize that another member of the team has just called in sick. Sharing information with your supervising nurse and other team members helps the health care team work well together so that everyone can enjoy a sense of satisfaction from a job well done.

Planning your time in home health care settings. Some home health care agencies give home health aides their assignments by telephone in the morning so that they can go directly to their first client's home. Other agencies require home health aides to report to the office in the morning to receive that day's assignment.

When providing care for clients in their homes, you have to use a different approach when planning your time. You may be assigned three or four clients a day, but you will have just one client to provide care for at one time.

Because your clients may live in different neighborhoods, you may be required to plan your travel time, as well as your caregiving time, with your supervisor or the scheduling nurse. You must consider factors such as how much time it takes to get from one client's home to another and how much traffic is on that route at that time of the day. Usually it is more efficient to visit clients in a logical geographic order, rather than to drive back and forth across town. The more time you spend in your car, the less time you have for providing care.

Unfortunately, a logical geographic order is not always possible. A client may have special needs, such as a treatment at a certain time, or an appointment, such as for physical therapy. These needs also must be considered, and you may have to adjust your schedule to accommodate these special needs. If you have a problem with scheduling, discuss the situation with your supervisor.

Resolving Schedule and Needs Conflicts

Mr. Rivera usually likes to receive his complete bed bath immediately after breakfast. But after breakfast today, he says he wants to rest for about a half hour. Knowing how important his needs are, you let him rest and plan to come back in a half hour to give him his bath. If you had written a schedule for the day and Mr. Rivera's needs changed, what would you do with that half hour's time?

Every day, no matter how well you plan things for yourself, people's needs change—and so does your schedule. You may ask, "Why bother to make a schedule if I can never stick to it?" The answer is that the schedule is an important tool that reminds you of *what* you have to do, *when* you must do it, and which things are most important for you to do.

Working in a health care setting is much like traveling by car. No

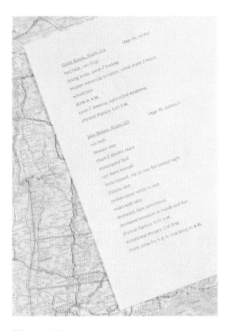

Figure 23-2
Think of your schedule as a road map that helps you "map" your route as you provide care.

matter how well you map out your trip, you are bound to make some detours along the way. Your schedule is like a map that helps you find an alternate route to your destination (Figure 23-2).

Staying in Control of Your Time

You have just finished helping Mr. Wilson brush his hair and shave. You're ready to leave his room to attend to the next thing on your schedule when he says, "Before you leave, could you do one quick favor for me?" You say that you would be happy to do something for him. Then he says, "Please make me a nice cup of tea and some dry toast. I'm hungry, but I just couldn't eat breakfast. I don't want to wait for an order to come up from the kitchen."

You want to be able to do this special task for Mr. Wilson, but you think to yourself that his quick favor is not going to be quick at all. You know that this task may take 20 minutes of your time. What can you do now? What could you have done to anticipate this situation? How would you handle a similar situation in the future?

Sometimes, unplanned events can be handled by taking charge of your time from the beginning. When you first go into Mr. Wilson's room, check to see what has to be done and let him know how long you are going to be there this time. Also, let him know when you plan to come back. Before you start your tasks in Mr. Wilson's room, ask him if he thinks he might need anything special. If, at the beginning of your time with Mr. Wilson, he says he wants tea and toast, you can adjust the time that you spend on other planned tasks to include his special request. If you wait until the end of your time with Mr. Wilson to find out that he has special needs, these last-minute requests may affect the rest of your schedule.

If you work in a private home, it is very important to let your client know when you will be leaving. By letting the person know in advance when you plan to leave, you may avoid having to deal with a request as you put one foot out the door.

If you communicate your plans and time requirements clearly to the person in your care, you may lessen the number of unplanned events during the day. What you say through verbal communication is important, and *how* you express it with your face and body through nonverbal communication is equally important. The following tips will help you remember to communicate your message clearly and, in the end, may save time:

❖ When you assist a person, even on a very busy day, try to be relaxed. Remember that the person in your care is your reason for being there. If you seem to be hurried and stressed, the person also may become stressed, which may require you to spend more time with him.

❖ Touch the person you provide care for, if touching is acceptable to him. Placing a hand on his shoulder or holding his hand is calming and helps the person know that you care. Showing the person that you care about him may help him feel more secure and help you spend your time more efficiently and effectively.

❖ When you help a person, take time to speak with him and really listen to what he has to say. Sometimes the simple act of stopping and listening to the person shows that you are available. This action can reduce his anxiety and perhaps even save you time in the long run.

Planning your time well, knowing how to adjust your schedule, and communicating your plans clearly to the person in your care may help you to control your time and, as a result, enjoy your job more and be more successful.

Nora's Day

In the following scenario, you can observe a day in the life of Nora Fuentes as she begins her second month of work as a nurse assistant at Morningside Nursing Home. The scenario does not provide all the possible types of decisions that you make as a nurse assistant, but it does show how one nurse assistant manages her time on one given day.

Nora arrives for work promptly at 7 A.M. She has been getting to know the residents at Morningside Nursing Home and is beginning to feel good about the way she performs her job. Some days, however, she finds it challenging to get everything done. Although she has been providing care for just five people, she knows that her load soon will increase to at least eight. She feels a need to focus on how she manages her time.

Morning Report

Today, in morning report, Nora learns that she has five residents in her care: Rachel Morgan (Figure 23-3), Victor Rivera (Figure 23-4), Jake Wilson (Figure 23-5), Shirley McDay (Figure 23-6 on p. 500), and Rodney Britten (Figure 23-7 on p. 500). Nora already knows four of these residents well, but Mr. Britten has been at the nursing home just a few days. She looks at the quick, abbreviated notes she has written during report and reads:

Rm. 121 *R. Morgan*—45—M.S. (un-bed)
   Can feed self (DR)
   Help c̄: bed bath—dressing—bedpan—transfer to WC—ROM
   Blurred vision—tires easily
   *PT—1 P.M.
Rm. 114 *V. Rivera*—78—stroke (un-bed)
   Help c: bed bath—dressing—elec razor— urinal (7, 9, 11, 1)— feeding (DR)—transfer to WC
   R-sided weakness—*ROM in A.M.
   *PT—1 P.M.
Rm. 120 *J. Wilson*—79—diabetes (un-bed)
   Can: dress—feed self (DR)—walk/cane—tub
   Help c̄: dentures—elec razor
   Sight—light perception—sensation: hands & feet
   *PT—10:30 A.M.   Rec.T—2 P.M.
   *Urine S&A early A.M.—diabetic diet

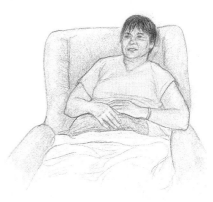

Figure 23-3
Rachel Morgan has multiple sclerosis. She lives in Room 121 at Morningside Nursing Home.

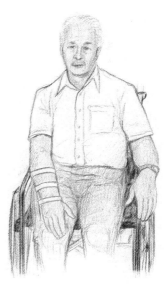

Figure 23-4
Victor Rivera had a stroke. He lives in Room 114 at the nursing home.

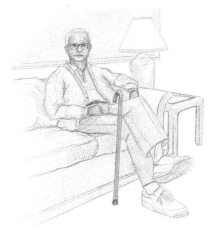

Figure 23-5
Jake Wilson has diabetes and lives in Room 120 at the nursing home.

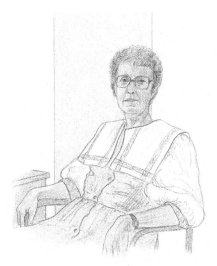

Figure 23-6
Shirley McDay, who has Alzheimer's disease, lives in Room 119 at the nursing home.

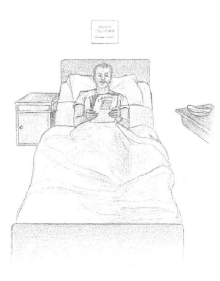

Figure 23-7
Rodney Britten has AIDS. Because of a staph infection in a wound, he is on "wound isolation" and lives in Room 124 and at the nursing home.

Rm. 119 *S. McDay*—55—Alzheimer's (un-bed)
    Can: feed self (DR)—OOB BR—walk c̄ assist
    Help c̄: tub—reminding her to use the toilet—incont. care—
    dressing
    Wanders A.M. & P.M.—rummages and hoards
Rm. 124 *R. Britten*—41—AIDS—wound isolation (oc-bed)
    Help c̄: bed bath—soft foods and liquids
    Vomiting and diarrhea
    *v.s. in A.M.
    NOTE: * Indicates that the task must be done at a particular time.

Planning the Day's Schedule

After reading the morning report, Nora creates a schedule for the day's activities like the one shown in Table 23-1.

She looks over her schedule and notes that she will need help lifting Rachel Morgan and Victor Rivera into and out of bed. Nora decides to talk to her friend Arthur Cid to see if he might be able to help her. Arthur has been working as a nurse assistant for 2 years, and Nora always learns so much from him. Arthur and Nora compare assignment sheets and realize that they are working in nearby rooms and that they both will need help with lifting, so they arrange to work together. They also realize that they both are assigned to the same lunch break.

Following the Schedule

Nora's first stop is Room 121, where she offers Rachel Morgan the bedpan. "I'll be back shortly to help you with your bed bath and dressing," Nora says to Mrs. Morgan before she leaves the room.

Nora's next stop is in Room 114. She offers Victor Rivera his urinal. Because Mr. Rivera had suffered a stroke and is on a bladder training program, he must be offered his urinal every 2 hours. "I'll be back with your breakfast tray, Mr. Rivera," Nora says.

She heads to Room 120. Because Jake Wilson is diabetic, he has to have his urine checked for sugar and acetone first thing in the morning. He knows the routine well and had first urinated earlier in the morning, and then later to provide a sample. Nora thanks him before asking how his favorite football team had done in the game last night. "The Redskins beat the Cardinals 34 to 10! You should have seen it!" Mr. Wilson says, his eyes sparkling. "I played some football myself when I was a young fellow." Using universal precautions, Nora tests the urine for sugar and acetone and records the results, which she later reports to her supervising nurse. "How are my 'levels' this morning?" asks Mr. Wilson.

Nora reassures Mr. Wilson that the test results are normal. She washes her hands and then walks with him to the tub room. While Nora helps Mr. Wilson with his dentures and shaving, they discuss his activities for the day. "Today's my session with the physical therapist," he says. "I want to be on time for her."

"Don't worry, Mr. Wilson," says Nora as she walks him back to his

Table 23-1   **Sample Caregiving Schedule**

	Rachel Morgan	Victor Rivera	Jake Wilson	Shirley McDay	Rodney Britten (Reverse Isolation)
7:00 A.M.	Bedpan	Urinal	Urine S&A Tub 7:15		V.S.
	Set up A.M. care, bed bath, help dress		Assist dentures/ shave	Tub 7:45 Help dress	A.M. care (gown/gloves)
8:00 A.M.	Rest				Tray setup
	Up to w/c to DR (need help)	Tray setup Assist feed	Assist walk to DR	Assist walk to DR	Assist feed Oc-bed
9:00 A.M.	Un-bed	Urinal			Rest
	DR—back	A.M. care, help dress, ROM	DR—back	DR—back	
10:00 A.M.	Rest in bed (need help) ROM	Up to w/c (need help) Un-bed	*10:30 PT Un-bed	Un-bed	
11:00 A.M.	Rest	Urinal		Check incont.	Check diar-rhea
11:30 lunch					
12:00 noon	Up to w/c to DR (need help)	Tray setup Assist feed	Assist walk to DR	Check incont. Assist walk to DR	Tray setup Assist feed Rest
1:00 P.M.	*1:00 w/c DR to PT	Urinal *1:00 PT	DR—back	DR—back	Check diar-rhea
2:00 P.M.	Rest in bed (need help)	Rest in bed (need help) Wife visits	*2:00 RecT	Check incont.	V.S.
3:00 P.M. Report Charting		Urinal			Check diar-rhea Remove trash and linens (need help)

room. "You'll be there on time." She then goes to Rachel Morgan's room to set up her A.M. care. "I think I can wash myself today, but it may take me awhile," Mrs. Morgan says. Nora smiles at her. "You just do what you can, Mrs. Morgan," she says at the door, "and I'll be back to help you finish your bed bath."

Nora puts on a gown and gloves before going into Mr. Britten's room to take his vital signs and provide A.M. care. Because of having AIDS, Mr. Britten developed a staph infection in an open wound on his arm and must remain in wound isolation until the infection is gone. "Hello, Mrs. Fuentes," Mr. Britten says quietly. Nora greets Mr. Britten and begins wrapping the blood pressure cuff around his unaffected arm. She asks him about his partner's trip to Australia. A smile

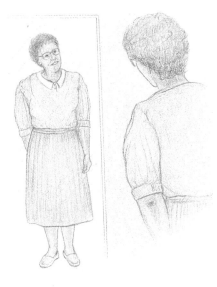

Figure 23-8
Her outfit may be unusual, but Mrs. McDay feels good about being able to select her own clothing.

tugs at the corners of his mouth. "Owen leaves for Sydney today," he says. "Would you believe I already miss him? He'll be gone for 2 whole weeks." Nora records Mr. Britten's vital signs, which are normal.

"Maybe he'll bring you a kangaroo," she says.

"If he does, I'll name it 'Nora'," he says with a grin.

Nora discards her gown and gloves and washes her hands before going to Room 119, where she greets Shirley McDay, who has Alzheimer's disease. "Hello, Mrs. McDay, I'm Mrs. Fuentes, your nurse assistant. Today is Tuesday, it's 7:45, and it's time for your morning bath," says Nora. After the bath, Nora helps Mrs. McDay get dressed. "I think I'll wear this outfit today," says Mrs. McDay, selecting a green blouse and an orange skirt from her closet. The blouse and skirt don't match, but Nora knows that green and orange are Mrs. McDay's favorite colors.

Wanting to say something positive, Nora says, "That blouse looks so nice on you." Mrs. McDay smiles shyly (Figure 23-8).

Then Nora returns to Mrs. Morgan's room to help her finish her bed bath and get dressed. Because Mrs. Morgan tires easily, Nora helps her get comfortable in her bed so that she can rest before going to the dining room for breakfast.

Next, Nora puts on a gown and gloves and enters Room 124 with Mr. Britten's breakfast tray. She suggests that he start eating the breakfast himself while she helps the other residents to the dining room for breakfast. Nora assures him that she will come back to help him finish his breakfast.

Nora removes and discards the gown and gloves and washes her hands before enlisting Arthur's help with getting Mrs. Morgan out of bed and into the wheelchair. As she pushes Mrs. Morgan to the dining room, she stops along the way and invites Jake Wilson and Shirley McDay to walk with her and Mrs. Morgan to the dining room.

After getting the three residents settled in the dining room, Nora takes a breakfast tray to Mr. Rivera who, until his condition worsened this week, had been eating regularly in the dining room. She helps him with his breakfast by placing her hand over his hand on the spoon. He has difficulty chewing and swallowing, so it takes a long time to help feed him. "My wife is coming to visit me today," says Mr. Rivera, dribbling oatmeal out of his mouth. "I can hardly wait." Nora gently wipes his chin and discusses the visit with him.

Observing universal precautions when she returns to Mr. Britten's room, Nora apologizes for taking so long. Much to her surprise, she finds that Mr. Britten has eaten all his breakfast by himself. "I'm so tired, I just want to sleep now," he says.

While Mrs. Morgan eats breakfast in the dining room, Nora changes the linens on her bed. Then she goes into Mr. Rivera's room and offers him the urinal. "One of these days I'm going to be regular like a clock," Mr. Rivera jokes. Nora helps him with his bed bath and helps him brush his teeth. While helping him dress, Nora encourages Mr. Rivera to fasten as many buttons with his "good hand" as possible. "You did more buttons today than you did yesterday," she says when he becomes tired. "You're really making good progress." Mr. Rivera beams. When Mr. Rivera is dressed, Nora helps him slowly complete his range-of-motion exercises.

On her way to the dining room, Nora smiles at Arthur, who is leading an elderly woman back to her room. In the dining room, Nora greets Rachel Morgan and wheels her to the elevator. "How was breakfast?" Nora asks. "Today they had pancakes, which I just love," says Mrs. Morgan. When they reach Room 121, Nora tells Mrs. Morgan that she'll be right back with someone to help transfer her into her bed. "All right, dear," says Mrs. Morgan. Nora steps into the hall and sees Arthur carrying bed linens. "Arthur, could you please help me transfer Mrs. Morgan into her bed?" she asks. "Comin' right up," says Arthur. "Let me just put these linens down in Mr. Lightfoot's room and I'll be right there."

After Mrs. Morgan is comfortably settled in bed, Nora heads back to the dining room where Mr. Wilson and Mrs. McDay have finished breakfast. As the three near the elevator, Mr. Wilson mentions that he's going to visit a friend on the second floor. Nora glances quickly at her watch and reminds him about his physical therapy appointment. "I'll be back in time," says Mr. Wilson. Nora walks Mrs. McDay back to her room.

"Is this my room?" Mrs. McDay asks as they near the supply closet.

"No, here we are," Nora says at the door to Room 119. She encourages Mrs. McDay to sit in a chair while she changes the linens on her bed. After the bed is made, Mrs. McDay climbs onto the bedspread and reaches for a magazine.

Nora sighs as she walks to Mr. Britten's room. She puts on a gown and gloves and enters the room. Mr. Britten is awake and is glad to see her. Nora gives him his bed bath, moving him as gently as possible to protect his fragile skin. She makes sure he is comfortable before leaving the room.

Getting Assistance

Nora heads toward Room 120 to see if she can find Arthur. He is in the room finishing Stephen Lightfoot's personal care. Arthur is ready to move Mr. Lightfoot out of bed, and he needs Nora's help. "Arthur, I'll help you move Mr. Lightfoot *and* change his bed if you will help me move Mr. Rivera and change his linens," Nora says.

"You've got a deal," says Arthur.

As Arthur and Nora lift Mr. Lightfoot into the bedside chair, he complains of extreme shortness of breath. First, Arthur makes sure that Mr. Lightfoot's oxygen tubes are not kinked anywhere. Then, so that Mr. Lightfoot doesn't hear, he quietly consults with Nora to see if she also noticed the blue color around his lips. Arthur decides to report Mr. Lightfoot's condition to his supervising nurse. First he takes Mr. Lightfoot's pulse and respiration and asks Nora to stay with him while he reports his vital signs and change in color to his supervising nurse.

After the supervising nurse attends to Mr. Lightfoot's breathing problem, Nora and Arthur go to Mr. Rivera's room at 10:15 (Figure 23-9). They move him into his wheelchair and change his bed. After leaving Mr. Rivera's room, Nora passes Mr. Wilson in the hall on the way to his physical therapy appointment. She then goes directly to Room 121 to help Rachel Morgan with her range-of-motion exercises. "Both of my arms are kind of stiff today," says Mrs. Morgan as they begin the exercises. Nora gently moves her wrists back and forth.

"We'll do everything slowly," she says to Mrs. Morgan, "and you tell me when to stop." After completing the exercises, Mrs. Morgan rests in her bed.

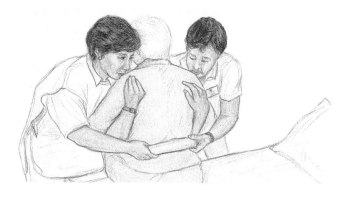

Figure 23-9
Nora and Arthur work well together. They know that they can always count on each other to be good team members.

Adjusting the Schedule

At 11:00 A.M., Nora finishes changing the linens on Mr. Wilson's bed when she remembers that it is time to offer Mr. Rivera the urinal again. "Gosh, I've gotta go check on Mr. Britten, too," she thinks to herself as she rushes toward Mr. Rivera's room. Halfway down the hallway, Nora notices that Mrs. McDay's call signal is on. "I'll be right there," she calls to Mrs. McDay. In her nervous state, Nora bumps into Arthur in the hall. "Arthur, I don't know what to do first!" she exclaims. "Mr. Rivera, Mrs. McDay, and Mr. Britten all need my help at the same time!"

"Calm down, Nora," says Arthur. "Let me see your schedule." Down the hallway, Mrs. McDay cries out for her mother. "I'll offer Mr. Rivera his urinal and then check on Mr. Britten while you take care of Mrs. McDay. Sounds like she really needs you," says Arthur.

"I don't know what I'd do without you!" Nora calls over her shoulder.

When Nora steps into Room 119, she sees that Mrs. McDay has wet the bed. Mrs. McDay rocks in her bed, scolding herself and picking at her bedspread. "I'm nothing but a baby! A baby!" she mutters under her breath.

Nora sighs to herself as she helps Mrs. McDay out of bed, removes the wet linens, and puts them in the hamper. As she helps Mrs. McDay wash and dress, she reassures her that the incontinence is not her fault and tells her that she doesn't mind helping her clean up.

She continues to comfort Mrs. McDay as she makes her bed. After a few minutes, Mrs. McDay asks, "Can I go to the dayroom?"

After helping Mrs. McDay to the dayroom, Nora goes to Room 124 and changes Mr. Britten's bed linens. She knows that he feels lonely in isolation and that he enjoys visiting with her while she provides care. On the other hand, Nora is scheduled for lunch at 11:30 and she's very hungry. She doesn't know how she's going to make it.

Controlling Time

After heating her soup in the microwave, Nora joins Arthur at a table where he is sipping a cup of coffee. It's 11:40 A.M. Nora has just 20 minutes to relax before she will have to begin taking people to the dining room and helping to feed lunch to the people in her care.

"I always seem to be running late," Nora says.

"Some days are like that," Arthur agrees. Then he suggests that they review Nora's schedule to see if she could have made any changes.

Arthur looks over Nora's schedule. "It seems to me that you have everything well organized," he says. "But people aren't like puzzle pieces, you know, that always fit into place. They don't always fit into our plans." Nora smiles.

"What do you do at home when things don't work out as planned with your kids' schedules?" Arthur asks.

Nora laughs, tells him about her crazy morning, and confesses that she tries to stay flexible and roll with the punches. "After Emmy threw up I just wanted to cry. But eventually everything works out, most of the time," Nora says.

Arthur laughs. "That's what they mean by experience being the best teacher," he says. "It takes awhile to learn how to balance the needs of each person with all the things that you have to get done. Do you think you could have done anything different this morning?" (Figure 23-10)

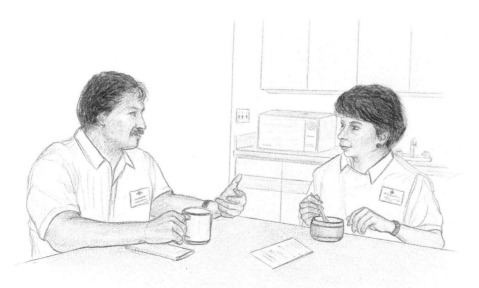

Figure 23-10
Arthur is right when he tells Nora that experience is the best teacher. As a seasoned nurse assistant, he knows that coping with conflicts and crises is part of an ordinary work day.

Nora thinks back on her morning. "I guess I could have checked on Mr. Britten before I did Mrs. Morgan's range-of-motion exercises. But, I didn't know that Mrs. McDay would need me just when I had to offer Mr. Rivera his urinal. I was so worried that I would mess up his bladder training program. I can't thank you enough for helping me today."

When Nora finishes talking, Arthur asks her what she has accomplished that morning. As Nora begins to list the many things that she accomplished, she begins to relax, realizing that she has successfully completed all her morning tasks. Feeling renewed, she goes back on the floor and helps everybody get lunch.

Focusing on Each Person in Your Care

It is 12:30 P.M. when Nora brings Mr. Britten his lunch tray. Instead of hurrying out, she stops to talk for a few minutes. Mr. Britten tells her about how hard it is for him to be in the nursing home while his partner is traveling on business. "I worry about him, and I would feel better if I were at home," he says. "He's the only friend and family I have."

"Owen sounds like a very special person. I hope I get to meet him," says Nora. She tells Mr. Britten that she'll be back later to check on him.

Nora stops by Rachel Morgan's and Victor Rivera's rooms to make sure that they are ready for their physical therapy appointments at 1:00 P.M. She offers Mr. Rivera his urinal before leaving.

At 1:15, Nora finds Mrs. McDay sitting by the window in her room. Nora asks her if she would like to talk for a while. Mrs. McDay looks up at Nora and yells, "I just want to be alone!" Then she begins to cry. Nora recognizes that Mrs. McDay is probably having a catastrophic reaction. The earlier incontinence has upset her more than Nora realized.

Nora walks over to Mrs. McDay, sits next to her, and speaks to her in a calm voice. After a while, Nora comments to Mrs. McDay that the brightly colored afghan spread across her lap is very pretty. Mrs. McDay smiles a little. "My sister made this afghan for me when I got married," she tells Nora (Figure 23-11).

Figure 23-11
Nora knows how important it is to take time out from her busy schedule to comfort Mrs. McDay, who is having a catastrophic reaction.

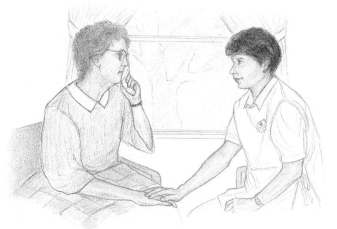

At a few minutes before 2:00 P.M., Nora stops in Room 120 to check on Mr. Wilson before his recreational therapy appointment. A physical therapy aide brings Mr. Rivera into his room and helps Nora move Mr. Rivera into his bed so that he can rest before his wife comes to visit. The physical therapy aide returns to the hall with Mrs. Morgan and again helps Nora as they transfer Mrs. Morgan out of the wheelchair and back into bed. "Those physical therapy sessions always wear me out," Mrs. Morgan says as Nora tucks the sheet around her shoulders. A few minutes later, Mrs. Morgan is fast asleep.

Nora's shift is over at 3:00 P.M. Before leaving, Nora and Arthur go to Mr. Britten's room. Nora checks his vital signs and then she and Arthur double-bag and transfer his soiled linens and trash. After saying good-bye to everyone, Nora completes her charting and makes her report to the team for the next shift. She includes a description of Mrs. McDay's catastrophic reaction in her report.

As she leaves the floor, Nora waves to Mr. Wilson, who is returning from recreation therapy. She smiles and feels very satisfied with herself.

On her ride home on the bus, she again meets her friend Sylvia. "Did your day get any better?" Sylvia asks.

"What? Oh, I barely thought about all that happened this morning," says Nora. "There was so much happening at the nursing home today. It's good for me to have a place of my own to go, where I can get away from all the responsibilities of being a single mother. Not that I don't have a mountain of responsibilities at work!

"I learned a lot today. I learned that people—me, my family, and the people in my care— aren't puzzle pieces that fit neatly into my plans — I also really saw the value of making a schedule. Finally, and perhaps most important, I learned how important it is to be relaxed and flexible."

Hillary's Day

Now, you have the opportunity to observe a day in the life of Hillary Bridges as she visits clients as a home health aide for Lewisford Home Health Care Agency. This scenario does not include all the possible types of decisions that you make as a home health aide, but it does illustrate how one home health aide manages her time on one given day.

At 8:00 A.M. Hillary parks her car and enters the Lewisford Home Health Care Agency office. She receives her assignments for the day, noting that she has two new clients, Mary Hill and her 3-month-old daughter Melissa. Hillary's supervisor reviews the new clients' cases with her and describes the family's needs. "The primary nurse will meet you at the Hills' home for an orientation and planning session at 2:30 P.M.," she tells Hillary.

When a Person Needs Your Company

Hillary's first stop, from 8:30 A.M. to 10:30 A.M., is with Mrs. Roth, a 73-year-old woman who has diabetes. In the past, Mrs. Roth con-

ADA
Abbreviation for **A**merican **D**iabetes **A**ssociation.

trolled her diabetes with a special diet. Recently, however, she has started taking an oral medication as well. During each visit, Hillary helps Mrs. Roth with personal care, monitors the **ADA** diet left by the nurse, and reminds her client to take her pill.

Mrs. Roth appears pleased for the company and starts talking to Hillary as soon as she walks in the door. "Oh, Mrs. Bridges, I'm so glad you're here," says Mrs. Roth. "Yesterday I was watching 'Abiding Light'—you know, that soap opera I love so much—and there was this new girl on there—Harry's girlfriend, I think—and she looked so much like you I just had to tell you. Did you ever do any acting? Then this commercial came on for that big department store downtown—you know, Trumbull's—and they have these darling dresses on sale that would look so nice on you, dear. Of course my sister was the best seamstress there ever was." Mrs. Roth and Hillary continue to talk as they check the contents of the refrigerator (Figure 23-12).

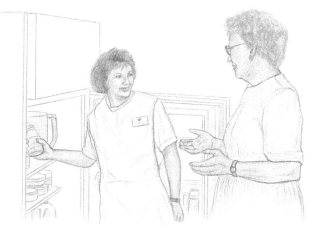

Figure 23-12
Home health care clients who live alone often are lonely. Hillary knows that Mrs. Roth is always glad to see her.

"Mrs. Roth, may I discard this custard?" asks Hillary, holding up a small glass bowl. "It looks like you've had it awhile."

"Heavens yes!" Mrs. Roth says. "I made that up the week before last and just forgot all about it."

"Tell me about what you've been eating, Mrs. Roth," Hillary says. Mrs. Roth shows Hillary her diet sheet, pointing to the red check marks she makes each time she eats something. Hillary praises Mrs. Roth for recording everything, then reminds her to take her medication.

Together, they make out a grocery list for Sandra, Mrs. Roth's niece, following the ADA diet. Sandra goes shopping for her aunt once a week. When the list is ready, Hillary completes the day's home maintenance tasks.

Hillary is almost out the door when Mrs. Roth says, "Dear, the little toe on my right foot is a bit sore. Maybe you could take a look at it." Hillary notices that Mrs. Roth is wearing soft slippers instead of the sturdy shoes she usually wears. Hillary asks Mrs. Roth to sit down and, upon examining her toe, discovers redness and the beginning of a small blister. She asks Mrs. Roth when she first felt the soreness.

Mrs. Roth says, "Last night." She seems very relieved when Hillary tells her that she'll call her supervisor. After Hillary explains the situation, her supervisor thanks Hillary for calling and says the primary nurse has an appointment tomorrow to check Mrs. Roth's condition and can look at her toe then. She tells Hillary to tell Mrs. Roth to keep wearing the soft slipper, keep her foot elevated, and keep her toe clean and dry until the primary nurse can assess the seriousness of the sore. Hillary relays the information to Mrs. Roth and then records her observations on Mrs. Roth's visit record. She reminds herself to ask early in her next visit if Mrs. Roth has noticed any changes in her health.

When Other Caregivers Are Delayed

Hillary's second stop, scheduled for 11:00 A.M to 1:00 P.M., is at the home of Tamara Frazier, who is recovering from an automobile collision. She recently has been discharged from the nursing home, where she had been in a coma, and is now confined to bed while her broken ankle bone heals. Ms. Frazier's fiancé Jim Thompson works during the day, so he cannot provide care for Ms. Frazier then.

When Hillary arrives, Mr. Thompson is waiting by the door with Carolyn, a friend who will stay with Ms. Frazier this afternoon. "Good morning, Ms. Bridges. It's nice to see you," says Mr. Thompson. He explains that Carolyn is ready to go to the eye doctor and has stopped by to leave her doctor's phone number and to assure him that she will come by to stay with Ms. Frazier after her appointment. "Hello, Mrs. Bridges," Ms. Frazier calls out weakly from the bedroom.

As usual, Ms. Frazier has a new joke for Hillary. Laughing, Hillary promises to repeat the joke to her other clients. It is only when Hillary begins to provide personal care that Ms. Frazier becomes serious.

"I was in the coma for so long—3 weeks, Jim tells me—and so much time went by and I wasn't a part of it. My sister in Ohio even had a baby while I was in the hospital. More than anything, I wish I could go back and recapture all that lost time," Ms. Frazier says sadly. Hillary sits down and comforts her client by taking time to listen.

She helps Ms. Frazier with her bed bath, then gently helps her through her range-of-motion exercises. At 1:00 P.M. Ms. Frazier's care is complete, and Hillary is ready to leave. Unfortunately, Carolyn has not yet returned. Ms. Frazier is also starting to worry. "What if something happened to her?" she asks.

Calling the doctor's office, Hillary learns that Carolyn's appointment has been delayed by an emergency. She will be out any minute and will soon be on her way home. Hillary explains the delay to Ms. Frazier and then calls her supervisor to get permission to leave.

"Hillary, remember that Clyde Vanson lives two doors down from Ms. Frazier and is listed on the emergency backup plan as a contact. Why don't you try calling him to see if he can come stay with Ms. Frazier," your supervisor suggests. Hillary asks Ms. Frazier if she would like her to call the neighbor to see if he can come over until Carolyn arrives (Figure 23-13).

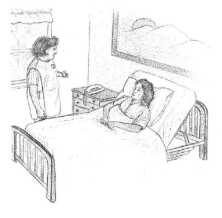

Figure 23-13
Hillary has to leave Tamara Frazier's house, but an emergency backup contact person is just a phone call away.

"Yes," says Ms. Frazier, "That would be nice." After making the call and waiting for Mr. Vanson to arrive, Hillary says her good-byes and leaves.

Taking Care of Her Own Needs

As she drives to pick up some lunch, Hillary thinks about Ms. Frazier. She feels sorry that she had to leave. "She really wanted to talk today," she thinks. "Maybe her neighbor is a good listener. I would have stayed, but I needed to leave so that I can eat lunch before driving all the way to the Hills.'"

Hillary sees a small park and decides to sit on a bench and eat her turkey sandwich and apple. Too often she has scolded herself for not taking time to take care of her own needs. She remembers how her instructor in the nurse assistant training course emphasized the importance of planning time for her own needs so that she doesn't get stressed on the job. She relaxes a bit, watching two squirrels chase each other up a tree.

Planning for a New Client

The primary nurse is with the new clients when Hillary arrives at 2:30 P.M. Mary Hill and her 3-month-old daughter Melissa live together in a small row house. Both have tested positive for HIV, and Mrs. Hill has been diagnosed with AIDS. The primary nurse works with Mrs. Hill and Hillary to begin creating a plan of care.

Hillary will visit the Hills for 2 hours, 3 days a week. Another home health aide will come on the other days. Mrs. Hill's mother now stays with her evenings and nights. Her sister works during the day but takes care of the weekly shopping and other needs on the weekends. Mrs. Hill's next-door neighbor learned universal precautions and comes over regularly to help with Melissa's diapering and feeding.

"Hillary, you will help provide personal care for both Mrs. Hill and Melissa, help with laundry and keeping the family's living areas clean, and prepare formula for Melissa and meals for Mrs. Hill. You also will monitor Mrs. Hill and Melissa for changes in their conditions and report any changes to me," the primary nurse explains.

When the plan of care is complete, the primary nurse leaves for her next appointment. Hillary spends the rest of her visit doing light housekeeping chores and preparing food and formula. She stops often to check on the baby, who smiles up at her from her playpen. While Hillary cleans and cooks, Mrs. Hill does not talk much. But as she finishes, Hillary notices her curled up on the couch with a sad look on her face.

"I wish I wasn't too weak to take care of my baby," says Mrs. Hill.

Hillary takes the baby out of her playpen and brings her over to her mother on the couch. Sitting next to her, Hillary places Melissa in Mrs. Hill's lap and helps position her comfortably. "She's such a pretty little one," Hillary says gently.

"I'm worried about a lot of things," Mrs. Hill says, looking at her daughter. "I don't have any way to support us. Plus, I don't know how much longer I'll be able to keep Melissa with me. Each day, it seems that I'm able to do less and less for her. I don't know what I would do if I didn't have such good friends and family to help me."

Hillary listens carefully to her client (Figure 23-14). When Mrs. Hill finishes talking, Hillary says, "If it's all right with you, I'm going to let my supervisor know about your concerns. There's a social worker at the Lewisford Agency. I think he can help you." Mrs. Hill smiles and nods her head. "I'd like that very much."

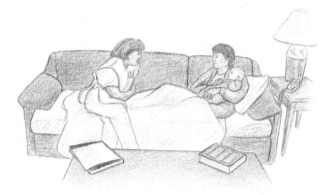

Figure 23-14
While listening carefully to her client's concerns, Hillary realizes that one of her agency's team members may be able to help Mrs. Hill.

Wrapping Up the Day

Hillary is a few minutes late reporting back to the office. Today, like every day on her job, Hillary has met unique challenges. She examined and reported Mrs. Roth's sore toe. Ms. Frazier's friend didn't come back on time, so Hillary arranged with her supervisor for an alternate plan. And she feels good about her first visit with Mary Hill and Melissa.

"Sounds like you handled everything very well," Hillary's supervisor says. "You've come a long way in the 5 months that you've been working here. Do you remember what it was like when you first went out on your own? You would call from a client's home every time something came up. Now you call only when you have to report something unusual. You stick to your schedule and make decisions when unexpected things come up. You made some really good decisions today."

Hillary agrees. Tomorrow she will face another challenging day. "See you in the morning," she says.

Fiction and Reality

Nora's and Hillary's days are fictional, although they may seem very real. They represent what a nurse assistant's day may be like. But no day—not your day, not the day of the person sitting next to you, not even Nora's or Hillary's day—is the same.

These situations show how two people, who have responsibilities that are similar to the ones that you may have, planned their days and controlled their time, yet responded to the needs of the people in their care. If you try to stay organized and plan your day, as well as remain flexible and responsive to situations as they arise, you too can manage your time effectively.

Information Review

Circle the correct answers and fill in the blanks.

1. Things that influence how you use your time are—
    a. The number of people in your care, their medical conditions, the kind of care they need, and their mobility.
    b. How many staff members are out sick and how many are playing hooky.
    c. How you spent your time before work and how well you coped with your prework activities.
    d. Whether you wore your watch and remembered to set the time correctly.

2. Your work day will go more smoothly if you plan a
    _____ of tasks that you must do.

3. When planning your schedule in hospital and nursing home care, you should consider (select two)—
    a. How many people have been assigned to your care.
    b. What you are wearing that day.
    c. What time your favorite program is on TV.
    d. How quickly and efficiently you can get the job done.

4. When you identify the most important tasks to be done and list them in order, you _____ the tasks.

5. When other co-workers ask for your assistance, you should—
    a. Stop whatever you are doing and help them.
    b. Refuse to help if your schedule doesn't allow time for such an interruption.
    c. Work this request into your schedule as best you can.
    d. Report the request to your supervising nurse.

6. If your day's assignment seems impossible to complete, you should—
    a. Do the best you can and don't worry about it.
    b. Ask for assistance from your co-workers.
    c. Speak to your supervising nurse immediately.
    d. Feel angry about being taken advantage of and leave at the end of your shift, even if the work isn't done.

7. When planning your schedule in the home health care setting, you must consider how much _____ it takes to get from one client's home to another and how much
    _____ is on that route at that time of day.

8. What is the best way to handle unexpected events? (Select two)
   a. Rearrange your schedule the best you can.
   b. Ignore the events.
   c. Ask for help, if you need it.
   d. Ignore your schedule for the rest of the day.

9. You now have the information to _____

   your time each working day, _____ your

   time if unplanned events occur, and _____
   clearly to help you stay in control of your time.

10. When other caregivers are delayed in the home health care set-
    ting, you should—
    a. Call your supervisor.
    b. Leave anyway so that you are not late for your next client.
    c. Before leaving, situate the client next to the telephone so
       that he can call for help if he needs it.
    d. Put a plan into place that you have previously worked out,
       such as calling a friend or neighbor to relieve you until the
       delayed caregiver returns.

Questions to Ask Yourself

1. How would you have planned your
   schedule if you were Nora? Were there
   some things that Nora could have
   communicated to the people in her care
   that would have helped her stay in control
   of her time?

2. You have established your schedule for the
   day at the hospital where you work. In
   your care are two people who need
   complete bed baths, one person who takes
   a tub bath, three people who take showers,
   and one person who can do her own
   partial bath. How would you schedule your
   time to do these baths?

3. You are serving dinner to the residents of a
   nursing home. You realize that Mr. Harris
   and Miss Yarnell both need a lot of
   assistance with eating tonight. You provide
   care for both of them and for one other
   person who needs help with eating. What
   would you do so that all of them can eat a
   hot dinner?

4. You arrive at a client's home at the
   appointed time and knock on the door. No
   one answers. What should you do?

5. You arrive at Mrs. Roth's house for your
   scheduled visit. You are concerned when
   you find Mrs. Roth tearful and distressed.
   She says she just received a letter telling
   her that her oldest and dearest friend died.
   You try to comfort her, but she pushes you
   away. "Please leave me alone. I don't want
   to be bothered," she says. When you ask
   about medication and diet, she gets very
   upset and cries out, "I said go away! Leave
   me alone!" What should you do?

6. Remembering the six principles of
   care—safety, privacy, dignity,
   communication, independence, and
   infection control—when and how did Nora
   practice these principles during the day?

Appendix A

❖ Glossary of Key Words ❖

The key words defined in this glossary include terms from this textbook, as well as from the American Red Cross *Skills for Caregiving* and the Instructor's Manual.

abbreviation (uh-bree-vee-AY-shun)   A shortened version of a word. An abbreviation is often made up of the first letters of several words.

abdominal (ab-DOM-in-uhl)   Pertaining to the abdomen, the part of the body between the ribs and groin.

abnormal (ab-NOR-muhl)   Not normal or regular.

abrasion (uh-BRAY-zhun)   A tiny cut or scrape.

abuse   (ah-BYOOS) Harm that occurs when a person is purposely hurt or mistreated.

acquired (uh-KWY-erd)   A condition that is not inherited and does not just happen to a person for an unexplained reason.

acquired immune deficiency syndrome (uh-KWY-erd/im-MYOUN/duh-FISH-uhn-see/SIN-drum)   A condition caused by the human immunodeficiency virus that results in a breakdown of the body's defense systems.

active range-of-motion exercise   The independent movement of a joint by a person who does not need assistance.

activities of daily living   Daily self-care activities that help keep a person independent and healthy.

ADA   Abbreviation for American Diabetes Association.

adapt (uh-DAPT)   To change a behavior to adjust to a certain illness or condition.

admit   To sign someone into a health care facility.

adolescence (add-uh-LES-ense)   The period between the ages of 12 and 20 when a person becomes more interested in sex and begins to have relationships with other people.

adolescent (add-uh-LES-ent)   A person between the ages of 12 and 20.

AIDS   An abbreviation for acquired immune deficiency syndrome. AIDS is caused by the human immunodeficiency virus (HIV), which

results in a breakdown of the body's defense systems.

airborne germs   Germs that are carried in the air by breathing, coughing, or sneezing.

alignment (uh-LINE-ment)   Correct positioning to keep the spine straight and to avoid any twisting, straining, pressure, or discomfort.

ambulation (am-byoo-LAY-shun)   The medical term for walking.

anal (A-nuhl)   Of or relating to the opening at the end of the rectum through which feces pass.

ancestor (AN-ses-ter)   A distant relative from whom a particular family descended.

ancestry (AN-ses-tree)   A family's history.

anesthetic (an-es-THET-ik)   A special medication that causes a loss of feeling in part or all of the body, as may be used during surgery.

angina pectoris (an-JY-nuh/PEK-tor-is)   The medical term for heart pain.

anonymous (uh-NON-uh-mus)   Not named or identified.

antibodies (AN-ti-bah-dees)   Special proteins or chemicals the body produces when an infection is present.

antimicrobial (an-ti-my-CROW-bee-uhl)   Capable of killing or slowing the growth of pathogens.

antiseptic (an-tuh-SEP-tik)   A substance that stops the growth of germs.

anxious (ANGK-shus)   The state of being extremely nervous or agitated.

appetite (AH-puh-tite)   The desire to eat and drink.

appropriate (ah-PRO-pree-it)   Right or correct for a given situation.

areola (uh-REE-oh-luh)   The dark area surrounding a woman's nipple.

arteriosclerosis (ar-teer-ee-oh-skluh-ROW-sis)   Hardening and thickening of the arteries.

artery (ARE-ter-ee)   Any of the branching blood vessels that carries oxygen-rich blood from the heart to all parts of the body.

514

asphyxiation (as-fik-see-AY-shun)   Suffocation caused by the lack of oxygen.

aspirate (AS-puh-rate)   To breathe in.

assertiveness (uh-SER-tiv-nes)   Communication that firmly expresses what the communicator wants.

atrophy (AH-tro-fee)   A condition in which a part of the body, such as the leg muscles, wastes away or shrinks due to disuse or inadequate nutrition.

auscultate (OS-kuhl-tate)   To listen for sounds produced by the body's organs.

axillary   Referring to the underarm. For example, an axillary temperature is taken in a person's underarm.

bed linens (LIN-ens)   Sheets, pillow cases, mattress covers, blankets, and bedspreads.

behavior (be-HAYV-yur)   The way a person acts or conducts himself.

bereavement care (buh-REEV-ment)   Care provided for people who are grieving after someone dies.

bill of rights   A list of rights and expectations of health care provided to a patient, resident, or client. A bill of rights may include the person's right to receive information about his care in a language he can understand, the right to refuse treatment, and the right to privacy, confidentiality, and continuing care.

biology   The science dealing with living organisms and vital processes.

bladder   A pouch that holds air inside the cuff of a sphygmomanometer. Also, a membranous sac in the body that holds fluid, such as the gallbladder or urinary bladder.

bloodborne disease   An illness that is easily transmitted or spread when the blood of an infected person comes into contact with the blood of another person.

blood pressure   Force exerted against the arteries as blood pumps from the heart into the body.

body fluids   Liquid substances produced by the body.

body image (IM-ij)   A person's attitude toward his body.

body mechanics   The way a person's body adjusts to keep its balance during movement.

body systems   Groups of organs that together perform one or more vital functions; for example, the nervous system.

botulism (BAH-chew-liz-um)   A severe type of food poisoning caused by bacteria found in improperly canned food and an impure honey. Untreated botulism can result in death.

brachial artery (BRAY-kee-uhl)   An artery in the arm at the inside bend of the elbow.

calorie (KAL-uh-ree)   A unit of heat or energy produced when the body uses food.

candidiasis (kan-de-DYE-uh-sis)   The growth of painful white patches in the mouth, throat, or the vagina caused by a fungus called *candida.*

cannula (KAN-you-luh)   A tube placed under the nostrils to deliver oxygen.

capillaries (KAP-uh-ler-ees)   Any of the small blood vessels with a slender, hairlike opening that attaches the end of an artery to the beginning of a vein.

carbon dioxide   A colorless, odorless gas that a person breathes out of the body through the respiratory system; a waste product of respiration.

cardiopulmonary resuscitation (kar-dee-oh-PULL-mon-air-ee/ree sus-suh-TA-shun)   Also known as CPR, a series of manual or mechanical procedures used to restore circulation and breathing after the heart and respiration have stopped.

care plan   A form used to record overall health care information.

CAT scan   Computerized axial tomography, a form of x-ray that produces a three-dimensional picture of sections of the brain or other parts of the body.

catastrophic reaction (kat-uh-STROF-ik)   Violent and sudden behavior that disrupts order.

catheter   A slender tube inserted into a cavity of the body. For example, a urinary catheter may be inserted into the bladder to remove urine.

cerebrovascular accident (suh-ree-bro-VAS-kyu-ler)   An interruption of blood flow to a part of the brain, which results in the death of a few or many brain cells.

certified (SER-tuh-fide)   Having skills that have been tested and approved.

cesarean section (suh-ZARE-ee-en/SEK-shun)   An operation in which the doctor makes a surgical incision in the mother's abdomen and through into the uterus, through which a baby is delivered.

chemical restraint (KEM-e-kuhl/re-STRAYNT)   A drug or medication that calms a person and changes his behavior.

chemotherapy (key-mo-THER-uh-pee)   Treatment with one or more drugs that stop cancer cells from multiplying.

cholesterol (ko-LES-ter-all)   A white, fatty substance that occurs naturally in the blood and tissues of the human body and that also is found in meat, egg yolks, liver, most dairy products, and animal fat.

chronic illness (KRAH-nik)   A long-lasting condition or illness that may occur again.

client (KLY-ent)   A person who receives health care at home.

clinic (KLIN-ik)   A hospital department that provides care to patients who do not need to stay overnight.

close-ended question   A question that requires a simple "yes" or "no" answer.

coagulation disorder (ko-ag-you-LAY-shun)   An illness identified by problems in the process of blood clotting.

coccyx (COCK-siks)   The "tailbone," or end of the spine.

cognitive (KOG-nuh-tiv)   Relating to thinking, understanding, remembering, believing, learning, and creating.

cognitive impairment (KOG-nuh-tiv/im-PARE-ment)   A condition that decreases a person's ability to think clearly.

comfort zone (KUM-fert)   The distance between one person and another that feels comfortable when communicating.

communication (kuh-myou-nuh-KAY-shun)   The process of giving and receiving information.

compassion (kum-PASH-un)   A feeling of sorrow for another person's hardship that leads to help.

complete bed bath   A personal care procedure in which all parts of a person's body are bathed while the person is in bed.

compression (kum-PRESH-un)   The act of pressing or squeezing together.

concentrated (KON-sen-tray-ted)   Containing a small percentage of water.

congestive heart failure (kun-JES-tiv)   A condition of the cardiovascular system in which weakened heart muscles prevent the heart from working effectively.

constipation   A condition of the bowels in which elimination of hard, dry stool is difficult or infrequent.

contagious   Readily transmitted from one person to another by direct or indirect contact.

contaminated (kun-TAM-in-ay-tid)   Containing dirt or disease-causing germs.

contracture (kun-TRAK-tyur)   A condition in which unused muscles cause a person's joints to become permanently bent.

COPD   An abbreviation for chronic obstructive pulmonary disease, a condition of the respiratory system that includes emphysema, asthma, and chronic bronchitis-diseases that are long term and interfere with the body's ability to breathe efficiently.

complete bed bath   A personal care procedure in which all parts of a person's body are bathed while the person is in bed.

coping (KOPE-ing)   The ability to deal with problems and difficulties.

cuff   The inflatable band of a sphygmomanometer that wraps around the arm.

culture (KUL-tyur)   The racial, ethnic, social, and religious principles that shape a person's thoughts and beliefs.

customs (KUS-tums)   Actions or practices that are done regularly by a group or family.

cuticles (KYU-tuh-kuhls)   The skin at the base of the fingernails and toenails.

CVA   An abbreviation for cerebrovascular accident.

cyanosis (si-uh-NO-sis)   The condition of having a blue or gray color, due to lack of oxygen in the blood.

dandruff (DAN-druff)   Flaking skin from the scalp.

decubitus ulcer (duh-KYOO-bi-tuhs/UHL-ser)   The medical term for a bedsore or pressure sore, caused by pressure or friction, which cuts off circulation. A decubitus ulcer can quickly progress into a deep, infected crater.

defecate (DEF-uh-kate)   To eliminate solid waste from the body.

dehydrated (dee-HI-dray-ted)   Not having enough water in the body.

demeaning (duh-MEEN-ing)   Something that lowers someone's dignity.

dementia (de-MEN-she-uh)   An incurable disorder of the brain in which there is a progressive loss of memory and other cognitive (thinking) functions.

depilatory cream (duh-PILL-uh-tor-ee)   A lotion that dissolves hair and removes it from the surface of the skin.

dermis   The sensitive layer of skin beneath the epidermis.

diabetes (dye-uh-BEE-tez)   A disease in which the pancreas does not secrete enough insulin and the body is not able to use all the carbohydrates, resulting in a high concentration of glucose in the blood.

diaphragm (DYE-uh-fram)   The thin, usually plastic, disk of a stethoscope that is placed on the skin to magnify body sounds.

diarrhea (dye-uh-REE-uh)   The frequent passage of liquid feces.

diastolic pressure   The pressure of the blood against the walls of the arteries when the heart relaxes. When a person properly measures blood pressure, this is the value determined by the point at which the pumping sound stops.

diet (DYE-it)   The foods and liquids that a person usually consumes.

digestion   The process of breaking down food into a form that can be absorbed by the body.

diluted (di-LOO-ted)   Containing a large percentage of water.

direct contact   A situation in which germs pass directly from one living thing to another living thing, for example, from one person to another.

disaster plan (di-ZAHS-ter)   A set of safety procedures to follow in case a natural disaster occurs.

discipline   An area of study or work.

disinfect (dis-in-FEKT)   To remove disease-causing germs.

disinfectant (dis-in-FEK-tunt)   A substance that destroys disease-causing germs.

disoriented (dis-OR-ee-en-ted)   A condition in which a person is unsure of who she is, where she is, and what day or time it is.

drawsheet   A bed sheet about 5 feet wide that is placed under a person, across the middle third of the bed. A drawsheet is useful in positioning and transferring procedures.

dysfunctional (dis-FUNK-shun-uhl)   Functioning in a way that is not normal.

dyspnea (disp-NEE-uh)   The condition of having difficult in breathing.

edema (uh-DEEM-uh)   Swelling of body tissue due to an accumulation of fluid.

eliminate (uh-LIM-uh-nate)   To get rid of.

emotional (ee-MO-shun-uhl)   Relating to how a person feels and how he expresses himself.

emotional abuse (ee-MO-shun-uhl/ah-BYOOS)   Harm that occurs when one person's words or actions make the other person feel bad about himself.

enema (EN-uh-muh)   A solution introduced into the rectum and lower colon to relieve fecal impaction or constipation.

engorgement (en-GORJ-ment)   A condition in which the breasts of a new mother become tightly swollen and sore due to her milk supply.

environment (en-VY-run-ment)   The surroundings in which a person lives.

epidermis (ep-uh-DER-mis)   The outer protective layer of skin.

epilepsy (EP-uh-lep-see)   An ongoing condition of the brain marked by changes in the level of consciousness and/or abnormal muscle or sensory activity.

episiotomy (uh-piz-ee-AH-tuh-mee)   An incision in the mother's perineum sometimes made during labor to widen the opening of the mother's vagina for easier delivery of the baby.

erection (uh-REK-shun)   A stiffening of the penis.

ESRD   An abbreviation for **e**nd-stage **r**enal **d**isease, a condition of the urinary system.

esteem (es-TEEM)   A high regard for someone.

ethical (ETH-e-kuhl)   That which is morally and professionally correct.

ethical dilemma (ETH-uh-kuhl/de-LEM-uh)   A problem or situation in which a nurse assistant must decide what is the correct, moral, and professional thing to do.

exploit (eks-PLOYT)   To take advantage of someone.

express   To press or squeeze out.

extend   To straighten.

fecal impaction   A condition of the bowels in which hard stool is wedged in the rectum.

feces (FEE-seez)   Solid body waste.

femoral artery (FEM-er-uhl)   An artery at the groin where the thigh meets the hip.

fetus (FEE-tus)   A developing human baby, from 12 weeks after conception until birth.

flex   To bend.

flossing   A part of mouth care in which dental floss is used to remove plaque and food particles from between the teeth. The procedure also stimulates the gums.

flow sheet   A form used to record health care information and track changes in a person's condition over a period of time.

fluoridated (FLOOR-uh-day-ted)   Containing fluoride, a chemical that helps decrease tooth decay. Toothpaste and drinking water often are fluoridated.

foreskin   The loose fold of skin that covers the end of the penis; part of the male reproductive system.

formula (FOR-myou-lah)   Milk-based or soybean-based liquid mixture given in bottles to babies.

Fowler's position   A position in which a person sits up with the head of the bed elevated for support.

frail   Very slender and fragile.

gait   The way a person walks.

gastrostomy tube   A device that a doctor inserts directly into a person's stomach through a surgical opening to provide liquid feeding.

gender (JEN-der)   A person's sex.

general hospital   A facility that provides care for people of all ages and with almost any type of illness or injury.

genitals (JEN-uh-tuhls)   The external sex organs between a person's legs.

germ   A tiny living organism that cannot be seen by the human eye. Some germs may cause infection and disease, others may be harmless, and some may even be useful.

glands   Groups of cells that manufacture secretions that are released and used in other parts of the body.

grooming   A personal care procedure in which one attends to a person's appearance by brushing the person's hair, providing nail care, shaving, and making the person neat and tidy.

handedness   The tendency to use one hand more frequently than the other.

hazard (HAZ-erd)   Something that is very dangerous.

HBV   An abbreviation for **hepatitis B virus**.

health care proxy (PROKS-ee)   A legal document that names a person to make health care decisions if the person receiving care is unable to.

health care team   A group headed by the person receiving care. Includes doctors, nurses, nurse assistants, therapists, secretaries, and other people involved in the caregiving process.

hemophilia (he-mo-FILL-e-uh)   A hereditary blood disease, occurring almost exclusively in males, in which the blood fails to clot and abnormal bleeding occurs.

hepatitis (heh-puh-TY-tis)   A disease or condition marked by an inflammation of the liver.

heritage (HAIR-uh-tij)   The culture passed on to a person through birth.

HIV   An abbreviation for **human immunodeficiency virus**.

HIV transmitter   See *transmitter.*

HIV wasting syndrome   An opportunistic condition characterized by the loss of 10 percent or more of total body weight over a short period of time.

home health aide   A nurse assistant who works in home health care.

home health care   Health care provided in private homes to people who do not need to stay in hospitals or nursing homes.

home health care agency   A health organization that employs home health aides and others who provide health care and other services to people in their homes.

homemaker   A home health agency employee who helps clients perform household tasks.

homicidal (hom-uh-SIDE-uhl)   A tendency to harm other people with the intent to kill.

hospice (HOS-pis)   A program of good medical and emotional care and support for people who are dying, as well as for their families.

hostile (HOS-tuhl)   Unfriendly.

human development (HUE-men/duh-VEL-up-ment)   The physical, social, emotional, and cognitive changes a person experiences as he grows older.

human immunodeficiency virus (im-you-no-duh-FISH-uhn-see)   The microscopic organism that causes AIDS.

human need   A basic requirement that enables a person to live healthily and happily.

hyperglycemia   An abnormally high amount of sugar in the blood.

hypoglycemia   An abnormally low amount of sugar in the blood.

immobile (im-MOW-bul)   Unable to move.

immune system   Part of the body that uses certain substances in the body to defend the body against germs, infection, and disease.

impaired   A condition in which something is diminished or weakened.

inappropriate (in-uh-PRO-pree-it)   Not right or correct for a given situation.

incapacitated (in-kuh-PAH-se-tay-ted)   Being unable to act for oneself.

incentive spirometer (in-SEN-tiv/spy-ROM-uh-ter)   A small device that encourages a person to take deep breaths to help clear his lungs after surgery.

incident (IN-suh-dent)   Anything unusual that happens and has the potential to cause harm.

incision (in-si-shun)   A cut made during surgery.

incontinence (in-KON-ti-nense)   The inability to control the release of urine or feces.

indirect contact   A situation in which germs pass from a living thing, such as a person, to an object and then to another person when that person touches the object.

infancy (IN-fan-see)   The first stage of life. The word "infant" means "unable to speak."

infection (in-FEK-shun)   A harmful condition caused by the growth of germs in the body.

infection control   Action taken to control the spread of germs. Infection control is one of the six principles of care.

infectious (in-FEK-shus)   Spreading or capable of spreading rapidly. Infectious germs are also described as communicable and contagious.

ingestion   The act of taking food into the body for digestion.

inpatient   A patient who must stay overnight in a hospital.

insertion site   The place on a person's body through which a nurse puts an IV needle.

intravenous (in-trah-VEE-nus)   In or into a vein.

isolation procedures (pro-SEE-dyurs)   Practices used to separate a person from others and prevent the spread of infection.

IV (eye-VEE)   An abbreviation for **intravenous**. An IV is a type of medical equipment that supplies medicine and other liquids to a person intravenously, or through a needle inserted into his veins.

Kaposi's sarcoma (KAH-poh-sees/sar-KO-muh)   A rare kind of skin cancer that may attack the skin, mucous membranes, and lymph nodes.

kidney failure   A condition of the urinary system that occurs when the kidneys no longer function and are unable to get rid of the body's waste products.

labia   Outer and inner folds of skin at the opening of the vulva; part of a woman's reproductive system.

legal right (LEE-gul)   A privilege that is protected by law.

life cycle (SI-kuhl)   The stages of aging and development experienced as a person grows older.

living will   A legal document, prepared by a person receiving care, that states how he would like his care to continue if he becomes unable to make health care decisions.

manometer (ma-NOM-eh-ter)   The gauge on a sphygmomanometer that measures systolic and diastolic blood pressure.

microorganisms (my-crow-OR-guh-niz-ums)   Tiny living things that can be seen only through the magnification of a microscope.

milk pools   Breast tissue that stores milk.

miter (MY-ter)   To square off the corners of bed linens by neatly tucking them under each other.

mobility (moe-BIL-uh-tee)   The ability to move.

modified side-lying position   A position in which a person lies partially to one side with his back supported.

modify   To change somewhat.

monitor (MON-e-ter)   To check regularly for the quality of a person's physical or emotional condition.

MS   An abbreviation for **multiple sclerosis**, a condition of the nervous system.

mucous membrane (MYOU-kus)   A thin layer of body tissue that lines body passages and cavities that communicate directly or indirectly with the outside, such as the inside of the mouth, nose, eyes, vagina, and rectum.

mucus   A slippery secretion produced by the mucous membranes, such as those in the mouth, digestive tube, and respiratory passages. Mucus protects the mucous membranes.

muscular dystrophy   A childhood disorder of the nervous system in which nerves in the muscles do not function, causing the muscles to become smaller and weaker.

myth   An idea that some people believe is true but that is not true.

nasogastric tube   A device that a nurse or doctor inserts into a person's nose and into his stomach to provide liquid feeding; also used to remove stomach contents.

nauseated (NAW-zee-ay-ted)   A feeling of sickness in the stomach.

navel (NAY-vuhl)   The area in the middle of the abdomen where the umbilical cord once was attached.

neglect (nuh-GLEKT)   Failure to provide proper care for someone.

NPO   An abbreviation that indicates that a person is to take nothing by mouth, including food and fluids.

nursing home   A facility that provides care for people who do not need to stay in a hospital, but who need medical care and assistance they cannot get at home.

nursing notes   Information documented by the nurse on a health care record or chart.

nurture (NUR-tyur)   To promote and encourage good care.

nutrient (NEW-tre-ent)   A substance that the body needs to grow, maintain itself, and stay healthy.

nutrition   The total of all the processes involved in taking in and using food and fluids for the health and maintenance of the body.

obesity (oh-BEE-suh-tee)   Having too much body fat.

OBRA '87 (OH-brah)   An abbreviation for the 1987 **O**mnibus **B**udget **R**econciliation **A**ct, which provides certain standards for nursing homes and home health care.

obstetric (ob-STET-rik)   A type of medicine or care provided for pregnant women, women who have just delivered babies, and their newborn children. The obstetric department includes the maternity ward.

obstruction (ob-STRUK-shun)   Something that blocks.

ombudsman (OM-buds-man)   A person who acts as a mediator between a resident and the nursing home. The ombudsman listens to the resident's concerns and complaints and resolves conflicts with the health care provider.

open-ended question   A question that requires more than a simple "yes" or "no" answer. An open-ended question encourages a person to talk.

opportunistic infection (op-por-too-NIS-tik)   An infection caused by germs that normally would not make a person sick. Any person whose immune system is weakened may develop opportunistic infections.

oral thrush   A fungus infection that produces sore patches in the mouth.

orally   Referring to the mouth. For example, an oral temperature is taken in a person's mouth.

orthopedic (or-tho-PEE-dik)   A type of medicine or care provided for people who have problems with their bones or joints.

osteoporosis (os-tee-oh-per-OH-sis)   A condition of the skeletal system in which the bones become weak and fragile.

outpatient   A patient who receives care in a hospital but does not need to stay overnight.

over-the-counter medicines   Medications, such as aspirin, cold remedies, laxatives, ointments, and eyedrops, that anyone can buy without a doctor's prescription.

oxygen   An odorless, colorless, tasteless gas that a person breathes into the body through the respiratory system; essential for maintaining life.

palpate   To examine by touching or feeling.

partial bed bath   A personal care procedure in which a person's face, hands, underarms, back, perineum, and buttocks are washed while the person is in bed.

passive range-of-motion exercise   The movement of a person's joint by another person.

pathogen (PATH-o-jen)   A harmful germ or microorganism that causes disease.

patient (PAY-shent)   A person who receives health care in a hospital.

pediatric (pee-dee-AT-rik)   A type of medicine or care provided for children under 18 years of age.

perception (pur-SEP-shun)   A person's awareness of his environment through his senses.

perineal care (per-uh-NEE-uhl)   A nursing procedure in which a person's body is cleaned from the genitals to the anus.

perspiration (pur-spi-RAY-shun)   Body waste eliminated through the skin.

physical (FIZ-uh-kul)   Relating to the body.

physical abuse (ah-BYOOS)   Harm that occurs when a person's body is purposely hurt.

physical neglect (ne-GLEKT)   Failure to provide proper physical care for someone.

physical restraint (re-STRAYNT)   A device that prevents a person from moving freely.

placenta (pluh-SEN-ta)   A blood-filled structure through which the unborn child receives oxygen and nourishment and through which it gets rid of carbon dioxide and its other wastes.

plaque (PLAK)   A sticky, colorless layer of bacteria that forms constantly on the teeth.

***Pneumocystis carinii* pneumonia (PCP)** (NEW-mo-sis-tis/kuh-REE-nee-eye/nuh-MO-ni-uh)   A parasitic lung infection that makes breathing very difficult. PCP is the leading cause of death for people who have AIDS.

pneumonia (nuh-MO-nyuh)   An infection in the lungs.

postoperative   After surgery.

postpartum   After childbirth.

precise (pree-SISE)   Another term for *exact.*

predictable (pree-DIK-tuh-bull)   Can be known in advance.

prefix (PREE-fiks)   The first part of a word that comes before the root word and changes the meaning of the root.

preoperative   Before surgery.

prescription medicines   Medications that can be sold only by the order of a doctor.

principles of care (PRIN-suh-puls)   Basic rules of caregiving that guide caregivers in making decisions about providing individualized care for each person.

prioritize (pry-OR-uh-tize)   To list items or tasks in order of importance.

procedure   A particular way of performing a task to achieve a desired result. Some procedures are minor (less complicated), and some are major (more complicated).

prompting   Using a simple statement to help someone remember.

prosthesis   A device that replaces a natural part of the body, such as an artificial limb (arm or leg).

radiation (ray-dee-AY-shun)   Treatment in which x-rays are focused on the part of the body where cancer cells are growing.

range of motion (ROM)   The amount of movement possible in a joint, such as the elbow, knee, or hip. Also, how far a person can move a joint comfortably.

recovery room   A room in a hospital used to observe and treat patients who have just had surgery.

rectal (REK-tuhl)   Of or referring to the lower portion of the large intestine just inside the anal opening.

referral process (re-FER-uhl)   A set of procedures that allows one member of the health care system to inform other members that a person needs their kind of specialized care.

regulation (reg-you-LAY-shun)   A rule that must be followed.

rehabilitation (re-huh-bil-uh-TAY-shun)   The process of regaining physical health.

resident (REZ-uh-dent)   A person who receives health care in a nursing home.

restorative services (ruh-STOR-uh-tiv)   Activities or devices that help a person improve, maintain, or regain physical functions.

restraint   Any device or chemical used to limit the movement of a person or control or mood or behavior.

root   The middle part, or base, of a word.

route (ROUT)   When referring to medications, this is the way the medication should be taken: for example, taken by mouth, applied as an ointment, or given as a rectal suppository.

safety survey (SUR-vay)   Examination of a home to make sure it contains no safety hazards.

saturated fat (SAH-tyur-ay-ted)   A form of fat found in meats, cheeses, dairy products, and certain vegetable oils, such as palm and coconut oil.

schedule (SKED-yule)   A written plan that lists the time and order of several tasks.

seizure (SEE-zhur)   A sudden attack of a disease or condition.

sexual abuse (SEK-shew-al/ah-BYOOS)   Harm that occurs when a person's body is mistreated for sexual reasons.

sexual harassment (SEK-shew-uhl/HAIR-as-ment)   Purposely annoying or threatening someone by not respecting his sex or sexuality.

sexuality (sek-shue-AL-uh-tee)   A basic human need for sexual pleasure and sexual expression.

shallow   Not deep.

sharps container   A sturdy box with a tight-fitting lid that cannot be punctured by sharp objects such as needles or razors. Use of a sharps container protects health care workers from injury and exposure to contaminated items.

shock   An abnormal condition that occurs when the flow of blood returning to the heart is inadequate for normal function, resulting in a lack of oxygen for all body organs and tissues.

side effect   An action, other than the intended action, caused by a drug. Usually this action is an undesired effect.

sign-off   A report prepared by a caregiver before going off duty that includes information about a person's treatment, condition, and needs. This report varies in the amount of detail from one health care facility to another.

social (SO-shul)   Relating to the way people interact with each other.

social façade (fuh-SAHD)   In a social setting, pretending to know or recognize an unfamiliar person or thing.

social reinforcement   Encouragement that emphasizes appropriate attitude and behavior.

specialized hospital   A facility that provides care for people with certain types of diseases or illnesses.

speculum (SPEK-you-lum)   An instrument used to examine a body passage or cavity.

sphygmomanometer (sfig-mo-ma-NOM-eh-ter)   An instrument used to measure blood pressure.

stage (STAYJ)   A defined and predictable period.

sterilize (STAIR-uh-lize)   To destroy all germs.

stethoscope (STETH-o-skope)   An instrument used to listen to body sounds.

stool   Another term for solid body waste, or feces.

suffix (SUH-fiks)   The last part of a word that comes after the root word and changes the meaning of the root.

suicidal (sue-uh-SIDE-uhl)   A tendency to intentionally and voluntarily harm oneself with the intent to take one's own life.

supine position (SUE-pine)   A position in which a person lies flat on his back.

surgeon (SER-jin)   A medical doctor who uses medical instruments to perform procedures to improve or restore a person's health.

suture (SUE-tyur)   The stitch used to join the edges of a cut or wound.

suture line   The seam of stitches created when an incision is closed.

symptom   Any change observed in a person's body or in the way it functions that may indicate an infection.

syncope (SING-kuh-pee)   A temporary loss of consciousness caused by a lack of blood flowing to the brain. It may occur because of fatigue, fear, pain, or blood loss.

syndrome (SIN-drom)   Several signs and symptoms that occur together and characterize a disease.

systemic herpes (sis-TEM-ik/HER-pees)   A type of infection caused by the herpes virus in which sores develop over the entire body, especially the hands, feet, and mouth.

systolic pressure   The pressure of the blood against the walls of the arteries when the heart pumps. When a person properly measures blood pressure, this represents the first sound heard as air is released from the cuff of the sphygmomanometer.

taboo (tah-BOO)   Forbidden.

TB   An abbreviation for **tuberculosis**.

terminal illness (TUR-muh-nul)   A serious illness or condition from which a person is not expected to recover.

theory (THEE-o-ree)   An explanation based on observation and reasoning.

therapeutic diet (ther-uh-PEW-tik)   A special diet that helps a person regain his health.

thready pulse   A condition in which the force of the pulse is very weak.

tradition (tra-DISH-uhn)   An inherited ritual or pattern of doing things.

transmitter   Something that sends or passes certain properties from one organism to another. Examples of HIV transmitters are blood, breast milk, fluid surrounding the spinal cord, semen, vaginal secretions, and any of the following fluids when they contain blood: feces, mucus, saliva, and urine.

tuberculosis (to-ber-cue-LOW-sis)   A contagious bacterial infection of the lungs.

turgor (TER-jer)   The ability of the skin to return to its normal shape when it is squeezed or gently pinched.

Type I diabetes (dye-uh-BEE-tez)   A form of diabetes in which the pancreas produces very little or no insulin. Also called juvenile onset or insulin-dependent diabetes.

Type II diabetes (dye-uh-BEE-tez)   A form of diabetes in which the output of insulin from the pancreas is inadequate for the body's needs. Also called maturity onset or insulin-independent diabetes, type II diabetes often develops later in life.

umbilical cord (um-BIL-uh-kuhl)   A tubelike structure arising from an unborn baby's navel that connects it to the placenta inside the mother. It carries nourishment to the baby and carries waste out of the baby.

unconscious (un-KON-shus)   A state of mind in which a person does not respond to the world around him.

universal precautions   Special infection control procedures that health professionals use to protect themselves and the people in their care from potentially infectious body fluids, such as blood.

urinary catheter (YUR-uh-nair-ee/KATH-uh-ter)   A small tube (ordered by a doctor) that is inserted (usually by a nurse or doctor) through the urethra into the bladder. A small balloon at the end of the tube on the bladder end is blown up, or inflated, to hold the tube in place. On the other end, the tube connects to a bag that collects the urine.

urinate (YUR-uh-nate)   To eliminate liquid waste from the body.

urine (YUR-in)   Liquid body waste.

valve   A device that controls the flow of air in an instrument such as a sphygmomanometer or fluid in an organ such as the heart.

vegan   A person who does not eat animal flesh, such as meat or fish, or animal products, such as eggs, cheese, or milk.

vegetarian   A person who does not eat animal flesh, such as meat or fish.

vein (VAYN)   Any of the blood vessels that carries blood from all parts of the body to the heart.

virus   A microorganism, smaller than bacteria, which depends on nutrients in a living cell to survive and reproduce.

vital   Necessary for life.

void   Another term for urinate.

vulnerable   Liable to be hurt.

walk-in clinic   A hospital department that provides care for patients who do not need appointments.

Appendix B

❖ Glossary of Word Elements ❖

Prefix	Prefix Meaning	Combined Form
a-, an-	without, not	an/esthesia (without sensation)
ab-, abs-	away, from	ab/duction (move away from)
ad-	toward, near	ad/duction (move toward)
anti-	against	anti/inflammatory (substance used to fight infection)
brady-	slow	brady/cardia (slow heart rate)
circum-	around	circum/oral (around the mouth)
contra-	against, opposite	contra/ception (preventing conception, or pregnancy)
de-	down, from	de/pendent (hanging down or below)
dis-	apart or two	dis/sect (cut apart)
dys-	abnormal, difficult, bad	dys/function (not functioning properly)
erythro-	red	erythro/cyte (red blood cell)
ex-	out, out of, from	ex/crete (discharge, get rid of)
hyper-	over, excessive	hyper/active (overly active)
hypo-	under, decreased	hypo/thyroid (underactive thyroid)
in-	within or not	in/continent (not able to control the release of urine or feces) in/dependent (not dependent)
mal-	bad, abnormal	mal/nourished (poorly fed)
non-	no, not	non/poisonous (not poisonous)

Prefix	Prefix Meaning	Combined Form
peri-	around, covering	peri/osteum (covering of the bone)
post-	after, behind	post/operative (after an operation)
pre-, or pro-	before, in front of	pre/operative (before an operation)
re-	again, back	re/port (speak or write about a previous event)
semi-	half	semi/conscious (half conscious or alert)
tachy-	fast, rapid	tachy/cardia (rapid heart beat)

Root	Root Meaning	Combined Form
arthr/o-	joint	arthr/itis (inflammation of the joint)
bronch/o-	bronchus, bronchi	bronch/itis (inflammation of the bronchus)
cephal/o-	head	en/cephal/itis (inflammation of the brain)
cholecyst/o-	gall bladder	cholecyst/ectomy (removal of the gall bladder)
col/o-	colon, large intestine	colo/stomy (surgical opening into the colon)
crani/o-	skull	crani/otomy (surgical opening into the skull)
cyan/o-	blue	cyan/osis (having a blue color)
cyst/o-	bladder	cyst-itis (inflammation of the bladder)
derma/o-	skin	derma/tology (study or science of the skin)
febr/i-	fever	febr/ile (having a fever)
gastri/o-	stomach	gastr/itis (inflammation of the stomach)
glyc/o-	sugar	glyco/suria (sugar in the urine)

Root	Root Meaning	Combined Form
gyn/e-	woman	gyne/cologist (one who studies diseases of women)
hem/a-	blood	hema/turia (blood in the urine)
hernia-	rupture	herni/orraphy (surgical repair of a hernia)
hyster/o-	uterus	hyster/ectomy (removal of the uterus)
lapar/o-	abdomen, or flank	lapar/otomy (surgical cut into the abdomen)
lith/o-	stone	chole/lith/iasis (having stones in the gallbladder)
mamm/o-, masto-	breast, mammary gland	mammo/gram (diagnostic picture of the breast)
men/o-	menstruation	pre/menstrual (before the menstrual period)
my/o-	muscle	my/algia (muscle pain)
narc/o-	numbness, stupor, or sleep	narco/tic (producing numbness, stupor, or sleep)
necr/o-	death	necr/osis (death of tissue or bone)
opthalm/o-	eye	opthalmo/scope (instrument for examining the eye)
oste/o-	bone	osteo/arthritis (inflammation of the bones and joints)
path/o-	disease	patho/gen (disease-causing organism or substance)
ped/o-	foot, child	ped/al (pertaining to the foot)
phleb/o-	vein	phleb/itis (inflammation of the veins)
pneum/o-	lung, air	pneumo/thorax (air in the chest cavity)
proct/o-	rectum	procto/scope (instrument for examining the rectum)
psych/o-	mind	psych/ology (study of the mind)
pulm/o-	lung	pulmon/ary (pertaining to the lung)

Root	Root Meaning	Combined Form
rect/o-	rectum	recto/stenosis (narrowing of the rectum)
renal-	kidney	reno/pathy (disease of the kidney)
septic-	poison, infection	septi/cemia (poison in the blood)
therm/o-	heat	thermo/therapy (application of heat for treatment)
thorac/o-	chest	thorac/otomy (surgical incision into the chest)
thromb/o-	clot	thrombo/lytic (destruction of a clot)
tox/o-, toxic-	poison	tox/emia (poisonous substance in the body)
ur/o-	urine	hemat/uria (blood in the urine)
urethr/o-	urethra	urethr/itis (inflammation of the urethra)
uter/o-	uterus	utero/vaginal (pertaining to the uterus and vagina)
vertebr/o-	spine, vertebrae	vertebr/al (pertaining to the spine)

Suffix	Suffix Meaning	Combined Form
-al	pertaining to	therm/al (pertaining to heat)
-algia, -algesia	pain	an/algesia (without pain)
-cide	kill	germi/cide (substance that kills germs)
-cise	cut	ex/cise (to cut out)
-ectomy	excision, removal of	append/ectomy (removal of the appendix)
-emia	blood condition	hypo/glyc/emia (low blood sugar)
-esthesia	sensation	an/esthesia (without sensation)
-gram	printed record	mammo/gram (diagnostic picture of a breast)

Suffix	Suffix Meaning	Combined Form
-graph	device for recording	electro/cardio/graph (machine for recording the activity of the heart)
-itis	condition of inflammation	phleb/itis (inflammation of the veins)
-iasis, -ism	having the characteristics or condition of	dwarf/ism (having the condition of, or being, a dwarf)
-meter	measuring instrument	thermo/meter (instrument that measures temperature)
-ology	the study or science of	neur/ology (the study or science of the nervous system)
-oma	tumor	hemat/oma (tumor caused by an accumulation of blood)
-orraphy	surgical repair of	herni/orraphy (surgical repair of a hernia)
-oscopy	examination of	gastro/scopy (examination of the stomach and abdominal cavity)
-ostomy	creation of an opening	colo/stomy (surgically created opening into the colon)
-otomy	surgical cutting	uter/otomy (surgical incision into the uterus)
-pathy	disease	cardio/myo/pathy (disease of the heart muscle)
-phasia	speaking	a/phasia (unable to speak)
-phobia	an exaggerated fear	photo/phobia (fear of or intolerance to light)
-photo	related to light	photo/graph (picture made by light)
-plegia	paralysis	quadri/plegia (paralysis of all four extremities)
-rrhage, -rrhagia	excessive flow	hemo/rrhage (excessive flow of blood)
-rrhea	profuse flow, discharge	rhino/rrhea (nasal discharge)
-scopy	examination using a scope (instrument to enable one to see)	endo/scopy (examination of internal cavities by the use of a scope)

Appendix C

❖ Abbreviations ❖

Abbreviations or shortened forms of words or phrases are frequently
used in health care facilities to save time and space when recording observations.
Some common ones are listed here, although their use may vary from one
facility to another. Ask your supervising nurse for a list of acceptable
abbreviations used in the facility where you work.

Abbreviation	Meaning
a.c.	Before meals
abd.	Abdomen
ad lib	As desired
ADL	Activities of daily living
Adm. (adm.)	Admitted or admission
A.M.	Morning
amb.	Ambulatory
amt.	Amount
b.i.d.	Twice a day
BM (bm)	Bowel movement
BP or B/P	Blood pressure
c̄	With
c/o	Complains of
Ca.	Cancer
Cath.	Catheter, catheterize
CBC	Complete blood count
cc	Cubic centimeter
CPR	Cardiopulmonary resuscitation
CVA	Cerebrovascular accident; stroke
dc (d/c)	Discontinue
DOA	Dead on arrival
DON	Director of nursing
dsg. or drsg.	Dressing
Dx.	Diagnosis
EKG	Electrocardiogram
ER	Emergency room
FBS	Fasting blood sugar
FF	Force fluids
fld.	Fluid
ft.	Foot or feet
h.s.	Hour of sleep; at bedtime
H_2O	Water
ht.	Height
I&O	Intake and output

Abbreviation	Meaning
in.	Inch
IV	Intravenous
Lab.	Laboratory
lb.	Pound
liq.	Liquid
LPN	Licensed practical nurse
LVN	Licensed vocational nurse
ml.	Milliliter
N.P.O.	Nothing by mouth
NA	Nurse assistant
neg.	negative
NKA	No known allergies
no., #	Number
noc(t)	Night
O.T.	Occupational therapy
O_2	Oxygen
OJ	Orange juice
OOB	Out of bed
oz.	Ounce
p.c.	After meals
p.o. (per os)	By mouth
per	By, through
P.M.	Afternoon
pm	As necessary
P.T.	Physical therapy
q	Every
q.d.	Daily
q.h.s.	Every night at bedtime
q.i.d.	Four times a day
q.o.d.	Every other day
qh	Every hour
q2h, q3h, etc.	Every 2 hours, every 3 hours, etc.
R	Rectal temperature
RN	Registered nurse
ROM	Range of motion
s̄	Without
S.O.B.	Short of breath
Spec. (spec.)	Specimen
SSE	Soap suds enema
Stat	Immediately
t.i.d.	Three times a day
TPR	Temperature, pulse, respiration
Tbsp.	Tablespoon
TLC	Tender loving care
tsp.	Teaspoon
U/a (U/A, u/a)	Urinalysis
VS (vs)	Vital signs
W/C	Wheelchair
wt. or wgt.	Weight

Appendix D

❖ Home Safety Checklist ❖

The following information is adapted from the American Red Cross brochure *Home Safety* (ARC 4104), which may be obtained free from your local Red Cross chapter. Use this form to evaluate your own home as well as your client's. If you are evaluating a client's apartment, you must still be concerned about hallways and the grounds of the building. Since you may be the only advocate for the person for whom you are giving care, you may have to talk to the apartment manager about hazardous conditions for your client.

Independent Living Series
Home Safety

Home accidents are a major cause of injury and death for all Americans. For those over 60, the risk of death and injury may be greater than for others.

People usually become less agile as they grow older. Their bones tend to become more porous and brittle and can break more easily. A simple fall can result in a serious, disabling injury. For these reasons, older people need to take special precautions to ensure a safe living environment.

Most accidents in the home can be prevented by the elimination of hazards. Using the checklists that follow, you can determine the safety level of your home. Place a check mark by each statement that applies to your home or to your habits in your home. Then review the unchecked boxes to determine what else you can do to make your home a safer place to live.

GENERAL

First, consider whether your home meets general safety standards. Place a check mark next to each of the following statements that apply:

[ ] Emergency numbers are posted by each telephone.

[ ] Appliances, lamps, and cords are clean and in good condition.

[ ] All electrical equipment bears the Underwriters Laboratories (UL) label.

[ ] A sufficient number of outlets are located in every room where they are needed. "Octopus" outlets—outlet extensions that can accommodate several plugs—are not used.

[ ] Overload protection is provided by either circuit breakers or fuses.

[ ] If the house contains do-it-yourself wiring, the wiring has been checked for safety. (A municipal electrical inspector or an electrical contractor can do this for you.)

[ ] Electrical service is of sufficient capacity to serve the house. It is up to code. (You can call your municipal electrical inspector to have the wiring in your house checked.)

[ ] The thermostat of the water heater is set at 110° F or lower to prevent accidental scalding.

[ ] Medications are stored in a safe place according to instructions on the label of the package or container.

[ ] Carpeting and rugs are not worn or torn.

[ ] Small, loose rugs have nonskid backing and are not placed in traffic areas.

[ ] Now, go through your home room by room.

KITCHEN

Consider whether your kitchen is safe.

[ ] The stove and sink areas are well lighted.

[ ] If you have a gas stove, it is equipped with pilot lights and an automatic cut-off in the event of flame failure. (Your local utility service representative can check this for you.)

[ ] The stove is not located under a window in which curtains are hanging.

[ ] The exhaust hood of the oven is provided with filters that can be easily removed for cleaning.

[ ] The kitchen exhaust system discharges directly outside or through ducts to the outside and not into the attic or other unused space.

[ ] Hazardous household agents are stored out of the reach of children.

[ ] Countertop space is ample to keep carrying and lifting to a minimum.

Now, consider your work habits in the kitchen.
Do you—

[ ] Turn pan handles away from other burners and the edge of the stove?

[ ] Avoid wearing garments with long, loose sleeves when cooking?

[ ] Keep hot pan holders near the stove?

[ ] Turn on the exhaust fan when using the stove?

[ ] Operate your microwave oven only when there is food in it?

[ ] Disconnect small appliances when you are not using them?

[ ] Keep knives in a knife rack or drawer?

[ ] Clear counter tops and work areas of all unnecessary objects?

[ ] Keep drawers and cupboards closed?

[ ] Use a stepladder or step stool rather than a chair to reach objects in overhead cabinets?

[ ] Wipe up grease or liquid spills at once?

STAIRWAYS AND HALLS

Consider whether your stairways and halls are safe.

[ ] Steps are in good condition and are free of objects.

[ ] Steps have nonskid strips, or the carpeting on them is securely fastened and free of fraying or holes.

[ ] Smoke detectors are in place in hallways and near sleeping areas.

[ ] Hallways are equipped with night-lights.

[ ] Hand rails are sturdy and securely fastened.

[ ] Balusters (banister supports) are close enough to prevent a small child from placing his head between. (If balusters are too far apart, you may attach a temporary barrier to eliminate the problem.)

[ ] Light switches are located at the top and bottom of stairways and at both ends of long hallways.

[ ] Doors do not swing out over stairsteps.

[ ] Clearance in the stairway provides adequate head room.

LIVING ROOM

Consider whether your living room is safe.

[ ] Electric cords are placed along walls—not under rugs—and away from traffic areas.

[ ] Chairs and couches are sturdy and secure.

BATHROOM

Consider whether your bathroom is safe.

[ ] The bathtub or shower has a nonskid mat or strips on the standing area.

[ ] Bathtub or shower doors are glazed with safety glass or plastic.

[ ] Hand bars are installed on the walls by the bathtub and toilet.

[ ] Towel bars and the soap dish in the shower stall are made of durable materials and are firmly installed.

[ ] Faucet and valve handles are unbreakable.

In the bathroom, do you—

[ ] Dispose of old medications safely?

[ ] Keep your radio, portable heater, and other electrical appliances away from the bathtub or shower area?

BEDROOM

Consider whether your bedroom is safe. In your bedroom, do you—

[   ] Keep a lamp or flashlight within reach of your bed?

[   ] Use a night-light to brighten the way to the bathroom at night?

OUTDOOR AREA

Consider whether your outdoor area is safe.

[   ] Steps and walkways are in good condition.

[   ] Handrails are sturdy and securely fastened.

[   ] Doorways are well lighted.

[   ] Porches, balconies, terraces, copings, window wells, and other elevations or depressions are protected by railings, are closed with banisters or accordion gates, or are otherwise protected.

[   ] Hedges, trees, or shrubs do not obscure the view of the street from the driveway or hide the presence of a child moving toward the driveway.

[   ] Garage doors are of a type that are easy for you to operate, even when snow is piled against them.

[   ] The house is equipped with a lightning rod system if it is situated in a relatively high, isolated place; antennas are grounded.

[   ] The garage is adequately ventilated.

[   ] Large trees are healthy and well maintained and have no dead limbs.

[   ] Swing-out (awning and casement) windows do not project over walks or other traffic areas.

When working outdoors, do you—

[   ] Store garden and lawn equipment and tools safely?

[   ] Avoid using flammable liquids other than charcoal lighter fluid to start fires for barbecuing?

[   ] Keep toxic materials (for example, pesticide and fertilizer) in their own containers, not in unlabeled jars or soft drink bottles?

Congratulations! You have just completed the first step in making your home a safer place to live. The Red Cross hopes you were able to check all or most of the boxes. If you have spotted deficiencies, you will want to correct them as soon as you can.

The American Red Cross is committed to the promotion of health and to helping Americans avoid injury and disease. Call your American Red Cross chapter today for information about health and safety courses—or about how you, too, can join this commitment by becoming an American Red Cross volunteer.

Appendix E

❖ Information Review Answer Key ❖

Note: Chapter 1, The Art of Caregiving, does not have
Information Review questions.

Chapter 2, Working in Health Care

1. hospitals, nursing homes, homes
2. d. Person receiving care
3. b. Dietitian
4. supervising nurse

Hospitals
1. patient
2. clinic
3. c. Admitting
4. a. Orthopedic department

Nursing Homes
1. c. Rehabilitation
2. resident
3. OBRA
4. cognitive impairment

Home Health Care
1. b. Home health aide
2. client
3. OBRA
4. a. Give medication

Chapter 3, Protecting People's Rights

1. right
2. c. Tell your supervising nurse about his concerns
3. a. Unopened
4. health care proxy
5. ombudsman
6. ethical
7. emotional abuse
8. d. Sexually abused
9. neglect
10. physical, chemical

Chapter 4, Understanding People

1. physical, social, emotional, cognitive
2. order, pattern
3. b. Her friends will think she is ugly
4. a. Older people can still learn things, but it may take a little longer than it once did
5. b. Tell him how interesting it must have been in those days and ask him some questions about it
6. physical, security, social, esteem, self-fulfillment
7. needs
8. sexuality
9. b. Tell the person firmly, but gently, that you do not like to be touched like that
10. d. Tell her that you can understand that it must feel strange to eat on a fasting day and encourage her to talk about it

Chapter 5, Communicating with People

1. sender, message, channel, receiver, confirmation
2. b. Ask for confirmation that the message was understood
3. b. Knock on the door, wait for a response, and introduce yourself
4. a. Nonverbal and written
5. d. Give his shoulder a squeeze and tell him he is doing a great job
6. d. Tell the daughter what you are doing and why you are doing it, and ask her to help with her mother's care
7. b. What she knows and how she takes care of her skin
8. a. Look at the different parts of the word, especially the root, to see if you know the meaning of any of the word's parts
9. care plan, flow sheet, nursing notes
10. a. Any change in a person's behavior or condition

Chapter 6, Keeping People Safe

1. d. Safety
2. back
3. a. Check to make sure it is working properly
4. c. Follow your employer's policies for fire alarms
5. b. Stop, drop, roll, and cool
6. a. Unplug appliances
7. check, call, care
8. partial, complete
9. c. Pale coloring and cool, moist skin
10. artery, vein

Home Health Care

1. c. Make a list of all safety hazards and correct those you can do immediately; discuss the remaining hazards with your supervising nurse
2. d. In a locked box in a well-lit hall closet
3. pillow

Chapter 7, Controlling the Spread of Germs

1. direct, indirect
2. cleaning, disinfecting, sterilizing
3. b. Hold them away from your uniform
4. b. Wash your hands
5. a. When you provide care for any person.
6. d. When you touch blood or other body fluids
7. sharps container
8. c. Wear gloves while providing care
9. a. The person has many infected dressings
10. gowns, masks, eyewear, gloves

Chapter 8, Measuring Life Signs

1. b. Vital signs
2. admitted, change
3. 97.6° F, 99.6° F
4. d. A fever
5. rhythm, force
6. brachial
7. a. Stethoscope
8. thumb
9. dyspnea
10. c. Respirations

Chapter 9, Positioning and Transferring People

1. bedsores, fat, muscle
2. b. Ears, elbows, and ankles and/or
   d. Coccyx and buttocks
3. a. A reddened area on the skin
4. c. At least every 2 hours
5. d. The person's mobility, level of independence, and ability to help
6. drawsheet
7. explain, help
8. Fowler's
9. back
10. brakes

Chapter 10, Assisting People with Personal Care

1. b. Personal needs, self-image, and independence
2. d. Rinse the person's mouth with diluted mouthwash before and after mouth care
3. c. Turn the person on his side so that he does not aspirate
4. front, back
5. chilled, privacy, dignity
6. d. By walking or by riding in a wheelchair or shower chair
7. c. Do not recap the razor; put it in the "sharps" container
8. weak
9. Safety
10. person, medication, time, route, amount

Chapter 11, Providing Care for the Person's Place

Bedmaking

1. b. Tell the person you would like to move something and ask her where to place it
2. c. Are used to prevent bedsores
3. b. Storing many linens in the person's room so that you don't have to go back and forth to get them
4. c. Use this time to talk and listen to the person
5. bottom sheet, drawsheet

Cleaning and Laundry

1. c. Ask your supervising nurse for instructions about whether to do the task

2. d. Disinfecting
3. b. ¼ cup of bleach to 1 gallon of water
4. your hands
5. plastic bag

Chapter 12, Eating for Health

1. c. All the food and liquid a person consumes
2. a. Carbohydrates
3. Fat
4. c. Full liquid
5. 48
6. high-protein
7. soft
8. d. Keep the head of the bed elevated for 30 minutes following a tube feeding
9. c. Frequent urination
10. a. Be patient, positive, and consistent

Home Health Care
1. c. Washing your hands with soap and water before handling food
2. ingredients, calories
3. Steaming

Chapter 13, Elimination

1. Drinking fluids
2. care plan
3. d. The inability to control the release of urine or feces
4. c. A chair with a toilet seat and a container to collect waste
5. toilet, 5
6. tract infection
7. perineal
8. a. Once daily
9. care plan
10. a. Abdominal pain and a diarrhea-like discharge from the anus

Children's Elimination Needs
1. b. Leave him for just a second to get supplies
2. c. Apply a self-adhesive collection bag

Chapter 14, Restorative Care

1. restorative
2. d. Encourage him to use a self-help eating utensil so that he can feed himself

3. self-help
4. a. Atrophied muscles
5. d. "It's so important for you to do these exercises to keep your joints flexible. Let's try to do them very slowly, and you can let me know when you need to rest or stop."
6. reinforces
7. prosthesis
8. b. Make sure it's turned off when the person isn't using it
9. clock
10. up

Chapter 15, Admitting, Transferring, and Discharging

1. admission
2. transfer
3. discharge
4. d. Possessions
5. vital signs
6. a. Belongings
7. roommate
8. b. Her clothing
9. discharge planner
10. nursing home, home

Chapter 16, Providing Care for People Who Have Specific Illnesses

1. d. Do active or passive range-of-motion exercises regularly
2. a. Pain in the lower legs
3. b. Sitting up
4. b. May have reduced sensation in his feet
5. c. Breathe deeply often during the day
6. d. Is spread by breathing in droplets that have been sprayed into the air by an infected person's coughing
7. a. Place the call signal within reach of the person's unaffected side
8. independence
9. changes, belongings, inner, medication
10. mucus
11. normal
12. infection

Chapter 17, Providing Care for People Who Have AIDS

1. c. Share needles with an infected drug user
2. a. A syndrome that has many signs and symptoms
3. human, virus
4. immune
5. condoms
6. infected
7. blood
8. opportunistic
9. all
10. condition
11. emotional
12. thrive

Chapter 18, Providing Care for People Who Have Alzheimer's Disease

1. cognitive impairment
2. Alzheimer's disease
3. communication
4. social façade
5. c. Return the missing items to their owners yourself, and try to determine when Mrs. McDay is most likely to wander into someone else's room and the reason why she behaves this way
6. b. Catastrophic reaction
7. c. Tell her that you can tell she is upset and offer to walk with her for a while
8. b. Help him into a reclining chair after dinner and put him in a quiet, dimly lit room
9. d. Placing a picture of her as a young woman on the door
10. a. "You both have such good taste in clothes. I think it's time for lunch now. Come with me."

Chapter 19, Restraints

1. physical, chemical
2. mind
3. OBRA, restraints
4. b. For life-threatening emergencies and medical treatments
5. asphyxiation

6. emotional
7. a. Place a large, dark circle on the floor in front of a doorway that leads to danger
8. 15 minutes
9. c. Every 2 hours, and more often if necessary
10. Any three of the following: leg restraints, arm restraints, wrist restraints, hand mitts, soft ties or vests, lap and wheelchair belts, safety bars, geri-chairs, chemical restraints

Chapter 20, Providing Care for People Having Surgery

1. c. Has pain after a surgical procedure
2. required
3. elective
4. anesthetic
5. b. Is closely watched for immediate complications
6. incentive spirometer
7. nasal cannula, mask
8. c. Some ice chips in a paper cup
9. d. Raise the foot of the bed so that the person's head is lower than his feet
10. a. They don't want to bother anyone

Chapter 21, Providing Care for Mothers and Newborns

1. physical, emotional
2. uterus
3. episiotomy
4. perineal
5. cesarean section
6. a. Physical and hormonal changes
7. b. Help keep the baby from getting sick
8. formula
9. neck, head
10. cord, circumcision

Chapter 22, Providing Care for People Who Are Dying

1. d. Age, culture, fulfillment, religion, and family and friends
2. a. Denial, anger, bargaining, depression, and acceptance

3. d. State that their doctors are wrong and have made a mistake
4. a. Encouraged to talk about their feelings and their needs
5. hospice
6. lividity
7. postmortem
8. respect
9. grief, pain
10. near death

Chapter 23, Managing Your Time

1. a. The number of people in your care, their medical conditions, the kind of care they need, and their mobility
2. schedule
3. a. How many people have been assigned to your care
    d. How quickly and efficiently you can get the job done
4. prioritize
5. c. Work this request into your schedule as best you can
6. c. Speak to your supervising nurse immediately
7. time, traffic
8. a. Rearrange your schedule the best you can
    c. Ask for help if you need it
9. plan, adjust, communicate
10. d. Put a plan into place that you have previously worked out, such as calling a friend or a neighbor to relieve you until the delayed caregiver returns

Bibliography

Chapter 3

A patient's bill of rights, Chicago 1975, American Hospital Association.

Downs M: Free-to-be in Vermont. In *Untie the elderly,* Kennett Square, Pa, 1990, The Kendall Corporation.

Home health care patient bill of rights/ responsibilities, Chatham, Mass, 1989, Chatham-Orleans Visiting Nurse Association.

Into aging, A commercially produced game no longer available, Thorofare, NJ, Slack Publishers.

U.S. Congress House: *Omnibus reconciliation act of 1987: conference report to accompany H.R. 3314,* 100th Cong, first session, Washington, DC, 1987, H. Rept. 100-495, pp 195-200.

Chapter 4

Carlson NR: *Discovering psychology,* Needham Heights, Mass, 1988, Allyn and Bacon.

Clemen S et al: *Comprehensive family and community health nursing,* New York, 1988, McGraw-Hill.

Ebersole E, Hess P: *Toward healthy aging: human needs and nursing response,* St. Louis, 1985, Mosby, p 573.

Kidd JR: *How adults learn,* Chicago, 1973, Follett.

Klevens C: *Material and methods in adult and continuing education,* Los Angeles, Klevens Publishing.

McVan B et al: *Patient teaching,* Springhouse, Pa, 1990, Springhouse.

Chapter 5

Clemen S et al: *Comprehensive family and community health nursing,* New York, 1988, McGraw-Hill.

Kidd JR: *How adults learn,* Chicago, 1973, Follett.

Klevens C: *Material and methods in adult and continuing education,* Los Angeles, 1983, Klevens Publishing.

McVan B et al: *Person teaching,* Springhouse, Pa, 1990, Springhouse.

Sorrentino SA, *Mosby's textbook for nursing assistants,* ed 3, St Louis, 1993, Mosby.

Will CA: *Being a long-term care nursing assistant,* ed 3, Englewood Cliffs, NJ, Brady–Prentice Hall.

Wilson MW: *Basic medical terminology concepts,* Englewood Cliffs, NJ, 1989, Brady–Prentice Hall.

Chapter 6

American Red Cross: *First Aid: Responding to Emergencies,* St. Louis, 1991, Mosby.

Child safety information was taken from American Red Cross child care course materials, "Preventing Injuries and Preventing Infectious Diseases."

Chapter 7

Charette S et al: *Infection control manual,* Ft. Smith, Ark, 1991, Beverly Enterprises.

Chapter 9

Beverly Enterprises: *Lift with care,* Redwood City, Calif, 1987, Visucom Productions.

Chapter 10

Badasch SA, Chesebro D: *Essentials for the nursing assistant in long-term care,* Albany, NY, 1990, Delmar Publishers.

Hogan J, Sorrentino SA: *Mosby's textbook for long-term care assistants,* St. Louis, 1988, Mosby.

Huber J, Apatz A: *Homemaker/home health aide,* ed 3, Albany, NY, 1989, Delmar Publishers.

Lewis LW, Timby BK: *Fundamental skills and concepts in patient care,* ed 4, Philadelphia, 1988, JB Lippincott.

Techniques for denture identification, Chicago, 1984, The American Dental Association Council on Prosthetic Services and Dental Laboratory Relations.

Wernig J, Sorrentino SA: *The homemaker/home health aide,* St. Louis, 1989, Mosby.

Will C, Eighmy J: *Being a long-term care nurse assistant,* ed 3, Englewood Cliffs, NJ, 1991, Prentice-Hall.

Chapter 12

American National Red Cross: *Better eating for better health,* Instructor's Guide, Washington, DC, 1984, American Red Cross.

American National Red Cross: *Family health and home nursing,* Washington, DC, 1979, American Red Cross.

Barton JA, Hertzler AA, Taper LJ: *Lesson 1, food for the preschooler: growth of the preschool child,* Publication 348-130, Blacksburg, Va, 1985, Virginia Cooperative Extension Service, p 1.

Barton JA, Hertzler AA, Taper LJ: *Lesson 2, food for the preschooler: the preschooler's diet,* Publication 348-131, Blacksburg, Va, 1985, Virginia Cooperative Extension Service, pp 1, 2, 5.

Barton JA, Hertzler AA, Taper LJ: *Lesson 3, food for the preschooler: development of food habits,* Publication 348-132, Blacksburg, Va, 1985, Virginia Cooperative Extension Service, pp 1-3.

Barton JA, Hertzler AA, Taper LJ: *Lesson 4, food for the preschooler: nutrition and dental health,* Publication 348-133, Blacksburg, Va, 1985, Virginia Cooperative Extension Service, pp 1-2.

Barton JA, Hertzler AA, Taper LJ: *Lesson 5, food for the preschooler: overweight/obesity in the preschool child,* Publication 348-134, Blacksburg, Va, 1985, Virginia Cooperative Extension Service, pp 1-2.

Barton JA, Hertzler AA, Taper LJ: *Lesson 6, food for the preschooler: iron deficiency in preschoolers,* Publication 348-135, Blacksburg, Va, 1985, Virginia Cooperative Extension Service, p 2.

Gerber Products Co: *Dietary guidelines for infants: special guidelines for babies less than two years of age,* Fremont, Mich, 1989, Gerber, p 15.

Guthrie HA: *Introductory nutrition,* St. Louis, 1989, Mosby.

Hale E: Good nutrition for your growing child. In *FDA Consumer,* Publication (FDA) 87-2218, Rockville, Md, 1987, US Department of Health and Human Services, p 3.

Hertzler AA: *Children's food behavior,* Publication 348-121, Blacksburg, Va, 1988, Virginia Cooperative Extension Service, pp 3-4.

Willis J: Good nutrition for the highchair set. In *FDA Consumer,* Publication (FDA) 86-2208, Rockville, Md, 1985, US Department of Health and Human Services, p 3.

Chapter 13

Blanchet KD, editor: *AIDS: a health care management response,* Rockville, Md, 1988, Aspen Publishers, p 135.

Chapter 14

Friedman, JA: *Home health care, a complete guide for patients and their families,* New York, 1986, WW Norton.

Jones ML: *Home care for the chronically ill or disabled child,* New York, 1985, Harper and Row.

Chapter 16

Arthritis Foundation: *Taking care: protecting your joints and saving your energy,* Atlanta, 1990, pp 3, 4.

Berkow R: *The Merck manual of diagnosis and therapy,* ed 14, Rahway, NJ, 1982, Merck.

Hegner BR, Caldwell E: *Nursing assistant; a nursing process,* ed 6, Albany, 1992, Delmar.

Chapter 17

American Red Cross: *A guide to home care for the person with AIDS,* Washington, DC, 1990, American Red Cross.

American Red Cross: *HIV/AIDS instructor's manual,* Washington, DC, 1992, American Red Cross, Chapter 12.

Quackenbush M, Sargent P: *Teaching AIDS: a resource guide on acquired immune deficiency syndrome,* Santa Cruz, Calif, 1986, Network Publications.

Chapter 18

French CJ, Morrison NL, Levine EB: *Understanding and caring for the person with Alzheimer's disease,* Atlanta, 1985, Alzheimer's Disease and Related Disorders Association.

Gwyther LP: *Care of Alzheimer's patients: a manual for nursing home staff,* Chicago, 1985, American Health Care Association and Alzheimer's Disease and Related Disorders Association.

Chapter 19

Miles SH: Escaping vest restraints: what we should do about "safety" devices that demoralize and kill. In Quality Care Advocate, Minneapolis, 1991.

Chapter 20

Potter PA, Perry AG: *Basic nursing theory and practice,* ed 2, St. Louis, 1991, Mosby.

Rosdahl CB: *Textbook of basic nursing,* ed 5, Philadelphia, JB Lippincott.

Schniedman R, Wander B: *Being a nursing assistant,* ed 6, Englewood Cliffs, NJ, 1991, Prentice Hall.

Smith DP et al: *Comprehensive child and family nursing skills,* St. Louis, 1991, Mosby.

Sorrentino SA: *Mosby's textbook for nursing assistants,* ed 2, St. Louis, 1987, Mosby.

Taylor C, Lillis C, Lenone P: *Fundamentals of nursing: the art and science of nursing care,* Philadelphia, 1989, JB Lippincott.

Chapter 21

American Red Cross: *HIV/AIDS instructor's manual,* Washington, DC, March, 1992, American Red Cross, Chapter 12.

American National Red Cross: *American Red Cross healthy pregnancy, healthy baby,* Washington, DC, 1991, American Red Cross.

American National Red Cross, in cooperation with the American Academy of pediatrics: *Preventing infectious diseases and caring for ill children,* Washington, DC, 1990, American Red Cross.

Maurano LW: Pediatric Home Care. In *Journal of Home Health Care Practice,* February 1989.

Chapter 22

Eidson T, editor: *The AIDS caregiver's handbook,* New York, 1988, St. Martin's Press, pp. 222-223.

Johnson JP, Goodwin M: *How to be a nurse aide in a nursing home,* Chicago, 1985, American Health Care Association.

Kalish RA: *Death, grief, and caring relationships,* ed 2, Pacific Grove, Calif, 1985, Brooks/Cole.

Kubler-Ross E: *Living with death and dying,* New York, 1981, Macmillan.

Kubler-Ross E: *On death and dying,* New York, 1969, Macmillan.

Kubler-Ross E: *Questions and answers on death and dying,* New York, 1974, Macmillan.

Little DW: *Home care for the dying,* Garden City, NY, 1985, Doubleday.

Credits

Figure 2-1 From Sorrentino SA: *Mosby's textbook for nursing assistants,* ed 3, St. Louis, 1992, Mosby.

Figure 6-4 From Sorrentino SA: *Mosby's textbook for nursing assistants,* ed 3, St. Louis, 1992, Mosby.

Figure 6-12 From American Red Cross: *Responding to emergencies,* St. Louis, 1991, Mosby.

Figure 6-13 From American Red Cross: *Responding to emergencies,* St. Louis, 1991, Mosby.

Figure 6-14 From American Red Cross: *Responding to emergencies,* St. Louis, 1991, Mosby.

Figure 6-15 From American Red Cross: *Responding to emergencies,* St. Louis, 1991, Mosby.

Figure 6-16 From American Red Cross: *Responding to emergencies,* St. Louis, 1991, Mosby.

Figure 7-9 From Sorrentino SA: *Mosby's textbook for nursing assistants,* ed 3, St. Louis, 1992, Mosby.

Figure 7-11 From Sorrentino SA: *Mosby's textbook for nursing assistants,* ed 3, St. Louis, 1992, Mosby.

Figure 8-3 From Sorrentino SA: *Mosby's textbook for nursing assistants,* ed 3, St. Louis, 1992, Mosby.

Figure 8-4 From Sorrentino SA: *Mosby's textbook for nursing assistants,* ed 3, St. Louis, 1992, Mosby.

Figure 8-8 From Sorrentino SA: *Mosby's textbook for nursing assistants,* ed 3, St. Louis, 1992, Mosby.

Figure 8-15 From Sorrentino SA: *Mosby's textbook for nursing assistants,* ed 3, St. Louis, 1992, Mosby.

Figure 8-16 From Sorrentino SA: *Mosby's textbook for nursing assistants,* ed 3, St. Louis, 1992, Mosby.

Unnumbered Figure 9-3 From Sorrentino SA: *Mosby's textbook for nursing assistants,* ed 3, St. Louis, 1992, Mosby.

Unnumbered Figure 9-4 From Sorrentino SA: *Mosby's textbook for nursing assistants,* ed 3, St. Louis, 1992, Mosby.

Unnumbered Figure 9-5 From Sorrentino SA: *Mosby's textbook for nursing assistants,* ed 3, St. Louis, 1992, Mosby.

Figure 11-2 Courtesy The Stryker Corporation, Kalamazoo, Mich.

Figure 11-3 From Sorrentino SA: *Mosby's textbook for nursing assistants,* ed 3, St. Louis, 1992.

Figure 11-6 From Sorrentino SA: *Mosby's textbook for nursing assistants,* ed 3, St. Louis, 1992.

Figure 13-4 From Sorrentino SA: *Mosby's textbook for nursing assistants,* ed 3, St. Louis, 1992, Mosby.

Figure 13-13 (1), (2), (3) From Sorrentino SA: *Mosby's textbook for nursing assistants,* ed 3, St. Louis, 1992, Mosby.

Figure 14-14 (1), (2), (3) From Sorrentino SA: *Mosby's textbook for nursing assistants,* ed 3, St. Louis, 1992, Mosby.

Figure 17-5 Redrawn from Quackenbush M, Sargent P: *Teaching AIDS: a resource guide on acquired immune deficiency syndrome,* Santa Cruz, Calif, 1986, Network Publications.

Figure 17-7 Reprinted by permission of The Names Project Foundation, Marcel Miranda III, photographer, 1988.

Figure 18-1 From National Institute on Aging.

Index

MISSION OF THE AMERICAN RED CROSS

The American Red Cross, a humanitarian organization led by volunteers and guided by its Congressional Charter and the Fundamental Principles of the International Red Cross Movement, will provide relief to victims of disaster and help people prevent, prepare for, and respond to emergencies.

ABOUT THE AMERICAN RED CROSS

To support the mission of the American Red Cross, over 1.3 million paid and volunteer staff serve in some 1,600 chapters and blood centers throughout the United States and its territories and on military installations around the world. Supported by the resources of a national organization, they form the largest volunteer service and educational force in the nation. They serve families and communities through blood services, disaster relief and preparedness education, services to military family members in crisis, and health and safety education.

The American Red Cross provides consistent, reliable education and training in injury and illness prevention and emergency care, providing training to nearly 16 million people each year in first aid, CPR, swimming, water safety, and HIV/AIDS education.

All of these essential services are made possible by the voluntary services, blood and tissue donations, and financial support of the American people.

FUNDAMENTAL PRINCIPLES OF THE INTERNATIONAL RED CROSS AND RED CRESCENT MOVEMENT

HUMANITY

IMPARTIALITY

NEUTRALITY

INDEPENDENCE

VOLUNTARY SERVICE

UNITY

UNIVERSALITY